sixth
EDITION

# THE MONT REID
# SURGICAL HANDBOOK

sixth
EDITION

# THE MONT REID
# SURGICAL HANDBOOK

The University of Cincinnati Residents
From the Department of Surgery
University of Cincinnati College of Medicine
Cincinnati, Ohio

**EDITOR-IN-CHIEF**

**Wolfgang Stehr, MD**

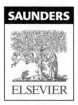

SAUNDERS

ELSEVIER

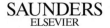

# SAUNDERS
ELSEVIER

1600 John F. Kennedy Blvd.
Ste 1800
Philadelphia, PA 19103-2899

THE MONT REID SURGICAL HANDBOOK, SIXTH EDITION ISBN: 978-1-4160-4895-4

---

### Notice

Knowledge and best practice in this field are constantly changing. As new research and experience broaden our knowledge, changes in practice, treatment and drug therapy may become necessary or appropriate. Readers are advised to check the most current information provided (i) on procedures featured or (ii) by the manufacturer of each product to be administered, to verify the recommended dose or formula, the method and duration of administration, and contraindications. It is the responsibility of the practitioner, relying on their own experience and knowledge of the patient, to make diagnoses, to determine dosages and the best treatment for each individual patient, and to take all appropriate safety precautions. To the fullest extent of the law, neither the Publisher nor the Editor assumes any liability for any injury and/or damage to persons or property arising out of or related to any use of the material contained in this book.

The Publisher

---

**Library of Congress Cataloging-in-Publication Data**
The Mont Reid surgical handbook / the University of Cincinnati residents from the Department of Surgery, University of Cincinnati College of Medicine ; editor-in-chief, Wolfgang Stehr. -- 6th ed.
    p. ; cm.
    Includes bibliographical references and index.
ISBN 978-1-4160-4895-4
1. Therapeutics, Surgical--Handbooks, manuals, etc. I. Reid, Mont. II. Stehr, Wolfgang. III. University of Cincinnati. Dept. of Surgery. IV. Title: Surgical handbook.
    [DNLM: 1. Surgical Procedures, Operative--Handbooks. WO 39 M7575 2008]
    RD49.M67 2008
    617.9--dc22

2008012874

*Acquisitions Editor:* Jim Merritt
*Developmental Editor:* Greg Halbreich
*Senior Production Manager:* David Saltzberg
*Design Director:* Louis Forgione

Printed in China

Last digit is the print number:   9   8   7   6   5   4   3   2   1

Working together to grow
libraries in developing countries
www.elsevier.com | www.bookaid.org | www.sabre.org

ELSEVIER   BOOK AID International   Sabre Foundation

# Contributors

**Steven R. Allen, MD**
Resident
Department of Surgery
UC College of Medicine
Cincinnati, Ohio

**Alexander J. Bondoc, MD**
Resident
Department of Surgery
UC College of Medicine
Cincinnati, Ohio

**Bryon J. Boulton, MD**
Resident
Department of Surgery
UC College of Medicine
Cincinnati, Ohio

**Eric M. Campion, MD**
Resident
Department of Surgery
UC College of Medicine
Cincinnati, Ohio

**Ondrej Choutka, MD**
Resident
Department of Neurosurgery
UC College of Medicine
Cincinnati, Ohio

**Callisia N. Clarke, MD**
Resident
Department of Surgery
UC College of Medicine
Cincinnati, Ohio

**T. Kevin Cook, MD**
Resident
Department of Surgery
UC College of Medicine
Cincinnati, Ohio

**Bradford A. Curt, MD**
Resident
Department of Neurosurgery
UC College of Medicine
Cincinnati, Ohio

**Benjamin L. Dehner, MD**
Resident
Department of Surgery
Division of Urology
UC College of Medicine
Cincinnati, Ohio

**Gerald R. Fortuna, Jr., MD**
Resident
Department of Surgery
UC College of Medicine
Cincinnati, Ohio

**Michael D. Goodman, MD**
Resident
Department of Surgery
UC College of Medicine
Cincinnati, Ohio

**R. Michael Greiwe, MD**
Resident
Department of Orthopaedic
     Surgery
UC College of Medicine
Cincinnati, Ohio

**Julian Guitron, MD**
Resident
Department of Surgery
Section of Cardiothoracic
     Surgery
UC College of Medicine
Cincinnati, Ohio

**Nathan L. Huber, MD**
Resident
Department of Surgery
UC College of Medicine
Cincinnati, Ohio

**Karen Lissette Huezo, MD**
Resident
Department of Surgery
UC College of Medicine
Cincinnati, Ohio

**Lynn C. Huffman, MD**
Resident
Department of Surgery
UC College of Medicine
Cincinnati, Ohio

**Thomas L. Husted, MD**
Resident
Department of Surgery
UC College of Medicine
Cincinnati, Ohio

**Angela M. Ingraham, MD**
Resident
Department of Surgery
UC College of Medicine
Cincinnati, Ohio

**Sha-Ron Jackson, MD**
Resident
Department of Surgery
UC College of Medicine
Cincinnati, Ohio

**Mubeen A. Jafri, MD**
Resident
Department of Surgery
UC College of Medicine
Cincinnati, Ohio

**Marcus D. Jarboe, MD**
Resident
Department of Surgery
UC College of Medicine
Cincinnati, Ohio

**Andreas Karachristos, MD, PhD**
Transplant Fellow
Department of Surgery
UC College of Medicine
Cincinnati, Ohio

**Dong-Sik Kim, MD**
Transplant Fellow
Department of Surgery
UC College of Medicine
Cincinnati, Ohio

**Renee Nierman Kreeger, MD**
Resident
Department of Anesthesia
UC College of Medicine
Cincinnati, Ohio

**Ryan A. LeVasseur, MD**
Resident
Department of Surgery
UC College of Medicine
Cincinnati, Ohio

**Jaime D. Lewis, MD**
Resident
Department of Surgery
UC College of Medicine
Cincinnati, Ohio

**Jocelyn M. Logan-Collins, MD**
Resident
Department of Surgery
UC College of Medicine
Cincinnati, Ohio

**Christopher A. Lundquist, MD**
Resident
Department of Surgery
UC College of Medicine
Cincinnati, Ohio

**Jefferson M. Lyons, MD**
Resident
Department of Surgery
UC College of Medicine
Cincinnati, Ohio

**Rian A. Maercks, MD**
Resident
Department of Surgery
UC College of Medicine
Cincinnati, Ohio

**Grace Z. Mak, MD**
Resident
Department of Surgery
UC College of Medicine
Cincinnati, Ohio

**Amy T. Makley, MD**
Resident
Department of Surgery
UC College of Medicine
Cincinnati, Ohio

**Joshua M. V. Mammen, MD**
Resident
Department of Surgery
UC College of Medicine
Cincinnati, Ohio

**Colin A. Martin, MD**
Resident
Department of Surgery
UC College of Medicine
Cincinnati, Ohio

**Rebecca J. McClaine, MD**
Resident
Department of Surgery
UC College of Medicine
Cincinnati, Ohio

**Benjamin C. McIntyre, MD**
Resident
Department of Surgery
UC College of Medicine
Cincinnati, Ohio

**Kelly M. McLean, MD**
Resident
Department of Surgery
UC College of Medicine
Cincinnati, Ohio

**Stacey A. Milan, MD**
Resident
Department of Surgery
UC College of Medicine
Cincinnati, Ohio

**Rajalakshmi R. Nair, MD**
Resident
Department of Surgery
UC College of Medicine
Cincinnati, Ohio

**Shannon P. O'Brien, MD**
Resident
Department of Surgery
UC College of Medicine
Cincinnati, Ohio

**Brian S. Pan, MD**
Resident
Department of Surgery
UC College of Medicine
Cincinnati, Ohio

**Prakash K. Pandalai, MD**
Resident
Department of Surgery
UC College of Medicine
Cincinnati, Ohio

**Charles Park, MD**
Resident
Department of Surgery
UC College of Medicine
Cincinnati, Ohio

**Parit A. Patel, MD**
Resident
Department of Surgery
UC College of Medicine
Cincinnati, Ohio

**Jonathan E. Schoeff, MD**
Resident
Department of Surgery
UC College of Medicine
Cincinnati, Ohio

**John D. Scott, MD**
MIS Fellow
Department of Surgery
UC College of Medicine
Cincinnati, Ohio

**Thomas W. Shin, MD**
Resident
Department of Surgery
UC College of Medicine
Cincinnati, Ohio

**Wolfgang Stehr, MD**
Resident
Department of Surgery
UC College of Medicine
Cincinnati, Ohio

**Janice A. Taylor, MD**
Resident
Department of Surgery
UC College of Medicine
Cincinnati, Ohio

**Ryan M. Thomas, MD**
Resident
Department of Surgery
UC College of Medicine
Cincinnati, Ohio

**Jonathan R. Thompson, MD**
Resident
Department of Surgery
UC College of Medicine
Cincinnati, Ohio

**Konstantin Umanskiy, MD**
Resident
Department of Surgery
UC College of Medicine
Cincinnati, Ohio

**Paul J. Wojciechowski, MD**
Resident
Department of Anesthesiology
UC College of Medicine
Cincinnati, Ohio

# Foreword

To the sixth edition

    The Surgical Residency Training Program at the University of Cincinnati has a long history of transforming medical students into capable, competent, and compassionate surgical leaders. Paramount to effective surgical leadership is a continuous commitment to the renewal and refinement of the scientific basis of clinical practice. Concrete evidence of our exceptional collective commitment is *The Mont Reid Surgical Handbook.* This sixth edition, composed on behalf of our residency and with faculty leadership and supervision, provides a comprehensive, user-friendly document to facilitate the state-of-the-art practice of surgery. The commitment and work ethic of these most exceptional resident authors are evident in the quality of every chapter.

    Having assumed the Christian R. Holmes Professor and Chair of the Department of Surgery at the University of Cincinnati College of Medicine in November 2007, I consider it a privilege to chair a department with such a great legacy. *The Mont Reid Surgical Handbook,* as much as any other achievement, is tangible evidence of our historical and ongoing commitment to excellence in the comprehensive missions of clinical service, education, and scholarship.

**Michael J. Edwards, MD, FACS**
**Christian R. Holmes Professor of Surgery**
**and Chairman of the Department of Surgery**
**University of Cincinnati Medical Center**
**Cincinnati, Ohio**
**2008**

# Foreword

To the first edition

Dr. Mont Reid was the second Christian R. Holmes Professor of Surgery at the University of Cincinnati College of Medicine. Trained at Johns Hopkins, he came to Cincinnati as the associate of Dr. George J. Heuer, the initial Christian R. Holmes Professor, in 1922, and became responsible for the teaching in the residency. He assumed the Chair in 1931 and died in 1943, a great tragedy for both the city and the University of Cincinnati College of Medicine. He was beloved by the residents and townspeople. A very learned, patient man, he was serious about surgery, surgical education, and surgical research. His papers on wound healing are still classics and can, to this day, be read with profit.

It was under Mont Reid that the surgical residency first matured. In his memory, the new surgical suite built in 1948 was named the Mont Reid Pavillion. Part of the surgical suite is still operational in that building, as are the residents' living quarters. *The Mont Reid Handbook* is written by the surgical residents at the University of Cincinnati hospitals for residents and medical students and thus is appropriately named. It represents a compilation of the approach taken in our residency program, of which we are justifiably proud. The residency program as well as the Department reflect a basic science physiological approach to the science of surgery. Metabolism, infection, nutrition, and physiological responses to the above as well as the physiological basis for surgical and pre-surgical interventions form the basis of our residency program and presumably will form the basis of surgical practice into the twenty-first century. We hope that you will read it with profit and that you will use it as a basis for further study in the science of surgery.

**Josef E. Fischer, MD**
**Christian R. Holmes Professor of Surgery**
**and Chairman of the Department of Surgery**
**University of Cincinnati Medical Center**
**Cincinnati, Ohio**
**1987**

# Preface

To the first edition
We can only instill principles, put the student in the right path, give him methods, teach him how to study, and early to discern between essentials and non-essentials.

**Sir William Osler**

The surgical residency training program at the University of Cincinnati Medical Center dates back to 1922 when it was organized by Drs. George J. Heuer and Mont R. Reid, both students of Dr. William Halsted and graduates of the Johns Hopkins surgical training program. The training program was thus established in a strong Hopkins mode. When Dr. Heuer left to assume the chair at Cornell University, Mont Reid succeeded him as chairman. During Reid's tenure (1931–1943), the training program at what was then the Cincinnati General Hospital was brought to maturity. Since then, the training program has continued to grow and has maintained the tradition of excellence in academic and clinical surgery which was so strongly advocated by Dr. Reid and his successors.

The principal goal of the surgical residency training program at the University of Cincinnati today remains the development of exemplary academic and clinical surgeons. There also is a strong tradition of teaching by the senior residents of their junior colleagues as well as the medical students at the College of Medicine. Thus, the surgical house staff became very enthused when Year Book Medical Publishers asked us to consider writing a surgical handbook which would be analogous to the very successful pediatrics handbook, *The Harriet Lane Handbook* (now in its 11th edition). We readily accepted the challenge of writing a pocket "pearl book" which would provide pertinent, practical information to the students and residents in surgery. The six chief residents for 1985–1986 served as editors of this handbook and the contributors included the majority of the surgical house staff in consultation with other specialists who are involved in the direct care of surgical patients and the education of residents and medical students.

The information collected in this handbook is by no means exhaustive. We have attempted simply to provide a guide for the more efficient management of prevalent surgical problems, especially by those with limited experience. Therefore, this is not a substitute for a comprehensive textbook of surgery, but is rather a supplement which concentrates on those things that are important to medical students and junior residents on the wards, namely the initial management of common surgical conditions. Much of the information is influenced by the philosophies advocated by the residents and faculty at the University of Cincinnati and thus reflects a certain bias. In areas of controversy, however, we have also provided other views and useful references.

The index has been liberally cross-referenced in order to provide a rapid and efficient means of locating information.

This handbook would not have been possible without the enthusiastic support and advice of our chairman, Dr. Josef E. Fischer, whose commitment to excellence in surgical training serves as an inspiration to all of his residents.

We would also like to acknowledge the invaluable advice provided by several of the faculty members of the Department of Surgery: Dr. Robert H. Bower, Dr. James M. Hurst, and Dr. Richard F. Kempczinski. The authors gratefully acknowledge the helpful input of Dr. Donald G. McQuarrie, Professor of Surgery at the University of Minnesota, for his review of each chapter in the handbook. Also we would like to thank Mr. Daniel J. Doody, Vice President, Editorial, Year Book Medical Publishers, for his patience and guidance in the conception and writing of this first edition of *The Mont Reid Handbook*.

None of this would have been possible were it not for the word processing expertise and herculean efforts of Mr. Steven E. Wiesner. His assistance in the typing and editing of the manuscript was invaluable.

Finally, this handbook is the result of the cumulative efforts of the surgical house staff at the University of Cincinnati as well as those residents who preceded us and taught us many of the principles that are so advocated in this book. We wish to thank all those who worked so diligently on this manuscript in order to make the first edition of *The Mont Reid Handbook* a reality.

**Michael S. Nussbaum, MD**
**Editor-in-Chief**
**Cincinnati, Ohio**
**1987**

# Special Comment

To the sixth edition

It is hard to believe that it has been 20 years since the first edition of the *Mont Reid Surgical Handbook* was published. In 1987, I was beginning my career as an academic surgeon, starting a clinical practice, performing experiments in the laboratory, studying for the American Board of Surgery Qualifying and Certifying Examinations, and completing the editing of the book that my five fellow chief residents and I had initiated in 1985. The inspiration for that first edition was our chairman at the time, Dr. Josef E. Fischer, whose dedication to excellence in surgical training was the motivation for our efforts. His successor, Dr. Jeffrey B. Matthews, continued the tradition through the last edition. Today I am the interim chair of the department, reviewing the most recent product of such efforts and hoping to carry on the commitment to surgical excellence of my predecessors. We at the University of Cincinnati remain very proud of this book and the legacy of surgical tradition that it represents.

Beginning with that first edition and continuing on through this sixth edition, the goal has been to produce an up-to-date handbook that can serve as a guide for efficient and effective management of common surgical problems. This remains a book that is written by residents for students and residents, and thus it continues to provide a fresh and practical approach to the care of the surgical patient. Dr. Wolfgang Stehr, the current editor-in-chief, and his fellow residents have provided a novel approach while relying on the traditional formula of delivering a comprehensive cross-section of relevant surgical problems as they are encountered in a surgical residency. *The Mont Reid Surgical Handbook* remains a tribute to all of the University of Cincinnati residents and faculty surgeons who have preceded us and inspired us to do our best for our patients.

**Michael S. Nussbaum, MD, FACS**
**Professor of Surgery and Interim Chairman**
**of the Department of Surgery**
**University of Cincinnati Medical Center**
**Cincinnati, Ohio**
**2007**

# Preface

To the sixth edition

We are proud to present the sixth edition of *The Mont Reid Surgical Handbook.* It has been 20 years since the book made its first appearance, and it continues to be a day-to-day companion to residents and medical students. During the past 20 years, the book has undergone multiple updates and improvements, and it continues to be a valuable and portable textbook for medical students and residents.

We are aware that in today's world of multimedia and the Internet, the role of a book may be less important, but we are convinced that there is no better way to foster an understanding of surgical pathologies, treatments and care for the patient, and understanding of the "big picture" than by reading a complete chapter in a textbook.

Once again this book is the work and product of the current residents at the University of Cincinnati Surgery Residency program. We have been given the opportunity to publish a new version of the *Handbook* every 3 to 4 years, which allows us to remain up-to-date and relevant, which for many other textbooks is impossible. As in years past, we did not attempt to create an exhaustive textbook of surgery; rather, we published a cross-section of relevant surgical problems as they are encountered in a surgical residency. To keep the book portable we have limited details on surgical procedures while expanding the section on bedside procedures.

We restructured the book by surgical subspecialties. The new structure allows the readers to find their questions answered under the surgical specialty that best fits the patient's problem. The book is designed to help students and residents understand surgical thinking, decision making, and surgical pathophysiology, and to allow them to find answers for questions on rounds, in the OR, and in standardized tests.

Wolfgang Stehr, MD
Editor-in-Chief
Cincinnati, Ohio
2008

# Acknowledgments

We want to thank the following faculty members of the University of Cincinnati for their time and help in reviewing the chapters for the sixth edition of *The Mont Reid Surgical Handbook*.

Syed A. Ahmad, MD

Richard G. Azizkhan, MD, PhD

J. Kevin Bailey, MD

David A. Billmire, MD

Karyn L. Butler, MD

Bradley R. Davis, MD

James F. Donovan, Jr., MD

Richard A. Falcone, Jr., MD, MPH

David R. Fischer, MD

Andrew D. Friedrich, MD

Michelle M. Gearhart, PharmD

Joseph S. Giglia, MD

John A. Howington, MD

Jay A. Johannigman, MD

W. John Kitzmiller, MD

Andrew M. Lowy, MD

Jeffrey B. Matthews, MD

Walter H. Merrill, MD

Mark Molloy, MD

Peter C. Muskat, MD

Raj K. Narayan, MD

Lindsey A. Nelson, MD

Michael S. Nussbaum, MD

Timothy A. Pritts, MD, PhD

Amy B. Reed, MD

Michael F. Reed, MD

Steven M. Rudich, MD, PhD

Elizabeth A. Shaughnessy, MD, PhD

Joseph S. Solomkin, MD

Sandra L. Starnes, MD

Jeffrey J. Sussman, MD

Amit D. Tevar, MD

Paul N. Uhlig, MD

John D. Wyrick, MD

Mario Zuccarello, MD

Special thanks go to April Dostie for her hard work and tremendous help in putting this book together. Steve Wiesner gets special acknowledgment for proofreading, as does Dr. Benjamin McIntyre for providing a significant number of the illustrations.

# Contents

## PART VI   Bariatric Surgery

## PART VII   Vascular Surgery

## PART VIII   Cardiothoracic Surgery

# PART I

# Surgical
# Education

Surgical
Education

# Surgical Education and Core Competencies

*Wolfgang Stehr, MD*

*Surgeons are trained, not born.*

## I. SURGICAL EDUCATION

### A. PAST 100 YEARS
1. Apprenticeship-style training (Halsted)
2. Key points: learning of medical knowledge and surgical skills through exposure, observation, and volume

### B. 21ST CENTURY
1. Challenges:
   a. Need to acquire medical knowledge and surgical skills
   b. New generation of residents: baby boomers making room for Generation X and Y
   c. Work hour restrictions
   d. Liability
2. Opportunities:
   a. Increased knowledge about adult education
   b. Computer-based simulators (minimally invasive surgery, endoscopy)
   c. Video and Internet as teaching adjuncts
3. New paradigms:
   a. Training focused on specialty (plastics, cardiothoracic, vascular, early specialization, 3y+3y programs)
   b. Disease-focused training (breast, endocrine, oncology)
   c. Trained surgeon educators
   d. Continuous personal development
      (1) Personal log-keeping of procedures, behaviors, experiences, and their outcomes
      (2) Critical assessment and development of an improvement plan
   e. Improvement of quality of life for residents
4. Current recommendations and goals:
   a. Medical students:
      (1) Structured curriculum on surgical rotations; dedication of department, faculty, and residents to education
      (2) Minimization of scutwork and integration in the care team
      (3) Development of insight into surgical pathologies and surgical decision making
      (4) Participation in surgical procedures, learning of basic surgical skills (suturing, knot tying, assisting in surgical procedures)

b. Residents:
  (1) Structured curriculum to provide knowledge in the principles of surgical diseases and patient care
  (2) Optimization of teaching conferences with didactic materials by trained surgeon educators
  (3) Optimal use of training aids and simulators to teach technical surgical skills
  (4) Minimization of scutwork and integration of physician extenders into the care teams (nurse practitioners, physician assistants)
  (5) Redesign of call schedules to comply with the 80-hour workweek requirements
  (6) Limiting fatigue to improve safety and promote better lifestyles for residents and their families
c. These recommendations have been developed and are backed by several surgical and medical associations including the American College of Surgeons (ACS), American Board of Surgery (ABS), Association of American Medical Colleges (AAMC), Accreditation Council for Graduate Medical Education (ACGME), and Residency Review Committee (RRC).

## II. CORE COMPETENCIES

### A. THE OUTCOME PROJECT
1. In 2001, the ACGME (www.acgme.org) implemented a curriculum and evaluation program covering six core competencies.
2. The goal was to provide evidence that residents are not only exposed to training, but to show that residents develop "know-how" and eventually can "show how."
3. The residency program must demonstrate that it has an effective plan that assesses resident performance throughout the program, and that it uses assessment results to improve resident performance.
4. Residents must be evaluated, and timely feedback must be provided to achieve progressive improvements in residents' competence and performance.

### B. THE SIX CORE COMPETENCIES
1. Patient care:
a. Patient management skills—collection of data, synthesis of data, clinical judgment
b. Technical skills—manual dexterity, mastery of fundamental technical skills, conduct of operations, bedside procedures
2. Medical knowledge:
a. Fund of fundamental surgical basic science and clinical knowledge
b. Application of knowledge to solution of clinical problems
3. Practice-based learning:
a. Notes, summaries, and operative reports are complete, concise, and completed on time.

b. Presentations at morbidity and mortality conference demonstrate mechanism of complication and ways to prevent complications in the future.

4. **Communication and interpersonal skills:**

a. Rapport with patients and families, effective communication with nurses, colleagues, consultants, and other members of the care team

b. Organized and succinct oral presentations

c. Effective teaching of junior residents and students

5. **Professionalism:**

a. Demonstration of initiative in caring for patients

b. Acceptance of appropriate level of responsibility

c. Honesty and reliability

d. Empathy and compassion

e. Team player

f. Professional appearance

6. **System-based practice:**

a. Familiarity with the medical care delivery system in which residents practice

b. Appropriate and effective use of clinical pathways

c. Cost-effective care without compromising quality

## RECOMMENDED REFERENCES

Accreditation Council for Graduate Medical Education—http://www.acgme.org

American Board of Surgery—http://home.absurgery.org

American College of Surgeons—http://www.facs.org

Association for Surgical Education—http://www.surgicaleducation.com

SURGICAL EDUCATION AND CORE COMPETENCIES

# PART II

# Perioperative Care

# Medical Record

*Christopher A. Lundquist, MD*

## I. SURGICAL HISTORY AND PHYSICAL EXAMINATION

### A. MEETING THE PATIENT

1. Initial contact
   a. KISS mnemonic: *K*nock. *I*ntroduce yourself. *S*crub your hands. *S*it down
2. Put patient at ease: Take time to ask the patient a personal, non-medical question before starting. Minimize all environmental distractions. Ensure that you and the patient are as comfortable as possible.
3. Listen to your patient. He or she is trying to tell you the diagnosis. As a general rule: Listen more, talk less, and interrupt infrequently. Ask the patient what his/her goals of treatment are so you can address them adequately.

### B. HISTORY

1. Chief complaint—in the patient's own words and in quotations
2. History of present illness
   a. Main symptom—helpful mnemonic: *OPQRST*
      **Onset:** When did it (main symptom) start? Was the onset gradual or acute? What was the patient doing when it started? Any previous similar episodes?
      **Position:** Where is it located? Is it focal or diffuse? Does it radiate? Has it migrated?
      **Quality:** What is it like? Is it sharp and stabbing? Dull and cramping? Has it changed?
      **Related symptoms:** Are there any other symptoms that could be related?
      **Severity:** How bad is it currently? How bad at onset? Has it worsened?
      **Timing/triggers:** What makes it better or worse? Eating? Position? Movement? How long does it last? How frequent? Is it constant or intermittent?
      Always conduct a comprehensive review of symptoms. The following factors require extra attention in general surgery:
   b. Fever/chills: Onset and severity help distinguish between inflammatory and infectious diseases.
   c. Emesis: Inspect vomitus when possible. What is its appearance? Is it bilious, feculent, or bloody? What is the volume? How often does this occur? Is it projectile? Is it associated with pain? With eating? With nausea? The relation among onset of abdominal pain, onset of vomiting, and quality of the emesis may indicate the level of obstruction.
   d. Bowel habits: Any change? Last bowel movement? Flatus? Stool consistency? Appearance? Intermittent constipation and diarrhea suggest colon cancer or diverticular disease, whereas constipation coupled with pencil-thin stools imply anal or rectal malignancies.

    e. Bleeding
      (1) A history of bleeding is the best predictor of perioperative bleeding.
      (2) Abnormal bleeding from any orifice must be evaluated carefully. Stool blood, whether gross or occult, is due to gastrointestinal (GI) malignancy until proved otherwise.
    f. Hematemesis or hematochezia: Is it clotted? Is it bright or dark red blood? Has it changed in any way? Its character helps discriminate between pathologic states. Coffee-ground vomitus is indicative of slow gastric bleeding. Dark, tarry stool is characteristic of upper GI bleeding. Acute-onset lightheadedness and diaphoresis are indicative of rapid GI blood loss.
    g. Jaundice: The rate of onset and the presence of clay-colored stools and dark urine help differentiate surgical from medical causative factors.
    h. Weight loss: Unintentional weight loss with normal appetite may indicate a malignant cause, whereas weight loss secondary to pain with eating suggests ulceration or intestinal ischemia.
    i. Trauma: Details must be established precisely.
    j. Medications: Inquire into which medications have been tried and their efficacy. Query the use of over-the-counter drugs and herbals, as well as opiates, nonsteroidal antiinflammatory drugs, diuretics, corticosteroids, antiepileptics/sedatives, and cardiac/respiratory drugs. Indicate dose, route, frequency, and duration of usage. Obtain a written record of current medications if possible.
  **3. Medical history: Always obtain prior operative reports, imaging/ laboratory studies, and discharge summaries. A comprehensive medical history is imperative in assessing patients for potential perioperative complications.**
    a. Chronic illnesses—diabetes mellitus, hypertension, coronary artery disease, chronic obstructive pulmonary disease, renal/hepatic/adrenal disease, hematologic disorders, malignancies, etc.
    b. Acute illnesses/hospitalizations—pneumonia, asthma attacks, diabetic ketoacidosis, biliary or renal colic
    c. Injuries/accidents—prior trauma
    d. Gynecological history—last menstrual period, history of sexually transmitted diseases, pregnancies
  **4. Surgical history**
    a. Type, date, hospital of surgery, and name of surgeon
    b. Indications for surgery—emergent vs. elective
    c. Prior difficulties with anesthesia; perioperative complications
  **5. Allergies—specific drug reaction (e.g., rash/hives, stridor, anaphylaxis)**
  **6. Social history—alcohol, tobacco, illegal drugs (Route? How much? How long? History of withdrawal?), and sexual history/orientation**
  **7. Family history—any surgical disorders are familial (e.g., colonic polyposis, multiple endocrine neoplasia syndromes, breast carcinoma)**

## C. REVIEW OF SYSTEMS

The system review must be formalized and methodical to ensure important details are not overlooked. Nutritional deficiencies (particularly recent acute fluid losses, weight loss, anorexia), chest pain, and dyspnea must be noted. Record pertinent findings.

## D. PHYSICAL EXAMINATION

1. Ensure patient comfort.
2. Develop a system. Develop a comprehensive yet systematic method of examination so that no detail is omitted. Ensure all tools are convenient and that lighting is optimal.
3. Assess the patient. Ensure that the patient is warm, pink, urinating, and talking. Look at the patient before the "laying on of hands."
4. Refer to Chapter 3 for a detailed description of pertinent physical findings associated with multiple surgical diseases.

## E. RECAP

Recapitulate to your patient your understanding of his or her problems and/or findings in the context of the patient's goals of therapy. Inquire further into any new findings. Allow the patient to clarify or correct any misconceptions. Have members of the patient's health-care team available at this time to ensure all constituents acknowledge these problems and goals.

## F. ANCILLARY STUDIES

1. Laboratory examination. Objectives of the laboratory studies are as follows:
a. Diagnose surgical disorders.
b. Confirm the suspected diagnosis and rule out alternative diagnoses.
c. Screen for diseases that may require preoperative treatment or may contraindicate elective surgery.
d. Screen for asymptomatic disease that may affect perioperative course (diabetes mellitus, adrenal insufficiency).
2. Routine laboratory studies
   Complete blood cell count $\pm$ differential
   Electrolyte profile, blood urea nitrogen/creatinine
   Coagulation profile (prothrombin time/international normalized ratio/ partial thromboplastin time)
   Urinalysis
   Electrocardiogram (>40 years of age or known history of cardiac disease)
   Hepatic profile for evaluation of specific diseases, known liver problems, or if hepatic surgery planned
3. Radiologic evaluation
A chest radiograph is indicated for most patients undergoing major surgery. Order special radiographs and studies in specific clinical situations. Provide radiologist with an adequate patient history, physical examination, and a specific reason for ordering each study.

## G. ASSESSMENT AND PLAN

Following a thorough history and physical examination, one should be able to assess the patient's problems and form a differential diagnosis, construct a problem list, and develop a diagnostic and therapeutic plan.

1. **Problem list:** List, from most to least important, the problems identified.
2. **Assessment:** An assessment includes a concise summary of relevant data that support the tentative conclusions and diagnosis. Delineate the thought process, including major decision-making points, deviations from the norm, alternative diagnoses, and complicating factors.
3. **Plan:** List specific diagnostic and therapeutic plans.

## H. EMERGENT HISTORY AND PHYSICAL EXAMINATION

Initial efforts should be directed toward resuscitating the patient. The routine history and physical examination must often be truncated.

1. **History:** The mnemonic is *AMPLE.*
   *A*llergies
   *M*eds
   *P*ast medical history
   *L*ast meal
   *E*vents preceding injury or illness
2. **Physical examination:** The mnemonic is *ABCDE.*
   *A*irway
   *B*reathing
   *C*irculation
   *D*isability
   *E*xposure

## II. PHYSICIAN ORDERS

Personally communicate all written and computer-entry orders to nursing staff to minimize ambiguity.

## A. ADMISSION: A HELPFUL MNEMONIC IS *ADCA-VAN-DIMLS.*

*A*dmit—admittance to ward or intensive care unit, surgery service/team, attending/resident/intern, contact pager number
*D*iagnosis—illness/disease
*C*ondition—excellent; good; fair; serious; critical
*A*llergies—specific symptoms
*V*ital signs
Frequency and need for neurologic/vascular checks
Parameters to notify physician
- Systolic blood pressure [SBP] <90, >180 mm Hg
- Diastolic blood pressure >110 mm Hg
- Pulse >110 or <60 beats/min
- Temperature >101.5° F
- Urine output <30 ml/h (<1 ml/kg/h in children)
- Change in neurologic/vascular status

- Increasing oxygen requirement
- Respiratory rate <10 or >30 breaths/min

Activity or position

Weight-bearing status

Elevation of head or foot of bed

Prevention of decubitus and thromboembolism (e.g., turn side to side every 2 hours, out of bed/ambulate with assistance three times a day)

Nursing orders

Strict intake and outputs

Blood glucose checks/sliding scale insulin parameters

Tube maintenance—nasogastric, feeding, urinary catheter, chest tube, drains

Wound care—dressing type and frequency

Monitors/arterial line/central venous pressure/intracranial pressure

Respiratory care—vent settings, supplemental oxygen parameters, ventilator settings, pulmonary toilet

Compression boots/sequential compression devices or thromboembolic disease stockings

Diet—nothing by mouth (NPO), clear liquid, regular, diabetic, special diets, tube feeds, total parenteral nutrition

IV fluids (e.g., D5 1/2 normal saline + 20 mEq KCl/L at 100 ml/h)

Medications (drug, dose, route, frequency, +/− as needed, hold parameters)

Helpful mnemonic—*ABCDEFGHI*

- *A*ntibiotics
- *B*owel regimen—stool softeners/laxatives
- *C*rying—analgesics
- *D*eep vein thrombosis prophylaxis—heparin subcutaneously
- *E*mesis—antiemetics
- *F*ever—antipyretics
- *G*I prophylaxis—H2 blockers vs. proton pump inhibitor (PPI)
- *H*ome medications
- *I*nsulin/itching—insulin/antipruritics

Laboratory tests

Special studies (radiographs, consults)

## B.  PREOPERATIVE

1. NPO after midnight (including tube feeds)
2. Adjust or hold insulin/hypoglycemics for NPO
3. IV hydration (D5 1/2 normal saline + 20 mEq KCl/L at 100 ml/h)
4. Perioperative antibiotics/stress dose steroids on call to operating room
5. Bowel prep
6. Labs
7. Type and screen/cross-match blood and blood products
8. Special studies

**2**

**MEDICAL RECORD**

## C. POSTOPERATIVE

1. Pain medications (epidural, patient-controlled analgesic, IV morphine, IV ketorolac tromethamine [Toradol])
2. Deep venous thrombosis prophylaxis
3. Perioperative antibiotic prophylaxis
4. GI prophylaxis
5. IV fluids/diet
6. Incentive spirometer/pulmonary toilet
7. Bowel regimen
8. Antiemetic, sleep, antipyretic, delirium tremens (DT) prophylaxis (as needed).

## III. NOTES

Date and time all medical record entries. Sign with name, service, and contact information.

## A. PREOPERATIVE NOTES

1. Preoperative diagnosis
2. Procedure planned
3. Surgeon/service
4. Anesthesia anticipated (general endotracheal, monitored anesthesia care [MAC], local, etc.)
5. Laboratory data
   a. Minor operations—complete blood cell count and urinalysis
   b. Major operations
      (1) Complete blood cell count, electrolytes, coagulation profile (partial thromboplastin time, prothrombin time)
      (2) Urinalysis
      (3) Electrocardiogram if patient is older than 40 or with cardiac risk factors
      (4) Chest radiograph if no recent radiograph or as indicated
      (5) Pulmonary function testing as indicated
      (6) Type and screen or cross-match as indicated (verify cross-match with blood bank)
      (7) Blood gases, hepatic profile, other laboratory studies, or specific radiographs as indicated by patient's comorbidities
6. Identify specific risk factors related to patient's cardiac, renal, pulmonary, hepatic, coagulation, and nutritional status.
7. Current medications or allergies
8. Preoperative order checklist
9. Blood/blood products to transfuse before surgery or on call to operating room
10. Antiseptic scrub
11. Prophylactic antibiotics/stress dose steroids on call to operating room
12. Special medications (e.g., steroids, insulin, antihypertensives, anticonvulsives)
13. NPO after midnight

14. IV fluids
15. Document that potential risks and benefits of intended operation have been explained, questions have been adequately answered, and patient (or guardian) has consented to the procedure. Ensure that signed consent is on the chart.

## B. POSTOPERATIVE NOTES

1. Subjective—patient concerns/complaints, oral intake, activity, nausea/emesis
2. Mental status—neurologic examination, pain control
3. Vital signs, urine, and drain output
4. Physical examination—inspection of surgical dressings and wounds
5. Postoperative laboratory data
6. Assessment of condition and plan

## C. PROGRESS NOTES

Use Weed's problem-oriented approach to medical records (see Recommended Reading).

1. Daily notes: Document current, newly identified, and potential problems. Include postoperative and hospital day number, antibiotic, or hyperalimentation day number.
2. *SOAP* notes.
   Subjective data (events overnight, patient complaints, nurse observations)
   Objective data (vital signs, physical examination, laboratory data)
   Assessment of condition
   Plan (Diagnostic studies, therapeutic changes, patient education/disposition)
3. Flow sheets: Adjuncts evaluate complex data as a function of time (e.g., hyperalimentation data, diabetes control, hemodynamic parameters).

## IV. DICTATIONS

Dictate immediately after an operation.

## A. OPERATIVE REPORT

1. Patient name
2. Patient medical record/account number
3. Date of procedure
4. Dictating physician
5. Attending surgeon
6. Assistants
7. Copies—to attending surgeon, assistants, billing office, referring physician
8. Preoperative diagnosis
9. Postoperative diagnosis—accuracy imperative for medical record and billing purposes
10. Procedure performed—dictate in list format

11. Complications
12. Specimens
13. Indications for surgery
a. Brief history: Document explanation of risks and benefits and acquisition of informed consent
14. Details of operation:
a. Patient position/anesthesia
b. Skin prep and draping
c. Type/location/technique of incision and course of dissection
d. Pathology/operative findings
e. Therapeutic approach/complications/blood transfusions.
f. Intraoperative consultations
g. Closure technique/dressings/drains
h. Sponge/needle/instrument count
i. Presence of attending surgeon (and if scrubbed)
j. Postoperative complications/disposition
k. Note: Provide a concise written note with visual aids immediately after all procedures to allow time for dictated operative reports to appear in the formal medical record.

## B.  DISCHARGE SUMMARY/DEATH SUMMARY
1. Patient name
2. Patient medical record number/account numbers
3. Date of admission/date of discharge
4. Dictating physician
5. Attending surgeon
6. Copies—to attending surgeon, dictator, billing office, referring physician
7. Discharge diagnoses
8. Operations/procedures performed
9. Consultations
10. Allergies
11. Discharge medications—current and any new medications
12. Indication for admission—history of present illness with pertinent preoperative physical findings, laboratory values, and studies
13. Hospital course
14. Condition on discharge—pertinent postoperative physical examination findings, laboratory values
15. Discharge instructions—diet and activity restrictions, follow-up appointments, and studies
16. Note: Dictated discharge summaries take time to appear in the patient's medical record. A simple written document with pertinent discharge information should be submitted with the medical record.

## V. BILLING

Patient billing is based on the medical record documentation. Perioperative detailing of comorbidities and complications may justify higher levels of billing. Medicare lists the minimal physical examination/patient interactions required for each organ system. A synopsis of the various levels is presented in Tables 2-1 and 2-2.

## VI. HEALTH INFORMATION PORTABILITY AND ACCOUNTABILITY ACT (HIPAA)

### A. PROTECTS PRIVACY OF PATIENT INFORMATION

### B. WHAT DOES HIPAA MEAN?

1. Disclosure of protected health information must be limited only to the minimum necessary for treatment.
2. Information may be shared as necessary to provide services.
3. Patient must sign a notice of privacy practices and give explicit permission to share any information outside of this system.
4. Research use requires special permission.
5. Identifying waste must be shredded and computer records protected.
6. Patient care may not be discussed in public places.

**2**

**MEDICAL RECORD**

### TABLE 2-1

#### COMPLEXITY OF H&Ps FOR BILLING PURPOSES

| | | | | |
|---|---|---|---|---|
| Problem focused | Brief HPI | 0 P/F/SH | 0 ROS | 1-5 examination elements |
| Expanded | Brief HPI | 0 P/F/SH | 0 ROS | 6 examination elements |
| Detailed | Full HPI | 1 P/F/SH | 2+ ROS | 12 examination elements |
| Comprehensive | Full HPI | 3 P/F/SH | 10+ ROS | 2 elements from any 9 organ systems |

HPI = history of present illness; P/F/SH = past/familial/social history; ROS = review of systems.

### TABLE 2-2

#### BILLING LEVELS FOR H&P DOCUMENTS

| Level | Decision Making |
|---|---|
| **New patient:** | |
| Level I: Problem focused | Straightforward |
| Level II: Expanded | Straightforward |
| Level III: Detailed | Low complexity |
| Level IV: Comprehensive | Moderate complexity |
| Level V: Comprehensive | High complexity |
| **Established patient:** | |
| Level II: Focused | Straightforward |
| Level III: Expanded | Low complexity |
| Level IV: Detailed | Moderate complexity |
| Level V: Comprehensive | High complexity |

## C. PROTECTED HEALTH INFORMATION
1. Demographic information
2. Physical or mental health information
3. Provision of health care
4. Payment of health care

## D. SHARING OF INFORMATION ALLOWED
1. To provide treatment
2. To obtain payment
3. For health care operations (e.g., quality assessment)
4. For research (with permission)
5. Incidental disclosure
6. In compliance with laws
7. For public health reporting
8. Law enforcement
9. To coroners and for organ donation

## E. PENALTIES
1. Civil
a. $100 per violation
b. Up to $25,000 per person
2. Criminal
a. Up to $250,000
b. Up to 10 years imprisonment

## VII. SUMMARY
### A. COMMUNICATION
Health-care team members use medical record documentation collectively to provide continuity to the patient's care. Your notes must effectively communicate your impressions of and plans for care of the patient.

### B. STANDARD DOCUMENTATION
A good rule of thumb is: If it is not recorded, it did not happen or you did not do it.
1. Admission history and physical examination
2. Daily SOAP notes
3. Procedure notes
a. All bedside procedures (e.g., wound debridement, central venous catheter placement)
b. Detailed findings and complications
4. Operative notes
   a. Preoperative note including consent
   b. Operative note dictated and written
   c. Postoperative note
5. Description of discussions with patients and patient families regarding care

6. Crucial occurrences: Document patient condition and treatments given/ordered when called to see patient for any concerning symptom.

7. Consultation notes: Review of patient history, physical examination, and pertinent laboratory studies and findings. Detail impressions, recommendations, and any discussions with patient, patient's family, and consulting physicians.

8. Discharge summary

## C. LITIGATION

Nothing can be defended without written legible documentation in the chart. Medical malpractice cases rely on proving dereliction of duty directly resulting in damage. Provide adequate documentation to illustrate adequacy of care.

### ACKNOWLEDGEMENT

*Special thanks to Dr. Paul Uhlig for advice and insight he provided during the writing of this chapter.*

### RECOMMENDED READING

Weed L: *Medical Records, Medical Education, and Patient Care: The Problem-Oriented Record as a Basic Tool.* Chicago, Year Book, 1970.

2

MEDICAL RECORD

# Physical Examination of the Surgical Patient

*Charles Park, MD*

Your senses of sight, hearing, touch, and smell can confirm or refute diagnostic hypotheses based on your patient's history and symptoms. The physical examination is methodical and done the same way each time. A well-documented examination may obviate the need for further diagnostic testing in surgical conditions such as a perforated viscus, appendicitis, and cholecystitis. In the trauma patient, the importance of constant reevaluation cannot be overemphasized to assure that new findings are not overlooked and to discover deterioration in previously noted findings.

**3**

## I. VITAL SIGNS

A temperature greater than 38°C or less than 36°C, a heart rate greater than 90 beats/min, and a respiratory rate more than 20 breaths/min are all criteria for defining a systemic inflammatory response.

### A. TEMPERATURE

1. Reference range: 36°C (96.8°F) to 38°C (100.4°F)—varies by age, time of day, and site of measurement.
2. Fever—greater than 38.6°C (101.5°F)
3. Hypothermia—less than 35°C (95°F)

### B. HEART RATE

1. Reference range: 60 to 100 beats/min for adults, 80 to 100 beats/min for children, and 100 to 120 beats/min for infants
2. Tachycardia is the most common vital sign change associated with early hypovolemic shock; however, tachycardia is present in less than half of patients in the supine position with moderate-to-severe blood loss.
3. Pain, hypoxia, stimulant drugs, and pregnancy may contribute to tachycardia.
4. Athletes, elderly adults, those taking beta-blockers, and those with neurogenic block are not as likely to become tachycardic.

### C. BLOOD PRESSURE

1. Reference range: systolic pressure 90 to 140 mm Hg, diastolic pressure 60 to 90 mm Hg for adults, systolic pressure 80 to 110 mm Hg for children
2. Palpable carotid, femoral, and radial pulses estimate a systolic blood pressure of at least 60, 70, and 80 mm Hg, respectively.
3. Mean arterial pressure [(diastolic blood pressure + 1/3 [systolic blood pressure − diastolic blood pressure]); reference range = 80–90 mm Hg] is a more consistent indicator of peripheral perfusion pressure than systolic pressure.

4. When in doubt, check blood pressure manually with a stethoscope and cuff.
5. Bilateral measurements should be compared.

**Pearl:** *An inappropriately small-sized cuff is a common source of error in blood pressure measurement. The <u>width</u> of the cuff should encircle at least half of the patient's upper arm or readings may be incorrectly high. Large cuffs read accurately.*

6. Significant orthostatic change
a. Heart rate increase of 30 beats/min
b. Systolic blood pressure decrease of 20 mm Hg
c. Dizziness on standing

**Pearl:** *A narrowed pulse pressure (systolic pressure − diastolic pressure) of less than 30 mm Hg may be an early indicator of hypovolemic shock or cardiac tamponade.*

## D. RESPIRATORY RATE
1. Reference range: 12 to 20 breaths/min for adults, 15 to 30 breaths/min for children
2. A rate of more than 20 breaths/min may reflect pain or systemic acidosis.
3. A rate of less than 12 breaths/min may reflect oversedation with narcotic pain medications.

## E. PULSE OXIMETRY
1. Accurate readings require a strong arterial pulse and good light transmission.
2. Hypotension, vasoactive medications, hypothermia, bright lights, and nail polish can result in spurious values.
3. Carbon monoxide or cyanide poisoning can lead to erroneously high $SpO_2$ values.

**Pearl:** *The pulse oximeter sensor should not be placed distal to the blood pressure cuff.*

## II. GENERAL APPEARANCE
The general appearance of a patient, particularly the face, can reveal the patient's level of consciousness, distress, mental status, nutritional status, and level of hydration.

## A. INSPECTION
1. Level of consciousness, mental state
a. Obtundation—sign of hypercarbia
b. Agitation or combativeness—sign of hypoxia
c. Anxiety level, diaphoresis

2. Facies and body habitus—indicator of nutritional state and intubation/surgical risk
a. Abnormal facies
b. Muscle mass (i.e., *temporal wasting*)
c. Obesity
3. **Skin**
a. Color
    (1) Pale, ashen skin may indicate anemia or poor peripheral perfusion.
    (2) Jaundice *(first appears on the frenulum, then sclera)*
        (a) Jaundice is seen with a total serum bilirubin of at least 2 to 3 mg/dl.
    (3) Redness may indicate inflammation of infectious or traumatic causative agent.
    (4) Blue-gray patches may be a sign of deadly infection.

**Pearl:** *The appearance of tender edema and erythema without clear boundaries may herald* **necrotizing fasciitis.** *The "finger test" can be performed under local anesthesia. Positive findings include: 1) lack of bleeding; 2) presence of "dishwater pus"; and 3) lack of tissue resistance to blunt finger dissection. Necrotic fascia appears gray.*

b. Integrity
    (1) Burns—estimate percentage surface area.
        (a) First degree—erythema, peeling of epidermis
        (b) Second degree—blisters with fluid collections, mottled pink/white surface
        (c) Third degree—white, cherry red or black; appears leathery, firm, depressed
        (d) Fourth degree—charred
    (2) Decubitus ulcer staging:
        (a) Stage 1—erythema
        (b) Stage 2—partial skin thickness loss
        (c) Stage 3—full-thickness skin loss
        (d) Stage 4—full-thickness skin loss and underlying tissue injury
    (3) Wounds
c. Petechiae (1–3 mm), purpura (>3 mm)—deep red or reddish purple, fading over time
d. Spider angiomata
    (1) Central arteriole surrounded by smaller vessels; does not blanch with pressure
e. Catheter sites (erythema, drainage)
f. Malignant lesions
    (1) Melanoma ABCDEs:
        (a) Asymmetry
        (b) Border irregularity

(c) Color variegation
(d) Diameter greater than 6 mm
(e) Elevation or history of enlarging size
(2) Basal cell
  (a) Pink, waxy papule with central ulcer and rolled, pearly borders
  (b) Common locations—inner aspect of nose, periorbital, upper lip, trunk
(3) Squamous cell
  (a) Ulcerated nodule, raised hyperkeratotic papules
  (b) Common locations—sun-exposed areas, lower lip, hands

**Pearl:** *The number and size of spider angiomas often correlate with the severity of liver disease. (Spider angiomas are seen in patients who are pregnant or who have severe malnutrition. Healthy people have less than three small lesions.)*

### 4. Signs of injury
a. Contusions, hemorrhage
b. Deformity
c. Lateralizing signs (i.e., *immobility*)

## B. PALPATION
### 1. Temperature
### 2. Skin turgor—volume status
a. Normal elastic skin over the back of the hand that is pinched and released resumes its customary shape; persistence of the fold is loss of turgor.
### 3. Edema
a. Note distribution. Interstitial fluid accumulates to the amount of ~5 kg before pitting edema is detectable.

## III. HEAD AND NECK
## A. INSPECTION
### 1. Skull, scalp, face
a. Lacerations, contusions, depressions
b. Fracture signs
  (1) Periorbital ecchymoses (raccoon eyes)
  (2) Retroauricular ecchymoses (Battle's sign)
c. Burn signs
  (1) Singed hair
  (2) Carbonaceous sputum
  (3) Erythematous, blistered, or leathery skin
  (4) These findings may herald respiratory failure from inhalation injury and airway edema.
### 2. Oropharynx
a. Foreign bodies, presence/stability of teeth, active bleeding
b. Dental occlusion

c. Mucous membranes—moisture, integrity, and color
d. *Mallampati scoring system*—predicts difficult intubation
   (1) Have the patient sit on the side of the bed and open his or her mouth widely, then protrude the tongue as far as possible without phonating.
   (2) Identify *visible* posterior oropharyngeal structures.
      (a) Classes I and II—soft palate, complete uvula. Low intubation failure rates are seen with these patients.
      (b) Class III—soft palate, base of uvula only
      (c) Class IV—only hard palate visible. Intubation failure rates may exceed 10% for these patients.

3. **Neck**
a. Trachea—deviation from midline position
b. *Jugular venous distension*
   (1) The pulsations of the right internal jugular vein are visible with proper patient positioning and lighting. Begin with the patient's trunk inclined at less than 30 degrees. The venous pulse is differentiated from the arterial by its double undulation and collapse during inspiration. Examine the internal rather than external jugular vein because there are no valves to interfere with pressure transmission. The arterial pulse is easily visible more medially and cephalad in the neck.
   (2) Neck veins may not be distended in the patient with hypovolemia.
c. Thyroid—have the patient swallow, then inspect for an ascending mass in the midline or behind the sternocleidomastoid muscle (SCM).

4. **Eyes**

**Pearl:** *In trauma, perform the eye examination before swelling makes it difficult.*

a. Acuity—the vital sign of the eye
b. Pupils—size and reactivity to light
c. Globe—position within orbit
d. Ocular mobility—exclude muscle entrapment.
e. Conjunctiva—pallor, hemorrhage
f. Foreign bodies, contacts

**Pearl:** *A dilated pupil or anisocoria (unequal pupil size) in a patient with decreasing consciousness may indicate a neurologic emergency resulting from increased intracranial pressure from bleeding.*

5. **Ears and nose**
a. Blood behind the tympanic membranes (hemotympanum)
b. Drainage of clear cerebrospinal fluid (otorrhea, rhinorrhea)
c. Inspect the nasal septum for bulging, bluish mass (hematoma), significant deviation.

3

PHYSICAL EXAMINATION OF THE SURGICAL PATIENT

## B.  AUSCULTATION
1. Airway assessment—clear speech indicates patency.
a. Gasping—oropharyngeal obstruction
b. Stridor—partial occlusion of trachea
2. Neck—carotid artery bruits

## C.  PALPATION
1. Neck
a. Crepitans, tracheal deviation
b. Carotid artery pulses
c. Suppleness versus rigidity
d. Cervical spine tenderness, presence of step-offs
e. Open wounds through the platysma should never be probed because of hemorrhage risk.

**Pearl:** *One third of patients with crepitans on palpation of the neck have an injury to the pharynx, esophagus, larynx, or trachea.*

2. Scalp—step-offs, open fractures
3. Face
a. Localized tenderness or step-offs on the forehead, periorbital region, zygomatic arch, mandible, or nasal arch
   (1) General facial fracture—press on the masseter muscles while patient is biting down; lack of pain indicates absence of fracture.
   (2) Test midface stability—grasp upper incisors and move anteroposterior.
   (3) *Tongue blade test* (sensitivity of greater than 95%)
      (a) Ask patient to bite down on a tongue blade; if examiner can break the blade in this position, a mandibular fracture is unlikely.
b. Paresthesia—note distribution.
4. Thyroid examination
a. Feel for tissue on the anterior surface of the tracheal rings.
b. Palpate the anterior surface of the lateral lobes through the SCM muscles with the patient's head inclined toward the side being examined to relax the muscles.
c. Use bidigital palpation to examine the lateral lobes, with one thumb pushing the trachea to one side while the other thumb and index finger feel deeply on either side of the SCM.

**Pearl:** *Thyroid cancer is found more often with firm, solitary nodules. Fixation to adjacent structures, vocal cord paralysis, and enlarged lymph nodes are associated with an increased risk for malignancy.*

## IV. CHEST

### A. INSPECTION

1. Bilateral chest wall expansion with inspiration
a. Localized bulging of thorax during expiration (flail chest)
2. Depth and frequency of respirations
3. Accessory muscle use (neck, upper abdomen)
4. Contusions/lacerations of chest wall
5. Breast
a. Erythema, edema, dimpling, nipple deviation, and/or ulceration should be noted. Leaning forward accentuates skin retraction.
b. Increased breast tissue around the nipple in male individuals (gynecomastia).

### B. AUSCULTATION

1. Technique
a. Have patient breathe through the mouth, more deeply and forcefully than usual.
b. Listen to the anterior apices and work caudally, comparing sequential symmetric points.
c. Repeat on the back.
2. In trauma, listen for good air movement at the nose and mouth.
3. Breath sounds
a. Absent/decreased.
   (1) High on anterior chest (pneumothorax)
   (2) Posterior bases (hemothorax/effusion)
b. Wheezing—short inspiration, long expiration with higher pitch (asthma or isolated bronchial obstruction)
c. Crackles (inspiratory at bases—atelectasis, pneumonia, pulmonary edema)
4. *Hamman's sign* (classically associated with a perforated esophagus)
a. Subcutaneous, mediastinal air causing precordial crunching with systolic beats

### C. PALPATION

1. Apply firm, steady pressure to the chest cage.
a. Clavicles
b. Sternum
c. Sternoclavicular, costosternal junctions
d. Intercostal spaces, rib segments
2. Crepitans, instability, step-offs, swelling and/or point tenderness
3. Breast examination
a. With the patient in the sitting position, support the patient's arm and palpate each axilla to detect adenopathy (see section IX).
b. Palpate each breast while the patient is supine with her ipsilateral hand placed behind her head.

3

PHYSICAL EXAMINATION OF THE SURGICAL PATIENT

c. Palpate the nipple for discharge.

d. Masses—location, size, shape, consistency, mobility, and tenderness

## D. PERCUSSION

1. Technique

a. The surface of the body is struck to emit sounds that vary in quality according to the density of the underlying tissue.

b. The middle finger of the nondominant hand is laid on the body surface and its distal interphalangeal joint is struck sharply with the tip of the middle finger of the dominant hand.

2. **Hyperresonance or dullness should be noted, particularly at the high anterior chest and posterior bases.**

## V. CARDIOVASCULAR

### A. INSPECTION

1. General—active hemorrhage

2. Heart—contusions or lacerations in the *precordial box* medial to the nipples, below the clavicles, and above the costal margin may indicate underlying injury.

3. Extremities

a. Acute arterial insufficiency

   (1) Pain

   (2) Pallor (mottling)

b. Chronic arterial insufficiency

   (1) Hair loss

   (2) Nail changes

   (3) Nonhealing skin breakdown

   (4) Ischemic ulcers

      (a) Location—tips of toes, malleolus, heel, metatarsal head, and dorsal arch

      (b) Borders frequently appear "punched out."

c. Impaired venous outflow

   (1) Brawny edema

   (2) Varicose veins

   (3) Hyperpigmentation

   (4) Indurative cellulitis

   (5) Painless ulceration

      (a) Location—superior and posterior to the medial malleolus. At this location, five to six perforators from the greater saphenous vein run from the superficial venous system to the deep posterior tibial vein.

d. Extremity thromboses

   (1) Ipsilateral swelling, erythema

## B. AUSCULTATION

1. Heart

a. Rate and regularity of paired heart sounds

b. Muffled sounds (emphysema, pericardial tamponade)
c. Murmurs
  (1) Timing—during systole or diastole
  (2) Location—where maximally heard and radiation
  (3) Pattern of sound intensity
2. **Extremities**
a. Bruits (stenosis, arteriovenous fistula)

## C. PALPATION
1. **Temperature**
2. **Pulse examination**
a. Regions
  (1) Carotid
  (2) Radial/brachial
  (3) Femoral
  (4) Posterior tibial/dorsalis pedis
b. Amplitude, contour, and upstroke
c. Compare bilaterally.
d. Thrill (arteriovenous fistula, arterial injury)
3. **Acute arterial insufficiency—4 *P*'s:**
a. Pulselessness
b. Poikilothermia
  (1) Fluctuation from core temperature of greater than 2°C because of ambient temperature change
c. Paresthesia (late finding)
d. Paralysis (late finding)
4. **Expanding or pulsatile hematoma**

**Pearl:** *In up to 20% of proven arterial injuries of an extremity, a distal pulse is palpable because of collateral circulation.*

5. **Venous insufficiency—Trendelenburg test of valve competence**
a. Have patient raise leg to drain venous system.
b. Apply tourniquet over the saphenofemoral junction and have patient stand.
c. Rapid filling of varicosities before tourniquet release indicates valve incompetence.
d. Rapid filling with release of tourniquet indicates incompetent saphenofemoral valve.
6. **Extremity thromboses: Physical signs have been shown to be quite unreliable in diagnosing deep venous thrombosis (risk factor history plus physical examination enables a diagnosis <50% of the time).**
a. Warmth in an isolated extremity
b. Palpable cord
c. *Homans' sign*—increased resistance/tenderness to foot dorsiflexion

PHYSICAL EXAMINATION OF THE SURGICAL PATIENT

3

**Pearl: *Ankle-brachial index*** *(ABI) is the highest ankle pressure divided by the highest brachial pressure on the ipsilateral arm, measured by a blood pressure cuff and Doppler instrument. A normal ankle/brachial index is slightly greater than 1. A patient with claudication or ischemia will have an ankle/brachial index less than 0.9. Pressure indices in other areas (i.e., wrist/brachial index) can be used to evaluate an extremity for occult vascular injury. A pressure index of less than 0.9 has 95% sensitivity and 97% specificity for major vascular injury. A pressure index of greater than 0.9 has a negative predictive value of 99%.*

## VI. ABDOMEN

Abdominal pain can often be a benign complaint but may herald serious acute pathology. Frequent reexamination, preferably by the same observer, is a key component to identifying evolving conditions of surgical import. Physical examination is critical to narrowing down the causative factor of your patient's abdominal pain. Approach the patient with gentleness, and make sure the patient is comfortably draped and supine before beginning the examination.

### A. INSPECTION

1. Patient attitude—critical
a. Laying still, resisting movement, with knees drawn up (peritonitis)
b. Restless (colic)
c. Writhing in pain (mesenteric vascular event)
d. Pain with coughing, movement, or Valsalva maneuver
2. **Abdominal contour, visible masses, visible peristalsis, engorged veins, bulging flanks**
3. **External signs of injury (i.e., ecchymosed seat belt sign), scars, striae, rashes, or jaundice**

**Pearl:** *A bluish umbilicus—Cullen sign—may occur as the result of retroperitoneal bleeding from any cause.*

4. **Distension—always significant; remember 6 *F*'s:**
a. Fat
b. Fluid
c. Flatus
d. Feces
e. Fatal growths
f. Fetus
   (1) Age of fetus may be estimated by uterine fundal height: If it is below the umbilicus, the fetus is 20 weeks or less and not viable.
5. **Bulges with coughing/straining, particularly near the pubic tubercle, umbilicus, and incision scar sites**
a. Indirect/direct inguinal hernia—above or at the level of the inguinal ligament

b. Femoral hernia—below the inguinal ligament, medial to the femoral arterial pulse

## B. AUSCULTATION
1. Hypoactive sounds can help to confirm ileus or inflamed bowel.
2. Postoperative bowel sounds are typically from small-intestine function; this does not indicate return of large-bowel function, which is better indicated by *flatus.*
3. Bruits

**Pearl:** *Hiccups can be a sign of gastric distension or diaphragmatic irritation such as a subdiaphragmatic abscess.*

## C. PALPATION
1. Ask the patient to localize the point of maximal tenderness and examine this region last.
2. Technique
a. Minimize abdominal wall resistance with gentleness; flexion of hips and knees will relax the musculature.
b. Initially, the entire abdomen should be palpated lightly as the patient's face is observed.
c. Place the entire palm and extended fingers of the hand on the surface of the abdomen; press the fingertips gently into the abdomen.
d. Deeper palpation can be performed by pressing the finger ends of the palpating hand with the fingers of the other hand. Keep the fingers relatively fixed on the skin and carry the wall of the abdomen in a gentle to-and-fro motion.
3. Guarding
a. Muscular increase in tone or rigidity—involuntary or voluntary
b. Early sign of peritoneal inflammation
4. Rebound tenderness
a. Painful response to the gentle depression and quick release of the abdomen
b. Indicates inflamed or irritated peritoneum
5. Murphy's sign
a. With fingers palpating the area of the gallbladder fossa, just beneath the liver edge, ask the patient to inspire deeply.
b. Inspiratory arrest from pain defines a positive sign.
c. In one series, the presence of Murphy's sign was 80% diagnostically accurate for acute cholecystitis. The predictive value of the test in elderly adults was significantly less.
6. Bulges
a. Palpate bulges with the patient standing relaxed, then coughing/straining, feeling for the edges of any abdominal wall defect. Estimate the defect size.

7. **Masses**
   a. Anatomy—nearly all masses arise from previously normal tissues.
   b. Spleen
      (1) With the patient supine, place the examining left hand underneath the patient's left rib cage, supporting upward, and use the right hand to palpate.
      (2) Using a light touch, depress the skin under the left costal margin.
      (3) An enlarged spleen is felt as a rounded edge that slips under the examiner's fingers at the end of inspiration.
   c. Liver
      (1) With the patient supine, place the examining left hand underneath the patient's right rib cage, supporting the 11th and 12th ribs; use the right hand to palpate.
      (2) When the patient inspires, the liver is palpable about 3 cm below the right costal margin in the midclavicular line.
      (3) Note tenderness, smoothness, nodularity
   d. Intramural versus intraabdominal can be distinguished if the mass is palpated while the abdominal muscles are tensed. An intraabdominal mass will move away from the palpating hand.
8. **Pulsation: The aortic bifurcation is at the level of the umbilicus; a pulsatile mass representing an abdominal aortic aneurysm is likely in the epigastrium.**
9. **Male inguinal hernia examination**
   a. Place the fingertip at the most dependent part of the scrotum and invaginate the slack scrotal wall to insert the finger into the subcutaneous (external) inguinal ring.
   b. If the ring is sufficiently relaxed, guide the finger laterally and cephalad through the canal and have the patient cough or strain. A hernia will cause an impulse to be felt on the end of the fingertip.
10. **Digital rectal examination**
   a. Inspect the skin of the perineum and perianal region for signs of local inflammation, sinuses, fissures, fistulas, or bulges.
   b. Press a gloved, lubricated finger on the anus. Slowly increase the pressure of the finger pad on the sphincter.
   c. When the external sphincter is felt to relax, rotate the finger into the axis of the canal and insert gently.
   d. Findings
      (1) Sphincter tone
      (2) Hemorrhoids
      (3) Masses/feces
      (4) Blood
      (5) Signs of injury—bony fragments, bowel wall integrity
      (6) Prostate position/palpability, shape, texture

### D. PERCUSSION
1. Technique (see IV.D)
2. Tympany—distended bowel
3. Dullness—mass or fluid
a. Liver span
   (1) Reference range: 6 to 12 cm in right midclavicular line, 4 to 8 cm in midsternal line.
   (2) Measure the vertical span of liver dullness in the right midclavicular line, percussing upward from below the umbilicus and downward from the nipple.
b. Bladder distension
c. *Ascites*—shifting flank dullness
   (1) With the patient supine, the level of flank dullness is percussed and marked on the skin. The patient is then turned to one side, and a new level of dullness is percussed.
       (a) Approximately 1 L of free fluid in the abdominal cavity is required to appreciate shifting dullness.
   (2) *Fluid wave test:* Press sharply with one hand while the other hand receives an impulse when placed against the opposite flank, with a perceptible time lag. Fat in the mesentery produces a similar wave, so the fat must be blocked by having the patient or an assistant press along the midline of the abdomen.
4. Rebound tenderness—painful response to percussion

**Pearl:** *The classic finding of "pain out of proportion to examination" is indicative of* **mesenteric ischemia.** *The pain is usually worsened by eating.*

## VII. GENITOURINARY
### A. INSPECTION
1. Signs of injury
a. Blood at the male penile meatus or female urethra, gross hematuria
b. Contusion, lacerations, ecchymoses on perineum
c. Scrotal hematoma

### B. PALPATION
1. Vaginal examination
a. Cervical discharge, cervical pain on movement
b. Palpation of uterine, ovarian masses
c. Lacerations, blood in vaginal vault

## VIII. MUSCULOSKELETAL
### A. INSPECTION
1. Skin
a. Color and perfusion
b. Lacerations, open wounds

2. **Limb deformity**
a. Shortening
b. Angulation
3. **Neuromuscular function**
a. Disability
b. Abnormal mobility
4. **Skeletal/ligamentous injury**

## B.  PALPATION

1. Identify localized bone tenderness or crepitans.
2. Pelvic fracture—instability or pain in response to gentle anterior-to-posterior compression at the anterior iliac crests and symphysis pubis; medial compression at hips.
3. Spine
4. Extremities
a. Pulse examination (see V.C.2.)
   (1) Doppler nonpalpable pulses and compare bilaterally.

**Pearl:** *The presence of palpable distal pulses does not exclude* **compartment syndrome.** *Pulselessness can, however, be a late finding.*

b. Joint stability
c. Impaired sensation
d. Weakness/paralysis
e. Limb viability—muscle turgor
   (1) Soft—likely viable
   (2) Doughy—likely ischemic
   (3) Rigid—probably nonviable
f. Compartment syndrome
   (1) Swollen and tense area of the extremity
   (2) Muscle(s) tender, with increased pain on passive flexion
   (3) Pain out of proportion to clinical findings
   (4) Paresthesia, then anesthesia will develop

**Pearl:** *In the lower extremity, weak dorsiflexion and numbness in the web space between the first and second toes are early signs of deep peroneal nerve deficit from compression in the anterior leg compartment.*

## IX. LYMPHATICS

The initial step when discovering an enlarged lymph node is to determine whether the adenopathy is localized or generalized by searching lymph-node basins in other regions of the body. Peripheral adenopathy is often an inflammatory response to trauma, and the extremity and region drained by the gland should be carefully examined.

## A. Inspection
1. Red streaks
2. Swelling—*lymphedema*
3. Lacerations, open wounds

## B. Palpation
1. Location
a. Cervical, occipital, epitrochlear, submandibular
b. Axillary
c. Supraclavicular—drains the head, arms, chest wall, and breast
d. Inguinal, femoral

**Pearl:** *The right supraclavicular node drains the* <u>lungs</u> <u>and</u> <u>esophagus</u>, *whereas the left side drains the* <u>abdominal</u> <u>cavity</u>. *Found behind the origin of the SCM, enlarged supraclavicular nodes are usually associated with malignancy or granulomatous disease.*

2. Size
a. Less than 1 cm—usually not significant
b. Greater than 2 cm—significant
3. Consistency
4. Tenderness
5. Fixed versus mobile

**Sister Mary Joseph node:** The Mayo brothers' head surgical nurse, whose name was Sister Mary Joseph, was credited with noticing periumbilical adenopathy in patients with advanced gastric cancer. (In the early part of the 20th century, the Mayo Brothers [William and Charles] founded their famous clinic in Rochester, Minnesota.)

## X. NEUROLOGIC

## A. INSPECTION
1. Mental status
a. Person
b. Place
c. Time
d. Situation
2. Papillary status (see III.A.4)
a. Size, reactivity, symmetry
3. Motor response (see Table 3-1)
a. Before the patient is sedated/paralyzed, ask the patient to hold up her fingers and move her toes.
b. If there is no compliance, check for localization response to painful central stimuli (sternal rub).
   (1) Flexor posturing (high brainstem injury)

**TABLE 3-1**

GLASGOW COMA SCALE SCORE

| Best Motor Response | | Verbal Response | | Eye-Opening Response | |
|---|---|---|---|---|---|
| Obeys commands | 6 | | | | |
| Purposeful (crosses midline) | 5 | Oriented speech | 5 | | |
| Withdraws | 4 | Confused speech | 4 | Spontaneous opening | 4 |
| Flexion | 3 | Inappropriate words | 3 | Opens to voice | 3 |
| Extension | 2 | Incomprehensible words | 2 | Opens to pain | 2 |
| No response | 1 | No verbal response | 1 | No response | 1 |

The Glasgow Coma Scale (GCS) scoring system is for use primarily in trauma situations. A patient with a perfect score (15) may still have hemiparesis and a life-threatening lesion. A GCS score of 8 defines a coma, or severe brain injury.

    (2) Extensor posturing (low brainstem injury)
    (3) No response (possible cervical spine injury)
  c. If there is right/left asymmetry in motor response, the *best* response is used to calculate the Glasgow Coma Scale score.
4. **Head/neck nerve testing**
  a. Accessory nerve—shoulder lift
  b. Facial nerve—squint eyes, show teeth
  c. Glossopharyngeal nerve—symmetric soft palate rise with gag reflex, normal swallow
  d. Hypoglossal nerve—midline position of protruded tongue
  e. Oculomotor nerve—eyeball movement in all directions
  f. Optic nerve—screen for visual field deficits
  g. Recurrent laryngeal nerve—clear voice, regular cough
  h. Trigeminal nerve—clenching of teeth, sensation on face
5. **Brachial plexus evaluation**
  a. Axillary nerve—abduction of arm
  b. Median nerve—ability to make a fist
  c. Musculocutaneous nerve—forearm flexion
  d. Radial nerve—wrist extension
  e. Ulnar nerve—abduction/adduction of fingers
6. **Brain death**
  a. Glasgow Coma Scale score of 3 (lowest possible score)
  b. Absent cerebral function
    (1) No response to stimuli above the neck. Complete loss of responsiveness, vocalization, and volitional activity.
  c. Absent brainstem function
    (1) Pupillary light reflex—pupil constriction with direct and consensual exposure to light
    (2) Corneal reflexes—blinking in response to touching of cornea

(3) Doll's eyes reflex—during passive rotation of a patient's head, movement of a patient's eyes in a direction opposite to the direction in which the patient's head is moved (**Note:** C-spine must be cleared)

(4) Vestibuloocular reflex—with the patient in the supine position, head elevated at 30 degrees, instill ~200 ml ice water into each external ear canal with careful observation for any eye movement or extremity response.

(5) Oropharyngeal (gag) reflex

(6) Apnea—an appropriate period of time is required for increase of serum $Paco_2$.

    (a) Hypercarbia with $Paco_2$ greater than 60 mm Hg for 30 seconds has been determined as "adequate stimulation" for respiratory drive.

d. No spontaneous ventilatory effort

e. No spontaneous and purposeful movement *(**Note:** Peripheral nervous system activity and spinal reflexes may persist after brain death.)*

f. These criteria are invalid in the presence of the following conditions: 1) drug and metabolic intoxication, 2) electrolyte imbalances or hyperosmolar coma, 3) hypothermia, and/or 4) hypotension.

**Pearl:** *Before examining a cardiac arrest survivor, ensure that all sedation and paralyzing medications have been discontinued, and note the administration of Advanced Cardiac Life Support medications (i.e., atropine) that cause findings such as dilated pupils. Patients who lack pupillary and corneal reflexes at 24 hours and/or have no motor response at 72 hours have an extremely small chance of meaningful neurologic recovery. Earlier prognosis, before 24 hours have passed from the time of cardiac arrest, should not be made by clinical examination alone.*

## RECOMMENDED READINGS

Booth CM, Boone RH, Tomlinson G, Detsky AS: Is this patient dead, vegetative, or severely neurologically impaired? Assessing outcome for comatose survivors of cardiac arrest. *JAMA* 291:870-879, 2004.

DeGowin RL, DeGowin DD: *DeGowin's Diagnostic Examination,* 7th ed. New York, McGraw-Hill, 2000.

McGee S, Abernathy WB, Simel DL: Is this patient hypovolemic? *JAMA* 281:1022-1029, 1999.

*Advanced Trauma Life Support for Doctors,* 7th ed. Chicago, American College of Surgeons, 2004.

PHYSICAL EXAMINATION OF THE SURGICAL PATIENT

3

# Preoperative and Postoperative Care

*Angela M. Ingraham, MD*

Perioperative care requires the identification and reduction of risk factors, whether patient or operation driven, that pose challenges to the patient's recovery from an operation. The patient's age, preoperative physiologic status, and the urgency and magnitude of the planned procedure are major determinants of operative morbidity and mortality. The perioperative goal is to identify the patients and organs that are at risk, estimate the net effect of all abnormalities on the outcome of an operation, and prevent current and future complications. This requires thought and at times interventions before, during, and after the patient undergoes an operation.

## I. NEED FOR OPERATION

### A. RELATIVE RISKS AND BENEFITS OF SURGERY

Determination of the relative risks and benefits of surgery requires consideration of the following factors:

1. Natural history of disease if left untreated
2. Benefit of surgical therapy versus medical therapy
3. Urgency of operation, which can limit the time available for preoperative preparation and risk reduction
4. Patient's physiologic reserve and overall ability to undergo anesthesia and operation
5. Potential complications of the procedure

## II. ASSESSMENT OF OPERATIVE RISK

### A. AGE

1. Elderly patients often have either limited reserves or impaired function of the major organ system.
2. True even for "healthy" septuagenarian: "There is nothing like an operation or an injury to bring a patient up to chronological age" (W. R. Howe).

### B. URGENCY OF OPERATION

1. In one study, emergent nature of the surgery doubled the risk for operative mortality in low- and moderate-risk patients.

### C. RELATION OF PHYSICAL STATUS TO ANESTHETIC MORTALITY

1. Impairment of more than one organ system and disease severity profoundly influences the risk for operative mortality. See the American Society of Anesthesiologists classification of physical status in Chapter 16.

## D. CARDIOVASCULAR RISK

1. Coronary artery disease, congestive heart failure (CHF), presence of arrhythmias, peripheral vascular disease, or severe hypertension
2. Goldman cardiac risk in noncardiac surgery
a. Computation of the cardiac risk index (Table 4-1)
b. General concepts (Table 4-2)
    (1) Class III and IV patients warrant routine preoperative cardiology consultation.
    (2) Class IV typically restricted to life-saving procedures only.
    (3) Twenty-eight of the 53 points are potentially correctable before surgery.
    (4) Index correctly classified 81% of the cardiac outcomes.

| TABLE 4-1 | | |
|---|---|---|
| COMPUTATION OF CARDIAC RISK INDEX | | |
| Category | Description | Score (Points) |
| History | Age >70 years | 5 |
| | Myocardial infarction within 6 months | 10 |
| Physical examination | S3 gallop or JVD | 11 |
| | Important valvular aortic stenosis | 3 |
| Electrocardiogram | Rhythm other than sinus or PACs or >5 PVCs/min at any time before surgery | 7 |
| Poor general medical status | $Po_2$ <60 or $Pco_2$ >50 mm Hg | 3 |
| | $K^+$ <3.0 or $HCO_3$ <20 mEq/L | |
| | BUN >50 or creatinine level >3 mg/dl | |
| | Abnormal SGOT | |
| | Chronic liver disease | |
| | Bedridden because of noncardiac cause | |
| Operation | Intraperitoneal, intrathoracic, aortic surgery | 3 |
| | Emergency surgery | 4 |

BUN = blood urea nitrogen; JVD = jugular vein distention; PAC = premature atrial contraction; PVC = premature ventricular contraction; SGOT = serum glutamic-oxaloacetic transaminase.

| TABLE 4-2 | | | |
|---|---|---|---|
| GOLDMAN CLASSIFICATION | | | |
| Class | Point Total | Major Complication (%) | Cardiac Death (%) |
| I | 0–5 | 0.6 | 0.2 |
| II | 6–12 | 3 | 1 |
| III | 13–25 | 11 | 3 |
| IV | ≥26 | 12 | 39 |

Adapted from Goldman L, Caldera DL, Nussbaum SR, et al: Multifactorial index of cardiac risk in noncardiac surgical procedures. *N Engl J Med* 297:845, 1977.

  (5) Criticism—assesses cardiac risks only and is based on mixed patient population (e.g., vascular patients have greater morbidity and mortality rates).

3. **1997 American College of Physicians Revised Cardiac Risk Index**

a. Provides no advice on how to work up patient before surgery, but stratifies into risk groups based on the following six variables:

  (1) High-risk surgical procedure
  (2) History of ischemic heart disease (excluding revascularization)
  (3) History of heart failure
  (4) History of stroke/transient ischemic attack
  (5) Preoperative insulin therapy
  (6) Preoperative serum creatinine concentration >2 mg/dl

b. New strategy based on the Revised Cardiac Risk Index (Table 4-3)

  (1) Patient with one to two risk factors—beta-blockade started perioperatively
  (2) Patient with three or more risk factors—perioperative beta-blockade more strongly indicated (if contraindicated or surgical risk seems excessive, cancel or defer surgery)
  (3) Patients who are difficult to assess—dobutamine stress echo (if negative, operative risk is low; if positive, confirms importance of perioperative β-adrenergic blockade)

4. **Additional information regarding perioperative beta-blockade can be found in the following reference: Fleisher L, et al. ACC/AHA 2006 Guideline Update on Perioperative Cardiovascular Evaluation for Noncardiac Surgery: Focused Update on Perioperative Beta-Blocker Therapy.** *J Am Coll Cardiol* 47:2343–2355, 2006).

## E. PULMONARY RISK (SEE III.C)

1. Risk factors include smoking (two-fold), chronic obstructive pulmonary disease (six-fold), advanced age, industrial exposures, preexisting pulmonary disease, thoracic or upper abdominal surgery, pulmonary hypertension, sleep apnea, and possibly obesity, although this relationship remains controversial.

2. Tests to identify pulmonary risk factors for nonthoracic operations include:

**TABLE 4-3**

REVISED CARDIAC RISK INDEX

| Class | Event/Patient | Event Rate | 95% CI |
|-------|---------------|------------|-----------|
| I | 0 RFs | 0.4 | 0.05–1.5 |
| II | 1 RF | 0.9 | 0.3–2.1 |
| III | 2 RFs | 6.6 | 3.9–10.3 |
| IV | 3 RFs | 11.0 | 5.8–18.4 |

CI = confidence interval; RF = risk factor. From Lee TH, Marcantonio ER, Mangione CM, et al: Derivation and prospective validation of a simple index for prediction of cardiac risk of major noncardiac surgery. *Circulation* 100:1043–1049, 1999.

a. Inability to blow out a match with unpursed lips from a distance of 20 to 25 cm
b. Shortness of breath during one to two flights of steps
c. $Pco_2$ greater than 45 mm Hg while inspiring room air, maximum breathing capacity less than 50% predicted, forced expiratory volume in 1 second ($FEV_1$) less than 2 L, pulmonary artery pressure greater than 30 mm Hg, $FEV_1$/forced vital capacity less than 65% predicted

## F. RENAL RISK

1. Renal insufficiency (blood urea nitrogen [BUN] >50 mg/dl; creatinine concentration >3 mg/day). Remember, however, that serum BUN and creatinine abnormalities are not seen until more than 75% to 90% of renal reserve is lost.
2. Greatest risk in acute renal failure

## G. HEPATIC RISK

1. Cirrhosis, hepatitis
2. Surgical mortality significantly increased in patients with bilirubin level greater than 2 mg/dl, albumin level less than 3 g/dl, prothrombin time greater than 16 seconds, presence of encephalopathy, and advanced Child–Pugh classification.
3. Mortality associated with noncardiac surgery is caused by high-output cardiovascular failure and low peripheral resistance.
a. Less than 5% of class A patients
b. Five percent to 10% of class B patients
c. Twenty percent to 50% of class C patients
d. Eighty percent mortality rate if blood ammonia greater than 150 μg/dl or albumin level less than 2.5 g/dl

## H. ENDOCRINE RISK

1. Diabetes mellitus
a. A growing body of literature suggests that tight glycemic control (glucose between 80 and 110 mg/dl) is beneficial (e.g., see Van den Berghe G, Wilmer A, Hermans G, et al: Intensive insulin therapy in the medical ICU. *N Engl J Med* 354:449–461, 2006).
b. Sixteen percent to 23% of patients experience development of diabetes mellitus in the perioperative period, most commonly after operations for vascular disease.
c. It is an independent predictor of postoperative myocardial ischemia among cardiac and noncardiac surgical patients.
d. Stress of operation causes secretion of epinephrine, growth hormone, glucocorticoids, and glucagon.
e. Anesthetic agents affect sympathetic tone, thereby decreasing insulin secretion.
2. Hyperthyroidism or hypothyroidism

## I. HEMATOLOGIC RISK
1. Thromboembolic disease (Table 4-4)
a. True prevalence is unknown and varies with the type of surgery, use and type of prophylaxis, and mode of diagnosis.
b. Without prophylaxis, fatal pulmonary embolism occurs in 0.1% to 0.8% of patients undergoing elective general surgery.
c. Risk factors for developing short-term (30-day) postoperative deep venous thrombosis:
   (1) Age older than 50 years
   (2) History of varicose veins
   (3) History of myocardial infarction
   (4) History of cancer
   (5) History of atrial fibrillation
   (6) History of ischemic stroke
   (7) History of diabetes mellitus
   (8) Other risk factors—previous deep venous thrombosis, heart failure, obesity, paralysis, and inherited conditions (factor V Leiden, prothrombin gene mutation, protein S deficiency, antithrombin deficiency)

## J. NUTRITIONAL-IMMUNOLOGIC RISK
1. Risk increased if severe malnutrition present—weight loss greater than 15% over previous 3 to 4 months, albumin level less than 3.0 g/dl, anergy to injected skin-test antigens, transferrin level less than 200 mg/dl.

## III. INTERVENTION TO REDUCE OPERATIVE RISK
### A. EMERGENT OPERATIONS
1. Procedure should not be delayed for most situations.
2. Exception is volume-depleted patients (e.g., those with intestinal obstruction, peritonitis, perforated viscus), who should undergo fluid and electrolyte repletion before induction of anesthesia.

### B. CARDIOVASCULAR
1. Coronary artery disease
a. Evaluated by electrocardiogram, exercise, or dipyridamole thallium scan, multigated acquisition, or echocardiogram. Coronary angiography may be indicated.
b. Coronary artery revascularization has been shown to decrease risk for postoperative myocardial infarction.
2. CHF
a. Risk factors for postoperative CHF are coronary artery disease, advanced age, and major operations.
b. Preexisting CHF should be optimally controlled (e.g., diuretics, digoxin).
c. Preoperative pulmonary artery pressure monitoring and intraoperative transesophageal echocardiogram can guide perioperative fluid management and monitoring of hemodynamic performance (i.e., need for fluids, inotropes, or vasodilators).

**TABLE 4-4**

RISK FOR THROMBOEMBOLIC EVENTS

| Risk Level | Surgical Parameters | Calf Vein Thrombosis | Proximal Vein Thrombosis | Clinical Pulmonary Embolism | Fatal Pulmonary Embolism |
|---|---|---|---|---|---|
| Low | Uncomplicated minor surgery in patients younger than 40 years with no clinical risk factors; require general anesthesia less than 30 minutes | 2% | 0.4% | 0.2% | 0.002% |
| Moderate | Any surgery in patients aged 40–60 years with no additional risk factors; major surgery in patients younger than 40 years with no additional risk factors and requiring general anesthesia longer than 30 minutes; minor surgery in patients with risk factors | 10–20% | 2–4% | 1–2% | 0.1–0.4% |
| High | Major surgery in patients older than 60 years old without additional risk factors or patients aged 40–60 years with additional risk factors; patients with myocardial infarction; medical patients with risk factors | 20–40% | 4–8% | 2–4% | 0.4–1% |
| Highest | Major surgery in patients older than 40 years with prior venous thromboembolism, malignant disease, or hypercoagulable states; patients with elective major lower extremity orthopedic surgery, hip fracture, stroke, multiple trauma, or spinal cord injury | 40–80% | 10–20% | 4–10% | 0.2–5% |

3. **Arrhythmias**
a. Optimal medical control required before surgery (see Chapter 11).
b. High-grade block and bradyarrhythmias may require preoperative temporary or permanent pacing.

4. **Hypertension**
a. No increased risk for nonlabile mild hypertension and diastolic blood pressure less than 110 mm Hg
b. Antihypertensive agents should be continued to time of surgery, except monoamine oxidase inhibitors (discontinue 2 weeks before surgery).
c. New-onset hypertension, severe hypertension with diastolic blood pressure greater than 110 mm Hg, systolic blood pressure greater than 250 mm Hg, or suspicion of unusual causes of hypertension should lead to further workup and treatment.
d. Check for evidence of end-organ deterioration (e.g., renal insufficiency, CHF).

## C. RESPIRATORY
1. **General principles**
a. Patient should discontinue smoking as long as possible before surgery.
b. Eight weeks of smoking cessation is required to have effect on postoperative morbidity.
c. Teach and use chest physical therapy, incentive spirometry, and deep-breathing exercises before surgery.
2. **Chronic obstructive pulmonary disease:** Initiate or continue use of bronchodilators (e.g., inhalants, theophylline), antibiotics, chest physical therapy, and steroids especially if significant airflow obstruction is present.
3. **Asthma:** If symptoms are persistent and $FEV_1$ and peak flow is less than 80% of previous best, optimize control with perioperative systemic corticosteroids.
4. **Pneumonia or acute bronchitis:** Delay elective surgery and treat with pulmonary toilet and antibiotics.
5. **Bronchiectasis:** Improve operative risk via preoperative expectorants, pulmonary toilet, incentive spirometry training, and antibiotics based on patient's cultures.

## D. RENAL
1. Identify and correct causes of renal insufficiency including, but not limited to, infection, uncontrolled hypertension, obstruction, dehydration, drugs (i.e., aminoglycosides).
2. Reduce azotemia with peritoneal dialysis or hemodialysis if needed.
3. Correct electrolyte abnormalities.
4. Optimize volume status—consider use of pulmonary artery monitoring.

## E. HEPATIC (SEE CHAPTER 45)
1. Abstain from alcohol, spironolactone, and furosemide with fluid restriction to control ascites; limit sodium to 0.5 to 2 g/day.

PREOPERATIVE AND POSTOPERATIVE CARE

4

## F. ENDOCRINE (SEE SECTION V AND CHAPTER 32)

1. Glucose control
   a. For patients with type I diabetes, minimize effect of fasting and ketosis by scheduling operations early in the day.
   b. Halve dose of long-acting insulin before surgery.
   c. Hold oral diabetic agents on the day of surgery because metformin, secretagogues, and sulfonylureas can be associated with lactic acidosis, hypoglycemia, and increased risk for perioperative myocardial infarction, respectively.

2. Steroids
   a. Indications
      (1) Preoperative for adrenalectomy
      (2) Known history of adrenal insufficiency
      (3) History of adrenal or pituitary surgery or surgery for renal cell carcinoma
      (4) Inflammatory bowel disease, steroid dependent
   b. Endogenous cortisol output
      (1) Normal unstressed adult—8 to 25 mg/day
      (2) Adult undergoing major surgery—75 to 100 mg/day
   c. Guide to steroid coverage
      (1) Correct electrolytes, blood pressure, and hydration if necessary.
      (2) Hydrocortisone phosphate or hemisuccinate—100 mg intravenous piggyback on call to operating room

## G. HEMATOLOGIC (SEE CHAPTER 13)

## H. NUTRITION (SEE CHAPTER 6)

1. If malnourished, recommend preoperative enteral or parenteral nutrition for a minimum of 4 to 5 or 14 days, respectively, to normalize short-turnover proteins (retinol-binding protein, prealbumin, and transferrin).

## IV. GENERAL PREOPERATIVE PREPARATION

### A. OVERALL ASSESSMENT AND DOCUMENTATION

1. For discussion of the patient, history, physical examination, indications for the procedure, informed consent, and preoperative note, see Chapter 2; for operative risk, see section II.

### B. PREOPERATIVE LABORATORY AND IMAGING EVALUATION

Although several studies have documented that many preoperative laboratory studies are not cost-effective, these preoperative studies are performed at many institutions.

1. Laboratory studies
   a. Complete blood cell count, urinalysis, electrolytes, BUN, creatinine, prothrombin time, partial thromboplastin time

b. Room-air arterial blood gas if at risk for respiratory insufficiency (see section II) or if prolonged postoperative ventilator support is anticipated

2. Radiographs—posteroanterior and lateral chest radiograph unless previously normal within the past 6 months or patient younger than 35 years

3. Electrocardiogram if patient older than 35 years or if otherwise indicated by cardiac history

## C. BLOOD ORDERS

1. Type and screen or type and cross-match for the number of units appropriate for the procedure

## D. SKIN PREPARATION

1. Hair removal is best performed the day of surgery with an electric clipper. Shaving the night before surgery is associated with an increased risk for infection.

2. Provide preoperative (night-before) scrub or shower of the operative site with a germicidal soap (e.g., Hibiclens, pHisoHex).

## E. PREOPERATIVE ANTIBIOTICS

1. When used, should have an established blood level at the time of initial skin incision. Administer preoperative antibiotics 30 minutes before incision.

2. Indications for prophylactic antibiotics

a. Clean procedures—most cardiac, noncardiac thoracic, vascular, neurosurgery, orthopedic, and ophthalmic procedures require cefazolin 1 to 2 g intravenously (IV) or vancomycin 1 g IV.

b. Clean/contaminated procedures—gastrointestinal/genitourinary tract, gynecologic, respiratory tract, head and neck procedures use cefazolin 1 to 2 g IV; for colorectal procedures, use oral neomycin and erythromycin, and cefoxitin or cefotetan 1 to 2 g IV.

c. Dirty procedure/ruptured viscus—cefoxitin or cefotetan 1 to 2 g IV with or without gentamicin 1.5 mg/kg every 8 hours IV, or clindamycin 600 mg IV every 6 hours and gentamicin 1.5 mg/kg every 8 hours IV.

d. Special consideration must be given to patients with prosthetic heart valves or history of valvular heart disease.

e. Redose the antibiotic if the operation lasts longer than 4 hours or twice the half-life of the antimicrobial agent.

f. Prophylactic antibiotics should not be continued beyond the day of the operation.

## F. BACTERIAL ENDOCARDITIS PROPHYLAXIS

1. Indications: Patients with the following conditions are particularly vulnerable to bacteriologic seeding during transient bacteremia:

a. Prosthetic valve
b. Congenital valve disease
c. Rheumatic valve disease
d. History of endocarditis
e. Idiopathic hypertrophic subaortic stenosis.
f. Mitral valve prolapse with murmur (Barlow syndrome)
2. **Antibiotic recommendations: Table 4-5 shows the use of antibiotics for endocarditis prophylaxis in dental, upper respiratory, genitourinary, and gastrointestinal procedures.**
a. Antibiotic prophylaxis as described in Table 4-5 is used for patients with valvular heart disease, prosthetic heart valves, most forms of congenital heart disease (but not uncomplicated secundum atrial septal defect), idiopathic hypertrophic subaortic stenosis, and mitral valve prolapse with regurgitation.
b. Oral regimens are more convenient and safer. Parenteral regimens are more likely to be effective; they are recommended especially for patients with prosthetic valves, those who have had endocarditis previously, or those taking continuous oral penicillin for rheumatic fever prophylaxis.
c. A single dose of the parenteral drugs is adequate for most dental and diagnostic procedures of short duration. However, one or two follow-up doses may be given at 8- to 12-hour intervals in selected high-risk patients.

## G. RESPIRATORY CARE

1. Preoperative incentive spirometry on the evening before surgery when indicated (upper abdominal operations, thoracic operations, predisposed to respiratory insufficiency)

| TABLE 4-5 | | |
|---|---|---|
| **PREVENTION OF BACTERIAL ENDOCARDITIS** | | |
| Drug | Adult Doses | Pediatric Doses |
| Oral amoxicillin | 3 g 1 hour before and 1.5 g 6 hours after procedure | 50 mg/kg 1 hour before and 25 mg/kg 6 hours after procedure |
| Oral erythromycin (if allergic to penicillin) | 1 g 2 hour before and 500 mg 6 hours after procedure | 20 mg/kg 2 hours before and 10 mg/kg 6 hours after procedure |
| IV/IM ampicillin | 2 g 30 minutes before procedure | 50 mg/kg 30 minutes before procedure |
| IV/IM gentamicin | 1.5 mg/kg 30 minutes before procedure | 2 mg/kg 30 minutes before procedure |
| IV vancomycin (if allergic to penicillin)* | 1 g 1 hour before procedure | 20 mg/kg 1 hour before procedure |

Prevention for dental, upper respiratory, genitourinary (GU), and gastrointestinal (GI) procedures.
*Add gentamicin to intravenous (IV) vancomycin for GI and GU procedures.
IM = intramuscular.

2. Bronchodilators for moderate-to-severe chronic obstructive pulmonary disorders

## H. BOWEL PREPARATION

The purpose of a bowel preparation is as follows: (1) to remove all solid and most liquid from the bowel, and (2) to reduce the bacterial population in anticipation of procedures or complications of procedures that may contaminate the wound and the peritoneal cavity. All patients are NPO (nothing by mouth) after midnight before the day of surgery.

1. **Nonbowel operation: Stomach decompression before induction of anesthesia by patient remaining NPO after midnight before surgery or by nasogastric suction**
2. Bowel operation
a. Bowel prep may be helpful if any of the upper or lower gastrointestinal tract is to be opened or if there is a risk for enterotomy (e.g., complicated ventral hernia repair).
b. Achlorhydria, gastric carcinoma, prolonged $H_2$ blocker usage, and obstructive peptic ulcer disease allow bacterial growth in the stomach. Consider using an oral antibiotic prep (e.g., neomycin) for gastric surgery in these patients.
c. Many variations exist, but all have the same goal of achieving a bowel movement before surgery that is liquid, clear, and free of any stool. For large- and small-bowel resection, the following is a standard bowel prep:
   (1) Clear liquid diet 48 hours before the procedure
   (2) Day before surgery:
   **10:00 AM**   45 ml Fleet Phospho-soda orally (PO) followed by 8 oz water
   **11:00 AM**   8 oz water PO
   **12:00 PM**   8 oz water PO
   **1:00 PM**   8 oz water PO and neomycin 500 mg and metronidazole 750 mg PO
   **2:00 PM**   8 oz water PO
   **3:00 PM**   neomycin 500 mg and metronidazole 750 mg PO
   **5:00 PM**   4 bisacodyl 5-mg tablets PO
   **7:00 PM**   1 bisacodyl 10-mg suppository by rectum
   **10:00 PM**   neomycin 500 mg and metronidazole 750 mg PO
   (3) If stool contains solid material, the patient can be given 1 bottle of magnesium citrate orally.

## I. ACCESS AND MONITOR LINES.
1. At least one 18-gauge intravenous line is needed for initiation of anesthesia.
2. Arterial catheters and central or pulmonary artery catheters are used when indicated (see Chapter 11).

## J. OTHER CONSIDERATIONS

1. Administer a maintenance rate of intravenous fluids beginning at midnight before the surgery.
2. Thromboembolic prophylaxis with sequential compression devices or heparin if greater risk
3. Maintenance medications (e.g., antihypertensives, cardiac medications, anticonvulsants) may be given the morning of surgery with a sip of water before routine operations.
4. Preoperative diabetic management; hold oral antihyperglycemic drugs.
5. Subacute bacterial endocarditis prophylaxis (see section V)
6. Perioperative steroid coverage (see section V)
7. The site for a stoma, if applicable, may be marked by the stomal therapist in elective situations, ideally at least 2 inches away from the skin fold at the level of the umbilicus.

## V. POSTOPERATIVE CARE

### A. PULMONARY

1. Postoperative pulmonary complications cause significant perioperative morbidity and mortality increasing hospital stay.
2. Complications include atelectasis, pneumonia, prolonged mechanical ventilation and respiratory failure, and worsening of underlying lung disease.
3. Operation-specific risk factors
   a. Incidence of complications increases with proximity of incision to the diaphragm.
   b. Duration of operation greater than 3 to 4 hours
   c. Type of anesthesia and half-life of neuromuscular blockade
4. Postoperative pulmonary care
   a. Early ambulation
   b. Aggressive pulmonary toilet (incentive spirometry, deep breathing, coughing)
   c. Adequate analgesia
      (1) Epidural analgesia in upper abdominal operations decreases incidence of pulmonary complications and length of hospital stay.
      (2) Advantages of epidural narcotics (morphine, fentanyl, sufentanil, hydroxymorphine)
         (a) Longer duration of action
         (b) Minimal sedation and respiratory depression
         (c) Minimal sensorimotor loss
      (3) Local anesthetic (bupivacaine, ropivacaine) may be added for shorter onset of action without risk for hypotension and motor blockade.
      (4) Pain can also be controlled via patient-controlled analgesia (PCA) to minimize narcotic use.

## B. HEMATOLOGY

1. Prevention of thromboembolism (Table 4-6)
a. Especially important in patients with cancer, elderly adults, and patients undergoing orthopedic procedures
b. Absolute contraindications to pharmacologic treatment—active bleeding, severe bleeding diathesis, platelet counts less than 20,000/$\mu$l, neurosurgery, ocular surgery within the past 10 days or intracerebral or subarachnoid hemorrhage within the past 48 hours
c. Relative contraindications to pharmacologic treatment—mild-to-moderate bleeding diathesis, platelet count 20,000 to 100,000/$\mu$l, brain metastases or recent major trauma, major abdominal surgery within the past 2 days, gastrointestinal or genitourinary bleeding within the past 14 days, infective endocarditis, malignant hypertension
d. Nonpharmacologic measures—early ambulation, graduated compression stockings that can be used on upper extremities, intermittent pneumatic compression (be cautious if patient has been immobilized or on bedrest for 72 hours because of the possibility of disrupting newly formed clots; do not use with lower extremity operations or injuries)

## C. RENAL

1. Hyperkalemia (>7.5 mEq/L) with electrocardiographic changes—IV calcium, one-half ampule of D50 followed by 10 units of insulin IV, one-half ampule of bicarbonate, 5 g sodium polystyrene sulfonate (Kayexalate) PO or enema
2. As BUN reaches 100 mg/dl, dysfunctional platelets may cause gastrointestinal bleeding, which further increases BUN.
3. Postoperative low urine output can have several causative factors—hypovolemia, depressed cardiac function, diuretic dependence, urinary retention, obstruction of Foley catheter.

## D. ENDOCRINE

1. Intensive glycemic control has become the standard of care because of its proven benefits, including reduced morbidity and mortality
a. American Diabetes Association Recommendations for Target Inpatient Blood Glucose Concentrations:
   (1) General surgical patient—random less than 180 mg/dl, fasting less than 90 to 126 mg/dl; better outcomes provide for lower infection rates
   (2) Cardiac surgery—less than 150 mg/dl; allowing for reduced mortality and risk for sternal wound infections
   (3) Critically ill—80 to 110 mg/dl
b. Methods for achieving strict glycemic control (80–110 mg/dl):
   (1) "Piggyback" infusion of regular insulin (50–100 units per 50–100 ml normal saline) with infusion rate (units per hour) calculated as serum glucose (mg/dl)/150 with sampling via an arterial line.

4

PREOPERATIVE AND POSTOPERATIVE CARE

**TABLE 4-6**

SIXTH CONSENSUS CONFERENCE ON ANTITHROMBOTIC THERAPY

| Condition | Risk (%) | Recommendation |
|---|---|---|
| **General Surgery** | | |
| Low risk | 3 | Early ambulation |
| Moderate risk | 29 | Unfractionated heparin: 5000 units subcutaneously given 2 hours before surgery and every 12 hours after surgery |
| | | LMWH: |
| | | Dalteparin, 2500 units 1–2 hours before surgery, then once daily |
| | | Enoxaparin, 2000 units before surgery, then once daily |
| High risk | 39 | Unfractionated heparin: 5000 units subcutaneously given 2 hours before surgery and every 8 hours |
| | | LMWH: |
| | | Dalteparin, 5000 units 10–12 hours before surgery, then once daily |
| | | Enoxaparin, 4000 units 10–12 hours before surgery, then once daily |
| Very high risk | 80 | 1. Unfractionated heparin at 5000 units subcutaneously given 2 hours before surgery and every 8 hours after surgery, dalteparin at 2500 units given 2 hours before surgery and every day, and intermittent pneumatic compression applied intraoperatively |
| | | 2. Dalteparin at 5000 units 10–12 hours before surgery, then once daily, and enoxaparin at 4000 units 10–12 hours before surgery, then once daily |
| | | 3. Perioperative warfarin to maintain INR of 2–3 |
| **Neurological Surgery/Trauma** | | |
| Acute spinal cord injury with leg paralysis | 40 | 1. Unfractionated heparin subcutaneously in doses adjusted to produce an activated partial thromboplastin time equal to 1.5 times the control value 6 hours after dose |
| | | 2. Enoxaparin at 3000 units twice daily |
| | | 3. Warfarin adjusted to an INR of 2–3 in the rehabilitation phase |
| | | 4. Intermittent pneumatic compression plus unfractionated heparin at 5000 units subcutaneously every 12 hours |
| Multiple trauma | 53 | Intermittent pneumatic compression until further bleeding is unlikely; then administer enoxaparin at 30 mg subcutaneously every 12 hours or warfarin adjusted to an INR of 2–3 |

INR = international normalized ratio; LMWH = low-molecular-weight heparin.
From Hirsh J, Dalen J, Guyatt G, American College of Chest Physicians: The Sixth (2000) ACCP Guidelines for Antithrombotic Therapy for Prevention and Treatment of Thrombosis. Chest 119:1S–2S, 2001.

(2) Length, type of surgery, and severity of glucose dysregulation determines need for intravenous insulin therapy.

2. **Steroids—guide to steroid coverage:**

a. Hydrocortisone phosphate or hemisuccinate—100 mg IV before surgery in postanesthesia care unit and every 6 hours for the first 24 hours

b. If progress is satisfactory, reduce dosage to 50 mg every 6 hours for 24 hours, then taper to maintenance dosage over 3 to 5 days. Resume previous fluorocortisol or oral steroid dose when patient is taking oral medications.

c. Maintain or increase hydrocortisone dosage to 200 to 400 mg/24 hours if fever, hypotension, or other complications occur.

d. If patient has potassium wasting, may switch to methylprednisolone (Solu-Medrol).

e. High-dose (300–600 mg/day) methylprednisolone regimens are potentially deleterious secondary to impaired wound healing, increased catabolism, electrolyte abnormalities, and increased infectious complications.

### E.  IMMUNOLOGIC/FEVER

1. **All pyrogens evoke a common mediator (interleukin-1), which alternates the activity of temperature-sensitive neurons in anterior hypothalamus.**

a. Internal thermostat is increased with blood temperature remaining relatively low, causing chills and shivering to increase blood temperature.

b. If set-point drops, a flush phase or crisis with vasodilation and sweating develops to rid body of heat.

2. **Common causes of fever are referred to as the five W's—wind (atelectasis), water (urinary tract infection), wound (wound infection), walking (thrombophlebitis), and wonder drugs (drug-induced fever).**

a. Within 24 hours—atelectasis or failure to clear pulmonary secretions

b. At 24 to 48 hours—respiratory complications, less likely catheter-related problems

c. After 48 to 72 hours—if previously afebrile, likely because of significant complication: bloodstream infection, thrombophlebitis, wound infection, urinary tract infection > pneumonitis, acute cholecystitis (acalculous if immobile or received large volumes of blood), idiopathic postoperative pancreatitis, drug allergy; *Candida* if receiving total parenteral nutrition (if blood cultures are negative but have Candida in another site, discontinue total parenteral nutrition line and start antifungal agent)

3. **If no systemic symptoms or supportive physical findings, no need to obtain routine chest radiographs, pan-cultures, or white blood cell counts.**

### F.  INTEGUMENTARY/WOUND COMPLICATIONS

1. **Wound infection**

a. Usually *Staphylococcus aureus* > hemolytic streptococci (3%), Enterococci, *Pseudomonas, Proteus,* or *Klebsiella*

   b. Incidence
     (1) Clean, atraumatic, uninfected wound—3.3% to 4%
     (2) Clean wounds without emergent operation, drained wounds, stab
        wounds—7.4%
     (3) Bronchus, gastrointestinal tract or oropharyngeal cavity entered—
        10.8%
     (4) Perforated viscera—28.3%
   c. Risk factors—advanced age, steroids, obesity, duration of operation,
     malnutrition
   d. Prevention—skin preparation (clip immediately before surgery), bowel
     preparation (most effective being mechanical preparation with clear
     liquids and cathartics), prophylactic antibiotics (given 15–30 minutes
     before the incision, keeping serum levels greater than the minimally
     inhibitory concentration throughout the operation), meticulous technique
     with minimal tissue destruction, temperature maintenance, appropriate
     drainage
   e. Usually present between the fifth and eighth postoperative day;
     however, necrotizing fasciitis (dishwater pus with Gram stain of mixed
     flora of gram-negative rods and gram-positive cocci) or clostridia
     myositis (crepitus, vesicles on the skin) can manifest within 24 hours
   f. Management of wound infections—depends on extent of destruction
     and type of infection, ranging from opening the incision to radical
     debridement; if surrounding cellulites and edema, antibiotics (Ancef IV
     or Keflex PO) are typically indicated.

**2. Wound hematomas**
   a. Caused by inadequate hemostasis
   b. Risk factors—anticoagulation, fibrinolysis, polycythemia vera,
     myeloproliferative disorders, decreased or inadequate clotting factors
   c. Cause pain and swelling with serosanguineous drainage
   d. If discovered early, return to operating room to evacuate hematoma and
     control bleeding
   e. If discovered late, apply heat, manage expectantly

**3. Wound dehiscence**
   a. Separation of the fascial layer
   b. Incidence rate—0.5% to 3.0%
   c. Usually caused by a technical error
   d. Heralded by serosanguineous, salmon-colored drainage from the wound
   e. Contributory factors—malnutrition, hypoproteinemia, morbid obesity,
     malignancy, uremia, diabetes, increased abdominal pressure, remote
     infection, and excessive suture material
   f. Treatment—fluid resuscitation, application of sterile dressing, early
     return to the operating room for repair

# Fluids and Electrolytes

*Bryon J. Boulton, MD*

## I. BASIC PHYSIOLOGY

### A. BODY FLUID COMPOSITION

1. Total body water (TBW)
   a. Composed of intracellular and extracellular fluid (ECF) compartments
   b. Fifty percent to 70% of total body weight
   c. Male (60%) greater than female (50%) percentage
   d. Adjusted for body habitus
      (1) In obesity, TBW is decreased by 10% to 20%.
      (2) In very thin individuals, TBW is increased by 10%.
      (3) In newborns, TBW is ~80% but decreases to ~65% by 12 months of age.

2. Intracellular fluid
   a. Thirty percent to 40% of total body weight
   b. Primarily found in muscle
   c. Principal cation is $K^+$, with smaller contributions from $Mg^{2+}$ and $Na^+$, and the principal anions are $HPO_4^-$ and negatively charged proteins.

3. ECF
   a. ECF = interstitial fluid + intravascular fluid.
   b. Interstitial fluid is 15% of total body weight.
   c. Intravascular fluid is 5% of total body weight.
      (1) Plasma volume is 50 ml/kg of body weight.
      (2) Blood volume is 70 ml/kg of body weight.
   d. Principal cation is $Na^+$, and principal anions are $Cl^-$ and $HCO_3^-$.

### B. SERUM OSMOLALITY AND TONICITY

1. Osmolality
   a. Defined as osmoles of solute particles per kilogram of water; basically as ions per unit volume
   b. Transcompartmental movement of water occurs because certain nonpermeable molecules cannot freely migrate through the semipermeable cell membrane, thus creating a gradient.
      (1) Compounds accumulating in ECF—$Na^+$ and glucose
      (2) Compounds accumulating in intracellular fluid—$K^+$, proteins, and organic acids
   c. Calculated by:

$$\text{Serum osmolality (mOsm/L)} = 2(Na^+) + \text{glucose}/18 + \text{blood urea nitrogen}/2.8$$

2. Tonicity
   a. Defined as the effect of particles on cell volume; only an impermeable solute ($Na^+$) can alter tonicity because a freely permeable solute cannot create an oncotic gradient
   b. The body attempts to regulate tonicity, not osmolality.

## C. FLUID AND ELECTROLYTE HOMEOSTASIS

### 1. Baseline requirements

a. Adult fluid requirements—35 ml/kg/day or 1500 ml/m$^2$/day; titrate to maintain urine output between 0.5 and 1.0 ml/kg/hr.

b. Adult electrolyte requirements

    (1) $Na^+$—100 to 150 mEq/day; 1 to 2 mEq/kg/day

    (2) $K^+$—50 to 100 mEq/day; 0.5 to 1 mEq/kg/day

    (3) $Cl^-$—90 to 120 mEq/day

    (4) $Ca^{2+}$—orally 1 to 3 g/day

    (5) $Mg^{2+}$—20 mmol/day

    (6) Phosphorus—20 to 30 mmol/day

### c. Pediatric hourly formula to determine fluid requirements

    (1) 0 to 10 kg = (4 ml × kg) per hour

    (2) 11 to 20 kg = 40 ml/hr + (2 ml for each kg over 10 kg) per hour

    (3) More than 20 kg = 60 ml/hr + (1 ml for each kg over 20 kg) per hour

<u>Example—25-kg child:</u>

(1st 10 kg) × 4 = 40

+ (2nd 10 kg) × 2 = 20

+ last 5 kg × 5 = 5

25 kg total = 65 ml/hr

d. Pediatric electrolyte requirements

    (1) $Na^+$—3 to 5 mEq/kg/day

    (2) $K^+$—2 to 3 mEq/kg/day

    (3) $Cl^-$—5 to 7 mEq/kg/day

    (4) See pediatric section for more details.

e. See specific chapters for fluid requirements/management of specific disease processes.

### 2. Fluid turnover and losses

a. Gastrointestinal (GI) tract

    (1) About 6000 to 9000 ml/day total secretion

    (2) Approximately 250 ml lost per day in stool

    (3) See Table 5-1 for specifics.

b. Renal

    (1) About 800 to 1500 ml/day lost

c. Insensible losses

    (1) Approximately 400 ml/m$^2$/day or 10 ml/kg/day for adults

    (2) Seventy-five percent via evaporate losses from skin and 25% via respiratory exchange

d. Abnormal losses

    (1) Fever—250 ml/day per degree centigrade of fever, or 15% increase in insensible losses for each degree centigrade above 37°C

**TABLE 5-1**

COMPOSITION OF GASTROINTESTINAL SECRETIONS

| Secretion | Volume in ml/24 hours (range) | Na, mEq/L (range) | K, mEq/L (range) | Cl, mEq/L (range) | HCO₃, mEq/L (range) |
|---|---|---|---|---|---|
| Salivary gland | 1500 (500–2000) | 10 (2–10) | 26 (20–30) | 10 (8–13) | 30 |
| Stomach | 1500 (100–4000) | 60 (9–116) | 10 (0–32) | 130 (8–154) | — |
| Duodenum | 140 (100–2000) | 140 | 5 | 80 | — |
| Ileum | 3000 (100–9000) | 140 (80–150) | 5 (2–8) | 104 (43–137) | 30 |
| Colon | — | 60 | 30 | 40 | — |
| Pancreas | — (100–800) | 140 (99–185) | 5 (3–7) | 75 (54–95) | 115 |
| Bile | — (50–800) | 145 (99–164) | 5 (3–12) | 100 (89–180) | 35 |

**FLUIDS AND ELECTROLYTES**

**5**

(2) Tachypnea—50% increase for each doubling of respiratory rate
(3) GI—diarrhea, fistula, tube drainage
(4) Third space losses—can be difficult to appreciate, often underestimated.
(5) Evaporation—ventilator, open abdomen, open wound
(6) Operative losses—can be estimated by:

# hours NPO (nothing by mouth) × baseline/maintenance intravenous fluid requirement

(preoperative deficient, if not replaced)

+ # hours of case × baseline/maintenance intravenous fluid requirement

+ operative blood loss

+ insensible losses − estimation guide:

1–3 ml/kg/hr for minor procedure

4–7 ml/kg/hr for intermediate procedure

8–12 ml/kg/hr for major procedure

## II. ELECTROLYTE DISTURBANCES

### A. SODIUM

1. Basic physiology
a. Reference serum levels between 135 and 145 mEq/L
b. Under renal regulation, and is the primary solute in determining plasma osmolality
2. Hyponatremia
a. Signs and symptoms—often asymptomatic until levels decline to less than 120 mEq/L or if levels acutely decline to less than 130 mEq/L
   (1) Central nervous system (CNS)—headache, fatigue, confusion, coma, seizures
   (2) GI—nausea, vomiting, diarrhea
   (3) M/S—weakness, muscle twitching, hyperactive deep-tendon reflexes
b. Diagnosis/causative factor
   (1) Begin by determining serum osmolality, glucose levels, and lipid levels.
   (2) Rule out isotonic hyponatremia (serum osmolality: 280–290 mOsm) due to pseudohyponatremia.
      (a) Pseudohyponatremia—occurs in the presence of hypertriglyceridemia or hyperproteinemia.
   (3) Sodium reduction can be calculated by multiplying the plasma triglyceride (mg/dl) level by 0.002 *or* by multiplying the protein levels greater than 8.0 g/dl by 0.25.

(4) Isotonic hyponatremia (serum osmolality: 280–290 mOsm) also occurs after infusions of isotonic glucose, mannitol, or glycine, or after transurethral resection of prostate (TURP).

(5) Next, rule out hypertonic hyponatremia (serum osmolality: >290 mOsm)—occurs after hypertonic infusions of glucose, mannitol, or glycine, or after TURP. Can also occur from hyperglycemia.

   (a) For each 100 mg/dl of serum glucose greater than 100 mg/dl, serum sodium is decreased by 3 mEq/L.

(6) Next, clinically determine the circulating volume to assist in differentiating between the forms of hypotonic hyponatremia (serum osmolality: <280 mOsm).

   (a) Hypovolemic hyponatremia can occur because of GI losses (vomiting, diarrhea, fistulas), skin losses (thermal injury), or renal losses (diuretics, diabetes insipidus, salt-wasting nephritis, peritoneal dialysis).

   (b) Isovolemic hyponatremia can occur because of water intoxication, iatrogenic causes, secretion of antidiuretic hormone, hypokalemia, drugs (sulfonylureas, carbamazepines, phenothiazines, and antidepressants), and reset thermostat.

   (c) Hypervolemic hyponatremia can occur because of congestive heart failure, nephrosis, liver failure, drugs (indomethacin, carbamazepines, vincristine, vinblastine, cyclophosphamide, and nicotine derivatives).

c. Treatment

(1) Correct the underlying disorder.

(2) The following formula can be used to estimate sodium deficit:

$$Na^+ \text{ deficit (mEq/L)} = (\text{desired } Na^+ \text{ level} - \text{actual } Na^+ \text{ level}) \times TBW$$

(3) Hypovolemic hyponatremia—replace deficit with 0.9% NaCl while monitoring frequent sodium levels to prevent too rapid of correction of subsequent hypernatremia.

(4) Water intoxication—corrects readily with simple fluid restriction (<1500 ml/day).

(5) Hypervolemic hyponatremia—most respond well to simple fluid restriction (<1500 ml/day); this may be assisted with a loop diuretic, with hourly replacements of $Na^+$ and $K^+$ while monitoring the levels.

(6) Isovolemic hyponatremia—usually corrects after addressing the underlying disorder.

(7) Caution should be used in aggressively treating the symptomatic patient. Rapid infusion of hypertonic saline solutions can result in central pontine myelinolysis. Serum sodium levels should not be corrected in an excess of 0.5 mEq/L/hr to avoid this devastating complication if the patient has been symptomatic for more than 48 hours. In the asymptomatic patient, correction rates can be administered safely at 1 to 2 mEq/L/hr.

3. **Hypernatremia**
   a. Always associated with a hyperosmolar state and occurs because of water loss in excess of salt loss; thus, there is a free water deficit, and hypernatremia is typically delineated according to the patient's ECF volume status.
   b. Signs and symptoms—rarely develop if $Na^+$ is less than 160 mEq and osmolality is greater than 320 mOsm, unless condition develops rapidly.
      (1) CNS—restlessness, irritability, delirium, mania, seizures, coma
      (2) Cardiovascular (CV)—tachycardia, hypertension
   c. Diagnosis/causative factor
      (1) Clinically assess extracellular fluid volume.
      (2) Hypovolemic hypernatremia—caused by loss of hypotonic body fluid such as insensible free water loss, GI losses, diuretics, diabetes insipidus.
      (3) Isovolemic hypernatremia—due to the same causative factors as hypovolemic, but is caused by improper correction.
      (4) Hypervolemic hypernatremia—most frequently iatrogenic (excessive administration of $Na^+$), but also seen in Conn syndrome, Cushing syndrome, steroid use, and congenital adrenal hyperplasia.
   d. Treatment—rapid reversal carries a high risk for cerebral edema and uncal herniation.
      (1) Address the underlying disorder.
      (2) Next, determine the free water deficit:

$$H_2O \text{ deficit} = (0.6 \times \text{kg of body weight}) \times [(\text{serum } Na^+ \text{ (mEq/L)}/140) - 1]$$

      (3) Begin by replacing half of the deficit in the first 24 hours, with the remainder in the following 2 or more days. Note that continued ongoing losses (urinary and insensible) need to be replaced concurrently.
      (4) Select a hypotonic fluid such as D5W.

## B. POTASSIUM

1. **Basic physiology**
   a. Normal serum levels are between 3.5 and 5.1 mEq/L, and it is the major intracellular cation.
   b. Changes in $K^+$ have significant effects on transmembrane potential, and hence cellular function.
   c. Fifty to 100 mEq ingested daily, 90% excreted in urine, 10% excreted in stool.
2. **Hypokalemia**
   a. Signs and symptoms—generally appear only after levels are less than 2.5 mEq/L and are primarily CV.
      (1) CNS—paresthesias, paralysis
      (2) CV—sensitization to digitalis and epinephrine, arrhythmias, electrocardiographic changes: low voltage, flattened T waves, ST-segment depression, prolonged QT interval, and prominent U waves

       (3) GI—constipation, ileus

       (4) M/S—weakness, cramps, myalgia, rhabdomyolysis

b. Causative factors

    (1) In surgical patient, GI (diarrhea, gastric drainage: vomiting/nasogastric tube), diuretics, and insulin administration

    (2) Redistribution to intracellular space; significant in metabolic alkalosis, insulin therapy, beta-blockers, catecholamines

    (3) Others—mucus-secreting colon tumors, magnesium deficiency, hyperaldosteronism, steroid use, anabolism, delirium tremens, hypothermia

c. Treatment

    (1) Ensure adequate renal function before beginning replacements.

    (2) Because $K^+$ is primarily intracellular, small decreases in serum $K^+$ represent significant decreases in total body stores. This deficit can be predicted in that for every 1-mEq/L decrease from the norm, there is a 100- to 200-mEq decrease in total body stores.

    (3) Treat the alkalosis and decrease $Na^+$ intake.

    (4) Enteral replacement preferred—40- to 100-mEq dosing.

       (a) Note: A banana has roughly 10 mEq $K^+$ per inch.

    (5) Parenteral replacement—used if patient cannot tolerate oral intake or if depletion is severe; only administer more than 10 mEq/hr peripherally of KCl or more than 20 mEq/hr of KCl in central line; may be increased to 40 mEq/hr if patient has cardiac monitoring and is in intensive care unit.

## 3. Hyperkalemia

a. Signs and symptoms

    (1) CV—peaked T waves, flattened P waves, prolongation of QRS, cardiac arrest, ventricular fibrillation

    (2) M/S—weakness, paresthesias

    (3) GI—nausea, vomiting, diarrhea, intestinal colic

b. Causative factors

    (1) Pseudohyperkalemia—can occur in hemolysis, thrombocytosis, and leukocytosis.

    (2) Redistribution into extracellular space; acidosis, insulin deficiency, reperfusion syndrome, tissue necrosis—crush injuries, burns, electrocution; beta-blocker therapy, digitalis intoxication, succinylcholine

    (3) Increased total body potassium—renal insufficiency (most common in surgical patient), diabetes, spironolactone, mineralocorticoid deficiency

c. Treatment

    (1) Mild hyperkalemia (<6.0 mEq/L and no electrocardiographic changes)

       (a) Remove exogenous sources.

       (b) Add a non–$K^+$-sparing diuretic (e.g., furosemide [Lasix]), and if possible, remove any medication that is capable of increasing potassium concentration.

    (2) Severe hyperkalemia (>6.0 and presence of electrocardiographic changes)
      (a) Temporizing measures (treatment for symptoms)
        (1) Calcium gluconate or calcium chloride—temporary cardiac stabilization
        (2) Inhaled $\beta$ agonists—causes the most rapid intracellular shift in $K^+$
        (3) D50W (50 g) and 10 units intravenously of regular insulin
      (b) Therapeutic measures (decreasing total body potassium)
        (1) Kayexalate—administered orally (20–50 g in 100–200 ml 20% sorbitol) or rectally (50 g in 200 ml 25% sorbitol)
        (2) Hydration and forced renal excretion with diuretics (e.g., Lasix)
        (3) Dialysis—definitive therapy in life-threatening hyperkalemia

**Mnemonic**—C Big K Di (see big K die)

<u>C</u>alcium, <u>B</u>eta agonists, <u>I</u>nsulin, <u>G</u>lucose, <u>K</u>ayexalate, <u>D</u>ialysis, Las<u>I</u>x

## C. CALCIUM

### 1. Basic physiology

a. Normal serum levels are 8.9 to 10.5 mg/dl, and serum ionized levels are 4.4 to 5.2 mg/dl.

b. Ninety-nine percent of total body calcium is stored in bone as hydroxyapatite crystals.

c. Calcium exists in several forms in serum: 45% as free ionized $Ca^{2+}$ (the only physiologically active form), 40% bound to proteins, and 15% bound to freely diffusible compounds.

d. Calcium metabolism is under the control of parathyroid hormone (increases $Ca^{2+}$ bone resorption and renal reabsorption) and vitamin D (increases $Ca^{2+}$ uptake from GI tract).

### 2. Hypocalcemia

a. Signs and symptoms (serum $Ca^{2+}$ level <8.0 mg/dl or ionized $Ca^{2+}$ level <4.0 mg/dl)
    (1) CV—QT prolongation, ventricular arrhythmias
    (2) M/S—cramping, paresthesias (first perioral/central, then extremities), tetany, increased deep-tendon reflexes
    (3) Chvostek's sign—facial muscle twitching after percussion over trunk of facial nerve
    (4) Trousseau's sign—carpal spasm after inflating blood pressure cuff for more than 3 minutes

b. Causative factors
    (1) Calcium sequestration—pancreatitis, rhabdomyolysis, packed red blood cell administration (citrate chelation)
    (2) If albumin is normal, check parathyroid hormone level.
      (a) Low parathyroid hormone—hypoparathyroidism, magnesium deficiency

(b) High parathyroid hormone—pancreatitis, hyperphosphatemia, renal insufficiency, fistulas, specific drugs (gentamicin, Lasix), pseudohypothyroidism, decreased vitamin D

c. Treatment
  (1) Oral management—appropriate in chronic hypocalcemia.
    (a) Calcium carbonate
      (1) Titralac—1 ml = 1 g $CaCO_3$ = 400 mg $Ca^{2+}$
      (2) Os-Cal—1 tablet = 1.25 g $CaCO_3$ = 500 mg $Ca^{2+}$
      (3) Tums—1 tablet = 0.5 g $CaCO_3$ = 200 mg $Ca^{2+}$
    (b) Phosphate-binding antacids improve GI absorption of $Ca^{2+}$.
    (c) Vitamin D—50,000 to 200,000 IU calciferol or other preparations; dihydrotachysterol, 1,25 dihydroxyvitamin $D_3$
  (2) Intravenous management—appropriate in acute hypocalcemia.
    (a) Not required in asymptomatic patient; 200 to 300 mg elemental $Ca^{2+}$ required to eliminate attack of tetany.
    (b) One gram calcium gluconate—contains 2.2 mmol $Ca^{2+}$.
    (c) One gram $CaCl_2$—contains 6.5 mmol $Ca^{2+}$.

## 3. Hypercalcemia

a. Signs and symptoms—"stones, bones, groans, and psychic overtones"
  (1) CNS—confusion, depression, psychoses, coma (psychic overtones)
  (2) GI—nausea, vomiting, anorexia, ileus, constipation, abdominal pains (groans)
  (3) Genitourinary—nephrolithiasis, polyuria (stones)
  (4) CV—hypertension, shortening of the QT interval
b. Causative factors
  (1) Hyperparathyroidism and malignancy are the most common causes.
  (2) Other causes—milk alkali syndrome (consumption of large amounts of milk and soluble alkali—i.e., antacids), hyperthyroidism, acromegaly, pheochromocytoma, medications (thiazides, vitamin A, vitamin D), granulomatous disease, adrenal insufficiency, Paget's disease of the bone, and prolonged immobilization
c. Treatment
  (1) Mild hypercalcemia (<12 mg/dl) can be treated with restriction of calcium intake and discontinuance of offending or contributing agents.
  (2) Severe hypercalcemia—requires prompt treatment.
    (a) Intravenous hydration—most patients are dehydrated; begin with 0.9% NaCl.
    (b) Oral or intravenous phosphate—inhibits bone resorption.
    (c) Diuresis with loop diuretic and aggressive intravenous hydration (>200 ml/hr)
    (d) Calcitonin—useful in treating hypercalcemia associated with malignancy or primary hyperparathyroidism; usual dose is 4 units/kg subcutaneously or intramuscularly every 12 to 24 hours.

**5**

**FLUIDS AND ELECTROLYTES**

(e) Mithramycin—useful in malignancy-associated hypercalcemia unresponsive to other treatments; usual dose is 15 to 25 μg/kg intravenously.

(f) Pamidronate—useful in malignancy-associated hypercalcemia; usual dose is 60 to 90 mg.

## D. MAGNESIUM

### 1. Basic physiology

a. Reference serum levels are 1.7 to 2.3 mEq/dl.

b. The kidney plays the greatest role in magnesium regulation.

c. Fifty percent of total body magnesium is found in bone, 49% is found in the intracellular space, and the remaining 1% can be found in the serum. Of the serum magnesium, 60% is in the ionized form, 25% is protein bound, and 15% is complexed with nonprotein anionic species.

d. Acute hypomagnesemia is usually accompanied by hypokalemia.

### 2. Hypomagnesemia

a. Signs and symptoms

   (1) CNS—mental status changes, seizures

   (2) CV—widening of QRS complex and T wave, prolongation of PR and QT intervals, ventricular arrhythmias

   (3) M/S—weakness, fasciculations, hyperreflexia, tremors, tetany

b. Causative factors

   (1) GI losses—diarrhea, malabsorption, vomiting, biliary fistulas

   (2) Genitourinary losses—diuresis, primary hyperaldosteronism, renal tubular dysfunction

   (3) Drugs—loop diuretics, cyclosporine, amphotericin B, aminoglycosides, and cisplatin

   (4) Others—parathyroidectomy, acute myocardial infarction, and burns

c. Treatment

   (1) Mild cases (asymptomatic and >1.0 mEq/ml)—oral replacement preferred.

      (a) Magnesium oxide—400-mg tablet = 20 mEq $Mg^{2+}$

      (b) Magnesium gluconate—500-mg tablet = 2.3 mEq $Mg^{2+}$

      (c) Magnesium chloride—535-mg tablet = 5.5 mEq $Mg^{2+}$

   (2) Severe cases (symptomatic or <1.0 mEq/ml)—intravenous replacement preferred.

      (a) In the presence of arrhythmias, 1 to 2 g $MgSO_4$ infused rapidly (5–15 minutes) followed by a continuous infusion of 1 to 2 g/hr.

      (b) Without symptoms, more than 4 to 8 g $MgSO_4$ infused at a rate of 0.5 g/hr may be required.

### 3. Hypermagnesemia

a. Signs and symptoms

   (1) CNS—mental status changes, paralysis ($Mg^{2+}$ >12 mEq), coma

   (2) CV—atrioventricular block, prolonged QT interval, hypotension, sinus bradycardia

     (3) GI—nausea, vomiting

     (4) M/S—loss of deep-tendon reflexes ($Mg^{2+}$ >8 mEq)

b. Causative factors

     (1) Rarely occurs in the face of normal renal function

     (2) Iatrogenic ($Mg^{2+}$ used to treat eclampsia), acute or chronic renal failure, administration of magnesium-containing antacids or laxative overuse, severe burns, crush injuries, rhabdomyolysis, severe metabolic acidosis, extracellular volume depletion

c. Treatment

     (1) Remove offending agents.

     (2) Calcium gluconate reverses some of the life-threatening symptoms (loss of deep-tendon reflexes, cardiac arrhythmias).

     (3) Intravenous hydration, correction of acid-base abnormalities, excretion with a loop diuretic, and dialysis in the patient with renal failure can be used.

## E. PHOSPHORUS

### 1. Basic physiology

a. Less than 1% of total body stores are found within the extracellular fluid compartment.

b. Normal serum concentrations are between 2.5 and 4.0 mg/dl.

c. It is under secondary control by a myriad of hormones that primarily control calcium metabolism and is primarily excreted by the kidneys.

### 2. Hypophosphatemia

a. Signs and symptoms

     (1) CNS—mental status changes, weakness, flaccid paralysis

     (2) CV—cardiac arrest

     (3) M/S—bone pain

     (4) Heme—platelet and granulocyte dysfunction

b. Causative factors

     (1) Increased renal loss—acid-base disturbances, acetazolamide, acute tubular necrosis, diabetic ketoacidosis

     (2) Decreased intestinal absorption—hypothyroidism, vitamin D deficiency, malabsorption, alcoholism, phosphate-binding antacids.

     (3) Total body redistribution—refeeding syndrome, total parenteral nutrition administration

     (4) Other—after severe burns

c. Treatment

     (1) Mild hypophosphatemia (>1.0 mg/dl)—oral Neutra-Phos 250 to 500 mg every 6 hours or Phospho-Soda 5 to 10 ml every 8 hours (Neutra-Phos contains 250 mg phosphorus/tablet, Phospho-Soda contains 129 mg phosphorus/ml) or intravenous $NaPO_4$ or $KPO_4$ 0.08 to 0.2 mmol/kg infused over 6 hours.

     (2) Severe hypophosphatemia (<1.0 mg/dl)—intravenous $NaPO_4$ or $KPO_4$ 0.16 to 0.24 mmol/kg infused over 6 hours is preferred.

### 3. Hyperphosphatemia

**5**

**FLUIDS AND ELECTROLYTES**

a. Signs and symptoms
   (1) M/S—tetany, soft-tissue calcification
b. Causative factors
   (1) Decreased renal excretion—renal failure
   (2) Total body redistribution—tissue trauma, acidosis
   (3) Others—antacids, vitamin D metabolites, postoperative hypoparathyroidism
c. Treatment
   (1) Restrict intake, increase excretion with intravenous hydration and diuresis (acetazolamide), and use phosphate-binding antacids ($AlOH_2$); lastly, hyperphosphatemia can be corrected with hemodialysis.

## III. PARENTERAL REPLACEMENT FLUID THERAPY

Table 5-2 demonstrates the composition of commonly used intravenous fluids.

### A. CRYSTALLOIDS

1. **Isotonic (lactated Ringer's solution [LR] and 0.9% normal saline [NS])**
a. Commonly used in volume resuscitation and used interchangeably, but the pH of 0.9% NS is less than LR; therefore, LR is the preferred fluid in a resuscitation where the patient is acidotic and does not have hyperkalemia, hyponatremia, hypochloremia, hypercalcemia, or an alkalosis. LR also is more similar to normal serum electrolyte composition, osmolality, and pH.
2. **Hypotonic (0.45% NS and D5W)**
a. Not used in resuscitation but commonly used to correct a free water deficit
3. **Hypertonic (3% NS)**
a. Has begun to have limited use as a volume expander in selected patient populations (some patients with head trauma); however, used primarily to correct symptomatic hyponatremia
4. **Maintenance intravenous fluid**
a. Most commonly used is D5 0.45% NS with 20 mEq KCl added; this is simply tailored to meet the daily basal metabolic requirements of an otherwise healthy patient.
b. Should be adjusted to the individual patient, for example, eliminating dextrose from the fluids of a patient with diabetes or potassium from a patient with renal insufficiency

### B. COLLOIDS

1. **Never been shown to be superior to crystalloids as a resuscitative fluid, only equivocal, and meta-analysis has revealed an increased mortality in patients where albumin was used as a volume expander; colloids also have not been shown to be cost-effective.**
2. **Albumin (100 ml of 25% and 500 ml of 5%)**
a. To be used cautiously, and not to be used in patients with an albumin level greater than 2.5 g/dl, total protein greater than 5 g/dl, or for supplementing serum albumin levels in patients with chronic disease

**TABLE 5-2**

REPLACEMENT THERAPY—PARENTERAL FLUIDS

| Solution | Na (mEq/L) | K (mEq/L) | Cl (mEq/L) | Base (mEq/L) | mOsm/L | Dextrose (g/L) | Kcal/L |
|---|---|---|---|---|---|---|---|
| D5W | — | — | — | — | 278 | 50 | 170 |
| D10W | — | — | — | — | 556 | 100 | 340 |
| D50W | — | — | — | — | 2780 | 500 | 1700 |
| 0.9% NaCl | 154 | — | 154 | — | 286 | — | — |
| 0.45% NaCl | 77 | — | 77 | — | 143 | — | — |
| 3% NaCl | 513 | — | 513 | — | 1026 | — | — |
| D5 0.9% NaCl | 154 | — | 154 | — | 564 | 50 | 170 |
| D5 0.45% NaCl | 77 | — | 77 | — | 421 | 50 | 170 |
| D5 0.2% NaCl | 39 | — | 39 | — | 350 | 50 | 170 |
| LR | 130 | 4 | 109 | 28 | 272 | — | 9 |
| D5 LR | 130 | 4 | 109 | 28 | 524 | 50 | 170 |

D5W = dextrose 5% in water; D10W = dextrose 10% in water; D50W = dextrose 50% in water; LR = lactated Ringer's solution.

**FLUIDS AND ELECTROLYTES**

**5**

b. Benefit has been shown in limited situations, for example, burn patients with hypoalbuminemia, resuscitation of a patient with cirrhosis.

c. Temporarily expands the intravascular volume at least 1:1 per milliliter infused because of ability to mobilize fluid from the interstitial space into the intravascular space.

**3. Dextran (Dextran 40 and 70)**

a. Synthetic glucose polymer that expands the intravascular volume by 1 ml for every milliliter infused, and is eliminated by the kidneys

b. Indicated as a volume expander and thromboembolism prophylaxis

c. Side effects include coagulopathy, laboratory test abnormalities, worsening renal function, and osmotic diuresis.

**4. Hetastarch (hydroxyethyl starch, 6% solution)**

a. A synthetic molecule that expands the intravascular volume 1 ml for every milliliter infused, and undergoes hepatic and renal elimination.

b. It can be used as a volume expander in shock.

c. Side effects include increased amylase and an osmotic diuresis, which can be misinterpreted as achieving adequate tissue perfusion, and worsening renal function.

## IV. ACID-BASE DISORDERS

### A. PHYSIOLOGY

1. Normal pH is 7.35 to 7.45; acidemia refers to a pH less than 7.35, and alkalemia refers to a pH greater than 7.45.

2. Acid-base balance is significant because most enzymatic reactions occur optimally only at a narrow pH range.

3. Primary buffer systems

a. Red blood cell bicarbonate-carbonate system is the most important and most rapid buffer system:

$$HCl + NaHCO_3 \leftrightarrow NaCl + H_2CO_3 \leftrightarrow H_2O + CO_2$$

b. Others playing a smaller role—intracellular proteins, organic phosphates, intracellular bicarbonate, and hemoglobin itself.

c. More than half the total body alkaline buffering capacity is found within the bone.

4. Compensation systems

a. Respiratory system eliminates volatile acids (primary = $CO_2$) generated during consumption of acid by the bicarbonate-carbonate system. As long as the respiratory system is not compromised, this system of acid elimination is inexhaustible.

b. Renal system is responsible for excretion of acids and both the recovery and generation of de novo bicarbonate.

### B. PRIMARY METABOLIC DISORDERS

1. Metabolic acidosis

a. Causative factors—it results primarily from the loss of alkali, accumulation of nonvolatile acids, or a decrease in the acid excretion from the kidneys.

b. Classification—it is characterized as either normal (hyperchloremic) anion gap or increased anion gap acidosis; normal anion gap = 3 to 12:

Anion gap = Na (mEq/L) − [Cl (mEq/L) + HCO$_3$ (mEq/L)]

(1) Increased anion gap—ketoacidosis, alcohol intoxication, lactic acidosis, renal failure, toxin ingestion (salicylates, paraldehyde, ethylene glycol, methanol)

**Mnemonic—MUDPILES:**

Methanol, Uremia, DKA, Paraldehyde, Ingestion, Lactic acidosis, Ethanol, Salicylates

(2) Normal anion gap (hyperchloremic)—renal tubular acidosis, potassium-sparing diuretics, hypoaldosteronism, diarrhea, biliary or pancreatic fluid losses, small-bowel fistulas, dilutional acidosis, carbonic anhydrase inhibitors, ureteral diversions.

**Mnemonic—USEDCRAP:**

Ureterostomy, Small-bowel fistulas, Extra chloride, Diarrhea, Carbonic anhydrase inhibitors, Renal tubular acidosis, Adrenal insufficiency, Pancreatic fistulas

c. Signs and symptoms
(1) Abdominal pain, nausea, vomiting
(2) Decreased cardiac contractility, peripheral vasodilation, bradycardia

d. Treatment
(1) Begin by correcting the underlying disorder.
(2) In trauma/surgical patients, a frequent cause of metabolic acidosis is lactic acidosis from inadequate tissue perfusion, which can be corrected simply by volume resuscitation.
(3) Without addressing the underlying disorder, the simple addition of bicarbonate will not correct the acidosis.
(4) With mild-to-moderate acidosis, the correction of the underlying disorder will correct the acidosis, and the excessive use of bicarbonate can lead to overcorrection (alkalosis), hypernatremia, hyperosmolarity, cerebrospinal fluid acidosis, and volume overload.
(5) For a pH less than 7.2 to 7.3, addition of an ampule or two of bicarbonate may be required; one ampule contains 50 mEq sodium bicarbonate.
(6) The exact bicarbonate deficit cannot be calculated, but it can be estimated with the following formula:

0.4 × wt (kg) × [desired bicarbonate − measured bicarbonate (mEq/L)]

(7) For severe acidosis, while addressing the underlying disorder, the addition of bicarbonate can be beneficial to increase the pH to greater than 7.2.

**2. Metabolic alkalosis**
a. Classified as either chloride responsive or chloride unresponsive, but caused by either acid loss or base gain, and aggravated by hypokalemia and volume contraction

5

FLUIDS AND ELECTROLYTES

(1) Chloride responsive—contraction alkalosis (commonly in the surgical patient from inadequate resuscitation), diuretic use, GI acid loss (vomiting or nasogastric tube), bicarbonate administration, villous adenoma

(2) Chloride unresponsive—severe hypokalemia, hyperaldosteronism, mineralocorticoid excess, renal failure, and chronic edema

b. Diagnosis

(1) Increased pH and bicarbonate, and may be associated with compensatory hypercapnia

(2) Urine chloride levels can be measured to help differentiate among the various causative factors. A urine chloride level less than 15 mEq/dl suggests chloride-responsive causative factors, whereas a urine chloride level greater than 15 mEq/dl indicates chloride-unresponsive causes.

c. Treatment

(1) Begin by addressing underlying causes. Volume expansion and correction of hypokalemia corrects most cases. Correction with 0.9% NS facilitates improvement because of its acidity and chloride contents.

(2) In refractory cases, the use of acetazolamide (Diamox 500 mg every 6 hours) will inhibit de novo synthesis and renal reabsorption of bicarbonate.

(3) In severe cases, administer acid-containing solutions such as $NH_4Cl$, lysine HCl, arginine HCl, or 0.1 N HCl.

(a) Calculate chloride deficit:

$$\text{wt (kg)} \times 0.4 \times [100 - \text{measured Cl (mEq/L)}]$$

(b) Administer over 24 hours with 0.1 N HCl.

## C. PRIMARY RESPIRATORY DISORDERS

### 1. Respiratory acidosis

a. Causative factor—it results primarily from an increase in $Pco_2$ secondary to inadequate ventilation.

(1) Causes of hypoventilation include respiratory center depression (a variety of causes including narcotics), chronic obstructive pulmonary disease, pulmonary disease, inadequate mechanical ventilation, and poor ventilation secondary to pain.

b. Diagnosis

(1) Decreased pH with an increased $Pco_2$; in chronic states, will see a compensatory increase in $HCO_3$.

c. Treatment

(1) Address underlying cause of hypoventilation.

(2) Improve minute ventilation—remove airway obstruction, pulmonary toilet, bronchodilators, avoidance of respiratory depressants, reversal of opioid narcotics and continuous positive airway pressure/bilevel positive airway pressure.

(3) Endotracheal intubation and mechanical ventilation if noninvasive measures fail; if intubated, increase minute ventilation (frequency and tidal volume).

(4) In chronic hypercapnia, particularly related to chronic obstructive pulmonary disease, hypoxemia becomes the agent driving the respiratory system; therefore, the patient's hypoxemia should not be fully corrected and the hypercapnia should be slowly corrected.

2. **Respiratory alkalosis**

a. Causative factor—it results primarily from a decrease in $Pco_2$ secondary to hyperventilation.

(1) Causes of hyperventilation include anxiety, pain, mechanical ventilation, CNS infections, metabolic encephalopathies, cerebrovascular accident, pulmonary embolism, hypoxia, congestive heart failure, pneumonia, cirrhosis, sepsis, closed head injury, toxins, pregnancy, and increased ventilation secondary to bronchospasm.

b. Diagnosis

(1) Increased pH with a decreased $Pco_2$

c. Treatment

(1) Address underlying disorder.

(2) Correct hypoxemia if present.

(3) If acutely symptomatic and not intubated, use a rebreathing device.

(4) In ventilated patients, decrease minute ventilation while maintaining $Pco_2$ no less than 30 mm Hg.

## D. MIXED ACID-BASE DISORDERS

1. Suspected any time pH is near-normal values with altered levels of $Pco_2$ and $HCO_3$ or when compensatory changes appear to be exaggerated or insufficient.

## E. EVALUATION OF ACID-BASE DISORDERS (TABLE 5-3).

1. Obtain simultaneous arterial blood gases and serum electrolyte panel (use Table 5-3 to assist in reading arterial blood gases).

2. Calculate anion gap.

3. Calculate expected compensation from chart and locate on acid-base nomogram.

4. If compensation is not within predicted values, a mixed disorder should be expected.

5. Correlate suspected diagnosis with clinical picture.

5

FLUIDS AND ELECTROLYTES

### TABLE 5-3

#### ACID-BASE DISORDERS

| Disorder | Primary Change | Secondary Change | Effect |
|---|---|---|---|
| Metabolic acidosis | $\downarrow HCO_3$ | $\downarrow Pco_2$ | Last 2 digits pH = $Pco_2$ |
|  |  |  | $HCO_3 + 15$ = last 2 digits pH |
| Metabolic alkalosis | $\uparrow HCO_3$ | $\uparrow Pco_2$ | $HCO_3 + 15$ = last 2 digits pH |
| Respiratory acidosis |  |  |  |
| Acute | $\uparrow Pco_2$ | $\uparrow HCO_3$ | $\Delta$ pH = 0.08 per 10 $\Delta$ in $Pco_2$ |
| Chronic | $\uparrow Pco_2$ | $\uparrow\uparrow HCO_3$ | $\Delta$ pH = 0.03 per 10 $\Delta$ in $Pco_2$ |
| Respiratory alkalosis |  |  |  |
| Acute | $\downarrow Pco_2$ | $\downarrow HCO_3$ | $\Delta HCO_3 = 0.2 \times \Delta$ in $Pco_2$ |
| Chronic | $\downarrow Pco_2$ | $\downarrow\downarrow HCO_3$ | $\Delta HCO_3 = 0.3 \times \Delta$ in $Pco_2$ |

### REFERENCES

Mulholland MW, et al: *Greenfield's Surgery Scientific Principles and Practice,* 4th ed. Philadelphia, Lippincott Williams & Wilkins, 2006, pp 214–238.

# Nutrition

*Jocelyn M. Logan-Collins, MD*

Surgical patients with malnutrition are two to three times more likely to have minor and major complications and a greater rate of mortality.

## I. NUTRITIONAL ASSESSMENT

**A. SCREENING: PREADMISSION NUTRITION SCREENING HAS THE POTENTIAL TO IMPROVE PATIENT OUTCOMES BY INCREASING NUTRIENT INTAKE BEFORE HOSPITAL ADMISSION AND REDUCING HOSPITAL STAY.**

1. Subjective global assessment
   a. Carefully performed history and physical examination to assess nutritional status
   b. Patients are defined as well-nourished, mild-to-moderately nourished, or severely malnourished using the following criteria:
      (1) Weight loss during previous 6 months—mild (<5%), moderate (5–10%), or severe (>10%)
      (2) Dietary intake—normal or abnormal based on changes in oral intake, including calories and nutrients
      (3) Gastrointestinal symptoms that impair deglutition or eating over previous 2 weeks—nausea, vomiting, diarrhea, dysphagia, and anorexia
      (4) Functional capacity—fully active, suboptimal function, or bedridden
      (5) Physical signs—subcutaneous fat loss in triceps and midaxillary line at lower ribs; muscle wasting in the temporalis muscle, deltoids, and quadriceps
   c. Those considered moderately or severely malnourished are at greater risk for mortality and delayed functional recovery regardless of acute illness severity, comorbidity, or functional dependence.
   d. Predictive value is equal to or better than laboratory data.
   e. Greater than 80% agreement when evaluated for interobserver variability
2. Biochemical indicators of malnutrition: No gold standard exists.
   a. Albumin
      (1) Reference range: 4–5 g/dl
      (2) Preoperative level <3.5 g/dl is a predictor of operative mortality and morbidity.
      (3) Long half-life (21 days)
      (4) Synthesis decreases with malnutrition.
      (5) Adequate indicator of malnutrition in absence of other causes of hypoalbuminemia (hepatic insufficiency, protein-losing nephropathy, or enteropathy)
      (6) Short-term fluctuations are not accurate in acutely ill surgical patients because concentrations are influenced by fluid redistributions during critical illness.

  b. Rapid-turnover proteins—shorter half-life, early indicator of nutritional depletion; decreasing levels suggest ongoing malnutrition.
    (1) Transferrin (half-life 8 days), prealbumin (2 days), retinol-binding protein (12 hours)
    (2) Increased sensitivity to changes in nutritional status (i.e., tends to return to normal with nutritional repletion)
    (3) Specifically reflect protein loss.
    (4) Erratic response to stress

**3. Nitrogen balance**
  a. 24-hour total nitrogen balance = intake − loss = (protein (g)/6.25) − (UUN + 4 g/day for estimated fecal and nonurinary nitrogen loss), where UUN represents urinary urea nitrogen collected over 24 hours.
  b. Requires accurate 24-hour urine collection and assessment of grams of nitrogen given daily

**4. Immunologic function: Malnutrition is associated with decreased cellular and humoral immunity.**
  a. Delayed cutaneous hypersensitivity—reflects cellular immunity
    (1) Anergy to antigens suggests malnutrition.
    (2) Anergy may also occur with cancer, severe infection, renal or hepatic failure, and after chemotherapy or radiation therapy.
  b. Total lymphocyte count <3000 suggests malnutrition.
  c. Complement levels, measurements of neutrophil function, and opsonic index (potency of leukocytes to phagocytize microorganism) may be useful measurements of response to infection but are not widely available for clinical use.

**5. Patients at risk: When all factors are considered, the two most important factors are likely recent weight loss and serum albumin level <3 g/dl. Other parameters are used for corroborative purposes.**

## II. NUTRITIONAL REQUIREMENTS IN STRESS
### A. BASIC CONCEPTS
**1.** Three sources of energy for bodily processes (normally carbohydrates and fat provide 85% of daily energy expenditure, with protein supplying 15%)
**2.** Glucose yields 4 kcal/g, dextrose 3.4 kcal/g, protein 4 kcal/g, and fat 9 kcal/g.
**3.** Brain, red blood cells, white blood cells, and renal medulla are dependent on glucose in early fasting. Other tissues can use fat as an energy source.
**4.** One gram of nitrogen equals 6.25 g protein.
**5.** Normal caloric needs are 25 to 30 kcal/kg/day, and normal protein needs are 0.8 to 1 g protein/kg/day.

6. Stressed, burned, or multitrauma patients may need as much as 50 kcal/kg/day and 2.5 g protein/kg/day.
7. Adequate calories in relation to nitrogen are needed to allow protein synthesis and minimize protein catabolism. Calorie/nitrogen ratios are as follows:
a. Most disease states—100–150:1
b. Uremic patients—300–400:1
c. Septic patients—100:1

## B. DETERMINATION OF CALORIC NEEDS

1. Rough estimate—35 kcal/kg/day
2. Calculate basal energy expenditure (BEE) using the Harris–Benedict equation:

$$BEE \text{ (men)} = 66 + 13.7W + 5H \ 6.8A$$

$$BEE \text{ (women)} = 655 + 9.6W + 1.8H \ 4.7A$$

where W = weight in kg, H = height in cm, and A = age
3. Calculate increase in energy needs imposed by illness or injury (BEE $\times$ activity factor $\times$ injury factor) using Calvin–Long injury factor:
a. Minor operation—1.2 (20% increase)
b. Skeletal trauma—1.35 (35% increase)
c. Major sepsis—1.60 (60% increase)
d. Severe thermal injury—2.10 (110% increase)
4. Calculate increase in energy needs imposed (activity factor):
a. Confined to bed—1.2
b. Out of bed—1.3
5. Indirect calorimetry—measurements of the patient's oxygen consumption and carbon dioxide production
a. Determines resting energy expenditure by measuring respiratory gas exchange (i.e., $O_2$ consumption, $CO_2$ production)
b. Gives index of fuel utilization:

$$RQ = V_{CO_2}/V_{O_2}$$

where RQ = respiratory quotient, $V_{CO_2}$ = carbon dioxide production, and $V_{O_2}$ = oxygen consumption
  (1) RQ of 0.8 to 1.0 is desirable.
  (2) RQ of $<0.7$ suggests ketogenesis (underfeeding).
  (3) RQ of $>1.0$ suggests lipogenesis (overfeeding).
    (a) Also spuriously induced by hyperventilation
c. Some RQs are listed:
  (1) Carbohydrate = 1.0
  (2) For mixed substrate = 0.8
  (3) Lipid = 0.70

## III. PERIOPERATIVE NUTRITIONAL SUPPORT

### A. PREOPERATIVE NUTRITIONAL SUPPLEMENTATION

1. The malnourished patient (at risk by subjective global assessment, low serum albumin, increased stress/metabolic demand as described in sections I and II) should receive preoperative nutritional support if undergoing elective major GI surgery.
2. Begins 7 to 10 days before surgery and includes enteral (preferred) or parenteral supplementation based on caloric requirements

### B. POSTOPERATIVE NUTRITIONAL SUPPLEMENTATION

1. In the malnourished patient, supplementation should be started as soon as possible after surgery and should continue for a minimum of 1 week.
2. A well-nourished patient should have a 5- to 7-day energy reserve such that starvation alone over this period, in the absence of severe injury or illness, should be tolerated.
   a. If oral intake is not adequate after this period, enteric tube feeds via nasoenteric feeding tube (preferred) or parenteral nutrition should be started.
3. If prolonged support is anticipated, a feeding gastrostomy or jejunostomy should be considered (see IV.C).

## IV. ENTERAL NUTRITION

If the gut works, use it!

### A. INDICATIONS

1. Prolonged period without caloric intake
2. Functional GI tract
3. Inadequate oral intake
4. Avoid gut mucosal atrophy, thereby preventing intestinal bacterial translocation and related sepsis.
5. In major burns and trauma, may decrease hypermetabolism

### B. SHORT-TERM SUPPLEMENTATION

1. For nasogastric or nasointestinal feedings, use small-bore (7–9 Fr) soft tubes to improve patient comfort
2. Nasogastric
   a. Adequate gastric emptying is required.
   b. Alert patient with intact gag reflex is necessary.
   c. Maintain gastric residuals <50% of total infusion over last 4 hours.
3. Nasointestinal (postpyloric)—patients with greater risk for aspiration (i.e., neurologic impairment, poor gastric motility)

### C. LONG-TERM SUPPLEMENTATION (>6 WEEKS)

1. Gastrostomy—placed operatively or percutaneously with endoscopic guidance
   a. Adequate gastric emptying is required.

b. Evidence of reflux or impaired gag reflex is a contraindication.
c. Intermittent bolus feeds or continuous infusion
**2. Jejunostomy—placed operatively**
a. Anticipate long-term enteral supplementation in patient for whom gastrostomy is contraindicated.
b. Requires continuous infusion
**3. Gastrojejunostomy**
a. Useful in patients with functional or mechanical gastric outlet obstruction
b. Allows external emptying of stomach if needed while feeding beyond the pylorus

## D.  PRODUCTS
**1. Oral supplements**
a. Indications—supplementation for inadequate caloric intake
b. Must be palatable (flavoring increases osmolarity and cost)
c. Examples—Ensure, Ensure Plus, Boost varieties, Sustacal, Carnation Instant Breakfast
**2. Tube feedings**
a. Blenderized (pureed) diet—primarily used with gastrostomy
b. Polymeric—Isocal, Osmolite, Jevity, Ultracal
    (1) Complete diet, with intact protein; generally lactose free
    (2) Isoosmolar, fairly well tolerated
    (3) 1 kcal/ml
c. High-caloric density (2 kcal/ml)—Magnacal, TwoCal HN
    (1) Complete diet, with intact protein; generally lactose free
    (2) Hyperosmolar—may provoke diarrhea
    (3) Patients with increased caloric needs and decreased volume tolerance
d. Monomeric—Vivonex T.E.N., Criticare HN
    (1) Amino acids with or without peptides as protein source
    (2) Requires no digestion
    (3) Essentially complete small-bowel absorption (low residue)
    (4) Hyperosmolar
e. Disease-specific formulas—most are of unproven benefit.
    (1) Renal failure—Amin-Aid, Nepro, Suplena
        (a) Elemental diet, essential L-amino acids, reduced nitrogen
        (b) Hyperosmolar, 2 kcal/ml
        (c) Best when administered by tube (not very palatable)
    (2) Acute or chronic hepatic failure—Hepatic-Aid II
        (a) Enriched with branched-chain amino acids (valine, leucine, isoleucine)
        (b) Low in aromatic and sulfur-containing amino acids
        (c) May be used as tube feeding or to supplement a protein-restricted oral diet
    (3) Immunomodulatory—Impact, AlitraQ

**6**

**NUTRITION**

(a) Enriched with immunostimulatory amino acids, lipids, and nucleic acids (see section VI)

## E. ADMINISTRATION

1. The position of the tube must be confirmed radiographically before use.
2. Elevate the head of the bed 30 degrees and check gastric residuals every 4 hours (>50% of total administered over the past 4 hours is considered high).
3. Metoclopramide (Reglan) 10 mg intravenously or orally every 6 hours may aid gastric emptying.
4. Most feeds can be started at 40 ml/h and advanced by 20-ml/h increments at 4-hour intervals as tolerated until goal rate is met.
5. If the infusion is stopped for any prolonged period, the tube must be flushed with water to prevent clogging (see IV.G.1).

## F. MAJOR COMPLICATIONS OF ENTERAL FEEDING

1. Aspiration pneumonia—may be minimized by jejunal feeding and by precautions indicated in section III.E.1
2. Feeding intolerance—evidenced by vomiting, abdominal distension, cramping, diarrhea. Treat by decreasing infusion rate or diluting feedings.
3. Diarrhea—defined as more than five stools per day
a. Rule out antibiotic-associated colitis.
b. Minimized by a continuous, appropriate administration schedule, assuming intact GI function and no pancreatic insufficiency
c. May be a symptom of too-rapid advancement of hyperosmolar tube feedings
d. Minimized by clean technique in formula preparation and administration (avoid bacterial overgrowth in formulation). Time limits on formula life and duration of administration should be observed.
e. Treatment: Depending on severity, one may either decrease administration rate or add an antidiarrheal agent when infectious cause is ruled out.
    (1) Kaolin pectin (Kapectolin) is safe to use even in infectious diarrhea.
    (2) Diphenoxylate (Lomotil) elixir 2.5 to 5 mg per gastrostomy tube every 6 hours as needed
    (3) Loperamide (Imodium) elixir 2 to 4 mg every 6 hours as needed
    (4) Psyllium seed (Metamucil) 1 package in 6 oz water twice daily (bulking agent)
f. Metabolic: In general, the metabolic complications of hyperglycemia and refeeding syndrome are the same as for parenteral nutrition (see V.J.3).

## G. TROUBLESHOOTING FEEDING TUBES

1. Clogged feeding tube
a. Ensure feeding tube is primarily used for feeds, that it is being flushed with water before and after use, and that all medications are swallowed or administered in elixir form when possible.

b. Sodium bicarbonate mixture from the pharmacy or cola (Coke or Mountain Dew) can break up insoluble material in the feeding tube.
   (1) Use a small syringe (1–3 ml) to administer the mixture into the feeding tube.
   (2) Allow the mixture to sit in the feeding tube for 5 to 20 minutes to give the clogged material time to disintegrate. Repeat if necessary.
c. A soft wire can sometimes aid in unclogging feeding tubes; however, it must be used with care because injury to the bowel from the wire can cause bleeding or perforation.

**2. Gastrostomy or jejunostomy tube has fallen out**
a. Attempt to replace feeding tubes must be performed as soon as possible to prevent granulation and closure of the stoma.
b. If tube was placed more than 6 weeks earlier, it can usually be replaced without radiographic guidance.
   (1) If the original size tube will not fit through the stoma, start out with a small red rubber or Foley catheter (e.g., 8 Fr) and gradually dilate the stoma to the desired size (lubrication jelly will help passage of the tube).
   (2) If the stoma is too small for an 8 Fr catheter, a soft wire can often be inserted under fluoroscopic guidance and the tract gradually dilated, thereby preserving the stomal tract.
c. If tube was placed less than 6 weeks earlier, it is ideal to replace it over a wire under fluoroscopic guidance.
   (1) If fluoroscopic guidance is not immediately available, the tube can be replaced gently through the stoma and advanced as long as there is minimal resistance (a small red rubber or Foley catheter can also be used).
   (2) Leave the tube in place to keep the stoma open (but do not use) until fluoroscopy is available or until its location can be confirmed with contrast radiography at the bedside.
d. If there is question about the location of the tube or if the tube was re-placed within 6 weeks of original stoma creation, Gastrografin contrast (20–30 ml) should be injected into the tube, followed immediately by plain-film abdominal radiograph to confirm placement before use.

## V. PARENTERAL NUTRITION
### A. INDICATIONS
1. Prolonged period without caloric intake
2. Enteral feeding contraindicated or not tolerated.
3. Presence of malnutrition

### B. ROLE IN PRIMARY THERAPY
1. Efficacy demonstrated in the following situations:
a. GI fistula—allows for total bowel "rest" while providing adequate nutrition. Rate of spontaneous closure is increased, but overall mortality is not affected.

b. Short bowel syndrome—maintain nutritional status until remaining bowel can undergo hypertrophy. This is the nonoperative strategy for long-term survival.

c. Acute tubular necrosis—mortality rate is decreased, with earlier recovery from renal failure. Hypercatabolism of renal failure is met by total parenteral nutrition.

d. Acute-on-chronic hepatic insufficiency—normalization of amino acid profiles results in improved recovery from hepatic encephalopathy and possibly decreased mortality.

**2. Efficacy not completely established for the following conditions:**

a. Inflammatory bowel disease: Crohn's disease limited to small bowel responds best; does not affect the course of ulcerative colitis, but allows for bowel rest and improved postoperative course when given before ileoanal pull-through operations.

b. Anorexia nervosa

## C. SUPPORTIVE THERAPY

**1. Efficacy established for the following conditions:**

a. Radiation enteritis

b. Acute GI toxicity caused by chemotherapeutic agents

c. Hyperemesis gravidarum

**2. Efficacy not yet established for the following conditions:**

a. Preoperative nutritional support for malnourished patients: Studies have shown improvement in metabolic end points but no statistically significant improvement in mortality or complication rate.

b. Cardiac cachexia

c. Pancreatitis

d. Respiratory insufficiency with need for prolonged ventilatory support

e. Prolonged ileus (>5 days)

f. Nitrogen-losing wounds

## D. INDICATIONS CURRENTLY UNDER INVESTIGATION

**1.** Cancer: Generally, nutritional support is indicated in patients undergoing antineoplastic therapy (e.g., surgery, radiation, chemotherapy) during times of ileus, GI mucosal damage, and other symptoms. The goal of nutritional support is weight maintenance, not weight gain.

## E. BASIC COMPOSITION OF FORMULATIONS (TABLES 6-1 AND 6-2)

**1.** Carbohydrate—Dextrose used exclusively in the United States. Concentrations range from 15 to 47%.

**2.** Amino acids—either balanced or disease specific (renal, hepatic, stress formulations)

**3.** Lipid emulsions

a. Available as 10% or 20% solutions (1 kcal/ml or 2 kcal/ml, respectively)

b. Infusion of 100 ml of 10% solution per week is adequate to prevent essential fatty acid deficiency.

**TABLE 6-1**

TOTAL PARENTERAL NUTRITION SOLUTION: COMPOSITION

| Type of Solution | Amino Acids | Glucose | Calories |
|---|---|---|---|
| Standard | 4.25% (42.5 g/L) | D-15 (150 g/L) | 510 kcal/L |
| | 5% (50 g/L) | D-25 (250 g/L) | 850 kcal/L |
| Renal | 1.7% (17 g/L) | D-47 (470 g/L) | 1598 kcal/L |
| Hepatic | 3.5% (35 g/L) | D-35 (350 g/L) | 1190 kcal/L |
| Peripheral | 3% (30 g/L) | D-10 (100 g/L) | 340 kcal/L |

**TABLE 6-2**

ADDITIONAL COMPONENTS TO TOTAL PARENTERAL NUTRITION SOLUTION

| Trace Elements (add to first bottle each day) | Dose | Type |
|---|---|---|
| Zn | 3.0 mg | |
| Cu | 1.2 mg | Stress formula |
| Cr | 12 µg | Hepatic formula |
| Se | 60 mg | Hepatic formula |
| Mn | 0.3 mg | |
| Vitamins | | |
| Multivitamin | 1 ampule every day (10 ml) | |
| K | 5 mg every week | For patients not requiring anticoagulants |

| Electrolytes and Insulin | Usual | Range |
|---|---|---|
| Na+ (mEq/L) | 20–80 | 0–150 |
| K+ (mEq/L) | 13–40 | 0–80 |
| Cl (mEq/L) | 10–80 | 0–150 |
| Ca2+ (mEq/L) | 4.7 | 0–10 |
| P (mmol) | 14 | 0–21 |
| Acetate (mEq/L) | 45–81 | 45–220 |
| Regular insulin (units/L) | 0–25 | 0–60 |

6

NUTRITION

   c. Check baseline measurements of serum triglycerides to avoid exacerbation of preexisting hypertriglyceridemia.
   d. Lipid emulsion substituted for carbohydrate calories in certain situations (decrease overall volume given, carbohydrate overfeeding, total parenteral nutrition hepatotoxicity)
   e. Safe to provide 20% to 60% of total calories as lipid
4. **Minor components**
   a. Vitamins—including 5 mg vitamin K weekly
   b. Trace elements—zinc, copper, chromium, manganese, selenium (see section VII for vitamin deficiencies)
   c. Insulin and electrolytes as necessary

## F. CENTRAL FORMULAS
1. Administration
   a. The tip of the catheter should reside within the superior vena cava; its location should be documented in the patient's chart.

b. Long-term catheters (Hickman, Port-A-Cath) may be placed in the superior vena cava to avoid catheter clotting.

c. Insertion of a central venous catheter for parenteral nutrition is never an emergency; the patient should be stable, well hydrated, and without serious coagulopathy.

**2. Standard central formula:** Most patients requiring parenteral nutrition can use formula containing 15% to 25% dextrose.

**3. Renal formulation**

a. NephrAmine (essential L-amino acids only)

b. Indicated in patients with acute renal failure who are not being dialyzed

c. Electrolyte composition offsets abnormalities in acute renal failure; useful in preventing increase in potassium level and blood urea nitrogen, and may delay dialysis.

d. Higher glucose base (D-47) serves to reduce volume.

e. Once the patient has converted to chronic dialysis, parenteral nutrition should be changed to standard.

**4. Hepatic formulation**

a. Indicated for patients with grade 2 (impending stupor) or greater (grade 3 = stupor, grade 4 = coma) hepatic encephalopathy

b. Hepatic formulation is enriched with 35% branched-chain amino acids, alanine, arginine, and reduced amounts of aromatic and sulfur-containing amino acids.

## G. PERIPHERAL PARENTERAL NUTRITION

**1.** Contains 3% amino acids in 10% dextrose

**2.** To provide adequate calorie/nitrogen ratio, the equivalent of 500 ml of 10% lipid emulsion should be administered with each liter of peripheral formulation to a maximum of 100 g fat/day. Monitoring lipid profile avoids hyperlipidemia.

**3.** Indicated in patients in whom central venous catheterization is contraindicated (Candida sepsis, blood dyscrasias, thrombosis)

**4.** Difficulties include increased cost and difficulties with long-term venous access caused by phlebitis from administration of hypertonic solution.

**5.** Peripheral parenteral nutrition may be indicated for 3 to 5 days of nutritional support in patients who may not be able to take an adequate oral intake and are thought to be at increased risk for complications of malnutrition.

**6.** Only major advantage is elimination of risks associated with central venous catheterization.

## H. INFUSION

**1.** Rate

a. All formulations begin at 40 to 50 ml/h with exception of renal formulation, which generally begins at 30 ml/h because of higher glucose content, and peripheral formulation, which begins at target rate.

b. Rate is increased in increments of 20 to 25 ml/h every 8 to 24 hours (if blood sugar is well controlled) until caloric needs are matched.

c. With renal formula, advance in increments of 10 ml/h each day.

**2.** With the exception of lipid emulsion, single-lumen catheters should not be used for any other infusion of maintenance fluid, medication, blood products, or central venous pressure readings.

## I. MONITORING

**1.** Vital signs every 6 hours for initial 24 to 48 hours

**2.** Fingerstick glucose determinations every 6 hours to monitor for hyperglycemia

**3.** Weight check every other day

**4.** Twice-weekly blood work—electrolytes, glucose, liver enzymes, calcium, phosphorus, prothrombin, partial thromboplastin time, complete blood cell count, short-turnover proteins, if available

## J. COMPLICATIONS

**1.** Technical (see Chapter 81)

**2.** Catheter sepsis—clinical sepsis in a patient receiving parenteral nutrition for whom no anatomic septic focus is identified and that resolves after removal of the catheter.

a. Administration of total parenteral nutrition independently increases the risk for catheter-related sepsis; therefore, meticulous line care is essential.

**3.** Metabolic complications

a. Disorders of glucose metabolism

   (1) Hyperglycemia (blood sugar >200 mg/dl)

      (a) Use of fatty acids and ketones during starvation can result in temporary insulin resistance when carbohydrates are introduced into the bloodstream

      (b) May be associated with either parenteral or enteral nutrition and may lead to hyperosmolar, hyperglycemic, nonketotic dehydration, with shock/death resulting if untreated

      (c) If blood sugar is >200 mg/dl, the rate of infusion of the formulation should not be increased; subcutaneous regular insulin should be administered acutely, and the amount of insulin in each liter of solution should be increased appropriately. Causes of sepsis should be ruled out.

   (2) Hypoglycemia—rare complication

      (a) If total parenteral nutrition is suddenly discontinued for any reason, intravenous administration of any 5% dextrose solution is sufficient to prevent hypoglycemia.

      (b) Rarely occurs with endogenous insulin response to high rates of infusion. Treat by slowing the infusion.

b. Liver dysfunction

   (1) Results from excess carbohydrates stored in liver as fat

   (2) Reversible, self-limited in adults

  c. Refeeding syndrome—can occur with the onset of parenteral or enteral nutrition in patients who are chronically malnourished or in a starved state

    (1) Hypophosphatemia

      (a) Results from intracellular shifts from increased insulin production

      (b) Increased adenosine triphosphate production, glycogenesis, and protein anabolism dramatically increase the demand for phosphates.

      (c) Extracellular levels can decline to less than 1 mg/dl within hours of initiating nutritional therapy.

      (d) Associated with muscle weakness, paralysis, seizures, coma, cardiopulmonary decompensation, and death

    (2) Hypokalemia and hypomagnesemia also occur as a result of increased adenosine triphosphate production and insulin-induced intracellular shifts.

    (3) At-risk individuals must be screened and fluid/electrolytes watched closely.

    (4) Supplementation with vitamins and electrolytes as soon as possible is necessary

      (a) Consider thiamine, folate, vitamin $B_6$ and zinc supplementation.

## VI. IMMUNONUTRITION

Nutritional deficits produce atrophy of lymphoid organs and impaired function, leading to infections. Addition of immune-enhancing supplementation may reduce infectious complications; however, there appears to be no mortality advantage.

### A. GLUTAMINE

1. Most abundant free amino acid in the body
2. Levels decrease during stress (used by kidney to form ammonia and improve acidosis)
3. Synthesized in muscle during catabolic states
4. Primary fuel for small intestinal enterocytes
5. Important for maintaining healthy intestinal mucosa
a. May protect mucosa after radiation therapy, chemotherapy, small-bowel resection
6. Provides fuel for macrophages, T cells

### B. ARGININE

1. Promotes T-cell proliferation, fibroblast proliferation

### C. OMEGA-3 FATTY ACIDS

1. Replace omega-6 fatty acids (an immunosuppressant)

### D. NUCLEOTIDES

1. Provide RNA for cell proliferation/immune function
2. If levels are decreased, there is decreased T-cell and IL-2 function.

## VII. NUTRIENTS/MACROMINERALS/MICRONUTRIENTS/VITAMINS

Nutrients, minerals, and vitamins; their deficiency-related symptoms; and daily required amounts are listed in Table 6-3.

### TABLE 6-3

NUTRIENTS/MINERALS/VITAMINS, SYMPTOMS OF DEFICIENCY, AND DAILY REQUIREMENT

| Essential Fatty Acids | Deficiency | Requirements | |
|---|---|---|---|
| Linoleic and linolenic acids | Scaly, erythematous skin rash | 30–50 g of lipid emulsion per week | |
| **Macrominerals** | **Deficiency** | **Daily Requirements** | |
| Calcium | Acute—tetany, paresthesias, hyperreflexia, seizures, mental status changes Chronic—rickets (children), osteomalacia (adults) | 800 mg | |
| Phosphorous | Muscle weakness, paresthesias, seizures, hemolytic anemia, impaired white blood cell function, tissue hypoxia | 800–1200 mg | |
| Magnesium | Hypocalcemia, tetany, ataxia, coma, psychosis, cardiac dysrhythmias, hypotension | 300–500 mg | |
| **Micronutrients** | | **Enteral** | **Parenteral** |
| Chromium | Glucose intolerance | 30 µg | 10–15 µg |
| Copper | Microcytic, hypochromic anemia | 0.9 mg | 0.3–0.5 mg |
| Iodine | Weakness, cold intolerance, facial swelling, pallor, hair-thinning, hoarseness, constipation | 150 µg | Not well defined |
| Iron | Microcytic anemia | 18 mg | Not routinely added |
| Manganese | Hair thinning | 2.3 mg | 60–100 µg |
| Selenium | Myositis, cardiomyopathy, collagen vascular disease | 55 µg | 20–60 µg |
| Zinc | Poor wound healing, perioral rash, hair loss, dysgeusia | 11 mg | 2.5–5 mg |
| **Water-Soluble Vitamins** | | | |
| Vitamin C | Bleeding gums, gingivitis, weakness of hair follicles | 1.2 mg | 3 mg |

Continued

6

NUTRITION

### TABLE 6-3—cont'd

**NUTRIENTS/MINERALS/VITAMINS, SYMPTOMS OF DEFICIENCY, AND DAILY REQUIREMENT**

| | | | |
|---|---|---|---|
| Vitamin $B_1$ (thiamine) | Anorexia, anemia, ataxia, polyneuritis, beriberi, Wernicke's encephalopathy | 1.2 mg | 3.6 mg |
| Vitamin $B_2$ (riboflavin) | Photophobia, soreness/burning of lips, tongue, mouth, "beefy red tongue" | 1.3 mg | 3.6 mg |
| Niacin | Pellagra (glossitis, dermatitis, scale erythematous rash, diarrhea, dementia | 16 mg | 40 mg |
| Folate | Megaloblastic anemia | 400 μg | 400 μg |
| Vitamin $B_{12}$ | Megaloblastic anemia, peripheral neuropathy | 2.4 μg | 5 μg |
| Vitamin $B_6$ | Dermatitis, glossitis, depression, confusion, convulsion | 1.7 mg | 4 mg |
| **Fat-Soluble Vitamins** | | | |
| Vitamin A | Xerophthalmia, immunodeficiency | 900 μg | 1000 μg |
| Vitamin D | Bone resorption, osteomalacia | 15 μg | 5 μg |
| Vitamin E | Neuromuscular dysfunction | 15 mg | 10 mg |
| Vitamin K | Bleeding coagulopathy | 120 μg | 1 mg |

# Wound Healing and Management

*Shannon P. O'Brien, MD*

*Wound healing is a complex process, and every surgeon should have an understanding of the basic principles and ways to maximize healing.*

## I. PHASES OF WOUND HEALING

Wound healing involves a complicated series of events that can be divided into three phases: inflammatory, proliferative, and maturation. Any disruption of the wound or general health of the patient can cause the process to start over or prolong a phase of healing.

### A. INFLAMMATORY (IMMEDIATE RESPONSE: 4 DAYS AFTER TISSUE INJURY)

1. *Hemostasis* (first response to injury) begins with vasoconstriction, which lasts for 5 to 10 minutes. *Platelets* release a number of cytokines (platelet-derived growth factor and transforming growth factor [TGF]-β) and glycoproteins (fibrinogen and fibronectin), which, together with kinins, complement, and prostaglandin, signal the initiation of *inflammation.*
2. *TGF-β* stimulates macrophage and lymphocyte chemotaxis and proliferation.
3. After hemostasis, histamine release causes vasodilation and increases vascular permeability to allow cellular migration into the wound.
4. The first cells to respond are *polymorphonuclear (PMN) leukocytes.* They arrive within a few hours and are the predominant cell type in early wound exudate. The role of PMNs is phagocytosis and wound debridement, but PMNs are *not* necessary in wound healing or collagen synthesis.
5. *Monocytes* follow closely behind the PMNs and are transformed into macrophages.
6. *Macrophages* are responsible for signaling normal fibroblast production.
   a. Predominant cell in wound exudate after the first 48 hours
   b. *Key choreographers* of wound healing: continue debridement and conclude the inflammatory response via cytokines and growth factors
   c. Secrete nitric oxide, which is bactericidal (particularly against *Staphylococcus aureus*)

### B. PROLIFERATIVE (4 DAYS TO 3 WEEKS)

1. Characterized by the migration and proliferation of fibroblasts and endothelial cells, and by the synthesis of collagen
2. *Fibroblasts* migrate into the wound and proliferate, stimulated by cytokines and growth factors (platelet-derived growth factor most importantly) secreted by macrophages and platelets. They secrete

proteoglycans and fibronectin, creating a temporary matrix. Most importantly, they synthesize collagen.

3. *Collagen,* produced by fibroblasts, replaces the temporary matrix. Its synthesis increases until 4 weeks after injury because of increasing numbers of fibroblasts in the wound and increased production per cell. Increased collagen equals increased tensile strength.

4. *Epithelialization* is the migration of keratinocytes across the wound to restore the barrier function of the skin. Epithelial cells increase their mitotic rate, release from the basement membrane, and creep across the open wound until they contact other keratinocytes. Contact inhibition stops migration.

   a. Partial-thickness wounds reepithelialize from the edges of the wound and from remaining epidermal appendages (i.e., hair follicles).

   b. Full-thickness wounds reepithelialize from wound margins only.

   c. Surgical incisions typically epithelialize within 48 hours.

5. *Angiogenesis* is the proliferation of endothelial cells to form capillary tubes. It occurs in response to vascular endothelial growth factor (VEGF), which is secreted by macrophages (for wound healing) and by keratinocytes (during epithelialization). Endothelial cells secrete *nitric oxide,* which increases VEGF secretion and causes vasodilation, which protects healing tissue from hypoxia and ischemia.

6. *Wound contraction* occurs when fibroblasts that are adherent within the wound change into *myofibroblasts* (TGF-$\beta$1 stimulates). Myofibroblasts have microfilaments similar to smooth muscle cells that contract to shrink wound.

7. Macrophages release cytokines and growth factors to guide fibroplasia, angiogenesis, and extracellular matrix synthesis.

## C. MATURATION (3 WEEKS TO 1 YEAR)

1. During this phase, overall collagen synthesis decreases until it reaches a point of *collagen homeostasis.*

2. Thin collagen fibrils are initially laid down parallel to the wound edge. As the wound matures, the fibers become thicker, cross-link, and are interwoven against tension lines, thus increasing the *tensile strength.* The tensile strength is greatest at approximately 60 days; then settles at about 80% of uninjured skin (never reaching the strength of normal skin).

3. Type I collagen makes up 90% of the collagen in normal skin, with type III collagen making up the remaining 10%. In granulation tissue, type III collagen makes up as much as 30%, then during the maturation phase that percentage returns to 10%, with type I collagen making up the rest.

4. Capillary ingrowth slows

5. The scar flattens and softens as it matures

## II. FACTORS THAT AFFECT WOUND HEALING

### A. OXYGENATION
1. Fibroblasts are $O_2$ sensitive and require partial pressure of oxygen ($P_{O_2}$) of 30 mm Hg, and can be stimulated to proliferate and synthesize collagen if $P_{O_2}$ >40 mm Hg.
2. Wound hypoxia, secondary to severe anemia or inadequate vascularity (ischemia), is the most common cause of wound infection.

### B. INFECTION
1. Prolongs inflammatory phase
2. Interferes with wound contraction, epithelialization, angiogenesis, and collagen deposition
3. Bacterial collagenases degrade collagen

### C. NUTRITION
1. Malnutrition: serum protein <2 g prolongs inflammatory phase, decreases fibroplasia, and therefore delays tensile strength
2. Vitamin C: essential cofactor in collagen synthesis (no benefit to supranormal levels of vitamin C)
3. Vitamin A: increases wound breaking strength

### D. STEROIDS
1. Inhibit wound macrophages, fibroplasia, angiogenesis, and wound contraction
2. Increase risk for infection

### E. SMOKING
1. Nicotine—vasoconstrictor—decreases cellular migration and oxygenation.
2. Increased partial pressure of carbon monoxide ($P_{CO}$) decreases $O_2$ carrying capacity of hemoglobin.
3. One cigarette results in vasoconstriction for 90 minutes.

### F. AGE
1. Tensile strength and wound closure rates decline with increasing age.

### G. FOREIGN BODIES
1. Include nonviable tissue
2. Prolong inflammation
3. Inhibit wound contraction, angiogenesis, and epithelialization

### H. EDEMA
1. Inhibits perfusion, and therefore inhibits healing

### I. CHEMOTHERAPY
1. Antimetabolites, cytotoxic agents, and steroids are commonly used.
2. Impaired immunity increases risk for infection and tissue repair failure.

WOUND HEALING AND MANAGEMENT

7

3. Little effect on healing if chemotherapy started 10 to 14 days after surgery

## J. RADIATION
1. Acutely, radiation causes stasis and occlusion in small vessels.
2. Fibroblast injury impairs proliferation, collagen synthesis, and tensile strength; injury to fibroblasts is permanent.
3. Progressive injury: tissues retain poor healing abilities forever

## K. DIABETES MELLITUS
1. Impairment to wound healing is multifactorial
a. Large vessel disease: atherosclerosis especially affects tibial and peroneal arteries
b. Increased edema secondary to increased venous pressure
c. Decreased $O_2$ delivery secondary to glycosylation of hemoglobin
d. Decreased phagocytosis

## L. GENERAL HEALTH
1. Obesity, coronary artery disease, chronic obstructive pulmonary disease, carcinoma, and renal or hepatic failure all impair healing potential

## III. TYPES OF WOUND CLOSURE
### A. PRIMARY CLOSURE
1. Closure of wound by direct approximation of wound edges

### B. SPONTANEOUS HEALING (HEALING BY SECONDARY INTENTION)
1. Closure by wound contraction and epithelialization

### C. TERTIARY HEALING
1. Delayed primary closure after allowing the wound to begin healing by secondary intention. May be performed any time after formation of granulation tissue, but may only be performed in clean/noninfected wound.

## IV. ADJUNCTS TO HEALING BY SECONDARY INTENTION
### A. NEGATIVE-PRESSURE TREATMENT (VACUUM-ASSISTED CLOSURE).
1. Exact mechanism unknown, but removes interstitial fluid and edema
2. Increases wound oxygenation and granulation tissue
3. Decreases inflammatory mediators and wound bacterial counts

### B. HYPERBARIC OXYGEN
1. Improves tissue oxygen tension via hyperoxygenation
2. Mitosis requires at least 30 mm Hg $O_2$, and chronic, nonhealing wounds usually have oxygen tensions in the 5 to 20 mm Hg range
3. Cannot aid healing if tissue not adequately perfused (ischemic)

## C. HYDROTHERAPY
1. Whirlpool therapy
2. Pulsed lavage treatment (4–15 psi): decreases bacterial count and cleans exudate
3. Never to be used on clean, granulating wounds

## V. MANAGEMENT OF SOFT-TISSUE WOUNDS

### A. TRAUMATIC WOUND PREPARATION
1. Fully evaluate patient, including ABCs; control wound hemorrhage with direct pressure.
2. Immune prophylaxis
a. *Tetanus* immunization should be considered for anyone with a traumatic open wound. It should definitely be given when a wound is high risk for a *Clostridium tetani* infection, including wounds that are deep, contaminated, and with devitalized tissue.
b. *Rabies* immunization is indicated for patients bitten by wild carnivorous animals. It is not indicated in bites by domestic animals that do not display symptoms of infection with the virus or for rodent bites.
3. Evaluate for fractures and foreign bodies with radiographs as indicated.
4. Anesthetize wound with local anesthetic (see Chapter 15).
5. Cleanse wound with Betadine or Hibiclens. Then irrigate wound profusely with normal saline.
6. Debride clearly devitalized tissue, clot, and foreign bodies. Be conservative with initial surgical debridement, particularly on the face where marginal-appearing tissue usually survives.
7. Explore wound carefully for neurovascular, tendon, bone, or joint injury.

### B. WOUND CLOSURE
1. Most traumatic wounds can be closed primarily if above steps are followed. Exceptions to this are infected wounds and human bites. If the wound cannot be closed, it should be packed loosely with normal saline–moistened gauze. This dressing should be changed every 8 to 12 hours as needed for debridement and to keep the wound moist.
2. Use anatomic structures (i.e., eyebrow, vermillion border, and so forth) as guides to align wound edges appropriately.
3. Wound edges should be reapproximated via deep dermal sutures, and these should minimize tension across the laceration. Using the minimum number of sutures to reduce tension is the goal, and using an absorbable monofilament (rather than braided) suture minimizes infectious risk.
4. Close skin edges using nonabsorbable monofilament suture in an interrupted technique. Exceptions to the nonabsorbable suture rule are wounds to mucosal surfaces and some pediatric hand injuries.

7

WOUND HEALING AND MANAGEMENT

## C. POSTOPERATIVE CARE

1. Keep wounds clean; may wash with soapy water 24 to 48 hours after closure. Open wounds may be washed with soapy water as well.
2. Wounds should be monitored for signs of infection.
3. Antibiotics are given to patients with wounds that were severely contaminated, infected, or caused by bites.
4. Antibiotic ointment to suture line every 12 hours for 2 days.
5. Sutures may be removed from face at 5 days, and all other areas at 7 to 10 days.

## D. WOUND DRESSINGS

1. The goal of a dressing is to protect the wound from further trauma and to create an environment that will maximize healing.
2. Intraoperatively placed dry dressings are typically left in place, after being applied under sterile conditions, for 48 hours. This allows for epithelialization to occur. Soiled dressings should be changed.
3. Treatment of partial-thickness or superficial wounds is application of antibiotic ointment and nonadherent dressings, which should be changed twice a day.
4. Wet to moist/dry dressings debride wound exudate and cellular debris, and prevent desiccation. Gauze is moistened with normal saline; however, if concerned for infection/contamination, particularly with *Pseudomonas,* use Dakin's solution (0.25% acetic acid). Dakin's solution delays healing but decontaminates well.
5. V.A.C. dressings are applied to open wounds to accelerate wound closure (see IV.A.) and are changed every other day.

## VI. MANAGEMENT OF WOUND COMPLICATIONS

### A. INFECTION

1. Postsurgical wound infections usually present approximately 3 days after surgery.
2. Symptoms are erythema, induration, exudate, fever, and lymphadenopathy.
3. Infections are typically caused by staphylococci (increasingly methicillin-resistant strains) or streptococci.
4. Risk increases with poor sterile technique, contaminated abdominal cases, prolonged OR time (more than 5 hours), and general conditions that adversely affect wound healing (listed earlier).
5. Treatment consists of antibiotics alone if there is only a cellulitis. If there is an abscess, drain it and excise all devitalized tissue.
6. *Necrotizing fasciitis* is a rapidly spreading infection that travels along the subcutaneous or fascial planes, or both. It is characterized by fever, wound crepitence, gray or dusky coloration of the skin, and rapid

progression. Treatment is early, aggressive surgical excision of affected tissue. It is usually a polymicrobial infection.

## B. SEROMA
1. A seroma is sterile serous fluid collection in operative dead space.
2. Best treated prophylactically with closed-suction drains, to be removed when output is low.
3. If a seroma forms, the fluid may be aspirated or a drain placed via ultrasound or computed tomography guidance using sterile technique. There is a small risk for infecting a sterile fluid collection when draining seroma; therefore, small seromas without signs of infection are usually safe to monitor and allowed to be resorbed.

## C. HEMATOMA
1. A hematoma is a collection of blood, a clot, or both.
2. The best treatment is prevention by appropriate intraoperative hemostasis.
3. Small hematomas may be followed closely for signs of infection and be allowed to resorb.
4. Larger hematomas usually require the wound to be opened in the operating room and irrigated, and any ongoing bleeding must be stopped. If there are no signs of infection, the wound may be closed again.

## D. DEHISCENCE
1. Superficial: separation of skin and subcutaneous fat
   a. If wound is clean, may clean and close again using sterile technique. May alternatively treat as open contaminated wound and allow closure by secondary intention
2. Fascial: separation of fascia
   a. Possibly secondary to technical failure but can be secondary to wound infection, pulmonary disease, hemodynamic instability, age >65 years, malnutrition, obesity, malignancy, ascites, steroid use, or systemic infection
   b. Mortality rate is 15% to 30%.
   c. Identified by rush of serosanguinous salmon-colored fluid
   d. Small fascial separation may be monitored closely with plan to repair hernia in future.
   e. If patient eviscerates, apply saline-soaked towels and repair fascia emergently in the operating room.
   f. In high-risk patients with poor fascia, multiple comorbidities, or chronic-steroid use, *retention sutures* can be placed to help support fascial closure. These are full-thickness bites of the abdominal wall and should be left in place for approximately 3 weeks.

## VII. HYPERTROPHIC SCARS AND KELOIDS

### A. HYPERTROPHIC SCARS

1. Characterized by wide, raised scars that remain within the original borders of injury
2. Occur within 4 weeks of injury
3. Usually resolve over time without treatment

### B. KELOIDS

1. Scar extends beyond the original borders of injury.
2. Occur within 1 year of injury
3. Recurrence rate is high (almost universal).
4. Epidemiology
   a. Most common in blacks—15:1 darkly pigmented skin/light skin ratio
   b. Uncommon in very young and elderly individuals
5. Histology
   a. Large bundles of collagen deposited in disorganized fashion
   b. Few macrophages, but many eosinophils and mast cells
6. Treatment
   a. Scars are often unsightly, but indication for treatment is chronic itching and skin breakdown.
   b. *Pressure therapy:* limits formation of keloids, especially in burn scars. It is not helpful in resolving keloids once formed.
   c. *Surgical excision:* inadequate treatment—keloid will recur
   d. *Surgical excision with steroids:* current treatment of choice
      (1) Excise keloid using sterile technique and immediately inject wound with steroids.
      (2) Then treat incision site with three monthly injections after surgery.
      (3) It is shown to improve recurrence rates.
   e. Surgical excision with radiation therapy
      (1) Excise keloid and treat with 15 to 20 Gy radiation within 24 hours.
      (2) Approximately five additional treatments are necessary.
      (3) Although it is a low radiation dose, there is some mild controversy regarding the risk of treating a benign tumor with radiation. Despite any controversy, this is an accepted practice for keloid management.

# Standard Precautions

*Parit A. Patel, MD*

Standard precautions, previously referred to as "universal precautions," are defined by the Centers for Disease Control and Prevention as a set of precautions designed to prevent transmission of human immunodeficiency virus (HIV), hepatitis B virus (HBV), and other blood-borne pathogens when providing first aid or health care. Blood and certain body fluids of all patients are considered potentially infectious for HIV, HBV, and other blood-borne pathogens.

8

## I. APPLICATIONS

### A. STANDARD PRECAUTIONS APPLY TO THE FOLLOWING BODY FLUIDS:

1. Blood—the most important source for HIV, HBV, and other blood-borne pathogens in terms of the occupational setting
2. Semen—not implicated in occupational transmissions because of relatively limited exposure in health-care settings
3. Vaginal secretions—rarely implicated in occupational transmissions because of relatively limited exposure and routine use of gloves during vaginal examinations
4. Cerebrospinal fluid
5. Synovial fluid
6. Peritoneal fluid
7. Pericardial fluid
8. Pleural fluid
9. Amniotic fluid

### B. STANDARD PRECAUTIONS DO NOT APPLY TO THE FOLLOWING BODY FLUIDS

Unless blood can be visualized in these fluids; it is recommended, however, that gloves be used while handling these materials:

1. Feces
2. Nasal secretions
3. Sputum
4. Sweat
5. Tears
6. Urine
7. Vomitus
8. Saliva—dental procedures are an exception and require implementation of standard precautions.

## II. GUIDELINES: OCCUPATIONAL SETTINGS

### A. AT THE BEDSIDE

1. Wash hands before and after each patient encounter.
2. Use gloves when anticipating being in contact with blood or other body fluids requiring the use of standard precautions, mucous membranes, and/or nonintact skin.
3. Remove gloves after each patient encounter.
4. Protective barriers such as masks, protective eyewear, and gowns should be worn during procedures where the potential for splatter or the generation of droplets of blood or other body fluids requiring standard precautions are anticipated.

### B. IN THE OPERATING ROOM

1. Wear gloves for all preoperative and postoperative patient contact.
2. Before the operation, scrub, gown, and glove according to standard techniques.
3. Wear protective eyewear with side shields at all times while in the operating room.
4. If an exposure occurs during the operation, **always** initiate the exposure protocol according to the institution at which the exposure occurred.
5. Immediately after the operation, remove the gown first and then the gloves, taking care to avoid exposure to contaminants.
6. Double-gloving is recommended when performing operations that are considered exposure prone or on patients whose body fluids are known to be infectious. There may be no benefit in terms of penetrating injury, but it does increase the penetrating force required to compromise the barrier.

### C. IN THE TRAUMA BAY

1. Gloves, eyewear with side protectors, mask, and gown should be used in all trauma resuscitation situations.

## III. RISKS OF NEEDLE-STICK/SHARP-INSTRUMENT INJURY

According to the Occupational Safety and Health Administration, annual needle-stick injuries in U.S. hospitals are estimated at 800,000. The Centers for Disease Control and Prevention states that most needle-stick injuries do not result in exposure to an infectious disease, and of those that do, most do not result in the transmission of infection. Nevertheless, needle-stick injuries may expose the health-care provider to blood-borne pathogens such as HIV, HBV, and/or HCV.

### A. HIV

1. Before the implementation of HAART (highly active antiretroviral therapy) after exposures, the data demonstrated the risk for seroconversion from a single percutaneous needle stick from HIV-infected blood

to be ≈0.3%. The risk for mucocutaneous exposures is ≈0.09%. Risk factors for serovconversion include visible contaminant on needle or instrument, depth of injury, placement of needle in a vessel, and health status of the patient (i.e., viral load).

## B. HEPATITIS B
1. Before the advent of the HBV vaccine for health care providers, studies demonstrated rates for HBV transmission from a single needle-stick exposure from an HBV-infected patient to range from 6% to 30%. HBV vaccination strategies have significantly decreased the incidence of HBV infections among health-care providers.

## C. HEPATITIS C
1. Epidemiologic studies of health care workers exposed to HCV from a needle stick or other percutaneous injury demonstrated that seroconversion to HCV is 1.8%.

## IV. CIRCUMSTANCES THAT LEAD TO NEEDLE-STICK INJURIES
A. SUDDEN MOVEMENTS OF THE PATIENT OR COWORKER
B. RECAPPING CONTAMINATED NEEDLES
C. TRANSFERRING BODY FLUIDS BETWEEN MEDICAL WASTE CONTAINERS
D. FAILURE TO ADEQUATELY DISPOSE OF CONTAMINATED NEEDLES IN THEIR APPROPRIATE CONTAINERS
E. DURING THE PROCESS OF DISPOSING CONTAMINATED NEEDLES

## V. DEFINITION OF EXPOSURE
A. PERCUTANEOUS INJURY WITH EITHER A CONTAMINATED NEEDLE OR SHARP OBJECT
B. CONTACT OF NONINTACT SKIN OR MUCOUS MEMBRANES WITH BLOOD OR OTHER INFECTIOUS FLUIDS (REFER TO I.A AND I.B)

## VI. POSTEXPOSURE PROTOCOL (OCCUPATIONAL SAFETY AND HEALTH ADMINISTRATION REQUIREMENTS)
A. PERCUTANEOUS AND MUCOCUTANEOUS EXPOSURES
1. Wash area immediately with soap and water; alcohol can be used for deeper and smaller injuries.
2. Mucous membrane exposures should be washed with copious amounts of water or saline.
3. Contact employee health office to report the incident.
4. Obtain consent from the source for blood testing, which includes HBsAg, HCV, and rapid HIV.
5. The health-care provider should also undergo blood testing for HBsAg (hepatitis B surface antigen), HBsAb (hepatitis B surface antibody),

HBcAb (hepatitis B core antibody), HCV, HIV, AST (aspartate aminotransferase), and ALT (alanine aminotransferase). For exposures from positive sources, repeat testing is recommended (HIV: 6 weeks, 12 weeks, and 6 months; HCV: 4–6 weeks and 4–6 months).

## B. POSTEXPOSURE PROPHYLAXIS (PEP)

1. HIV: For a high-risk source, PEP should be initiated within 1 to 2 hours or after the rapid HIV result. According to Centers for Disease Control and Prevention guidelines, two nucleoside reverse transcriptase inhibitors should be used for lower risk exposures. Higher risk exposures require one or more additional drugs. PEP can reduce the risk for seroconversion by approximately 80%.
2. HBV: Unvaccinated health-care providers should receive the first dose of HBV vaccine series regardless of source HBV status. HBIg can also be given for exposures from sources that are HBV-positive.
3. HCV: No PEP is recommended for such exposures. Interferon has not proved to be effective for PEP.

## VII. COMPLIANCE

A. EDUCATE HEALTH-CARE PROVIDERS ON STANDARD PRECAUTIONS.
B. HAVE PROTECTIVE EQUIPMENT READILY AVAILABLE FOR USE.
C. LEAD BY EXAMPLE. PHYSICIANS AND OTHER HEALTH-CARE PROVIDERS ARE MORE LIKELY TO EXERCISE STANDARD PRE-CAUTIONS IF COMPLIANCE IS DEMONSTRATED BY THEIR PEERS.
D. ENFORCE ADHERENCE OF STANDARD PRECAUTIONS.

# Coagulopathies in Surgery

*Rebecca J. McClaine, MD*

## I. COAGULATION CASCADE (FIG. 9-1)

## II. MEDICAL HISTORY TO DETERMINE RISK FOR BLEEDING

A. **FAMILY HISTORY OF COAGULOPATHY**

B. **PERSONAL HISTORY**

1. Postoperative or postprocedural bleeding/hemarthrosis/intramuscular bleeds (indicates coagulation factor disorder) and/or easy bruising/mucosal bleeding (indicates platelet disorder)

C. **MEDICAL HISTORY OF LIVER FAILURE (CIRRHOSIS)**

D. **MEDICATIONS**

1. Nonsteroidal antiinflammatory drugs, aspirin, warfarin (coumadin), clopidogrel (plavix)

## III. LABORATORY TESTS

A. **PROTHROMBIN TIME (PT)**

1. Evaluates production of vitamin K–dependent factors (II, VII, IX, X); indicates function of extrinsic pathway. Increased when functional volume of one or more factors is <50% (reference range, 12–14 seconds).

B. **ACTIVATED PARTIAL THROMBOPLASTIN TIME (aPTT)**

1. Evaluates function of intrinsic pathway. Increased when functional volume of one or more factors is <50% (reference range, 40–60 seconds, varies by laboratory).

C. **ACTIVATED CLOTTING TIME**

1. Similar to aPTT but designed to measure clotting time with large amounts of heparin in blood. Correlates linearly with concentration of heparin in blood; used during cardiopulmonary bypass.

D. **INTERNATIONAL NORMALIZED RATIO**

1. Developed because of laboratory variations in PT results caused by variations in thromboplastin (PT test reagent) activity; used to modulate warfarin therapy (reference, 1.0).

E. **BLEEDING TIME**

1. Evaluates platelet function and blood vessel integrity (reference range, 2.5–5.5 minutes); assessed with small cut on patient's skin.

F. **THROMBIN TIME**

Measures polymerization of fibrinogen.

9

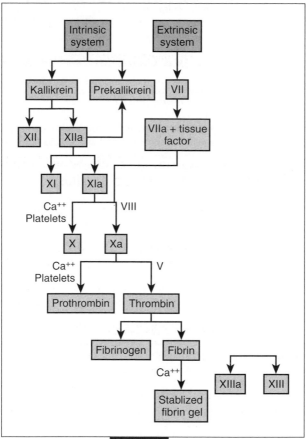

**FIG. 9-1**
Coagulation cascade.

## G. FIBRINOGEN: AFFECTS aPTT AND PT WHEN <50 MG/DL.

### IV. CONGENITAL BLEEDING DISORDERS

### A. HEMOPHILIA A

X-linked deficiency of factor VIII, intrinsic pathway dysfunction with increase of aPTT

1. For surgery, require 75% to 100% factor VIII activity for 7 to 10 days perioperatively.
2. One factor VIII unit contains 1% factor VIII activity.

3. Dose of factor VIII concentrate (must be dosed every 12 hours): [desired factor VIII activity (%) − current factor VIII activity (%)] × [total plasma volume (ml)/100] = number of units to be infused.
4. Can also treat with desmopressin 0.3 μg/kg intravenous daily (induces release of von Willebrand factor from endothelial cells, increasing levels of factor VIII).
5. Can treat with cryoprecipitate if other therapies are not available.

## B. HEMOPHILIA B (CHRISTMAS DISEASE)

X-linked deficiency of factor IX, intrinsic pathway dysfunction with increase of aPTT

1. For surgery, requires 75% to 100% factor IX activity for 7 to 10 days perioperatively.
2. A total of 1.5 factor IX units contain 1% factor IX activity, then use formula above; must be dosed every 18 hours.

## C. VON WILLEBRAND DISEASE

Autosomal dominant deficiency in functional von Willebrand factor, which is a subendothelial protein with two functions: (1) binder of platelets to endothelium, and (2) carrier for factor VIII.

1. Treat with 0.3 μg/kg desmopressin intravenous daily; will see effect in 30 to 90 minutes; must wait 24 hours between doses to allow levels to recover.
2. Some factor VIII concentrate solutions also contain von Willebrand factor.
3. May be treated with cryoprecipitate in severe refractory cases.

## D. THROMBASTHENIA (GLANZMANN DISEASE), BERNARD–SOULIER SYNDROME

Absence of platelet surface proteins necessary for binding and aggregation.

1. Treat with platelet transfusion.

## V. ACQUIRED BLEEDING DISORDERS

### A. VITAMIN K DEFICIENCY

Caused by warfarin use, poor nutrition, reduction of normal flora, total parenteral nutrition, and biliary obstruction.

1. Treat with vitamin K, 10 mg intravenous or subcutaneous once (correction in 6–8 hours). May also give vitamin K, 10 mg orally, with correction in 24 hours.
2. Treat with fresh frozen plasma (FFP) infusion for immediate correction (duration 8–12 hours).

### B. HYPOTHERMIA

Activity of all coagulation factors and platelets severely impaired at temperatures <34°C.

COAGULOPATHIES IN SURGERY

9

## C. LIVER FAILURE

Caused by decreased synthesis of vitamin K–dependent clotting factors and factor V (including fibrinogen with advanced disease). Correct with FFP (will not correct with vitamin K).

## D. CHRONIC RENAL FAILURE

Causes platelet dysfunction secondary to uremia. Treat with desmopressin, dialysis, or chronic, low-dose estrogen therapy.

## E. DISSEMINATED INTRAVASCULAR COAGULATION

Caused by concurrent coagulation and clot lysis in small vessels (consumptive coagulopathy).

1. Can occur with sepsis, trauma, obstetric complications, malignancy, burns, anaphylaxis, infection
2. Laboratory—increased PT, aPTT, bleeding time; decreased platelets, fibrinogen; increased fibrin degradation products (D-dimer)
3. Coagulation cascade activated in small vessels, leading to fibrin deposition. Results in consumptive coagulopathy, consumptive thrombocytopenia, hemolytic anemia, local tissue ischemia, followed by hemorrhage.
4. Treat with transfusions to correct specific deficits; do not transfuse platelets until $<50,000$ mm$^3$.

## F. ACQUIRED THROMBOCYTOPENIA

1. Decreased production because of folate/B$_{12}$ deficiency, leukemia, radiation, chemotherapy, acute ethanol intoxication, and viral infection
2. Shortened survival because of immune thrombocytopenia, thrombotic thrombocytopenic purpura, disseminated intravascular coagulation, and hemolytic uremic syndrome. Treat with steroids, intravenous immunoglobulin, or plasmapheresis with guidance by hematologist
3. Transfuse platelets for clinical bleeding or procedure.

## G. HEPARIN-INDUCED THROMBOCYTOPENIA—SPECIAL CASE OF DRUG-INDUCED IMMUNE THROMBOCYTOPENIA

1. Caused by formation of antibodies to heparin-platelet factor 4 complexes, which binds to platelets, causing clumping (consumptive thrombocytopenia, venous thrombosis 70%, arterial thrombosis 15%)
2. Suspect with platelet count $<100,000$/mm$^3$, or 50% reduction in patient receiving heparin.
3. Usually seen within 5 to 7 days of starting heparin therapy but may occur more quickly on reexposure to heparin
4. Occurs less frequently with use of low-molecular-weight heparin
5. Diagnosis by assay for antibodies (heparin-induced thrombocytopenia panel)
6. Treat with alternate method of anticoagulation to prevent further thrombosis (argatroban or lepirudin)

## VI. MEDICATIONS

### A.  ANTIPLATELETS

**1.** Aspirin

a. Inhibits platelet aggregation and degranulation by **irreversibly** preventing production of thromboxane $A_2$ by cyclooxygenase

b. Hold for 7 days before procedure.

**2.** Nonsteroidal antiinflammatory drugs

a. Inhibit platelet aggregation and degranulation by **reversibly** preventing production of thromboxane $A_2$ by cyclooxygenase

b. Hold for 2 days before procedure.

**3.** Clopidogrel (Plavix)

a. Inhibits platelet aggregation by **irreversibly** inhibiting platelet binding of adenosine diphosphate (ADP) and ADP-mediated activation of glycoprotein IIb/IIIa complex

b. Hold for 5 to 7 days before procedure.

**4.** Transfuse platelets for immediate correction of medication effects.

### B.  HEPARINS

**1.** Unfractionated heparin

a. Enhances inhibitory effects of antithrombin III on thrombin and factor Xa

b. Administered as continuous intravenous infusion to keep aPTT between 1.5 and 2.5 times upper limit of normal

c. Surgical procedures may take place with aPTT <1.3 times upper limit of normal.

**2.** Low-molecular-weight heparin

a. Enhances inhibitory effects of antithrombin III on factor Xa; more stable therapeutic anticoagulation than unfractionated heparin, thus routine monitoring is not required

b. Increased effects seen in renal failure.

c. Monitor anti–factor Xa activity (not aPTT) to determine therapeutic effect.

**3.** Hold therapeutic doses of heparin and low-molecular-weight heparin 8 to 12 hours before procedures.

**4.** For immediate correction, administer 1 mg protamine intravenously for every 100 units of heparin most recently administered, halved for each hour since last heparin dose (less effective in counteracting LMWH).

### C.  WARFARIN

**1.** Inhibits vitamin K cycle (production of factors II, VII, IX, and X)

**2.** Administered orally and dose adjusted to keep international normalized ratio of 2.0 to 3.0

**3.** Operation safe for international normalized ratio <1.5.

**4.** Hold warfarin 5 to 7 days before procedure.

**5.** For urgent procedure, administer 10 mg vitamin K orally once (effects in 24 hours).

**6.** For emergency, administer 10 mg vitamin K intravenously or subcutaneously once (effect in 6–8 hours) and FFP (immediate effect).

### D. DIRECT THROMBIN INHIBITORS

1. Administered as continuous intravenous infusion
2. No known reversing agents
3. Lepirudin
   a. Titrated for aPTT ratio (patient's measured aPTT/laboratory median reference aPTT value) of 1.5 to 2.5
   b. Renally excreted, so increased effects seen with renal insufficiency
4. Argatroban
   a. Reversible inhibitor of thrombin
   b. Administered as intravenous infusion and monitored by aPTT
   c. Increased effects seen in hepatic failure
   d. Discontinue infusion 2 to 4 hours before procedure (aPTTs usually return to reference levels within this time frame).

# PART III

# Surgical Intensive Care

# Shock

*Gerald R. Fortuna, Jr., MD*

Shock is not hypotension but rather a state of inadequate tissue delivery of oxygen and nutrients necessary for normal tissue and cellular functioning, leading to cellular hypoxia and death.

## I. PATHOPHYSIOLOGY

Inadequate oxygen delivery in relation to local oxygen demand results in the conversion from aerobic to anaerobic metabolism. This results in the production and accumulation of lactic acid, and the development of metabolic acidosis. If this state persists, cellular adenosine triphosphate is depleted, sodium and potassium leave the cell, and the cell membrane loses its potential. With continued energy depletion, cellular death occurs.

**10**

## II. HEMODYNAMIC CONSIDERATIONS

Appropriate management of the patient in shock is a basic and essential skill required by all surgeons, and it consists of modifying intravascular volume. This requires an understanding of basic hemodynamic relation and an understanding of how modifying preload, afterload, and myocardial contractility in the various forms of shock causes changes to intravascular volume to be effective.

### A. IMPORTANT RELATIONSHIPS

1. MAP = CO × SVR, where MAP = mean arterial pressure, CO = cardiac output, and SVR = systemic vascular resistance
2. CO = HR × SV, where CO = cardiac output, HR = heart rate, and SV = stroke volume
3. Stroke volume is determined by preload, myocardial contractility, and afterload.
4. For a given end-diastolic volume, stroke volume increases with increased myocardial contractility and decreased afterload.
5. The Frank–Starling curve relates left ventricular end-diastolic volume (LVEDV; preload) to stroke volume. Up to a certain level (the "flat" portion of the curve), increased preload leads to increased stroke volume, with subsequently increased cardiac output. With the exception of septic shock, all other forms of shock have a low cardiac output.

### B. PRELOAD

1. Preload is a measure of the filling of the ventricle and, theoretically, is an indication of the left ventricular end-diastolic volume.
2. As an alternative, the central venous pressure (CVP) can be used as an indirect measurement of central blood volume except when there is right ventricular dysfunction. For this reason, in many elderly patients with cardiac disease or pulmonary dysfunction, CVP is an inaccurate assessment of left-sided filling volume.

3. Pulmonary artery (Swan–Ganz) catheters measure pulmonary capillary wedge pressure, an estimation of left ventricular end-diastolic pressure, which in turn should reflect left ventricular end-diastolic volume. These assumptions may be inaccurate in patients with mitral valve disease, aortic insufficiency, pulmonary venous pathology, and altered left ventricular compliance. Optimal pulmonary capillary wedge pressure is 8 to 15 mm Hg, but this varies with the individual.

## C. AFTERLOAD

1. Afterload is defined as the resistance against which the heart muscle must contract or pump against.
2. Afterload can be estimated by calculating the systemic vascular resistance (SVR). This can be done using the following formula:

$$SVR = [(MAP - CVP) \times 80]/CO$$

where MAP = mean arterial pressure, CVP = central venous pressure, and CO = cardiac output.
3. By reducing afterload, cardiac output can be optimized for a given preload and contractility. This is especially useful in cardiogenic shock where there is reduced myocardial function. A reduction in afterload in this setting can greatly improve cardiac output.
4. Patients with hypovolemia may demonstrate increased afterload caused by compensatory peripheral vasoconstriction to maintain adequate blood flow to vital organs. Reducing afterload in this setting is inappropriate until steps to correct volume status have been completed.
5. In neurogenic shock, an inappropriate decrease in afterload caused by loss of vasomotor tone is present. A decreased afterload is also present in septic shock, together with inappropriate vasodilation and relative hypovolemia. In these instances, vasopressors are often used to improve vascular tone to help maintain adequate perfusion. Vasopressors are addressed later in this chapter.

## D. MYOCARDIAL CONTRACTILITY

1. Defined as the strength of myocardial contraction at a given preload and afterload
2. Determined by velocity of shortening, force of contraction, and length of displacement
3. Affected by changes in myocardial perfusion
4. Compromised myocardial contractility is the chief pathology in primary cardiogenic shock. Treatment is directed toward increasing myocardial function with various inotropic agents.

## E. VASOACTIVE AGENTS

1. Inotropic agents and vasopressors

Note: *These agents should not be used as a substitute for adequate volume resuscitation.*

a. Dopamine—effects are dose dependent.
   (1) 3 to 5 $\mu$g/kg/min (renal dose)—renal artery vasodilation may enhance splanchnic perfusion and promote diuresis.
   (2) 5 to 10 $\mu$g/kg/min—stimulation of cardiac $\beta$ receptors, with increased contractility and cardiac output. Increased heart rate is seen with increasing dosage.
   (3) >10 $\mu$g/kg/min—increasing $\alpha$-adrenergic effects, with increased mean arterial pressure and SVR caused by peripheral vasoconstriction
b. Dobutamine—synthetic dopamine analog with $\beta_1$ and $\beta_2$ effects; also acts as a mild vasodilator in addition to its inotropic effects; usual dosage is 5 to 15 $\mu$g/kg/min.
c. Amrinone—phosphodiesterase inhibitor with inotropic effects; also reduces afterload, increases cyclic adenosine monophosphate.
d. Norepinephrine (Levophed)—exerts both $\alpha$ and $\beta$ effects. $\beta$ effects predominate at lower doses, with increased heart rate and contractility; dose-dependent increases in $\alpha$ effect seen, with vasoconstriction at increasing dosages.
e. Epinephrine—at lower dosages (0.01 $\mu$g/kg/min), there are $\beta_1$-mediated increases in heart rate and contractility. Vasoconstriction occurs with increasing dosages. Concerns about increased myocardial oxygen demands may limit its usefulness in adults.
f. Phenylephrine (Neo-Synephrine)—$\alpha_1$ effect (vasoconstriction)
g. Vasopressin—direct vasoconstrictor without ionotropic or chronotropic effects, may result in decreased cardiac output and splanchnic flow. Typical doses range from 0.01 to 0.04 unit/min.

**2. Vasodilators**
a. Nitroglycerin—primary effect is venodilation via direct action on vascular smooth muscle; increases venous capacitance.
b. Nitroprusside—acts directly on both arterial and venous smooth muscle.

**10**

**SHOCK**

## III. SHOCK STATES

Blalock (1934) divided shock states into four basic categories, based on causative factor: (1) hypovolemic, (2) septic, (3) neurogenic, and (4) cardiogenic shock. With some additional subcategories, these divisions are still useful. The basic hemodynamic profiles of each type of shock are outlined in Table 10-1 and are described in greater detail in this section.

## A. HYPOVOLEMIC SHOCK
**1. Subdivided into hemorrhagic, traumatic, and nonhemorrhagic (e.g., burn shock)**
Signs and symptoms depend on degree of volume depletion, rapidity of volume depletion, duration of shock, and the body's compensatory reactions. Severity of hemorrhagic shock and clinical presentation can be stratified according to the amount of fluid lost. Although the classifications presented in Table 10-2 are generally applied to hemorrhagic shock, they are useful in estimating volume depletion.

| TABLE 10-1 | | | | | |
|---|---|---|---|---|---|
| HEMODYNAMIC PROFILES IN SHOCK | | | | | |
| Type of Shock | HR | CVP | PCWP | CO | SVR |
| Hypovolemic | ↑↓ | ↓ | ↓ | ↓ | ↑ |
| Septic | | | | | |
|   Hyperdynamic | ↑ | ↓ | ↓ | ↑ | ↓ |
|   Hypodynamic | ↑↓ | ↑↓ | ↑↓ | ↓ | ↑ |
| Neurogenic | ↑ | ↓ | ↓ | ↓ | ↓ |
| Cardiogenic | ↑↓ | ↑ | ↑ | ↓ | ↑ |

CO = cardiac output; CVP = central venous pressure; HR = heart rate; PCWP = pulmonary capillary wedge pressure; SVR = systemic vascular resistance.

**Note:** *Inebriated patients or patients with cirrhosis maintain skin perfusion despite inadequate cardiac indices, making early shock difficult to assess. In addition, young patients, who have particularly effective compensatory responses, may be able to maintain a normal blood pressure and heart rate up to the point of cardiovascular collapse and arrest. It is important to recognize early signs of shock in these patients.*

a. Hemorrhagic shock
   (1) Remember ABCs—establish airway; ensure adequate oxygenation and ventilation.
   (2) Control of external hemorrhage, if present
   (3) Intravenous access and administration of crystalloid, preferably lactated Ringer's solution. Lactate buffers hydrogen ions from ischemic tissues that are washed out with reperfusion.
   (4) Blood products as needed. Historically a 3:1 rule (1 unit packed red blood cells for every 3 L crystalloid) was the predominant guideline. Recent data from the war in Iraq and the use of whole blood for resuscitation has shifted this dogma to earlier administration of blood products. Now most major trauma facilities in the United States use a 1:1 transfusion protocol (1 unit packed red blood cells [PRBC], 1 unit fresh frozen plasma, 6 pk platelets, etc.).
   (5) Operative control of hemorrhage if necessary
   (6) Avoid hypothermia.
b. Traumatic shock
   (1) Initially caused by both internal and external volume losses, such as loss of blood or plasma externally from wound or burn surface or loss of blood or plasma into the damaged tissues; worsened by plasma extravasation into tissues distal to injured areas.
   (2) Débridement of ischemic or nonviable tissue may be necessary.
   (3) Immobilize fractures to prevent further tissue damage.
   (4) Pulmonary artery catheterization may be necessary for fluid management, especially in elderly patients.
c. Nonhemorrhagic shock
   (1) Similar to hemorrhagic shock, except that blood transfusion is usually not necessary

**TABLE 10-2**

CLASSES OF HYPOVOLEMIC SHOCK

| Class | Amount of Blood Loss (ml) | Blood Loss (%) | Heart Rate Pressure (beats/min) | Blood Pressure | Pulse | Respiratory Rate (breaths/min) | Urinary Output (ml/h) | Mental Status |
|---|---|---|---|---|---|---|---|---|
| I | <750 | <15 | <100 | Normal | Normal to ↑ | 14–20 | >30 | Slightly anxious |
| II | 750–1500 | 15–30 | >100 | Normal | → | 20–30 | 20–30 | Mildly anxious |
| III | 1500–2000 | 30–40 | >120 | → | → | 30–40 | 5–15 | Anxious, confused |
| IV | >2000 | >40 | >140 | → | → | >35 | Negligible | Confused, lethargic |

(2) Examples include third-space losses in bowel obstruction, gastrointestinal losses from diarrhea, emesis, biliary drainage, pancreatic fistula, and burns.

(3) Once the initial resuscitation effort with normal saline or lactated Ringer's solution is over, replacement fluids should be crystalloid with appropriate electrolyte composition of fluid lost. Usually D5 1/2 normal saline + 10 mEq KCl/L for gastrointestinal losses proximal to ligament of Treitz; lactated Ringer's for losses distal.

## B. SEPTIC SHOCK

1. Implies hemodynamic instability caused by host inflammatory response to infection

2. Local response to infection includes rubor, calor, dolor, and tumor. Systemic responses in this setting include vasodilation, altered mental status, fever, capillary leak, and organ dysfunction.

3. Host mediators implicated in pathogenesis of septic shock include multiple cytokines (e.g., tumor necrosis factor-$\alpha$ and interleukin-1), reactive oxygen radicals, vasoactive peptides, the complement cascade, and platelet-activating factor.

4. May result from infection with gram-positive or gram-negative bacteria, fungi, virus, or protozoa, initiating inflammatory, metabolic, endocrinologic, and immunologic pathways

5. Response (see Table 10-1) may be hyperdynamic (compensated) or hypodynamic (uncompensated).

6. Gram-positive—massive fluid losses secondary to dissemination of potent exotoxin, often without bacteremia

a. Causative organisms include *Clostridium, Staphylococcus,* and *Streptococcus* spp.

b. Characterized by hypotension with normal urine output and unaltered mental status. Acidosis is infrequent.

c. Generally, the prognosis is good with treatment.

d. Treatment—intravenous fluids to correct volume deficit, appropriate antibiotics, surgical drainage, or débridement, if necessary

7. Gram-negative—initiated by endotoxins in cell walls of gram-negative bacteria.

a. Causative organisms—gastrointestinal flora, including coliforms and anaerobic bacilli, for example, Klebsiella, Enterobacteriaceae, Serratia, and Bacteroides

b. Common sources in order of decreasing frequency—urinary tract, pulmonary, alimentary tract, burns, and soft-tissue infections. Always be suspicious for line sepsis.

c. Endotoxin, or lipopolysaccharide, in the outer membrane of gram-negative bacteria can elicit marked host inflammatory response even in the absence of viable bacteria.

8. Treatment

a. Early identification of source of infection and appropriate antibiotic treatment

b. Foley catheter to monitor urine output
c. Invasive hemodynamic monitoring
d. Intravenous fluid resuscitation to achieve normal filling pressures
e. Vasopressors, inotropes as needed, first-line therapy consisting of norepinephrine or dopamine followed by the addition of vasopressin
   (1) Should avoid use of vasopressin in patients with cardiac index <2 to 2.5 L/min and should be used with caution in patients with cardiac dysfunction
   (2) Doses of vasopressin >0.04 unit/min have been associated with myocardial ischemia, significant decreases in cardiac output, and cardiac arrest.
f. In patients who remain hypotensive after adequate fluid resuscitation and remain on vasopressor therapy, treatment with intravenous corticosteroids (hydrocortisone 200–300 mg/day) for 7 days in 3 to 4 divided doses or by continuous infusion should be considered until an appropriate stim test for adrenal insufficiency can be completed.
g. Recombinant human activated protein C or drotrecogin alfa (Xigris) is recommended in patients at high risk for death and an Acute Physiology and Chronic Health Evaluation II (APACHE II) score of >25 with sepsis-induced multiple organ system failure, septic shock, or sepsis-induced acute respiratory distress syndrome. The patient should also have no absolute contraindications related to bleeding risks.
   (1) During severe sepsis, the inflammatory response is closely related to procoagulant and endothelial activation.
   (2) Treatment with recombinant human activated protein C, an endogenous anticoagulant with antiinflammatory properties, for 72 hours has been shown in a large, multicenter, randomized, controlled trial to improve survival in patients with multiorgan system failure from sepsis.
h. Support of individual organ systems
i. Newer therapies directed at specific inflammatory mediators of sepsis include antibodies against lipopolysaccharide and modulation of host cytokines and mediators; these therapies have met with mixed results in clinical and animal trials, likely because of the redundancy of the inflammatory cascade.

9. **Fungal—causative organisms are commonly *Candida* spp.**
a. Seen in neutropenic, immunosuppressed, multitrauma, or burn patients
b. Risk factors include parenteral nutrition, invasive monitors, and broad-spectrum antibiotics.
c. When *Candida* organisms reach the intravascular compartment, widespread dissemination can occur.
   (1) Fungi lodge in the microcirculation, forming microabscesses.
   (2) Characterized by high fevers and rigors
   (3) Blood cultures negative in 50% of patients
   (4) Ophthalmologic evaluation may show evidence of ocular involvement in dissemination.

d. Treatment—antifungal agent, for example, amphotericin B
10. Human immunodeficiency virus infection with its ever-increasing prevalence and its effects on the immune system should always be of consideration when dealing with trauma patients who are in septic shock with an unknown source.

## C. NEUROGENIC SHOCK
1. Usually results from spinal cord injury, regional anesthetic agent, or autonomic blockade. Diagnosis is based on history and neurologic examination.
2. Mechanism
a. Loss of vasomotor control
b. Expansion of venous capacitance bed with peripheral pooling of blood
c. Inadequate ventricular filling
3. Manifestations
a. Warm, well-perfused skin
b. Low blood pressure
c. Low or normal urine output
d. Bradycardia may be present if adrenergic nerves to heart are blocked.
4. Treatment
a. Correct ventricular filling pressure with intravenous fluids
b. Vasoconstrictors to restore venous tone (vasopressin, phenylephrine [Neo-Synephrine], etc.)

**Note:** *Vasculature to those parts of the body with an intact autonomic nervous system may constrict excessively, resulting in ischemia to vital organs or necrosis of fingers.*

c. Trendelenburg position if necessary
d. Maintain body temperature

## D. CARDIOGENIC SHOCK
Differentiate between myocardial dysfunction from primary (e.g., myocardial infarction) and from secondary (e.g., compressive) causative factors.
1. Primary myocardial dysfunction
a. Includes myocardial infarction, dysrhythmias, valvular dysfunction, and myocardial failure
b. Treatment
   (1) Identification and correction of hemodynamically significant arrhythmias
   (2) Optimization of filling pressures (pulmonary capillary wedge pressure should be >15 mm Hg)
   (3) If SVR is increased, initiate afterload reduction with nitroglycerin or nitroprusside.
   (4) If SVR is low or normal, initiate inotropic support with dopamine, dobutamine, phenylephrine, vasopressin, or amrinone.

(5) In practice, afterload reduction and inotropic support are often performed concurrently.

(6) If inotropic support fails, consider intraaortic balloon pump or ventricular assist device.

(7) In the setting of acute myocardial infarction, consider interventional cardiac catheterization, percutaneous catheter-based interventions, thrombolytic therapy, or surgical treatment.

(a) In the SHOCK trial, early use of percutaneous coronary intervention was crucial, showing a 50.3% mortality rate in patients with cardiogenic shock receiving percutaneous coronary intervention vs. 63.1% in patients treated medically.

(b) Surgical intervention with coronary artery bypass grafting is indicated in patients who do not respond to treatment with percutaneous coronary intervention.

2. **The newest paradigm in cardiogenic shock revolves around the activation of inflammatory cytokines stimulating nitric oxide synthase to produce an increase of nitric oxide and peroxynitrite.**

a. This leads to systemic vasodilation and decreased peripheral vascular resistance, and potentiates the development of gram-negative septic shock.

(1) In response, a promising new treatment is the inhibition of inducible nitric oxide synthase by L-NMMA. This is being currently studied by the SHOCK-2 trial, a large, multicenter, randomized trial.

3. **Secondary myocardial dysfunction, also known as obstructive shock**

a. Includes tension pneumothorax, cardiac tamponade, vena cava obstruction, and pulmonary embolus

b. Treatment of the underlying problem should alleviate shock.

c. In the setting of trauma, distended neck veins should suggest secondary myocardial dysfunction (cardiac compression) and should be acted on immediately. Absence of distended neck veins does not rule out cardiac compression in the patient with hypovolemia. Distention may become evident only after adequate fluid resuscitation.

(1) Common causes

(a) Tension pneumothorax—shift of trachea to uninvolved side, decreased breath sounds, distended neck veins. This is not a radiographic diagnosis! These findings should prompt the immediate needle decompression of the affected lung fields by inserting a 16-gauge or larger Angiocath in the second intercostal space midclavicular line. Insertion of a chest thoracostomy tube should promptly follow.

(b) Cardiac tamponade—hypotension, muffled heart sounds, distended neck veins (Beck's triad); low voltage on electrocardiogram and enlarged cardiac silhouette on chest radiograph (classic "water bottle" shape). In this situation, pericardiocentesis should be performed promptly at the bedside or a pericardial window performed in the operating room.

(2) Associated findings may include pulsus paradoxus (decline in systolic blood pressure >10 mm Hg with inspiration) and Kussmaul's sign (increase in CVP with inspiration [infrequently present]).

(3) Treatment is by fluid administration and correction of underlying mechanism.

    (a) Tension pneumothorax: Decompress with 14-gauge angiocatheter in 2nd intercostal space, midclavicular line; definitive treatment by chest tube placement in 5th intercostal space, anterior axillary line.

    (b) Acute cardiac tamponade: If hemodynamically stable, perform pericardiocentesis or pericardial window. (Trinkle maneuver: Make a 5- to 10-cm upper abdominal incision starting over the xiphoid. The xiphoid process can be excised with heavy Mayo scissors to aid exposure. Use blunt dissection in the preperitoneal space to expose the pericardium. Alice clamps are used to grasp the pericardium, which is then pulled downward into the operative field away from the myocardium. The pericardium is then incised with heavy scissors, exposing the pericardial space and pericardial fluid, which can then be evacuated.) If the patient is hemodynamically unstable, consider prompt operative thoracotomy or sternotomy.

## E. HYPOADRENAL SHOCK/ADRENAL INSUFFICIENCY

1. Adrenal cortical hormones provide natural resistance to shock during times of stress and injury.
2. A reduction in blood volume and chemistry of these hormones can mimic hypovolemic shock.
a. Leads to decreased capillary tone and permeability
3. Can be verified by checking cortisol levels <15 mg/dl
a. Can also be measured after an adrenocorticotropic hormone stimulation test.
    (1) Any measurement less than 5 mg/dl or less than a 9-mg/dl increase would constitute deficiency.
b. The diagnosis is difficult due to the relative lack of classic Addisonian symptoms, and a high degree of suspicion is needed.
4. Corrected by administering physiologic doses of steroids.

## IV. ORGAN RESPONSE TO SHOCK
## A. MICROVASCULAR DYSFUNCTION

1. Vasoconstriction to selectively decrease perfusion to dermal, renal, muscle, and splanchnic vascular beds to keep adequate perfusion to central organs such as the brain and heart
2. Capillary endothelial layer is usually compromised in shock states.
a. Circulating inflammatory mediators, byproducts of infection, lipopolysaccharide, thrombin, tumor necrosis factor-$\alpha$, interleukin-1, nitric oxide, and endotheliin-1 all cause capillary leak.
b. Exact mechanism is still not clear, and the only current treatment is early resuscitation of volume status, rapid elimination of infectious and

necrotic tissue, and vasopressors for ionotropic support if cardiopulmonary function is compromised.

## B. NEUROENDOCRINE RESPONSE

1. An involuntary response originating from the hypothalamus, autonomic nervous system, and endocrine glands.
2. Initiated by hypoxia, hypotension, and hypovolemia as detected by baroreceptors and chemoreceptors throughout the body.
3. With activation of the sympathetic response, epinephrine and norepinephrine is released.
4. Catecholamines released systemically alter insulin and glucose metabolism, ultimately increasing the availability of glucose for metabolism as part of the "fight-or-flight" response.
5. Hyperglycemia results from increased glycogenolysis, gluconeogenesis, and decreased pancreatic insulin release.
6. The anterior pituitary is stimulated by the hypothalamus, causing an increase in adrenocorticotropic hormone, which in turn stimulates the release of cortisol and aldosterone from the adrenal cortex.
7. Increased levels of cortisol cause increases in gluconeogenesis, lipolysis, and decreased peripheral use of glucose and amino acids.
8. The pancreas produces less insulin whereas glucagon production is increased. This causes an increase in hepatic gluconeogenesis.
9. This simultaneous and combined response results in stress-related hyperglycemia and refraction to insulin.
10. The renin-angiotensin system is also stimulated, causing an increase in the resorption of sodium, resulting in low-volume, concentrated urine.
11. Vasopressin is also released by the posterior pituitary, causing an increase in water resorption in the distal renal tubules.

## C. INFLAMMATORY RESPONSE

1. Shock triggers a massive systemic inflammatory response (SIRS).
a. Activated monocytes and polymorphonuclear cells, platelets, endothelial cells, and macrophages are main players.
   (1) These cells generate loads of amplifying inflammatory mediators with widespread physiologic consequences.
2. Coagulation cascade is triggered.
3. Leaky vessels cause extravasation into noninjured tissues away from the primary site of injury.
4. Creates a hyperdynamic inflammatory response that can lead to SIRS, acute respiratory distress syndrome, and multiorgan system failure.

## D. PULMONARY

1. The lungs are the most sensitive organ to injury and usually the first organ system to fail, leading to the development of acute respiratory distress syndrome.

10

SHOCK

2. Normally triggered and perpetuated by the above inflammatory changes and interleukin-8 generated from systemic responses to injury from hypoperfused tissues elsewhere in the body
3. Ultimately leads to a decrease in compliance, surfactant abnormalities, and alveolar collapse
   a. Functional residual capacity decreases and pulmonary insufficiency develops.
   b. Increase in pulmonary vascular resistance; increase in cardiac workload leading to more strain of the cardiopulmonary systems

### E. RENAL
1. Hypotension during the early phases of injury cause renal vasoconstriction.
   a. An increase in the afferent arteriole resistance causes a decrease in glomerular filtration rate together with an increase in aldosterone and vasopressin.
   b. Persistent oliguria can lead to acute tubular necrosis (ATN) and multiorgan system failure.

## IV. MULTIORGAN DYSFUNCTION SYNDROME

### A. DEFINITION
Multiorgan dysfunction is a syndrome of progressive but potentially reversible dysfunction involving two or more organs or organ systems that arises after resuscitation from an acute disruption of normal homeostasis.

### B. CAUSES
1. Can result from prolonged or inadequately controlled shock
2. Is the most common cause of mortality in the surgical intensive care unit

### C. PREVENTIVE MEASURES
1. Hemodynamic support—maintenance of adequate tissue oxygenation and substrate delivery
2. Nutritional support—provision of adequate nutrition and reversal of catabolism
3. Prevention of infection—maintenance of optimal antimicrobial defenses and prompt antimicrobial therapy at first sign of infection

# Cardiopulmonary Monitoring

*Thomas L. Husted, MD*

*It should be clearly recognized that arterial pressure cannot be measured with precision by means of sphygmomanometers.*
—American Heart Association, Committee for Arterial Pressure Recording, 1951

The goal of cardiopulmonary monitoring is to assess the adequacy of the cardiac and pulmonary systems in meeting the metabolic needs of the patient. Although these goals may appear simple, this monitoring can become amazingly complicated in practice. The most important idea to grasp is that no single measurement can exist in isolation; all data must be considered with other data and the presentation of the patient. The ideal monitor is noninvasive, reliable, and conveys physiologic information in "real time." Often, in critically ill patients, noninvasive monitoring is either unreliable or inaccurate and invasive monitoring is required.

**11**

## I. MONITORING

### A. VITAL SIGNS

1. Evaluation of pulse, blood pressure, temperature, respiratory rate, and urine output—the simplest parameters to measure and record
2. Assessment of vital signs at periodic intervals is usually adequate for the stable patient; the critically ill patient requires closer evaluation on a more frequent schedule, and continuous assessment is the ideal situation.

### B. MONITORING TECHNIQUES: NONINVASIVE AND INVASIVE

1. Noninvasive monitoring: The ideal monitor is noninvasive while being completely accurate and reliable. Because medicine has not advanced to this level we must rely on imperfect measurements and assumptions.
   a. Continuous cardiac monitoring—electrocardiogram demonstrates heart rate and rhythm while alerting to ischemia (S-T segment analysis).
   b. Apnea monitoring—follows respirations.
   c. Pulse oximetry—measures transcutaneous capillary $O_2$ saturation.
   d. Capnography—measures end-tidal $CO_2$.
   e. Sphygmomanometer—measures peripheral arterial blood pressure.
   f. Doppler ultrasonography—assesses nonpalpable pulses.
2. Invasive monitoring: Although often considered the gold standard of physiologic monitoring, specific distinction must be made between those values that are measured directly and those that are calculated or assumed.
   a. Arterial catheter—directly measures peripheral blood pressure and waveform while providing access for blood gas sampling.
   b. Central venous catheter—measures central venous pressure and central access.

   c. Pulmonary artery (PA) catheter—measures cardiac and pulmonary pressures while providing a calculated estimate of cardiac performance.
3. In practice, a combination of noninvasive and invasive monitoring is usually required in the critically ill patient. (For a description of the technical placement of invasive monitoring catheters, see later sections of this handbook.)

### C. INDICATIONS FOR INVASIVE MONITORING
1. Complex or lengthy surgical procedures with anticipated large volume fluid shifts
2. Hemodynamic instability
3. Issues with fluid management or unexpected response to fluid challenge
4. Deteriorating pulmonary or cardiac function
5. Surgical procedure or complex trauma in patient with baseline compromise of cardiac, pulmonary, or renal function

## II. NONINVASIVE GLOBAL ASSESSMENT
### A. URINE OUTPUT
1. Urine output is a good indicator of overall status. In general, a surgical patient who is able to maintain an hourly urine output of 30 to 50 ml/hr has adequate circulating volume, perfusion pressure, and cardiac capacity.
2. Hourly urine output reflects circulating levels of antidiuretic hormone and aldosterone more than degree of renal perfusion.
3. Adequate levels are usually 0.5 ml/kg/hr in adults, although normal urine output does not independently indicate that the patient is healthy.

### B. SKIN TEMPERATURE
1. Temperature is directly correlated with cutaneous blood flow and indicates adequacy of overall perfusion.
2. If skin temperature is within 2°C of ambient temperature (unusually low), then perfusion is critically low; if the skin temperature is maintained at normal or increased, this is evidence that the heart can generate a fairly robust output.

## III. PULMONARY MONITORING
### A. APNEA MONITORING
Detects chest wall motion by sensing a change in the electrical impendence across the chest wall; alarms are usually set to detect bradypnea or apnea.

### B. PULSE OXIMETRY
1. Noninvasive method to measure capillary hemoglobin saturation using a light absorption technique.
2. The lighted probe is usually attached to body areas with capillary beds near the skin surface (e.g., fingernail bed, earlobe, nasal ala).

3. It will not function predictably under conditions of hypoperfusion, hypothermia, or obstructions to light pulse (e.g., stained fingernails).

## C. CAPNOGRAPHY
1. Direct measurement of end-tidal carbon dioxide in exhaled air
2. Continuous measurement of end-tidal carbon dioxide is an indicator of adequate tidal volume and clearance of metabolic by-products.
3. Once calibrated to an arterial blood gas, end-tidal $CO_2$ monitoring is useful to determine trends in $CO_2$ production and clearance.

## D. ARTERIAL BLOOD GAS
1. Allows determination of oxygen delivery and consumption and clearance of metabolic waste products
2. A reflection of oxygenation, ventilation, and acid-base status
3. A complete discussion of blood gas interpretation is beyond the scope of this chapter (see Recommended References for more details).

## IV. HEMODYNAMIC MONITORING
### A. ARTERIAL BLOOD PRESSURE (NONINVASIVE)
1. Indirect measurement of arterial blood pressure is made by sphygmomanometer or ultrasonic blood pressure monitor. These methods work best on euvolemic patients.
2. Cautions:
a. Cuff size is important in a large arm.
   (1) The entire principle of sphygmomanometry is based on the assumption that pressures in the cuff are equal to pressures in the encompassed artery, which may be incorrect in obese or diabetic patients.
   (2) Small arms and large cuffs present much less of an error in pressure.
b. Nearly all noninvasive methods to determine blood pressure are unreliable in patients with hypovolemia or hypotension.
c. Mean arterial pressure (MAP) is the most reliable and accurate measurement taken by most cuff methods.
   (1) The MAP is measured directly using the oscillometric technique, and the systolic and diastolic pressures are calculated from an algorithm.
   (2) If the blood pressure values are suspect, rely on the MAP as the most accurate reading; normal MAP is 90 to 100 mm Hg.

## B. ARTERIAL BLOOD PRESSURE (INVASIVE)
Arterial catheters provide a direct measure of arterial blood pressure and arterial access for blood sampling. Direct measurement of intravascular pressure is recommended for all patients requiring careful monitoring of arterial pressure.
### 1. Indications for placement of arterial catheter
a. Labile blood pressure requiring vasoactive or cardiotonic drugs
b. Require frequent arterial blood sampling (>3 times/day)
c. Any potential instability (e.g., undergoing major surgery or recent trauma)

d. Management of one failing organ system that might precipitate failure in another organ system

**2. Information obtained from arterial catheterization**

a. Arterial pressure: The pressure waveforms are a synthesis of harmonics of the ejection pressure of the ventricular stroke volume into the elastic arterial tree.

b. Although the actual blood pressure in the small peripheral arteries is rarely of clinical importance, the MAP is a useful surrogate for the central aortic root pressure; this pressure is of paramount importance because it is the driving pressure for end-organ perfusion; normal MAP is 90 to 100 mm Hg.

c. Access for arterial blood sampling: Periodic blood gas samples, samples for blood cultures, periodic glucose level monitoring, arterial levels of ammonium, and a multitude of other analyses can be obtained from the reliable arterial access provided from an arterial catheter.

**3. Cautions**

a. The pressure-transducer must be properly flushed, attached to the pressure bag, leveled, and zeroed to obtain predictable and reliable measurements.

b. Fluid-filled recording systems can produce artifacts caused by resonance, waveform distortion, and presence of air in the system.

c. Correction of arterial blood pressure as measured by arterial catheter is NOT the end point for resuscitation of a severely ill or injured patient. Other parameters must be taken into account to assess global organ and tissue perfusion.

## C. CENTRAL VENOUS PRESSURE

**1. Indications for placement of a central venous catheter**

a. Infusion of hypertonic solutions (e.g., total parenteral nutrition, 3% saline)

b. Infusion of vasoactive or cardiotonic substances requiring immediate perfusion

c. Need to monitor central venous and right-sided cardiac pressures

d. Access to central venous blood samples

**2. Information obtained from a central venous catheter**

a. Permits measurement of central venous and right-sided cardiac pressures (normal CVP is 2–8 mm Hg)

b. Allows periodic sampling of central venous blood

**3. Cautions**

a. As with all centrally placed catheters, there is risk for placement (pneumothorax, hemothorax, arterial puncture, among others) and risk for maintenance (central venous catheter infection).

b. CVP measurements should be made at end expiration to minimize the effects of respiration.

c. As with all pressure monitors, the true goal is to understand cardiac volumes despite measuring pressures. Without knowledge of the cardiac compliance (rarely known), the directly measured pressures are useful only to follow trends and response to therapy.

d. Correlation with left-sided cardiac measurements. CVP generally correlates with systemic intravascular volume and correlates well with left-sided preload volume, until significant left ventricular dysfunction (left ventricular ejection fraction <40%).

e. The pressure-transducer unit is important to be properly assembled and accurately zeroed to reliably measure CVP independent of time and observer variability.

## D. PA PRESSURE

The power of the PA catheter is not based on its ability to generate information, but rather on the clinician's ability to understand that information.

**1. Indications for placement of PA catheter**

a. Questionable cardiac function (recent myocardial infarction, known myocardial dysfunction, etc.)

b. Questionable pulmonary function (acute respiratory failure, noncardiogenic pulmonary edema, etc.)

c. Acute systemic illness (sepsis, peritonitis, severe trauma, minor trauma in elderly patient, etc.)

d. Questionable fluid status (acute renal insufficiency, inappropriate response to fluid challenge, etc.)

**2. Information obtained from a PA catheter**

a. Left-sided cardiac filling pressure (occlusion pressure) in addition to right-sided cardiac filling pressure (CVP)

b. Cardiac output and stroke volume by thermodilution technique

c. Pulmonary pressures (pulmonary systolic/diastolic pressures) and pulmonary artery occlusion pressure; reference range is 5 to 15 mm Hg

d. Right ventricular end-diastolic volume

e. Sampling of mixed venous oxygen saturation

　(1) Mixed venous oxygen saturation ($Svo_2$) provides an index of tissue perfusion and oxygenation. Increasing $Svo_2$ correlates positively with cardiac output and tissue perfusion, and negatively with systemic shunt states (e.g., sepsis and hepatic failure).

　(2) Although $Svo_2$ cannot reflect changes in regional perfusion, a decreasing $Svo_2$ is a generally ominous sign. Knowledge of the $Svo_2$ will also allow calculation of arteriovenous oxygen content and physiologic shunt ($Q_{sp}/Q_t$), both of which can assist in managing respiratory failure.

f. Specialized catheters allow atrial, ventricular, or atrioventricular sequential cardiac pacing.

**3. Cautions**

a. The directly measured values from a PA catheter are as follows:

　(1) Body temperature

　(2) Central venous pressure (CVP)

(3) Pulmonary systolic and diastolic pressures (PAS and PAD)
(4) Pulmonary capillary occlusion pressure (pulmonary artery occlusion pressure or wedge)
(5) Right ventricular end-diastolic volume (RVEDV)
(6) Cardiac output (CO)
(7) If equipped, continuous mixed venous oxygen saturation

All other data from a PA catheter are calculated and, therefore, are of best utility to assess trends.

b. Pulmonary artery occlusion pressure is an estimation of left-heart filling pressure. However, pulmonary artery occlusion pressure is not actual left ventricular preload; it is an extrapolation, requiring several assumptions, of left-heart filling volume. Cardiac disease states such as changes in myocardial compliance or valvular disease may lead to inaccurate measurements.

c. Respiratory failure requiring high levels of positive end-expiratory pressure increases intrathoracic measurements (including all measurements and calculations obtained from PA catheter) to an unknown and unpredictable degree; all measurements should be made at end expiration.

d. For patients with low cardiac output, right-sided cardiomegaly, unusual anatomy, or accessed from the left internal jugular vein, it may be difficult to achieve proper placement of the catheter. Persistence and fluoroscopy may be helpful.

e. Arrhythmias are not unusual during placement of a PA catheter (in fact, they are reassuring because they indicate the catheter is in the heart and not some other location). If these arrhythmias are sustained or life-threatening, removal of the catheter and reassessing the need for the catheter is usually wise.

## V. CARDIAC MONITORING

Continuous cardiac monitoring is nearly universal in critically ill patients, with easy recognition of tachycardia, bradycardia, and life-threatening arrhythmias.

### A. RATE

Bradycardia is less than 60 beats/min and tachycardia is greater than 100 beats/min.

### B. RHYTHM

Although *regular* and *irregular* describe the basic rhythm, further investigation may reveal whether the rhythm is hemodynamically significant, sustained, or life-threatening.

### C. WAVES, INTERVALS, AND SEGMENTS

Although a comprehensive discussion of electrocardiographic interpretation is beyond the scope of this handbook, there are specific electrocardiographic changes to which the surgeon should be alert.

1. ST-segment changes may be the only indication of ischemia or infarction.
a. ST-segment depression is seen in subendocardial myocardial infarction and myocardial ischemia.
b. ST-segment elevation is seen in transmural myocardial infarction.
2. T-wave changes are seen in transient ischemia and electrolyte abnormalities.

## RECOMMENDED REFERENCES

Holcroft JW, Anderson JT. Cardiopulmonary monitoring. *ACS Surgery: Principles and Practice*. WebMD, 2003. www.webmd.com 2007.

Kellum JA, Puyana JC. Acid-base disorders. *ACS Surgery: Principles and Practice*. WebMD, 2006. www.webmd.com 2007.

Section III hemodynamic monitoring. In Marino PL (ed): *The TCU Book,* 2nd ed. New York: Lippincott Williams & Wilkins, 1998.

## APPENDIX: IMPORTANT FORMULAS

**Cardiac output (CO):**

$$CO = HR \times SV$$

$$HR = \text{heart rate}; SV = \text{stroke volume}$$

$$\text{Reference range} = 4\text{--}8 \text{ L/min}$$

**Arterial content of oxygen ($Cao_2$):**

$$Cao_2 = (1.39 \times Hg \times Spo_2) + (Pao_2 \times 0.0031)$$

$Hg$ = hemoglobin level; $Spo_2$ = arterial oxygen saturation; $Pao_2$ = arterial partial pressure of oxygen

$$\text{Reference value} = 18 \text{ ml/dl}$$

**Oxygen delivery ($DO_2$):**

$$DO_2 = Cao_2 \times CO \times 10$$

$Cao_2$ = arterial content of oxygen; $CO$ = cardiac output

$$\text{Reference value} = 1000 \text{ ml/min}$$

11

CARDIOPULMONARY MONITORING

# Mechanical Ventilation

*Thomas L. Husted, MD*

*Development in most fields of medicine appears to occur
according to sound scientific principles. However, exceptions can
be found, and the development of mechanical ventilatory support
is one of them.*

—J. Rasanen

The goal of mechanical ventilation is to facilitate gas exchange for tissue
oxygen delivery, provide ventilation for removal of carbon dioxide, unload the
work of the respiratory muscles, and minimize the detrimental effects of both
endotracheal intubation and mechanical ventilation. The procedures and
indications for endotracheal intubation, tracheostomy placement, and crico-
thyroidotomy are addressed later in this handbook.

**12**

## I. DETERMINING NEED FOR MECHANICAL VENTILATION
### A. AIRWAY INSTABILITY
1. From operation, head injury, intoxication, among other causes, usually
   only requiring temporary support

### B. RESPIRATORY FAILURE
1. From acute respiratory distress syndrome, chronic obstructive pulmonary disease, pulmonary edema, among other causes, usually requiring prolonged support

### C. GUIDELINES
1. The first indication is consideration of intubation.
2. Intubation is NOT a sign of weakness.
3. Ventilation is not "addictive."
4. Remember, mechanical ventilation is a support measure, not a cure
   for cardiopulmonary disease.

## II. VENTILATION VERSUS OXYGENATION
### A. VENTILATION
1. The purpose of ventilation is to excrete $CO_2$, a function of minute
   ventilation (selected on the ventilator with respiratory rate and tidal
   volume [$V_T$]). Minute ventilation ($V_E$) has two components, alveolar
   ventilation ($2/3$ of $V_T$) and dead space ventilation ($1/3$ of $V_T$); normal $V_E$
   is 6 L/min, driven at brainstem by $Paco_2$ and pH.

### B. OXYGENATION
1. Oxygenation is a function of ventilation and perfusion (V/Q)
   matching, evaluated by calculating alveolar-arterial (A-a)

gradient ($PAo_2 - PAo_2$), where $Fio_2$ is the fraction of inspired oxygen:

$$[PAo_2 = Fio_2 \times (\text{barometric pressure} - P_{H2O}) - Pao_2/RQ]$$

Reference range is 8–12 mm Hg

Estimate: P/F ratio ($Pao_2/Fio_2$), which at sea level is $100/0.21 = 500$.

## III. NONINVASIVE POSITIVE PRESSURE VENTILATION

### A. POSITIVE PRESSURE VENTILATION
1. Provided via face mask with either continuous positive airway pressure or bilevel positive airway pressure

### B. INITIAL SETTINGS
1. Usually 5 cm $H_2O$ positive end-expiratory pressure (PEEP) and 5 to 10 cm $H_2O$ pressure support

### C. ADVANTAGES
1. Most studies have described advantages of noninvasive positive pressure ventilation in patients with immediately reversible causes of respiratory insufficiency (exacerbations of chronic obstructive pulmonary disease or cardiogenic pulmonary edema).

### D. RESERVED
1. For those patients who have a presumed temporary respiratory insufficiency from a rapidly reversible cause (narcotic overdose, multiple rib fractures, exacerbations of congestive heart failure, or chronic obstructive pulmonary disease)

## IV. CONVENTIONAL MECHANICAL VENTILATION

Several parameters may be manipulated to limit the functions of the ventilator; however, the most common and default arrangement is time trigger (mandatory ventilation) or flow trigger (spontaneous ventilation), volume cycled, and pressure limited for each breath.

### A. MODES OF VENTILATION
1. Volume control ventilation: Either physician or patient determines respiratory rate; once triggered (time or flow), the ventilator will deliver a preselected volume. Often poorly tolerated by awake patients, there is a risk for increased airway pressures if the pulmonary compliance is decreased.
2. Pressure control ventilation: Either physician or patient determines respiratory rate; once triggered (time or flow), the ventilator will deliver a preselected pressure, which will result in a variable volume depending

on the pulmonary compliance. Pressure control ventilation is useful for poorly compliant lungs to decrease the risk for barotrauma, although it may lead to increased $Paco_2$ (permissive hypercapnia).

3. Pressure support ventilation: The simplest form of pressure-limited ventilation, it is used to augment spontaneous breathing, not to provide full ventilatory support. The patient triggers both respiratory rate and inspiratory time at a physician-selected pressure support. Exhalation occurs passively. This mode most closely resembles spontaneous unassisted breathing and should be the mode of choice in the patient with a spontaneous respiratory drive.

## B. MANDATORY VERSUS SPONTANEOUS VENTILATION

1. Assist control: Ensures delivery of a minimum (mandatory) $V_E$ but also allows additional patient-triggered (spontaneous) breaths; each breath, regardless of the trigger (time or patient initiated) is completely supported to desired volume or pressure. Major limitation is that agitated patients may become hyperventilated (with respiratory alkalosis or development of auto-PEEP) if the respiratory rate is rapid.

2. Intermittent mandatory ventilation: Only a selected number of breaths are fully supported to desired volume or pressure; additional breaths are reliant on patient effort with delivered pressure support. Often used as a bridge to spontaneous respirations, but experience has demonstrated this to be a suboptimal approach to liberation from the ventilator. Intermittent mandatory ventilation can reduce the risk for respiratory alkalosis and auto-PEEP.

3. In patients who are breathing rapidly during assist/control ventilation and show evidence of respiratory alkalosis or auto-PEEP, a change to intermittent mandatory ventilation should prove beneficial; however, in patients with respiratory muscle weakness or cardiac dysfunction, assist/control should be favored.

## C. VENTILATOR STRATEGIES

1. Oxygenation

a. $Fio_2$: This parameter is usually adjusted initially when a patient has difficulty oxygenating (decreased $Spo_2$ [arterial saturation as measured during pulse oximetry] or $Pao_2$). Although $Fio_2$ <60% is well tolerated, prolonged periods at >60% can result in nitrogen washout, resorption atelectasis, increased pulmonary shunt, and pulmonary fibrosis.

b. PEEP: Used to prevent alveolar collapse during expiration and preserve functional residual capacity. PEEP of 5 cm $H_2O$ may simulate the closed glottis in normal respiration. Increasing PEEP may be helpful for recruitment of alveoli and to optimize the V/Q interface (if more alveoli are open and oxygenated, then more oxygen can diffuse into the blood). An important caveat is that increasing PEEP can have detrimental hemodynamic effects (see later). Best PEEP is best determined using stepwise increases in PEEP and assessing the

**12**

**MECHANICAL VENTILATION**

effects on oxygen delivery ($DO_2$), not simply aiming for increased arterial oxygenation.

2. Ventilation

a. An initial ventilator setting of respiratory rate of 12 to 15 breaths/min and $V_T$ of 5 to 8 ml/kg should ensure adequate clearance of $CO_2$.

b. If $Paco_2$ level remains increased, increasing the respiratory rate to 20 to 24 breaths/min will likely correct the hypercapnia while preserving a reasonable pulmonary airway pressure. If this maneuver does not correct the hypercapnia, consider excessive production of $CO_2$ as a complicating factor (obtain metabolic cart to assess for overfeeding; see later).

c. When all maneuvers fail and $CO_2$ level continues to increase, remember there is little physiologic detriment if the pH remains greater than 7.20.

## D. LIBERATION FROM MECHANICAL VENTILATION

1. Nurse- or respiratory therapist–driven protocols with daily spontaneous breathing trials (SBTs) have shown the best results in early liberation from mechanical ventilation.

2. Weaning strategies: When the clinical scenario improves (patient is awake, able to take spontaneous breaths, and arterial oxygenation is acceptable [$Pao_2$ >80 mm Hg on $Fio_2$ 40%] with minimal ventilatory support [$Fio_2$ <50% and PEEP $\leq$ 5 cm $H_2O$]), then the process of liberation begins.

3. SBTs: Best determined daily over 30 minutes with the patient breathing through the ventilator circuit with minimal PEEP only; the patient will determine respiratory rate, $V_T$, and minute ventilation. If arterial blood gas shows acceptable values ($Pao_2$ >80 mm Hg and with acceptable pH), then the patient is ready for extubation.

4. Rapid shallow breathing index: Another parameter used is the rapid shallow breathing index. If frequency/$V_T$ is <105, then a high likelihood exists that the patient is ready for extubation (e.g., respiratory rate of 20 and $V_T$ of 0.500 L = rapid shallow breathing index of 40). If the patient passes the SBT, then seriously consider extubation.

5. Failure of SBT is demonstrated by tachypnea, increased work of breathing, dysrhythmias, or hemodynamic instability.

## E. FAILURE TO LIBERATE FROM MECHANICAL VENTILATION

If the patient does not pass the SBT, it is important to determine why the patient did not pass.

1. Mental status: Patients should be awake and alert for best success of liberation.

2. Airway protection: Patients should be able to protect the airway by coughing, swallowing secretions, and calling for help.

3. Secretion control: Excessive secretions may further compromise a tenuous airway.

4. Respiratory muscle fatigue: This usually requires 24 hours of rest on ventilator with respiratory rate of 20 to 25 breaths/min to completely off-load the work of breathing.

5. Electrolyte abnormalities: Phosphorus and magnesium in particular can contribute to continued ventilator dependence.
6. It is usually best medicine to wait 24 hours before attempting another SBT after a failed SBT.

## V. EFFECTS ON CARDIAC PERFORMANCE

A. **ENDOTRACHEAL INTUBATION AND MECHANICAL VENTILATION PLACE IMPORTANT PHYSIOLOGIC DEMANDS ON PATIENTS.**
B. **THE SHIFT FROM NEGATIVE-PRESSURE TO POSITIVE-PRESSURE VENTILATION CAN COMPROMISE PRELOAD BY:**
1. Decreasing the pressure gradient for venous inflow into the thorax
2. Reducing ventricular distensibility, thus decreasing ventricular filling during diastole
3. Compressing the pulmonary veins, thus increasing right heart after-load, possibly to the extent that it dilates the right heart, shifts the ventricular septum, and thus decreases left ventricular chamber size (known as ventricular interdependence)

C. **POSITIVE-PRESSURE VENTILATION**
1. Can decrease afterload by augmenting the pressure gradient between the left ventricle and the extrathoracic outflow tract (decreases left ventricular transmural pressure)

D. **THE EFFECTS OF POSITIVE-PRESSURE VENTILATION ON CARDIAC PERFORMANCE**
1. Tend to reduce ventricular filling during diastole but enhance ventricular emptying during systole. These effects can be countered in most hypovolemic patients with fluid administration. However, patients with cardiac failure will not respond to fluid administration.

## VI. NEED FOR TRACHEOSTOMY

In patients who repeatedly do not pass the SBT, consideration should be given to tracheostomy to decrease the complications associated with long-term endotracheal intubation (tracheal stenosis, ventilator associated pneumonia, prolonged intensive care unit stay, etc.). Another group of patients to be considered for tracheostomy is patients with a high likelihood of requiring prolonged mechanical ventilatory support. It is our policy to perform early (<7 days) bedside percutaneous tracheostomy as often as possible in these patients.

## VII. VENTILATOR CAUTIONS

A. **ACUTE LUNG INJURY IS DEFINED AS FOLLOWS:**
1. P/F ratio <300
2. In theory from excessive alveolar pressures (barotraumas) or excessive alveolar volume (volutrauma)

3. Results in poor oxygenation
4. Postulated that acute respiratory distress syndrome–type lung protection strategies may be of benefit

### B. ACUTE RESPIRATORY DISTRESS SYNDROME IS DEFINED AS FOLLOWS:

1. P/F ratio <200
2. Acute onset
3. Bilateral chest infiltrates on chest radiograph
4. No evidence of cardiac failure component (pulmonary capillary wedge pressure <18 mm Hg)

### C. ACUTE LUNG INJURY/ACUTE RESPIRATORY DISTRESS SYNDROME TREATED WITH PROTECTIVE LUNG STRATEGY

1. Limit lung volumes to 8 ml/kg
2. Limit pulmonary plateau pressure to 30 cm $H_2O$
3. Use PEEP to limit $Fio_2$ to 0.60
4. Transient levels of increased PEEP can be used to recruit additional alveoli

### D. VENTILATOR-ASSOCIATED PNEUMONIA

1. Evidence of pneumonia after 3 to 5 days of mechanical ventilation
   a. Fever
   b. Increased white blood cell count
   c. Purulent sputum production
   d. New infiltrate on chest radiograph
2. The previous criteria combined with bronchoscopically obtained specimen with >100,000 colonies/ml
3. Protocol-driven therapy: Initial broad-spectrum antimicrobials and deescalation of therapy when culture results dictate a specific organism and sensitivities

### VIII. PEARLS

### A. STANDARD INITIAL VENTILATOR SETTINGS:

Assist/control rate: 12
$V_T$: 8 ml/kg
Pressure support: 10 cm $H_2O$
PEEP: 5 cm $H_2O$
$Fio_2$: 0.60
Obtain arterial blood gas in 30 to 60 minutes and make appropriate changes

Normal inspiratory/expiratory ratio is 1:3, with 15 breaths/min; this is 1 second of inspiration and 3 seconds of expiration. $Pao_2$ >60 mm Hg usually equates to $SPo_2$ >90%

## FURTHER READING

Section VII Mechanical Ventilation. In Marino PL (ed): *The ICU Book,* 2nd ed. New York, Lippincott Williams & Wilkins, 1988.

Sena MJ, Nathens AB: Mechanical ventilation. In *ACS Surgery: Principles and Practice,* 2005. WebMD.

# Blood Component Therapy

*Rebecca J. McClaine, MD*

## I. GENERAL TOPICS

### A. FORMULAS

1. Total blood volume (TBV) = 70 ml/kg total body weight (80 ml/kg for newborns)
2. Total volume red blood cells (RBCs) = TBV × hematocrit
3. Total plasma volume = TBV × (1 − hematocrit)

### B. TYPING AND CROSS-MATCHING

1. Typing—serologic compatibility established for donor and recipient A, B, O, and Rh groups
2. Cross-matching—to ensure compatibility of blood product to be infused. Test mixes donor's RBCs and recipient's serum, drawn less than 72 hours before test takes place.

### C. MASSIVE TRANSFUSION IS DEFINED AS TRANSFUSION OF >2500 TO 5000 ML IN 24 HOURS.

### D. ADMINISTRATION GUIDELINES

1. Allow 30 minutes for frozen products to thaw or for cold products to be warmed. Products should be warmed to 33°C to 35°C before or during infusion.
2. Ensure patient has appropriate intravenous access.
3. Before administration of blood product, the patient's name, medical record number, blood product ordered, blood type, and product's expiration date should be checked, usually by two people together.
4. Use standard blood filter to remove clots or large aggregates of cells.
5. Check vital signs at minimum before beginning infusion, 15 minutes into infusion, and after completion of transfusion of each unit.

## II. WHOLE BLOOD

### A. TBV = 70 ML/KG = 5 L IN 70-KG MALE INDIVIDUAL

### B. SPECIFICS OF TRANSFUSION

1. Must be ABO identical, cross-match required
2. Banked whole blood usually stored in 500-ml units
3. Stored at 4°C in citrate, phosphate, dextrose preservative for up to 21 days
4. Contains all blood components
   a. Poor source of platelets, which lose function after stored for 24 hours in whole blood
   b. Clotting factors stable in whole blood, except factors V and VIII
   c. In RBCs, intracellular 2,3-diphosphoglycerate (DPG) and adenosine triphosphate are reduced during storage, shifting the hemoglobin dissociation curve to the left (more affinity for oxygen).

d. During storage, pH decreases; lactate, ammonia, and potassium increase.

## C. INDICATIONS
1. Used during mass trauma situations in military, usually supplied by fresh donations
2. Burn surgery—used perioperatively when large losses of blood, platelets, and bleeding factors are expected.

## D. AUTOLOGOUS BLOOD
1. May be collected before surgery for perioperative use
a. Up to 5 units may be collected over 40 days before surgery.
b. Erythropoietin is given to hasten generation of blood cells.

## E. FRESH WHOLE BLOOD
1. (Administered within 24 hours of donation) rarely used because it must be administered untested for infectious disease because of time constraints.

## III. RED BLOOD CELLS

## A. REFERENCE RBC VOLUMES
1. 26 ml/kg (1.8 L for 70-kg male individual) for male patients, 24 ml/kg (1.7 L for 70-kg female individual) for female patients
2. Measured using chromium-tagged erythrocytes, which is cumbersome and not often performed clinically
3. Approximated clinically using hematocrit (40–54% in male individuals, 38–47% in female individuals) and hemoglobin (13.5–18.0 g/dl in male individuals, 12.0–16.0 g/dl in female individuals)
4. After acute episode of blood loss of 1000 ml (20% of TBV), hematocrit value will be 3% less in 1 hour, 5% less in 24 hours, 6% less in 48 hours, and 8% less in 72 hours.

## B. SPECIFICS OF TRANSFUSION
1. Ideally, ABO identical, cross-match required
a. For emergency transfusions, type-specific and O-negative RBCs are equally safe for transfusion.
b. After 4 units of O-negative blood, risk for hemolysis significantly increases.
2. One unit of packed red blood cells (pRBCs) has volume of 250 to 350 ml.
3. Stored at 4°C in citrate, phosphate, dextrose preservative is viable for 21 days
4. Contains concentrated whole blood, hematocrit 60% to 65%
a. Effects on intracellular adenosine triphosphate and DPG are lessened but not eliminated.

b. Leukocyte-reduced pRBCs are standard in most Western countries, although in the United States, controversy exists as to cost-effectiveness of measure.

5. Transfusion of 1 unit pRBCs should increase hematocrit value 3% to 4% in adults. In children, transfusion of 10 ml/kg pRBCs should increase hemoglobin level by 2 g/dl.

## C. INDICATIONS

1. Trauma: During resuscitation, when vital signs do not stabilize after transfusion of 2 L crystalloid, this indicates blood loss of >30% of blood volume, and transfusion of 2 units pRBCs is indicated.
2. pRBCs should not be transfused for treatment of chronic anemia or anemia of pregnancy. Chronic anemia may be treated with iron or erythropoietin, and transfusion is rarely required because patients have adjusted to low hemoglobin level.
3. Absolute hemoglobin "trigger" for pRBC transfusion is <6 g/dl; pRBCs rarely are needed for hemoglobin level >10 g/dl.
4. In the intensive care unit setting, transfusion should be based on evidence of impaired oxygen delivery ($DO_2$) to tissues, rather than on hemoglobin or hematocrit measures.
   a. Decreased oxygen uptake ($VO_2$ <100 ml/min/m$^2$), increased oxygen extraction ratio ($O_2ER$ >0.5), or hyperlactatemia in the presence of normovolemia and normal cardiac output may be used as an indication for transfusion.
   b. $DO_2$ should be measured 15 minutes after transfusion of 1 to 2 units pRBCs. If no improvement in $DO_2$, $VO_2$, or $O_2ER$ is seen, no further transfusions are indicated at that time.
5. In patients with history of coronary artery disease, cerebrovascular insufficiency, or significant cardiac dysfunction, hemoglobin "trigger" may be increased to <7 g/dl, based on previous practice of transfusing for hemoglobin level <10 g/dl in this population. Neither practice has been validated by prospective trial.
6. Prophylactic preoperative pRBC transfusion based on expected intraoperative blood loss is not indicated.
7. Intraoperative blood loss >20% of TBV (1 L) usually is replaced with combination of crystalloid, pRBCs, and fresh frozen plasma (FFP).

## D. AUTOLOGOUS RBC COUNT

1. Cell salvage (CellSaver)—blood collected from cavities uncontaminated by malignant cells or infectious agents intraoperatively, centrifuged, and washed to contain only RBCs. Must be used within 4 hours of collection.

**13**

BLOOD COMPONENT THERAPY

## IV. PLATELETS

**A. REFERENCE PLATELET COUNTS RANGE FROM 150,000 TO 400,000/MM³; 50,000/MM³ IS REQUIRED FOR NORMAL HEMOSTASIS.**

**B. SPECIFICS OF TRANSFUSION**

1. ABO compatibility preferred, Rh type unimportant, no cross-match required

   a. Patients who undergo frequent transfusions can develop antibodies to transfused platelets or other proteins, significantly decreasing effectiveness of transfusion.

   b. When refractoriness develops, human leukocyte antigen–matched platelets often are used.

2. Package consists of 6 units (each ~50 ml) pooled from individual donors (6 times increased risk for transmission of infectious disease).

3. Stored at 20°C to 24°C; should be used within 120 hours of donation

4. Each packet contains stable clotting factors (except factors V and VII) from 1 to 2 units of FFP.

5. Each packet increases platelet count by 5000 to 10,000/mm³.

**C. INDICATIONS FOR TRANSFUSION**

1. Clinical bleeding with functional platelet counts less than 50,000/mm³ (i.e., transfusion of normal platelets may be necessary to overcome congenital or acquired disorders causing abnormal platelet function)

2. Correction of functional platelet count to 50,000/mm³ in preparation for surgical procedure, to 30,000/mm³ in preparation for lumbar puncture or central line placement

3. No role for prophylactic transfusion as routine accompaniment to massive transfusion of pRBCs or FFP, but expect dilutional decrease in platelets after transfusion of 10 units of other products

4. No role for prophylactic transfusion for any platelet count without clinical bleeding

5. Functional platelet count is measured by bleeding time; bleeding time longer than two times upper limit of normal with clinical bleeding is indication for platelet transfusion.

## V. FRESH FROZEN PLASMA

**A. REFERENCE VALUES**

1. Prothrombin time—12 to 14 seconds; activated partial thromboplastin time—40 to 60 seconds (varies by laboratory); international normalized ratio—1.0 to 1.3

**B. SPECIFICS OF TRANSFUSION**

1. ABO compatibility required, Rh type unimportant, no cross-match required

2. Aliquoted into 250 ml units from whole blood

3. Frozen to −18°C within 8 to 24 hours of collection, may be stored for 24 hours at 1°C to 6°C
4. Contains 200 units of all coagulation factors (1 unit/ml), estimated 40% recovered function after transfusion
   a. Factors V and VII less stable than vitamin K–dependent factors, begin depreciating after thawing
5. Estimated 10% increase in all functional factors with 4 units FFP

## B. INDICATIONS

1. Correction of clinical coagulopathy with abnormal laboratory values (prothrombin time >1.5 times reference value, activated partial thromboplastin time >2 times reference, international normalized ratio >2.0)
2. Expect coagulopathy during transfusion of multiple units of pRBCs, with need for FFP transfusion. New trauma protocols suggest transfusion of units of pRBCs and FFP in 1:1 ratio.
3. Immediate reversal of warfarin
4. Treatment of coagulopathies because of liver failure or disseminated intravascular coagulation
5. Treatment of congenital coagulation factor deficiencies if no specific component therapies available

## VI. CRYOPRECIPITATE

### A. NORMAL FIBRINOGEN LEVELS ARE 200 TO 400 MG/DL, NORMAL FUNCTION VALUES ARE >150 MG/DL.

### B. SPECIFICS OF TRANSFUSION

1. ABO compatibility preferred but not required, Rh type unimportant, no cross-match required.
2. One pooled "unit" contains six 15- to 20-ml units from individual donors.
3. Made from precipitate of thawed FFP, must be transfused within 4 hours.
4. Each individual unit contains 80 to 150 units factor VIII/von Willebrand factor, 250 to 350 mg fibrinogen (pooled "unit" contains 5–6 times these amounts).
   a. Fibrinogen in 1 unit FFP equals amount in 2 units cryoprecipitate.
5. One pooled unit increases fibrinogen by about 50 mg/dl.

### C. INDICATIONS

1. Correction of clinical coagulopathy with fibrinogen concentration <80 mg/dl
2. Expect fibrinogen deficiency after massive transfusion of other blood products.
3. May be given for hemophilia A, von Willebrand's disease if no specific component therapies available

**13**

**BLOOD COMPONENT THERAPY**

## VII. TRANSFUSION REACTIONS

### A. IMMUNE MEDIATED

1. Acute hemolytic reaction occurs when recipient plasma contains antibodies to donor RBCs because of ABO incompatibility (pRBCs, whole blood).
   a. 1:250,000 to 1:1,000,000 transfusions
   b. Characterized by immediate fever, chills, dyspnea, back pain, bleeding, and shock initially, with renal failure occurring later in course. Anesthetized patients may experience only hypotension or bleeding.
   c. Treat with volume expansion, diuresis, and urine alkalinization after immediately stopping transfusion. Reaction can occur after transfusion of only 10 ml; severity increases with amount transfused.
   d. Hemoglobinemia (pink plasma) and hemoglobinuria will occur within minutes. Decreased haptoglobin indicates hemolysis. Direct agglutination test (Coombs' test) will be positive as long as residual incompatible RBCs persist in circulation.
   e. Delayed hemolytic reaction can occur 2 to 10 days after transfusion when recipient's antibody titer recovers; reaction characterized by mild anemia and hyperbilirubinemia.

2. Febrile nonhemolytic reaction occurs when recipient plasma contains antibodies to leukocytes in donor unit (pRBCs, whole blood).
   a. 1:100 transfusions
   b. Characterized by 1°C increase in body temperature 1 to 6 hours after start of infusion
   c. Stop transfusion until hemolytic reaction is ruled out by absence of hemoglobinemia or hemoglobinuria, rule out other causes of fever.
   d. Reduced occurrence when leukocyte-reduced pRBCs are used

3. Allergic reaction to donor components (any transfusion)
   a. Characterized by itching, urticaria, wheezing, angioedema
   b. Treat with antihistamines, acetaminophen, and continue transfusion. Premedicate for future transfusions and used washed, leukocyte-reduced products.
   c. Patients with history of IgA deficiency without history of transfusion may have an anaphylactic reaction.

4. Alloimmunization to RBCs, leukocytes, platelets, or other protein components (human leukocyte antigen class I antigens) can occur after multiple transfusions (especially with human leukocyte antigen–unmatched products).
   a. No immediate complications, but sensitizes patient and increases risk for adverse event during future transfusions
   b. Can prevent by using all ABO-matched products and washed/leukocyte-reduced pRBCs

5. Transfusion-related acute lung injury occurs when donor antibodies attack recipient leukocytes, leading to immune complex deposition in pulmonary capillary beds (any transfusion).

a. 1:5000 transfusions
b. Presents as pulmonary edema, acute respiratory distress syndrome–like syndrome, secondary to rapid increase in pulmonary capillary permeability, usually within 2 to 6 hours of infusion
c. Treat supportively; may require intubation and mechanical ventilation for 2 to 4 days while insult resolves.

**6. Graft-versus-host disease occurs in immunocompromised patients when donor leukocytes attack recipient tissues (pRBCs, whole blood).**
a. Characterized by multiorgan system failure; mortality rate >90%
b. Stop transfusion; supportive treatment. Use of leukocyte-reduced, irradiated blood reduces occurrence.

## B. NONIMMUNOLOGIC REACTIONS

**1. Transmission of infectious disease same for whole blood, pRBCs, and FFP**
a. Human immunodeficiency virus transmission: 1:200,000 to 1:2,000,000 transfusions
b. Hepatitis B transmission: 1:30,000 to 1:250,000 transfusions
c. Hepatitis C transmission: 1:30,000 to 1:150,000 transfusions
d. Reports of cytomegalovirus, Epstein–Barr virus, and West Nile virus transmission

**2. Bacterial contamination occurs rarely, most often in platelets because they are stored at higher temperature (1:12,000 transfusions).**

**3. Multiple retrospective studies suggest link between transfusion and rates of nosocomial infection, pneumonia, length of stay, and mortality.**
a. One theory suggests that recipient leukocytes become tolerant because of infusion of donor leukocytes with similar but nonidentical human leukocyte antigen patterns.
b. Another theory suggests that donor leukocytes or components released during transfusion down-regulate recipient leukocyte response.

**4. Hemosiderosis occurs with repeated pRBC transfusion.**
a. Each unit of pRBCs contains 250 mg iron.
b. Treated with deferoxamine, which chelates iron to promote its excretion

**5. Potassium abnormalities are caused by alterations in normal action of the sodium-potassium pump in pRBCs.**
a. Initial hyperkalemia during transfusion because pRBC pumps are inactive during storage, leading to increased potassium in supernatant of unit
b. Often followed by hypokalemia because pumps in transfused RBCs become active and drive extracellular potassium into cells

**6. Hypocalcemia is caused by citrate preservative in all blood products complexing with ionized calcium for excretion. Usually transient, self-limited effect, unless multiple transfusions are being performed.**

13

BLOOD COMPONENT THERAPY

## RECOMMENDED REFERENCES

Practice guidelines for perioperative blood transfusion and adjuvant therapies: an updated report by the American Society of Anesthesiologists Task Force on Perioperative Blood Transfusion and Adjuvant Therapies. *Anesthesiology* 105:198–208, 2006.

Silliman CC, Ambruso DR, Boshkov LK: Transfusion-related acute lung injury. *Blood* 105:2266–2273, 2005.

Spahn DR, Rossaint R: Coagulopathy and blood component transfusion in trauma. *Br J Anaesh* 95:130–139, 2005.

# Surgical Infection

*Alexander J. Bondoc, MD*

## I. DEFINITIONS

### A. SURGICAL INFECTION
1. A process that typically requires operative treatment or results from operative therapy.

### B. SOURCE CONTROL
1. Foremost principle behind the management of surgical infection
2. Entails eradication of an infectious source so that host defenses, often in conjunction with antibiotic therapy, are able to restore normal function

**14**

### C. NONOPERATIVE-ASSOCIATED INFECTIONS
1. Body cavity infections
a. Disruption of the enteric stream
   (1) Primary peritonitis—intraabdominal infection without organ derangement
   (2) Secondary peritonitis—infection caused by anatomic derangement
b. Suppurative pericarditis
c. Empyema
2. Confined tissue, organ, or joint infections
a. Abscess
b. Devitalized tissue
c. Septic arthritis
3. Foreign body/prosthetic–related infections

### D. POSTOPERATIVE INFECTIONS
1. Wound infection
2. Abscess
3. Other hospital-acquired infections—removal of indwelling devices, antibiotics often sufficient.
a. Hospital-acquired pneumonia, ventilator-associated pneumonia
b. Urinary tract infection
c. Catheter-related bloodstream infection

## II. DETERMINANTS OF INFECTION

### A. MICROBIAL FEATURES
1. Virulence of organism—dependent on multiple factors
a. Organism cell structures
b. Toxin production
c. Antimicrobial resistance
2. Number of organisms present (inoculum)

## B. HOST DEFENSE—OFTEN REDUNDANT AND INTEGRATED
1. Tissue barriers—either mucosal or epithelialized
2. Respiratory system
a. Mucous secretion
b. Ciliary system
c. Pulmonary macrophages
3. Gastrointestinal—center for global immunity
a. Stomach
   (1) $10^2$ to $10^3$ colony-forming units (CFU)/ml
   (2) Highly acidic environment with relatively low motility
b. Small intestine
   (1) $10^5$ to $10^8$ CFU/ml
   (2) Largest immune tissue in the body given mucosal-associated lymphoid tissue
c. Large intestine
   (1) $10^{11}$ to $10^{12}$ CFU/ml
   (2) Combination of endogenous and enteropathic organisms
4. Immune system—both innate and acquired

## C. SURGICAL TECHNIQUE/PREVENTION OF INFECTION
1. Antibiotic prophylaxis
a. Prevention of surgical infection
b. Indications
   (1) Based on the National Nosocomial Infection Surveillance system (Table 14-1)
   (2) Risk index score ranges from 0 to 3.
   (3) Operations causing bone manipulation, injury
       (a) Orthopedic surgery
       (b) Cardiac surgery
c. Duration of treatment often a one-time dose; otherwise, no longer than 24 hours
2. Removal of hair with clippers and not a razor
3. Gentle handling of tissue
4. Removal of devitalized tissue, blood, and other substances that promote microbe growth
5. Appropriate drain use
6. Avoidance of excessive cautery
7. Performance of anastomoses with minimal tension and adequate blood supply
8. Maintenance of euglycemia

## D. DIAGNOSIS
1. History and physical examination (see cases later in this chapter)
2. Laboratory tests
a. Complete blood cell count with differential

**TABLE 14-1**

NATIONAL NOSOCOMIAL INFECTION SURVEILLANCE SYSTEM
FOR DETERMINING PREOPERATIVE ANTIBIOTIC USE

| Criterion | Significant Value | Comments |
|---|---|---|
| American Society of Anesthesiologists (ASA) preoperative assessment | Class 3, 4, or 5 | **ASA 1**—normal healthy patient<br>**ASA 2**—patient with mild systemic disease with no functional limitations<br>**ASA 3**—moderate systemic disease with limitations<br>**ASA 4**—severe systemic disease that is a constant threat to life<br>**ASA 5**—patient is not expected to survive with or without surgery in 24 hours |
| Degree of operative contamination | Contaminated or dirty | **Clean** (class I)—no infection present<br>**Clean/contaminated** (II)—hollow viscus is opened in a controlled fashion<br>**Contaminated** (III)—extensive bacterial spillage caused by violation of sterile technique or gross spillage<br>**Dirty** (IV)—traumatic wounds with delay in treatment or presence of necrotic tissue |
| Duration of operation | x hours | x is dependent on the type of operation being performed |

(1) White blood cell (WBC) count greater than 12,000 or less than 6000 cells/$\mu$L
(2) Differential left shift indicates predominance of neutrophils and immature neutrophils (e.g., bands).
(3) Neutropenia or thrombocytopenia in overwhelming sepsis
b. Arterial blood gas or renal panel—evaluate pH or $HCO_3$ for signs of sepsis.
**3. Imaging**
a. Radiography
(1) Chest radiograph—may demonstrate pneumonia or intraperitoneal free air.
(2) Abdominal radiograph—may demonstrate bowel obstruction or pneumatosis.
b. Ultrasound
(1) Useful for evaluating the biliary system
(2) Also useful for evaluating gynecologic disorders

c. Computed tomography scan
   (1) Most sensitive and specific modality for intraabdominal processes
   (2) May aid in percutaneous treatment of intraabdominal pathology
4. **Specimen collection**
a. Blood cultures
   (1) Two peripheral cultures or one peripheral and one from a central venous catheter if in place
   (2) Obtain aerobic and anaerobic cultures
   (3) Obtain Gram stain for preliminary goal-directed antibiotic therapy
b. Aspiration of fluid
c. Tissue sample—surgical or sterile samples preferred
d. Wound or fluid swab—much less reliable and more prone to contamination than laboratory tests or imaging
e. Urine and sputum cultures
f. Viral specimens
   (1) Immunofluorescence of scraped cells
   (2) Immunologic studies of serum
   (3) Quantitative polymerase chain reaction
   (4) Qualitative
g. Fungal infections
   (1) Gram stain
   (2) Tissue biopsy

## III. PRINCIPLES OF THERAPY
### A. SOURCE CONTROL
The foremost principle of surgical infection
1. Incision and drainage of fluid collections
2. Debridement of necrotic tissue and foreign bodies
3. Removal of contaminated foreign bodies
4. Diversion of the enteric stream

### B. WOUND MANAGEMENT
1. Primary skin and fascial closure should be achieved when possible; sometimes it cannot be achieved.
a. Shock and generalized edema
b. Fecal contamination
2. Dressing care
a. Moist dressings for open skin with closed fascia
b. Vacuum-assisted closure device once wound is clean
c. Temporary abdominal closures may be necessary for an open abdomen.

### C. ANTIBIOTIC THERAPY (TABLE 14-2)
1. Types of antibiotics
a. Bacteriostatic—prevention of bacterial growth and multiplication without killing; reliance on host defense mechanisms to clear infection
b. Bactericidal—kills bacteria; must be used in immunocompromised patients.

## TABLE 14-2

### ANTIMICROBIAL AGENTS

| Antibiotic Class | Mechanism of Action (MOA) | Microbial Target/Side Effects |
|---|---|---|
| *Penicillins* | *All are bactericidal; use a β-lactam ring that inhibits cell wall synthesis* | |
| Penicillin G, V | | Streptococcus pyogenes and Clostridia species |
| Methicillin, nafcillin, oxacillin, dicloxacillin | Resistant to β-lactamase enzyme | Staphylococcus aureus and epidermidis |
| Ampicillin and amoxicillin | Enhanced ability to penetrate cell walls | Enterococcus and gram-negatives |
| Piperacillin, carbenicillin, mezlocillin, and ticarcillin | | Gram negatives, especially Pseudomonas, and some anaerobic species |
| Ampicillin-sulbactam, amoxicillin-clavulanate, ticarcillin-clavulanate, piperacillin-tazobactam | Penicillin/β-lactamase inhibitor combinations | Covers gram-positives, gram-negatives, and anaerobes. Does not cover MRSA |
| *Cephalosporins—5% to 10% allergic cross-reactivity with penicillin-allergic patients* | *All are bactericidal with a similar MOA to penicillins but with additional side chains* | *MRSA and enterococci are resistant to all cephalosporins* |
| 1st generation (cefazolin, cephalexin) | | Gram positives |
| 2nd generation (cefuroxime, cefoxitin, cefuroxime) | | Gram positives and gram negatives |
| 3rd generation (ceftriaxone, cefotaxime) | | Multidrug resistant gram negative aerobes, including nosocomial infections |
| 4th generation (cefepime) | | Broad gram positive and gram negative coverage , including Pseudomonas |
| *Monobactams— aztreonam* | *Bactericidal; monocyclic β-lactam* | *Only gram negative anaerobes including Pseudomonas* |
| *Carbapenems— imipenem/cilastin,\* meropenem* | *Bactericidal and stable against β-lactamase* | *Broadest spectrum antibiosis. Diphtheroids, P. maltophilia, and Proteus mirabilis are resistant* |

*Continued*

**TABLE 14-2—cont'd**

ANTIMICROBIAL AGENTS

| Antibiotic Class | Mechanism of Action (MOA) | Microbial Target/Side Effects |
|---|---|---|
| Aminoglycosides— gentamicin, tobramycin, amikacin, kanamycin | Bactericidal; inhibition of the 30S ribosomal subunit | Aerobic gram negative enterics. Dosing is 5–7 mg/kg/24 hrs or 1.7 mg/kg every 8 hrs. Side effects include non-reversible ototoxicity and nephrotoxicity. Synergistic with penicillins |
| Trimethoprim and sulfonamides | Combination is bactericidal by inhibiting folate and pyrimidine synthesis, respectively | Wide gram negative and gram positive coverage. First-line drug for uncomplicated UTIs and effective against Pneumocystis carnii and Nocardia. MRSA sometimes sensitive to combination of TMP/ SMX and rifampin |
| Fluoroquinolones 2nd generation (ciprofloxacin) 3rd generation (gatifloxacin) 4th generation (moxifloxacin) | Bactericidal; inhibition of DNA gyrase | High blood levels with oral administration and good tissue penetration. Good gram negative coverage including complicated UTIs and in-traabdominal infections |
| Tetracyclines— tetracycline and doxycycline | Bacteriostatic; inhibition of the 30S ribosomal subunit | Used with ceftriaxone against STDs. MRSA often sensitive. Do not use in children or lactating mothers as drugs can cause dental discoloration and depressed bone growth |

**TABLE 14-2—cont'd**

ANTIMICROBIAL AGENTS

| Antibiotic Class | Mechanism of Action (MOA) | Microbial Target/Side Effects |
|---|---|---|
| Macrolides—erythromycin, azithromycin, clarithromycin | Bacteriostatic (bacteriocidal for some gram positives); inhibition of the 50S subunit | Good coverage of gram positives and causes of atypical pneumonia including, Legionella, Mycoplasma, and Chlamydia. Also used as a motilin agonist |
| *Other antibacterials* | | |
| Vancomycin | Bactericidal; inhibition of cell wall synthesis | Broad coverage of gram positives, including MRSA. Not absorbed orally, so can be used as a second-line agent for *Clostridium difficile* colitis |
| Linezolid | Bactericidal; inhibition of the 50S ribosomal subunit | Often reserved for vancomycin-resistant organisms |
| Metronidazole | Bactericidal; inhibition of DNA replication | Coverage of anaerobes, a few gram negatives, amoebae, and trichomonads. First-line agent for *Clostridium difficile* colitis |
| Clindamycin | Bacteriostatic; inhibition of the 50S ribosomal subunit | Gram positives and anaerobes. More effective than penicillins in preventing toxic shock syndrome by preventing exotoxin synthesis. Can often cause *Clostridium difficile* colitis |
| *Antituberculosis agents* | | |
| Isoniazid | Bactericidal; inhibition of the synthesis of the mycolic acid component of the cell wall | Hepatotoxicity |
| Rifampin | Bactericidal; inhibition of RNA polymerase | Induction of the cytochrome P450 system (decreases the half life of drugs such as warfarin, oral hypoglycemics, and anticonvulsants) |

14

SURGICAL INFECTION

*Continued*

**TABLE 14-2—cont'd**

ANTIMICROBIAL AGENTS

| Antibiotic Class | Mechanism of Action (MOA) | Microbial Target/Side Effects |
|---|---|---|
| Pyrazinamide | Unknown | Hepatotoxicity |
| Ethambutol | Unknown | Decreased visual acuity and color vision loss |

**Antifungals**

| | | |
|---|---|---|
| Polyenes (amphotericin B) | Fungicidal; binds to ergosterol, increasing cell wall permeability | The standard for disseminated candidiasis. Lipid-based formulations often have a better side effect profile and allow for higher dosing. Major toxicity is renal, which is reversible if stopped. Can also cause anemia and an acute febrile reaction. |
| Azoles (clotrimazole, miconazole, fluconazole, itraconazole, voriconazole) | Fungicidal; blocks ergosterol synthesis by blocking the cytochrome P450 system | Fluconazole is the preferred agent to amphotericin B in hemodynamically stable patients with susceptible isolates given its safer side effect profile. Voriconazole has increased activity against *albicans species* as compared with fluconazole. It also has activity against resistant *glabrata* and *krusei* species |
| Echinocandins (Caspofungin, micafungin) | Fungicidal; inhibition of $\beta$1,3-glucan synthase | As effective as amphotericin B in disseminated candidiasis. Very safe side effect profile |
| Flucytosine | Fungicidal; inhibition of DNA/RNA synthesis | Synergistic with amphotericin B. Used for severe *Candida* and *Cryptococcus* infections. Resistance develops rapidly |

**TABLE 14-2—cont'd**

ANTIMICROBIAL AGENTS

| Antibiotic Class | Mechanism of Action (MOA) | Microbial Target/Side Effects |
|---|---|---|
| Nystatin | Fungicidal; binds to ergosterol, increasing cell wall permeability | Too toxic to use parenterally. Used prophylactically in immunosuppressed patients or those on broad-spectrum antibiotics to prevent overgrowth of *Candida* |
| *Antivirals* | | |
| Anti-herpesviridae agents | | |
| Acyclovir | Guanine analogue that must be phosphorylated by a viral-specific thymidine kinase | Targets herpes simplex and varicella zoster. Not effective against CMV because it lacks thymidine kinase. Adverse effects are minimal |
| Valacyclovir, famciclovir | Guanine analogue that must be phosphorylated by a viral-specific thymidine kinase | Similar profile to acyclovir but with increased serum drug levels after oral administration |
| Ganciclovir | Guanine analogue that must be phosphorylated by a viral-specific thymidine kinase | Only used to treat CMV in immunocompromised hosts given its significant side effect profile, including reversible neutropenia and thrombocytopenia |
| Interferon-$\alpha$ | A cytokine that induces an antiviral state | Treatment of hepatitis B and C. Relapse rate is high (hepatitis B, 50%; hepatitis C. 75–80%). If used in combination with IFN, response rates improve |

*Cilastin prevents breakdown in the kidney.

**14**

**SURGICAL INFECTION**

**2. Selection of antibiotics**
a. Empiric choices
   (1) Based on likely organism and source
   (2) Reserve broad spectrum for patients who have health care–associated infections.
**3. Specific choices**
a. The use of antibiogram for possible hospital-acquired infection is crucial for institution-specific antibiotic sensitivities.
b. Deescalate antibiosis if possible as relevant culture and sensitivity data become available.
c. Other factors
   (1) Adequate dosage in renal failure
   (2) Adequate tissue perfusion
   (3) Tissue-specific penetration
   (4) Minimize side effects
   (5) Maximize host defense
d. Consider treatment failure after 48 to 72 hours of antibiosis without clinical improvement.
**4. Complications of antibiotic therapy**
a. Drug toxicity
   (1) Drug fevers, rashes, or anaphylaxis on initiation
   (2) Neurologic complications, gastrointestinal symptoms, renal dysfunction, blood/bone marrow dyscrasias, visual and auditory losses
b. Emergence of multidrug-resistant strains
c. Superinfection with opportunistic microorganisms (e.g., *Clostridium difficile,* fungus)

**Case Scenario:** *A 56-year-old man with a medical history significant for insulin-dependent diabetes mellitus, hypertension, and diverticulitis presents to the emergency department with a 2-day history of worsening abdominal pain, anorexia, and fever. On evaluation, his vital signs are as follows:*

Tmax 101.9°, HR 118, RR 36, BP 104/78

## IV. DIAGNOSIS
### A. HISTORY
**1. Characteristics of abdominal pain**
a. *Time of onset*—2 days
b. *Provoking and palliative factors*—pain with touch and while riding in the car to the emergency department
c. *Quality*—sharp, deep inside his abdomen
d. *Radiation*—throughout his abdomen
e. *Severity*—7 or 8/10 on a scale of 10

2. Other possible associated symptoms
a. Nausea/vomiting
b. Change in stool—diarrhea, bloody stool
c. Fever
d. Loss of appetite
3. Medical history
a. System-specific history—diverticulitis. No history of cholecystitis, appendicitis, or pancreatitis.
b. Medical comorbidities—diabetes, hypertension
c. Immunosuppressive disorders—for example, human immunodeficiency virus, previous organ transplant
4. Surgical history—laparoscopic sigmoid colectomy 6 days ago. No previous abdominal trauma.
5. Allergies/medications—no known allergies. Currently taking metoprolol, NPH insulin, and lisinopril
6. Social history—nonsmoker, quit 10 years ago. Drinks alcohol socially. No recent travel.

## B. PHYSICAL EXAMINATION
1. General—review of vital signs, ill-appearing, obvious discomfort
2. Cardiovascular/pulmonary—rule out other possible sources of abdominal pain.
3. Abdomen—examined in 4 stages
a. *Inspection*—no signs of bruising
b. *Auscultation*—bowel sounds absent
c. *Percussion*—distended, tympanic
d. *Palpation*—focal tenderness in the left lower quadrant

## C. LABORATORY VALUES
1. Complete blood count—WBC count of 16,000/mm$^3$ with 82% band forms
2. Amylase—70 units/L
3. Lipase—60 units/L
4. Liver panel
a. Alkaline phosphatase concentration—45 IU/L
b. Aspartate aminotransferase/alanine aminotransferase—20/40 IU/L
c. Total/direct bilirubin level—1.0/0.4 μmol/L
5. Urinalysis—no WBC or bacteria. No presence of leukocyte esterase or nitrites.

## D. SOURCE CONTROL
1. Percutaneous drainage
a. If the fluid is walled off and has become an abscess
2. Operative drainage
a. And diversion of the enteric stream—if there is evidence of uncontrolled colonic perforation and/or fecal peritonitis

14

SURGICAL INFECTION

## E. EMPIRIC THERAPY
1. See Table 14-3
2. Start broad and tailor antibiotic therapy as appropriate.

## F. FOLLOW-UP CARE: INDICATION OF THERAPY EFFICACY
1. Resolution of fever and pain
2. Return of gastrointestinal function
3. Normalization of WBC
4. Interval improvement on follow-up computed tomography scan

## V. SEPSIS (FIG. 14-1)

### A. SYSTEMIC INFLAMMATORY RESPONSE SYNDROME
1. Definition—a generalized response of the innate immune system to any number of physiologic stressors including, but not limited to the following:
a. Infection
b. Trauma
c. Burns
d. Sterile inflammatory processes (e.g., pancreatitis)
2. Classical clinical criteria
a. Body temperature—more than 38°C or less than 36°C
b. Heart rate—more than 90 beats/min
c. Blood pressure—systolic blood pressure less than 90 mm Hg or mean arterial pressure less than 70 mm Hg

### TABLE 14-3

INITIATION OF ANTIBIOTIC THERAPY FOR INTRAABDOMINAL INFECTION

| Type of Therapy | Agent(s) Recommended for Mild-to-Moderate Infections | Agent(s) Recommended for High-Severity Infections |
|---|---|---|
| **Single agent** | | |
| beta-lactam/beta-lactamase inhibitor combinations | Ampicillin/sulbactam, ticarcillin/clavulanate | Piperacillin/tazobactam |
| Carbapenems | Ertapenem | Imipenem/cilastatin, meropenem |
| **Combination regimen** | | |
| Cephalosporin based | Cefazolin or cefuroxime + metronidazole | Third/fourth-generation cephalosporin + metronidazole |
| Fluoroquinolone based | Ciprofloxacin, levofloxacin, moxifloxacin or gatifloxacin, each + metronidazole | Ciprofloxacin + metronidazole |
| Monobactam-based | | Aztreonam + metronidazole |

From Solomkin JS, Mazuski JE, Baron EJ, et al: Guidelines for the selection of anti-infective agents for complicated intra-abdominal infections. *Clin Infect Dis* 37:998, 2003.

d. Hyperventilation with respiratory rate greater than 20 breaths/min or arterial partial pressure of carbon dioxide ($Paco_2$) less than 32 mm Hg

e. WBC count greater than 12,000 cells/$\mu$L or less than 4000 cells/$\mu$L

3. Realistically, there are multiple other clinical and laboratory indicators of systemic inflammatory response syndrome, including organ dysfunction variables (e.g., hypercreatininemia or oliguria) and tissue perfusion variables (e.g., hyperlactatemia or base deficit).

## B. SEPSIS AND SEPTIC SHOCK

1. Definitions

a. Sepsis—systemic inflammatory response syndrome with evidence of an infectious causative agent

b. Severe sepsis—sepsis with associated end-organ dysfunction

c. Septic shock—sepsis with arterial hypotension despite adequate fluid resuscitation

2. **Cell-based pathophysiology—as with other shock states, sepsis causes cell hypoperfusion.**

a. Aerobic metabolism fails and production of adenosine triphosphate becomes impaired.

b. Anaerobic metabolism leads to lactate production and relative acidemia.

c. Hypoxia and acidemia lead to global cellular metabolic dysfunction and eventual cell death.

3. **Organ-based pathophysiology**

a. Cardiovascular

   (1) Decreased peripheral vascular resistance and increased capillary leak caused by systemic proinflammatory cytokines

   (2) Decreased preload caused by peripheral venodilation

   (3) Increased cardiac index driven primarily by tachycardia

b. Respiratory

   (1) Acute lung injury—neutrophil-moderated injury secondary to pneumonia or other infectious processes

   (2) Acute respiratory distress syndrome caused by capillary leak and cytokine activation

c. Immune

   (1) Proinflammatory cytokines

      (a) Tumor necrosis factor-$\alpha$—released by macrophages and T cells.

      (b) Interleukin-1$\beta$ (IL-1$\beta$)—both local and systemic stimulation

      (c) IL-2—activates other lymphocyte subpopulations.

      (d) IL-6—end-organ dysfunction

   (2) Antiinflammatory cytokines

      (a) IL-10

   (3) Complement system

   (4) Neutrophil (polymorphonuclear neutrophils) activation

d. Endocrine

   (1) Hypothalamic—pituitary axis activation

      (a) Adrenal

**14**

**SURGICAL INFECTION**

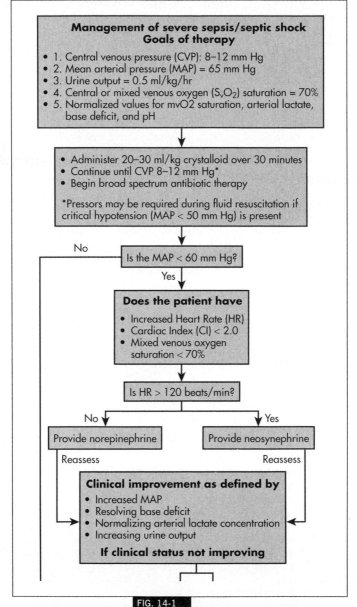

### FIG. 14-1
Management of sepsis.

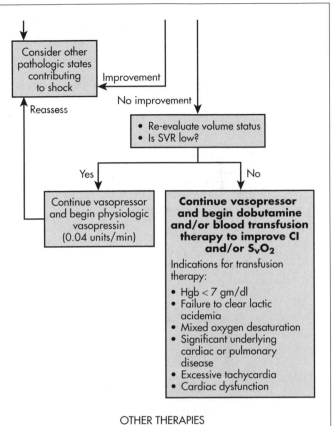

Consider other pathologic states contributing to shock

Improvement

No improvement

Reassess

- Re-evaluate volume status
- Is SVR low?

Yes

No

Continue vasopressor and begin physiologic vasopressin (0.04 units/min)

**Continue vasopressor and begin dobutamine and/or blood transfusion therapy to improve CI and/or $S_VO_2$**

Indications for transfusion therapy:

- Hgb < 7 gm/dl
- Failure to clear lactic acidemia
- Mixed oxygen desaturation
- Significant underlying cardiac or pulmonary disease
- Excessive tachycardia
- Cardiac dysfunction

OTHER THERAPIES

- Steroid therapy (hydrocortisone) for possible adrenal insufficiency
- Tight glycemic control (80–100 g/dl)
- Ventilator tidal volumes (6 ml/kg of ideal body weight) per ARDS net criteria with a concurrent goal of end-inspiratory pressures < 30 cm $H_2O$
- Recombinant activated Protein C for patients with Acute Physiology and Chronic Health Evaluation (APACHE) II score = 25 who meet all other criteria
- Deep vein thrombosis prophylaxis
- Stress ulcer prophylaxis
- Enteral nutrition if GI system allows

FIG. 14-1—cont'd

Management of sepsis.

(1) Increased cortisol release

(2) Increased epinephrine release

(b) Increased antidiuretic hormone and vasopressin release

(2) Renin-angiotensin-aldosterone system activation

(3) Hyperglycemia

(a) Increased glucagon and catecholamine secretion, which leads to decreased serum insulin in early sepsis

(b) Peripheral insulin resistance in late sepsis

e. Hematologic

(1) Leukocytosis/leukopenia

(2) Activation/up-regulation of the coagulation cascade → disseminated intravascular coagulopathy

(3) Thrombocytopenia

f. Neurologic—mental status changes (e.g., delirium)

4. **Infectious causative agents**

a. Bacterial

(1) Gram-positive organisms (e.g., *Staphylococcal* sp)

(a) Now the most prevalent cause of sepsis

(b) Soluble immunogenic factors

(1) Peptidoglycan—forms the basis of the cell wall.

(2) Lipoteichoic acid

(2) Gram-negative organisms (e.g., enteric organisms, *Pseudomonas*)

(a) Most often caused by bacilli species

(b) Soluble immunogenic factor

(c) Lipopolysaccharide

b. Fungal

(1) There was a 207% increase in incidence of fungal sepsis from 1979 to 2000.

(2) Often related to nosocomial, opportunistic infections in immunocompromised hosts

c. Viral—seen in immunocompromised patients, most notably recipients of solid organ allografts.

## VI. COMMON SOURCES OF INFECTION IN THE SURGICAL PATIENT

**A. POSTOPERATIVE FEVER/INFECTION (SEE CHAPTER 4)**

**B. COMMON SOURCES OF INFECTION**

1. Urinary tract infection—2% to 16% of patients with indwelling catheters will experience development of a urinary tract infection each day. Up to half of patients who require a Foley catheter for 5 or more days will experience development of a urinary tract infection.

a. Diagnose by urinalysis (leukocyte esterase, nitrite positive and >10 WBC/high-powered field) and culture of more than $10^5$ CFU.

b. Discontinue Foley catheter if possible; if not, change catheter.

c. Antibiosis as appropriate

d. Candiduria without fungemia does not necessitate antibiosis.

2. **Catheter-related infections**

a. Catheter-site infection
  (1) Redness, tenderness, purulence, and lymphangitis at the site
  (2) Removal of the catheter is sufficient
b. Catheter-related bloodstream infection—more than 200,000 cases/year
  (1) Most commonly coagulase-negative staphylococci, *Staphylococcus aureus,* aerobic gram-negative bacilli, and *Candida albicans*
  (2) Diagnosis
    (a) Blood cultures—one culture peripherally and one culture via the catheter. Predictive for infection if:
      (1) Catheter blood colony count 5- to 10-fold greater than peripheral
      (2) Catheter blood culture positive at least 2 hours earlier than peripheral.
    (b) Catheter cultures
      (1) Qualitative catheter cultures—positive Gram stain
      (2) Quantitative catheter cultures—when positive, more specific than qualitative cultures
        (a) Semiquantitative—$\geq 15$ CFU is diagnostic.
        (b) Quantitative—$\geq 10^2$ CFU is diagnostic.
  (3) Management
    (a) Remove catheter if peripheral access placed.
    (b) If central access necessary, place new line at a different site.
    (c) Provide antibiotics if highly suspicious for bloodborne dissemination (Table 14-4).
    (d) If only the catheter has significant growth and blood cultures are negative, antibiotic use is governed by local site evaluation.

## 3. Pneumonia
a. Clinical diagnosis
  (1) Macroscopically purulent sputum
  (2) Fever
  (3) Leukocytosis
  (4) Oxygen impairment
  (5) Infiltrate on chest radiograph
b. Bacteriologic diagnosis—presence of pathogens in respiratory secretions obtained via lower respiratory tract sampling.
  (1) Qualitative—Gram stain and culture
  (2) Quantitative—able to count CFUs in addition to culture. Can discriminate between colonization and pathologic infection.
c. Treatment—initial broad-spectrum antibiosis with resultant tailoring per sensitivities.
d. Ventilator-associated pneumonia—occurs in 9% to 27% of intubated patients.
  (1) More stringent diagnostic criteria
    (a) $10^5$ organisms on bronchioalveolar lavage
    (b) Forty-eight to 72 hours after endotracheal intubation
  (2) Antibiotic treatment

**TABLE 14-4**

**CATHETER-RELATED SEPSIS**

| Uncomplicated | Complicated |
|---|---|
| As demonstrated by positive blood and catheter cultures | As demonstrated by:<br>Septic thrombosis<br>Endocarditis<br>Osteomyelitis or other metastatic seeding<br>Intravascular prosthetic device |

**TREATMENT**

| | |
|---|---|
| Coagulase-negative *Staphylococcus* infection—5–7 days vancomycin or semisynthetic penicillin if isolate sensitive<br>*S. aureus*—14 days of beta-lactam if not methicillin-resistant *S. aureus;* vancomycin otherwise<br>Gram-negative bacilli—10–14 days of systemic antibiotics with activity against *Pseudomonas*<br>*Candida*—14 days of fluconazole in patients who are hemodynamically stable; otherwise, amphotericin-B or if patient has received fluconazole in the last 14 days | Systemic antibiotic therapy for 4–8 weeks depending on type of organism, site of infection, and response to therapy |

Adapted from Mermel LA, Farr BM, Sherertz RJ, et al: Guidelines for the management of intravascular catheter-related infections. *Clin Infect Dis* 32:1257–1260, 2001.

     (a) Monotherapy often sufficient for patients on the ventilator less than 7 days

     (b) More aggressive combination therapy may be necessary for patients at risk for multidrug-resistant organisms such as *Pseudomonas,* the extended-spectrum β-lactamase–producing organisms (*Klebsiella*, *Serratia*, and *Enterobacter*), and methicillin-resistant *Staphylococcus aureus.*

**4. *C. difficile* (pseudomembranous) colitis—mortality rate is 6% to 30% when pseudomembranous colitis is present.**

a. Overgrowth of *C. difficile*, a gram-positive, spore-forming rod that is an obligate anaerobe

     (1) Antibiotics cause alterations in normal colonic flora. All antibiotics have been implicated (most notably, clindamycin, third-generation cephalosporins, and fluoroquinolones).

     (2) Mucosal damage caused by two exotoxins, A and B, possibly via disruption of intestinal epithelial cytoskeleton. An epidemic strain described in 2005 identified a deletion in a pathogenicity locus gene, *tcdC,* which may increase toxin production.

     (3) Binary toxin clostridium difficile toxin (CDT)—questionably pathogenic itself but may potentiate the action of toxins A and B. It has been implicated in *C. difficile* epidemic strains.

       (4) Pseudomembranes—dead epithelial cells, WBCs, fibrin, and mucus

b. Clinical manifestations
    (1) Watery, often nonbloody diarrhea
    (2) Fever, leukocytosis, and abdominal pain may be present.
    (3) Often 5 to 10 days after antibiotic initiation
    (4) Can range from diarrhea to fulminant colitis.

c. Diagnosis: Know what assays your laboratory uses!
    (1) Cell cytotoxicity assay is the gold standard but labor intensive and inefficient.
    (2) Enzyme-linked immunosorbent assay for exotoxins A and B is becoming more sensitive and specific.

d. Treatment
    (1) Antibiotics for treatment
       (a) Metronidazole—first-line treatment and oral is preferred dosage route. Initiate 2 to 3 days after onset of symptoms if patients fail to respond. More recently, greater failure (22%) and recurrence (33%) rates have been reported.
       (b) Vancomycin—second-line treatment because of cost and potential development of resistance. Oral formulation is the only effective dosage form because it is not absorbed and stays inside the gastrointestinal lumen. Recommended in the following patients:
          1. Those who are critically ill, unable to tolerate metronidazole (Flagyl), pregnant, or younger than 10 years
          2. Those who did not respond to initial metronidazole therapy
          3. Those whose organisms were metronidazole resistant
    (2) Adjunct therapies
       (a) Bacitracin—as effective as vancomycin in isolated cases.
       (b) Nitazoxanide—early results demonstrate equivalence to metronidazole. Further studies are ongoing.
       (c) *Lactobacillus* and *Saccharomyces boulardii*—reconstitutes normal colonic flora. Can be saved for recurrent disease.
       (d) Anion exchange resins lack clinical efficacy and may bind oral antibiotics. A new resin, tolevamer, is currently being tested.
    (3) Avoid antiperistaltic agents.
    (4) Recurrence rate—occurs 8% to 50% of the time. Recurrence predicted by the following factors:
       (a) New exposure to antibiotics, especially multiple antibiotics
       (b) Age older than 65 years
       (c) Severity of underlying illness
       (d) Low serum albumin levels ($<2.5$ g/dl)
       (e) Stay in the intensive care unit
       (f) Hospitalization for 16 to 30 days

e. After a single recurrence, repeat metronidazole. After a second, give oral vancomycin. Both of these can be tapered over 6 weeks to prevent further recurrence.

**14**

**SURGICAL INFECTION**

    f. Prevention—strict contact isolation and sanitization, including hand washing, is important for prevention of transmission. Alcohol-based hand washes DO NOT destroy spores.

5. Other sources—pulmonary embolus, drug fevers, sinusitis (in patients with endotracheal, nasogastric, or nasoenteric tubes), perirectal abscess, acalculous cholecystitis (in critically ill, burn, or chronically NPO [nothing by mouth] patients)

**Case Scenario:** *A 64-year-old man with a history of diabetes presents to the emergency department with right shin redness and swelling after he scraped his knee on a sidewalk when he tripped and fell.*

## VII. DIAGNOSIS

### A. HISTORY
1. Characteristics of pain
a. *Onset*—5 days of pain
b. *Provocative factors*—pressure applied to the area and prolonged standing worsen pain.
c. *Palliative factors*—none
d. *Quality of pain*—aching throughout
e. *Radiation of pain*—into his foot and calf
f. *Severity*—4 to 6 on a scale of 10
2. Other possible associated symptoms
a. Fever
b. Other classic soft-tissue symptoms
    (1) Pain (dolor)
    (2) Warmth (calor)
    (3) Swelling (tumor)
    (4) Redness (rubor)
    (5) Loss of function (functio laesa)
3. Medical history
a. System-specific history—previous history of left hand cellulitis
b. Medical comorbidities indicate overall health status and susceptibility to infection—diabetes, asthma with recent hospitalization for exacerbation, coronary artery disease.
4. Surgical history—none significant
5. Allergies/medications—allergy to penicillin; currently taking metformin, glyburide, metoprolol, hydrochlorothiazide, steroid taper, albuterol, and ipratropium bromide (Atrovent)
6. Social history—one pack per day smoker, drinks alcohol daily

### B. PHYSICAL EXAMINATION
1. General—review of vital signs, appears malnourished
2. Pulmonary—bilateral wheezes

3. Extremities—2 × 2-cm area of induration and swelling over the right mid tibia. There is an associated 5 × 6-cm erythematous area surrounding it.
4. Neurologic—intact knee and ankle range of motion in the affected limb

### C. LABORATORY VALUES
1. Complete blood count—WBC count of 11,000/mm$^3$ with 60% band forms
2. Amylase—70 units/L
3. Lipase—60 units/L
4. C-reactive protein—110 mg/L

### D. SOURCE CONTROL
1. Incision and drainage of the lesion with daily packing and dressing changes
2. Trace the area of cellulitis to follow resolution of infection.
3. Send fluid cultures.

### E. ANTIBIOTIC
1. Broad-spectrum antibiosis given history of diabetes, steroid use, and tobacco use until sensitivities return

## VIII. SKIN AND SOFT-TISSUE INFECTIONS

### A. FOCAL INFECTIONS
1. Cutaneous abscesses
a. Furuncle or "boil"—abscess in a sweat gland or hair follicle
b. Carbuncle—multilocular suppurative extension of a furuncle into adjacent subcutaneous tissue; usually caused by staph infection
c. Impetigo—intraepithelial abscesses, usually caused by staph or strep
2. Pyoderma gangrenosum—rare
a. Painful, raised pustule with necrotic center that progresses to spreading ulceration
b. Sixty percent to 80% are associated with an underlying disease—inflammatory bowel disease, polyarthritis, or leukemia.
c. Treat with local wound care and antibiosis. Must treat underlying condition.

### B. DIFFUSE NONNECROTIZING INFECTIONS
1. Cellulitis
a. Nonsuppurative inflammation of subcutaneous tissues
b. Presents with redness, swelling, pain, often fever and chills
c. Strep and staph infections are most common. Gram-negative rods may be present, especially in patients with diabetes.
d. Failure to improve after 72 hours of antibiotics suggests abscess formation or necrotizing process, requiring incision and drainage.
2. Lymphangitis
a. Inflammation of lymphatic channels manifested by erythematous streaks

14

SURGICAL INFECTION

| TABLE 14-5 | |
|---|---|
| **ANTIBIOTIC THERAPY IN SOFT-TISSUE INFECTIONS** | |
| Type of Infection | Antibiotic |
| Mixed infection, i.e., both gram-positive and -negative organisms, as well as anaerobes (often occurs in diabetic and immunosuppressed patients) | Piperacillin/tazobactam, imipenem, ertapenem; the addition of vancomycin may be necessary until MRSA has been eliminated |
| Gram-positive skin organisms | First-generation cephalosporins, amoxicillin/clavulanate |
| Gram-negative organisms | Fluoroquinolones |
| Methicillin-resistant *Staphylococcus aureus* (MRSA) | Bactrim, doxycycline, linezolid depending on resistance patterns |
| *Clostridium perfringens,* group A *Streptococcus* | High-dose intramuscular penicillin |

b. Often accompanies cellulitis and is associated with strep.
c. Regional lymphadenopathy is usually seen.
d. Appropriate antibiosis is often sufficient.

3. **Erysipelas**
   a. Acute spreading streptococcal cellulitis and lymphangitis
   b. Also responds well to antibiosis

## C. DIFFUSE NECROTIZING INFECTIONS (TABLE 14-5)

1. **Nonclostridial**
   a. A spectrum of life-threatening necrotizing infections, including:
      (1) Necrotizing fasciitis
      (2) Fournier's gangrene—necrotizing fasciitis of the perineum
      (3) Gram-negative, synergistic, necrotizing cellulitis
   b. Causal organisms are anaerobic strep, staph, and *Bacteroides.*
   c. Characterized by erythematous skin, edema at the margins, crepitus, and possible hemodynamic instability because of sepsis
   d. Diagnosis—serosanguineous exudates, necrotic fascia, and Gram stain
   e. Treatment—emergent wide debridement to viable tissue and broad-spectrum beta-lactam antibiotics. Consider adding clindamycin to decrease toxin production.

2. **Clostridial**
   a. Often caused by *perfringens* species
   b. Occurs in the immediate postoperative period (postoperative days 0–1)
   c. Indicated by murky discharge from the wound
   d. Treatment—emergent debridement and high-dose intramuscular penicillin

# PART IV

# Anesthesia

# Local Anesthesia

*Rian A. Maercks, MD*

Local anesthetics may simplify the treatment of many surgical ailments without the risks of general anesthesia. The surgeon should have an understanding of the risks, benefits, and appropriate applications. Understanding anatomy and the limits of regional anesthesia is paramount to appropriate clinical use.

## I. INJECTABLE AGENTS

### A. AGENTS

1. Amides include a second *i* in their name (i.e., lidocaine) and are not typically associated with allergy. Esters do not contain a second *l* and are associated with allergic reactions.
2. Lidocaine and bupivacaine (Marcaine) are the most commonly used agents for surgical procedures.
   a. Lidocaine provides 1 to 2 hours of anesthesia, whereas Marcaine provides 5 to 7 hours.
   b. Remember the pneumonic "357 Magnum" (a popular hand gun)—3-5-7 corresponds to the maximum dose (in mg/kg) of bupivacaine, lidocaine, and lidocaine with epinephrine, respectively.
   c. Epinephrine delays systemic absorption and increases the dose that is well tolerated.
3. Commonly used agents
   a. Procaine (Novocain, Planocaine)—dosage: 14 mg/kg; duration: 0.5 hour
   b. **Lidocaine** (Xylocaine, Xylotox)—dosage: **5 mg/kg, 7 mg/kg with epinephrine;** duration: 1 to 2 hours
   c. Mepivacaine (Carbocaine, Polocaine)—dosage: 7 mg/kg; duration: 1 to 2 hours
   d. Tetracaine (Pontocaine, Pantocaine)—dosage: 1.5 mg/kg; duration: 2 to 3 hours
   e. **Bupivacaine** (Marcaine)—dosage: **3 mg/kg;** duration: 5 to 7 hours
4. Standard solution: For the majority of emergency room procedures, a solution of 0.5% lidocaine with 1:5 bicarbonate should be prepared. This solution works well, application is well tolerated, and has easy dosing. One milliliter of solution (5 mg) can be given per kilogram of body weight. A 70-kg patient can receive 70 ml local anesthesia. This solution will avoid adverse effects, as a stock solution of 1% to 2% can get to toxic doses quickly in a multitrauma patient.
   a. In a 10-ml syringe, add:
      5 ml 1% lidocaine
      3 ml injectable saline
      2 ml $HCO_3$ solution
5. For short- and long-term pain control, a solution of 0.5% lidocaine and 0.25% Marcaine is preferred.

a. Simply combine 1% lidocaine with 0.5% Marcaine 1:1.
b. Four milliliters 1% lidocaine, 4 ml 0.5% Marcaine, and 2 ml 8.4% $HCO_3$ in a 10-ml syringe yields 8 ml of this solution for dosing purposes.

### B. MECHANISM-PHASIC BLOCK (STIMULATED CHANNELS) OF SODIUM CHANNELS

1. Only uncharged forms enter peripheral nerves; thus, locals perform better in alkaline environments. Infected and inflamed fields can be treated more effectively by alkalinizing the solution with $HCO_3$ (see application). Once the agent reaches the cytoplasm, the ionized form is able to block sodium channels.

### C. TOXICITY

1. Central nervous system toxicity is biphasic, initially excitatory with lowering of seizure threshold. Further increase in levels causes central nervous system depression with drowsiness, unconsciousness, and cardiac arrest.
2. First sign of central nervous system toxicity is often perioral numbness and visual disturbances. Discontinue procedure if these symptoms ensue, and prepare to treat seizure with 100% $O_2$, benzodiazepines, and airway control.
3. Cardiac toxicity is caused by much greater levels of local than central nervous system toxicity. Bupivacaine (Marcaine) is an exception. Bupivacaine has a high affinity for Purkinje fibers and can cause arrhythmias such as ventricular fibrillation that are refractory to treatment. For this reason, special care is taken to avoid intravascular injections when bupivacaine is used.

## II. TECHNIQUES

Before injecting local anesthetic in traumatic injuries, be sure to perform and document a detailed sensory examination.

### A. FIELD BLOCKS

A field block involves blocking nerves circumferentially around the periphery of a wound. It is useful for wounds without a specific nerve or nerves that can be blocked directly. Ideally, a bicarbonate-containing solution should be used to minimize pain on application and improve efficacy near abscesses and acidic environments. A subcutaneous wheal should be created on entering the skin. Allow the wheal to dissect ahead of the needle. In this manner, the patient should not feel much more than on stick.

### B. NERVE BLOCKS FOR THE FACE

1. Supratrochlear and supraorbital nerve block
a. The supraorbital and supratrochlear nerves and extensions of the frontal branch of the first division of the trigeminal after it exits the

supraorbital fissure. Together, they supply sensory innervation to the anterior scalp.

b. The supraorbital foramen can be located at the superior orbital rim above the pupil in midline gaze. Palpate the foramen while retracting the brow laterally.

c. Enter the lateral aspect of the middle third of the brow and aim for the foramen.

d. Inject 2 ml at this point. Keep your other hand at the orbital rim to protect the orbit. Advance the needle, continuing a wheal until the nasal bone is contacted; 2 to 5 ml of desired local agent should be used.

## 2. Infraorbital nerve block

a. The infraorbital nerve is an extension of the second division of the trigeminal. It provides sensation to the lower eyelid, upper lip, the tip and lateral aspect of the nose, and part of the nasal septum.

b. The infraorbital foramen can be located just below the midpoint of the pupil in midline gaze. Digital palpation causes pain (try it on yourself).

c. An intraoral route is generally preferred; inject a wheal into the gingivobuccal sulcus just above the maxillary first premolar. While palpating the foramen externally, advance the needle to contact maxilla adjacent to the foramen. Keep a finger firmly on the foramen to protect the orbit. Aspirate first!

d. Inject 1 to 2 ml while your external digit feels the wheal expand. If perioral or intraoral lacerations are present, engage the foramen by injecting percutaneously above the foramen.

## 3. Complete V3 block

a. There are multiple approaches to anesthetize the inferior alveolar nerve through intraoral injections. The preferred approach to access the nerve high in its course is percutaneous. This is preferable in trauma to the mouth and mandible because intraoral injection may not be tolerated by the patient.

b. Just below the zygoma, the sigmoid notch of the mandible can be palpated 2.5 cm anterior to the tragus. Ask the patient to open and close his or her mouth; the condyle will bump against your finger.

c. Administer a subcutaneous wheal at the midpoint of the sigmoid notch.

d. With a long fine-gauge needle, such as a 25-gauge spinal needle, enter straight through the anterior portion of the sigmoid notch and advance until it hits the pterygoid plate. Note the needle position and retract the needle almost out of the skin. Advance the needle to the same depth, aiming 1 cm posterior to the previous point of pterygoid contact. ASPIRATE! Inject 3 to 4 ml.

e. The anesthetized area includes most of the cheek from the preauricular area to the mandibular border, the mandible to midline.

f. Alternatively, the intraoral Gow–Gates approach can be completed (considered safer for the neophyte). With the patient's mouth maximally opened, identify the maxillary second molar. The syringe should angle

**15**

**LOCAL ANESTHESIA**

such that it crosses the contralateral oral commissure. Advance the needle approximately 2.5 cm until the condyle is encountered, and aspirate. Withdraw 1 mm and advance superiorly. Aspirate again and, if negative, inject 2 to 3 ml of local.

4. **Mental nerve block/mental plus block**
a. The mental foramen varies in position from 1 cm distal to 1 cm mesial to the second mandibular bicuspid.
b. Effective blocks are achieved by engaging the nerve within 1 cm of the foramen. An intraoral approach is preferred. Apply lateral traction on the lower lip near the canine. The nerve is sometimes visible or palpable through the mucosa while on traction.
c. Injection of 2 ml submucosal in this area provides anesthesia to the ipsilateral lower lip.
d. To anesthetize the chin, the distal branches of the mental nerve and the mylohyoid branches must be addressed. This can be done by inserting the needle anterior to the canine and passing the inferior border of the mandible. Inject 2 ml using a fanning technique. This block can be referred to the mental plus block. These regions are all covered by a V3 block.

5. **Dorsal nasal block:** The dorsal nasal nerve, a branch of the anterior ethmoidal, emerges at the inferior border of the nasal bone approximately 6 mm from midline. Bilateral injection at these points anesthetizes the nasal tip and cartilaginous dorsum.

6. **Zygomaticotemporal and zygomaticofacial block.**
a. The zygomaticotemporal and zygomaticofacial nerves exit foramens on the concave lateral orbital rim. They are addressed by palpating the zygomaticofrontal suture and inserting a needle 0.5 cm inferior to the suture and 1 cm posterior to the superolateral orbital rim.
b. Aiming 1 cm below to the lateral canthus, the zygoma is encountered; 2 to 3 ml of local anesthesia is injected while withdrawing the needle.
c. Area of anesthesia includes the temporal scalp abutting the area of supraorbital innervation and the zygomatic arch. The zygomaticofacial block includes a wedge of the lateral malar check area overlying the zygoma.

7. **Great auricular nerve**
a. To identify the greater auricular nerve, have the patient turn his or her head against your hand placed on the ipsilateral forehead.
b. At the midpoint of the SCM 6.5 cm from the inferior aspect of the external auditory canal, the nerve can be reliably located.
c. Inject 2 ml of local anesthesia just over the muscle at this point. Anesthesia is provided to the lower third of the ear, postauricular skin, and a variable area of the tragus down toward the mandibular angle. The ear should be addressed as a field block because there are multiple nerve contributions. Injecting a large wheal anterior and posterior connecting with each other will anesthetize the entire ear.

## C.  UPPER EXTREMITY

When performing nerve blocks, do not use more than gentle pressure on injection to avoid intraneural injection. Patients may describe shooting pain/paresthesias if the needle enters the nerve. If this occurs, reposition the needle before injecting. Although it is unlikely to compromise perfusion, using epinephrine in the hand and fingers is advised against.

### 1.  Digital block

a. Provides anesthesia for fingers from base to tip by blocking the digital nerves bilaterally.

b. Start by injecting a wheal to either side of the base of the proximal phalanx of the finger to be anesthetized.

c. Insert the needle adjacent to the phalanx while the index finger of your other hand palpates the volar surface of the hand in the trajectory of the needle.

d. Advance the needle until you feel the needle tent the volar skin.

e. Inject a 2-ml wheal and slowly remove the needle, delivering another milliliter.

f. Next, without exiting the skin, create a wheal across the dorsum of the finger and repeat the procedure through anesthetized skin to bathe the contralateral digital nerve.

### 2.  Wrist block—provides complete hand anesthesia

a. Targets the median and ulnar nerves and the dorsal sensory branch of the radial nerve.

b. Depending on the area of injury or procedure, only parts of the wrist block may be necessary. The distributions of the median, ulnar, and radial nerves are outlined below.

### 3.  Median nerve block

a. The median nerve sits just below and radial to the palmaris longus under the flexor retinaculum.

b. Injection landmarks include the palmaris longus if present and the flexor carpi radialis at the wrist crease.

c. Inject a subcutaneous wheal to anesthetize the skin; then advance the needle through the fascia. A "click" may or may not be noted.

d. Advance at a 45- to 60-degree angle, aiming at the base of the fourth finger to contact the bone of the distal carpal row.

e. Withdraw the needle about 2 mm, aspirate, and inject 2 to 4 ml local anesthesia with gentle pressure. If the local does not flow freely, reposition the needle.

f. Injecting in a fanning manner by performing initial injection, then repeating, aiming toward the third digit, may improve success.

### 4.  Ulnar nerve block

a. The ulnar nerve sits between the flexor carpi ulnaris and the ulnar artery.

b. The flexor carpi ulnaris can be easily identified by having the patient forcefully flex the wrist.

**15**

**LOCAL ANESTHESIA**

c. The preferred approach is to enter the ulnar (medially) aspect of the wrist just dorsal (deep) to the flexor carpi ulnaris after administering a skin wheal.

d. Insert the needle 5 to 10 mm, aspirate, and inject 3 to 5 ml of local anesthesia. An additional 2 ml is useful subcutaneously to block cutaneous branches to the hypothenar area.

5. Radial nerve block

a. The dorsal sensory branches of the radial nerve are multiple and less predictable than the other nerves described.

b. To anesthetize the radial portion of the hand, use a subcutaneous field block from the radial styloid to the radial dorsum of the wrist; approximately 5 ml is required.

## III. TOPICAL AGENTS

### A. COCAINE

1. Cocaine was the first widely used local anesthetic.
2. Added benefit of vasoconstriction for hemostasis, that is, closed reduction of nasal fractures
3. Systemic toxicity cardiovascular collapse
4. Application

a. Cocaine should be used in all closed reductions of nasal fractures that can be safely completed at bedside.

b. On neuropatties 1 × 3 inches

c. Place neuropatties saturated with 4% cocaine solution into bilateral nares directed superiorly. Systemic absorption is minimized with this technique. Allow 5 to 10 minutes for mucosal anesthesia and vasoconstriction. Technique may be repeated once.

d. Never apply cocaine directly to mucosa because systemic absorption is rapid.

e. May combine this technique with a nasal block (see later).

### B. TOPICAL SKIN AGENTS

These are used in many pediatric institutions. The rather unpredictable level of anesthesia and long-term requirements limit their usefulness.

1. TAC (tetracaine 0.5%, adrenaline 0.05%, cocaine 11.8%)—effective on face and scalp in 10 to 30 minutes. Not effective on intact skin. Theoretical concern with cocaine absorption in open wounds has limited its use.

2. LET (lidocaine 4%, epinephrine 0.1%, tetracaine 0.5%)—more cost effective and improved safety over TAC. Effective in 20 to 30 minutes applied to lacerations. Not recommended for use on lacerations greater than 6 cm or complicated wounds.

3. EMLA (eutectic mixture of local anesthetics)—consists of 25 mg/ml lidocaine, 25 mg/ml prilocaine, a thickener, an emulsifier, and distilled water adjusted to a pH level of 9.4. EMLA is approved for use on intact nonmucosal surfaces. It provides anesthesia in 90 minutes. A liposomal preparation has a more rapid onset and efficacy.

# Conscious Sedation

*Renee Nierman Kreeger, MD*

As the world of medicine expands and, with it, the ability to perform less invasive procedures, the necessity for understanding and being able to administer conscious sedation becomes paramount for nearly all practitioners. It is no longer solely the role of the anesthesiologist to provide sedation and analgesia for patients undergoing less complex, but still painful or stimulating procedures. One must be familiar with the pharmacology, physiology, and techniques necessary to safely deliver sedation.

## I. INTRODUCTION
### A. DEFINITION
1. Sedation is "a minimally depressed level of consciousness that retains the patient's ability to independently and continuously maintain an airway and respond appropriately to physical stimulation and verbal commands" (American Dental Association Council on Education).
2. Comprises a continuum from minimal sedation to general anesthesia (American Society of Anesthesiologists Guidelines) (Table 16-1)

### B. APPLICATIONS (SELECTED)
1. Emergency department procedures
2. Central venous line insertions
3. Chest tube insertions

## II. PREPROCEDURAL EVALUATION
### A. HISTORY
1. General history and review of systems, including tobacco, alcohol, and drug use history
2. Previous anesthetics and any adverse outcomes
3. Airway abnormalities (e.g., obstructive sleep apnea, severe snoring, stridor, previous tracheostomy)
4. Rheumatoid arthritis
5. Chromosomal abnormalities and/or syndromes (e.g., Down's syndrome)
6. Gastroesophageal reflux disease/hiatal hernia
7. Obesity
8. Adequate intravenous (IV) access in situ

### B. AIRWAY EXAMINATION
1. General assessment of patient (e.g., body habitus, presence of cervical collar)
2. Mallampati examination (Fig. 16-1)
3. Mouth opening (adults should have 3- to 4-cm distance between upper and lower incisors)

**TABLE 16-1**

| | Minimal Sedation (Anxiolysis) | Moderate Sedation/Analgesia (Conscious Sedation) | Deep Sedation/Analgesia | General Anesthesia |
|---|---|---|---|---|
| Responsiveness | Normal response to verbal stimulation | Purposeful* response to verbal or tactile stimulation | Purposeful* response after repeated or painful stimulation | Unarousable, even with painful stimulus |
| Airway | Unaffected | No intervention required | Intervention may be required | Intervention often required |
| Spontaneous ventilation | Unaffected | Adequate | May be inadequate | Frequently inadequate |
| Cardiovascular function | Unaffected | Usually maintained | Usually maintained | May be impaired |

*Because sedation is a continuum, it is not always possible to predict how an individual patient will respond. Hence practitioners intending to produce a given level of sedation should be able to rescue patients whose level of sedation becomes deeper than initially intended.

Modified from document developed by the American Society of Anesthesiologists (ASA); approved by the ASA House of Delegates, October 13, 1999.

4. Thyromental distance (distance from thyroid cartilage to mandible; should be at least 5 cm in adults)
5. Neck extension
a. Assess for any cervical spine abnormalities or disorders associated with atlantooccipital instability.

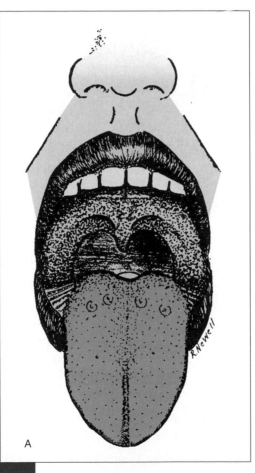

A

**FIG. 16-1**

Mallampati classification: class I—faucial pillars, soft palate, and uvula are visible; class II—faucial pillars and soft palate are visible, and uvula view is obstructed by base of tongue; class III—only soft and hard palates are visible; and class IV—only hard palate visible.

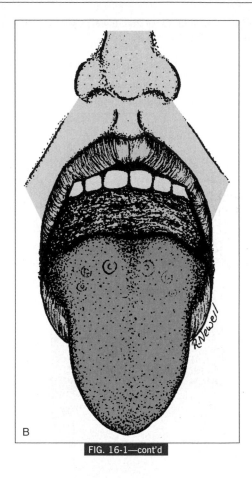

B

FIG. 16-1—cont'd

   b. Lack of extension or significantly reduced extension may indicate
      difficulty with direct laryngoscopy.
**6. Any craniofacial/bony abnormalities**
a. Receding mandible
b. High, arched palate
c. Syndromes (e.g., Pierre Robin, Treacher Collins)
**7. Dentition**
**8. Facial hair (presence of a beard or other significant facial hair may
   signal difficult mask ventilation)**

C. **AMERICAN SOCIETY OF ANESTHESIOLOGISTS FASTING GUIDELINES (TABLE 16-2)**
1. Need to follow for all elective procedures
2. May be modified in emergency situations at discretion of practitioner

## III. MONITORING
A. **BEST ACHIEVED BY SOMEONE OTHER THAN PERSON PERFORMING PROCEDURE**
B. **CLINICAL ASSESSMENT**
1. Most important monitor
2. Needs to be ongoing
3. Examples: respiratory status, general well-being, color, among others

C. **BLOOD PRESSURE**
D. **PULSE OXIMETRY**
E. **ELECTROCARDIOGRAM**
F. **CAPNOGRAPHY (USUALLY WITH DEEP SEDATION OR GENERAL ANESTHESIA ONLY; NOT AVAILABLE IN ALL PATIENT CARE AREAS)**
G. **APPROPRIATE ALARMS ON MONITOR**
H. **SUPPLEMENTAL OXYGEN**

**16**

**CONSCIOUS SEDATION**

---

**TABLE 16-2**

SUMMARY OF FASTING RECOMMENDATIONS
TO REDUCE THE RISK FOR PULMONARY ASPIRATION*

| Ingested Material | Minimum Fasting Period (hr)[†] |
|---|---|
| Clear liquids[‡] | 2 |
| Breast milk | 4 |
| Infant formula | 6 |
| Nonhuman milk[§] | 6 |
| Light meal[‖] | 6 |

*These recommendations apply to healthy patients who are undergoing elective procedures. They are not intended for women in labor. Following the guidelines does not guarantee complete gastric emptying.
[†]The fasting periods noted apply to all ages.
[‡]Examples of clear liquids include water, fruit juices without pulp, carbonated beverages, clear tea, and black coffee.
[§]Because nonhuman milk is similar to solids in gastric emptying time, the amount ingested must be considered when determining an appropriate fasting period.
[‖]A light meal typically consists of toast and clear liquids. Meals that include fried or fatty foods or meat may prolong gastric emptying time. Both the amount and type of foods ingested must be considered when determining an appropriate fasting period.

## IV. AVAILABILITY OF EMERGENCY MEDICAL EQUIPMENT AND PERSONNEL

A. **IMMEDIATE ACCESS TO SUCTION, BAG-MASK VENTILATION, INTUBATION MATERIALS, DEFIBRILLATOR, AND EMERGENCY (ADVANCED CARDIAC LIFE SUPPORT) MEDICATIONS**

B. **ANESTHESIA OR OTHER TRAINED AIRWAY STAFF IN CLOSE PROXIMITY**

## V. TRAINING IN AIRWAY MANAGEMENT

A. **ABILITY TO PROVIDE ESCALATING LEVELS OF AIRWAY SUPPORT**

B. **EXPERIENCE IN CONTROLLED SETTING WITH SKILLED EXPERTS**

C. **KNOWLEDGE OF AIRWAY ADJUNCTS AND THEIR APPROPRIATE USE**

## VI. MEDICATIONS

A. **NARCOTICS**

1. Used for both analgesia and sedation
2. All produce dose-dependent respiratory depression, with increased risk in those at extremes of age.
3. Other common side effects include but are not limited to orthostatic hypotension, pruritus, nausea and vomiting, constipation, and urinary retention.
4. Titrate to desired effect using small, incremental dosing.
5. Doses provided are for adults; see pediatric literature for pediatric dosing.

a. Morphine sulfate:
   (1) Prototypic narcotic
   (2) Dose: 2 to 5 mg IV
   (3) Peak effect in 20 to 30 minutes

b. Fentanyl (Sublimaze):
   (1) 100 times more potent than morphine
   (2) Dose: 25 to 50 $\mu$g IV
   (3) Onset in 1 to 3 minutes
   (4) Chest wall rigidity at large doses

c. Hydromorphone (Dilaudid):
   (1) Approximately five times more potent than morphine
   (2) Dose: 0.2 to 0.4 mg IV
   (3) Onset in approximately 15 minutes; peaks at 1 hour
   (4) Lacks histamine release associated with morphine

d. Meperidine (Demerol):
   (1) 1/10 as potent as morphine
   (2) Dose: 12.5 to 50 mg IV
   (3) Helpful with postoperative shivering

## B. BENZODIAZEPINES
1. Enhance affinity of receptors for $\gamma$-aminobutyric acid
2. Produce sedation and anterograde amnesia
3. Side effects: respiratory depression, disorientation
4. CAUTION: May potentiate sedative effects of narcotics; may have paradoxic or exaggerated effects in patients at extremes of age.
5. Titrate to desired effect using small incremental dosing.
6. Doses provided are for adults; see pediatric literature for pediatric dosing.
a. Midazolam (Versed):
   (1) Initial dose of 0.5 to 2 mg IV
   (2) Onset within 30 to 60 seconds
   (3) Peak effect at 3 to 5 minutes
   (4) Duration of sedation (varies): 15 to 80 minutes
   (5) Metabolized by cytochrome P-450 system
b. Diazepam (Valium):
   (1) Dose: 2 to 5 mg IV
   (2) Slower onset (1–3 minutes)
c. Lorazepam (Ativan):
   (1) Dose: 0.5 to 1 mg IV
   (2) Slow onset (5–15 minutes)

## C. NONBARBITURATE ANESTHETIC DRUGS (ONLY INCLUDED TO MAKE REVIEW COMPLETE; SHOULD BE USED ONLY BY TRAINED ANESTHESIA PROVIDERS).
1. Propofol (Diprivan):
a. Potent IV sedative
b. No analgesic properties
c. Use not recommended for light-to-moderate sedation
   (1) Causes profound, rapid decline in level of consciousness, producing a state of general anesthesia if not carefully titrated
   (2) Practitioners must be able to rescue patient from any level of sedation, including general anesthesia, to administer.

## VII. REVERSAL MEDICATIONS
### A. NALOXONE (NARCAN)
1. Opioid antagonist
2. Dose: 40 to 100 $\mu$g IV (adult dose)
3. Side effects: pulmonary edema, tachycardia, hypertension, arrhythmias, nausea/vomiting, **pain**
4. CAUTION: Short duration of action (30–45 minutes) makes redosing often necessary.

### B. FLUMAZENIL (ROMAZICON)
1. Benzodiazepine competitive antagonist
2. Initial dose: 0.01 mg/kg IV (maximum, 0.2 mg)

16

**CONSCIOUS SEDATION**

3. Subsequent doses of 0.005 to 0.01 mg/kg/dose to maximum cumulative dose of 1 mg administered at 60-second intervals.
4. Side effects: acute anxiety, hypertension, tachycardia
5. CAUTION: Duration of action is 30 to 60 minutes, necessitating redosing.

## VIII. RECOVERY AND DISCHARGE

### A. GENERAL PRINCIPLES

1. Patients must remain in areas where monitoring is feasible.
2. Patients should be monitored closely at intervals determined by the practitioner until discharge criteria is met (see later).
3. Personnel capable of recognizing and managing complications must be present at all times.

### B. DISCHARGE GUIDELINES

1. Vital signs are stable and within acceptable limits for individual patient.
2. Patient is alert and oriented or at baseline mental status.
3. Sufficient time has elapsed since last medication or reversal agent dosage to allow for recovery.
4. Outpatients must have appropriate guardian to escort home and remain with patient for at least 24 hours.
5. Outpatients must receive written instructions for care at home, diet, restrictions, and so forth.

## RECOMMENDED REFERENCES

Mallampati RS, Gatt SP, Gugino LD, et al: A clinical sign to predict difficult tracheal intubation: A prospective study. *Canadian Anaesthetists Society Journal* 32:429–434, 1985.

Practice Guidelines for Preoperative Fasting and the Use of Pharmacologic Agents to Reduce the Risk of Pulmonary Aspiration: Application to Healthy Patients Undergoing Elective Procedures: A Report by The American Society of Anesthesiologists Task Force on Preoperative Fasting. *Anesthesiology* 90:896–905, 1999.

Practice Guidelines for Sedation and Analgesia by Non-anesthesiologists. *Anesthesiology* 96:1004–1017, 2002.

# General Anesthesia

*Paul J. Wojciechowski, MD*

Although an anesthesiologist plays an integral role in the perioperative management of patients, the surgeon should be familiar with the various anesthesia techniques and their potential impact on the surgical patient. Communication between the surgeon and the anesthesiologist is paramount to improved perioperative outcomes.

## I. PREOPERATIVE ASSESSMENT AND PREPARATION

### A. SURGICAL INTERVENTION OR PROCEDURE BEING PERFORMED

1. Careful attention must be paid to verification of site.

### B. CHART REVIEW

1. Previous anesthetic records
a. Review for history of difficult airway, success of specific techniques, and intraoperative complications.
2. Consults from medicine, cardiology, or anesthesia departments

### C. HISTORY

1. Medical and surgical histories
a. Has the patient received general or regional anesthesia in the past?
2. Anesthesia history
a. History of malignant hyperthermia
b. Family history of malignant hyperthermia
c. History of postoperative nausea and vomiting (PONV)
d. History of difficult intubation
3. Current medications
a. Special attention paid to anticoagulants, beta-blockers, antihypertensives, diuretics, oral hypoglycemics, and antidepressants, especially monoamine oxidase inhibitors
4. Drug allergies (including latex)
5. Review of systems
a. Particular attention should be paid to pulmonary and cardiovascular history, including an assessment of functional status with documentation of level of activity.
6. Fasting status–"NPO status" (see Chapter 16 for American Society of Anesthesiologists Guidelines)

### D. PHYSICAL EXAMINATION

1. Vital signs, including height and weight
2. Airway examination
a. Size of tongue versus pharynx (Mallampati classes I-IV; see Chapter 16)
b. Cervical spine mobility

c. Anterior mandibular space—distance from the notch of the thyroid cartilage to the tip of the mentum (thyromental distance) while the head is maximally extended; <6 cm (receding mandible, short muscular neck) increases the risk for difficulty encountered during intubation

d. Dentition—noting loose, chipped, cracked teeth and dentures or dental appliances

3. Neurologic examination
4. Cardiovascular examination—noting murmurs, S3 gallop, jugular venous distention
5. Respiratory examination
6. Abdominal examination
7. Examination of regional anesthesia site (if applicable)
a. Locating surface anatomy and noting abnormalities including signs of localized infection

## E.  LABORATORY DATA
1. Complete blood cell count if history of anemia or ongoing bleeding
2. Electrolytes, blood urea nitrogen, and creatinine for patients with a history of renal disease or currently taking diuretics
3. Prothrombin time, international normalized ratio, and partial thromboplastin time if patient is taking anticoagulants or has history of coagulopathy

## F.  RADIOLOGY, CARDIOLOGY, OTHER PREOPERATIVE TESTING
1. Plain radiographs, computed tomography, magnetic resonance imaging, ultrasound
2. Echocardiogram, exercise or chemical stress test, electrocardiogram, cardiac catheterization results
3. Pulmonary function tests

## G.  ASSESSMENT
1. Detailed problem list including pertinent anesthetic, surgical, and medical issues
2. Assign American Society of Anesthesiologists Physical Classification Status using Emergency designation if appropriate:
   I —healthy patient
   II —patient with mild systemic disease
   III —patient with severe systemic disease
   IV —patient with severe systemic disease that is a constant threat to life
   V —moribund patient who is not expected to survive without the operation
   VI —declared brain-dead patient whose organs are being removed for donor purposes (classification is available online at: www.asahq.org)

## H.  ANESTHETIC PLAN
1. Determine appropriate anesthetic technique (see section II).
2. Determine whether invasive monitoring (arterial line, central venous

line, pulmonary artery catheter, transesophageal echocardiography, etc.) is necessary.
3. Decide on method for postoperative pain control (intravenous [IV] narcotics, epidural, nerve block).
4. Make preliminary decision on patient's postoperative destination (postanesthetic care unit or intensive care unit).
5. Determine whether special equipment is necessary (double-lumen ETT, fiberoptic bronchoscope, etc.).
6. Explain associated risks and benefits to patient/guardian, and document conversation in the chart.

### I. INDICATIONS FOR DELAYING OR POSTPONING ELECTIVE SURGERY
1. Uncontrolled medical disease (cardiac, respiratory, hepatic, renal, endocrine)
2. Upper respiratory infection
3. Patient noncompliance with fasting guidelines
4. Informed consent not obtained

### J. PREOPERATIVE PREPARATION
1. IV access (at least 18 or 20 gauge); may need more than one
2. Placement of invasive lines, epidurals, among others
3. Administer preoperative medications (see later).

### K. PREOPERATIVE MEDICATION GOALS
1. Anxiety relief, sedation, analgesia, amnesia
2. Control oral and bronchial secretions.
3. Increase gastric pH and decrease gastric secretions; antiemetic effects.
4. Preparation for airway manipulations (aerosolized lidocaine, viscous lidocaine)

## II. INTRAOPERATIVE MANAGEMENT
### A. EQUIPMENT
The equipment listed in this section should be present whenever an anesthetic is administered. This list is not comprehensive and additional equipment may be necessary depending on the patient and clinical situation.
1. Standard monitors
a. Noninvasive blood pressure
b. Pulse oximetry
c. Electrocardiogram—leads II and V5
d. Capnography
e. Oxygen analyzer
f. Temperature
2. Anesthesia machine
a. Suction
b. Spare oxygen tank

### 3. Airway
a. Laryngoscope handles (short and long)
b. Laryngoscope blades (Miller 2 and 3; Macintosh 3 and 4)
c. Oral airways—multiple sizes
d. Endotracheal tubes—multiple sizes
e. Stylets
f. Nasal airways
g. Oxygen delivery devices (nasal cannulas and face masks)
h. Ambu bag
i. Stethoscope

## B. TECHNIQUES OF ANESTHESIA
### 1. General anesthesia
a. Inhalational versus IV induction
b. Airway—nasotracheal versus orotracheal versus laryngeal mask airway versus mask
c. Maintenance—inhalational versus IV
d. Analgesia
e. Neuromuscular blockers
f. Reversal of neuromuscular blockers
### 2. Regional anesthesia
a. Spinal
   (1) Injection of local anesthetic into subarachnoid space
   (2) Level of anesthesia—controlled by specific gravity of injected mixture, contour of the spinal canal, and patient position
   (3) Complications—diminished sympathetic tone, vasodilation, hypotension, decreased cardiac output, spinal headache, hypoventilation (thoracic level), total spinal (block above C3), urinary retention
   (4) Contraindications—coagulopathy, infection at insertion site, neurologic dysfunction, hypovolemia, patient refusal
b. Epidural
   (1) Injection of local anesthetic into potential space bordered by dura mater and spinal canal periosteum (level of placement depends on surgical site and dermatomal coverage needed)
   (2) Complications—hypotension, infection (superficial or epidural space), epidural hematoma, local anesthetic toxicity (larger volume needed in epidural space), intravascular injection local anesthetics (epidural space has extensive venous plexus)
   (3) Contraindications—coagulopathy, infection at insertion site, neurologic dysfunction, hypovolemia, patient refusal
c. Combined spinal/epidural
Combined spinal/epidural anesthesia takes advantage of the beneficial aspects of both, that is, a rapid, reliable block with spinal anesthesia and the ability to supplement the block and provide postoperative pain relief with an epidural.

d. Caudal—injection of local anesthetic at S5 through sacrococcygeal ligament

e. Peripheral nerve blocks; local/field blocks with or without sedation

3. **Monitored anesthesia care**

a. Sedation

b. Analgesia

c. Monitoring

4. **Bier block (IV regional anesthesia)**

a. Excellent for forearm, hand, or foot procedures

b. Usually limited to 1 hour

c. Double-pneumatic tourniquet applied above elbow (or calf)

d. Initially inflate above venous pressure to distend vein, then venipuncture with 22-gauge IV line.

e. Release tourniquet, exsanguinate extremity with elevation and wrap with elastic bandage, and inflate distal tourniquet then proximal tourniquet.

f. Inject catheter with 0.5% lidocaine injection.

g. With onset of tourniquet pain (at 45 minutes), inflate distal tourniquet and release proximal tourniquet for slow release of lidocaine into systemic circulation.

## C. INTRAOPERATIVE COMPLICATIONS

Anesthesiologists are trained to recognize and prevent hemodynamic, respiratory, airway, and other difficulties that could potentially lead to intraoperative catastrophes.

1. **Hemodynamic**

a. Hypotension (bleeding, hypovolemia, etc.)

b. Hypertension

c. Tachycardia

d. Bradycardia

e. Arrhythmia

2. **Respiratory**

a. Hypoxia

b. Hypercarbia

c. Bronchospasm

3. **Airway**

a. Difficult airway

b. Airway trauma from intubation

c. Pulmonary aspiration of gastric contents

d. Laryngospasm

4. **Malignant hyperthermia**

Malignant hyperthermia is characterized by a hypermetabolic state and has a genetic predisposition. It is presumed that a defect in the calcium release channel sustains greater concentrations of calcium in the myoplasm, causing persistent skeletal muscle contraction after administration of succinylcholine or volatile anesthetics, or both. Definitive diagnosis is by muscle biopsy.

a. Prophylaxis—avoid malignant hyperthermia-triggering drugs in patients with suspected family history.
b. Clinical signs
  (1) Masseter rigidity after succinylcholine administration
  (2) Unexplained tachycardia and tachypnea
  (3) Arrhythmias
  (4) Cyanosis
  (5) Metabolic or respiratory acidosis, or both (increased end-tidal $CO_2$ is an early sign)
  (6) Fever is a late sign (may reach 107°F).
c. Treatment
  (1) Terminate anesthetic agent and administer nonmalignant hyperthermia-inducing agent.
  (2) Notify surgeon and request termination of the surgical procedure when possible.
  (3) Dantrolene—start with 2.5 mg/kg up to total 10 mg/kg.
  (4) Hyperventilate with 100% $O_2$.
  (5) $NaHCO_3$—guided by arterial pH
  (6) Hyperkalemia—treat with $NaHCO_3$, insulin (0.15 mg/kg), 20% dextrose.
  (7) Initiate active cooling—cooled saline, cold gastric lavage, surface cooling
d. Late complications
  (1) Consumptive coagulopathy
  (2) Acute renal failure
  (3) Hypothermia
  (4) Pulmonary edema
  (5) Skeletal muscle swelling
  (6) Neurologic sequelae

## III. PHARMACEUTICALS
### A. IV ANESTHESIA
IV anesthetics may be used as induction agents, supplemental anesthetic agents, or sole anesthetic agents.
1. Barbiturates—act at γ-aminobutyric acid receptor
a. Thiopental
  (1) Onset—immediate; awakening occurs secondary to redistribution
  (2) Side effects—respiratory depression, peripheral vasodilation, hypotension, tachycardia; use with caution in patients with coronary artery disease and hypovolemia; decreases cerebral blood flow and intracranial pressure
  (3) Contraindicated in patients with porphyrias
b. Methohexital
  (1) Side effects—myocardial depression, hypotension
2. Etomidate—acts at γ-aminobutyric acid receptor

a. Onset—rapid onset for induction and intubation
b. Side effects—adrenocortical suppression with multiple doses, myoclonus, pain on injection
c. Organ effects—cardiovascular stability maintained; potent cerebral vasoconstrictor; induction dose may not cause apnea
3. **Ketamine—acts at *N*-methyl-D-aspartate, opioid, and other receptors**
a. Dissociative anesthesia with good analgesia; acts as a bronchodilator and maintains airway reflexes; does not relieve visceral sensation; useful for brief anesthetic procedures (e.g., burn dressing changes)
b. Side effects—apnea with rapid administration, tachycardia, hypertension, increased cardiac output and myocardial oxygen demand; cerebral vasodilator and may increase cerebral blood flow and intracranial pressure; emergence hallucinations prevented by pretreatment with a benzodiazepine.
4. **Propofol—acts at γ-aminobutyric acid receptor**
a. IV hypnotic with immediate onset and rapid return with minimal central nervous system effects
b. Metabolism—conjugation in the liver to inactive metabolites that are excreted by the kidney; extrahepatic metabolism
c. Pharmacokinetics not changed by hepatic or renal failure
d. Uses—induction of anesthesia, sedation, antipruritic effect, anticonvulsant effects
e. Side effects—pain on injection; decreases mean arterial pressure; apnea
5. **Narcotics**
Narcotics are used for analgesia and sedation. Morphine, fentanyl, hydromorphone, and meperidine are common agents. See Chapter 16 for more detailed information on the pharmacology of these agents.
6. **Benzodiazepines**
Benzodiazepines provide good anterograde amnesia, anxiolysis, and sedation, and act as an anticonvulsant. Midazolam, diazepam, and lorazepam are common agents. See Chapter 16 for more detailed information on the pharmacology of these agents.

## B. NEUROMUSCULAR BLOCKING DRUGS

Patients must be adequately anesthetized before administration of neuromuscular blocking drugs because they are without analgesic or anesthetic effects. The choice of neuromuscular blocking agent depends on the desired speed of onset, duration of effect, route of elimination, and potential side effects. Clinically, the degree of neuromuscular blockade is monitored by visually monitoring a twitch response after electrical stimulation of a peripheral motor nerve (ulnar or facial nerve branch).
1. **Depolarizing agents—mimic the action of acetylcholine, producing depolarization of the postjunctional membrane**
a. Succinylcholine
    (1) Onset of action—30 to 60 seconds; duration less than 10 minutes; metabolized by pseudocholinesterase

    (2) Side effects—may cause hyperkalemia and subsequent dysrhythmias in patients with severe muscle denervation (i.e., burns, crush injury, spinal cord injury); can cause bradycardia and hypotension, as well as postoperative muscle pain (secondary to fasciculations); potent trigger of malignant hyperthermia

**2. Nondepolarizing agents**

Nondepolarizing agents are classified clinically as long-, intermediate-, and short-acting. They compete with acetylcholine for postjunctional receptors and prevent changes in membrane ion permeability.

a. Pancuronium
    (1) Renal and hepatic elimination
    (2) Side effects—interacts with halothane to increase ventricular irritability; may cause tachycardia and hypertension because of vagolytic effect

b. Atracurium
    (1) Metabolism—ester hydrolysis and Hoffmann elimination; can use in hepatic or renal failure
    (2) Side effects—its metabolite laudanosine may build up and cause seizures

c. Vecuronium
    (1) Biliary and renal excretion
    (2) Fewer cardiovascular effects than other neuromuscular-blocking agents

d. Rocuronium
    (1) Onset of action—1 minute (only rapid-onset nondepolarizing agent)

e. Cisatracurium
    (1) Hoffmann elimination—pH and temperature-dependent degradation
    (2) No adverse hemodynamic effects

## C. REVERSAL OF NEUROMUSCULAR BLOCKADE

Nondepolarizing agents can be antagonized by anticholinesterase drugs. Atropine or glycopyrrolate should be added to block muscarinic side effects (e.g., salivation, bronchospasm, and bradycardia).

**1. Edrophonium: Always use with atropine because onset and duration are similar**

**2. Neostigmine: Always use with glycopyrrolate**

**3. Pyridostigmine**

## D. INHALATIONAL ANESTHESIA

Minimum alveolar concentration is the minimum concentration of anesthesia that prevents movement in 50% of patients in response to a noxious stimulus (skin incision). Speed of onset depends on alveolar partial pressure (Pa) of the anesthetic, blood solubility, cardiac output, and alveolar-to-venous partial pressure difference.

1. **Nitrous oxide**
a. Nonflammable and odorless (good patient acceptability); rapid recovery with low potency; decreases minimum alveolar concentration of volatile agents
b. Complications—diffusion hypoxia (provide $O_2$ after surgery to prevent hypoxia), expansion of air-filled cavities, for example, bowel (dangerous in bowel obstruction), pneumothorax
2. **Sevoflurane**
a. Rapid induction and emergence, inhalational induction
b. Complications—decreases systemic vascular resistance and arterial blood pressure, interacts with $CO_2$ absorbers (soda lime, barium lime) to produce compound A that is potentially toxic to the kidneys
3. **Isoflurane**
a. Complications—pungent, not suitable for inhalational induction; decreased systemic vascular resistance and arterial blood pressure; increased heart rate
4. **Desflurane**
a. New inhalation agent with rapid induction and rapid recovery (similar to that of $N_2O$)
b. Hemodynamic effects similar to isoflurane
c. Complications—sympathetic activation with rapid increases in concentration

# E. LOCAL ANESTHETICS
1. **Uses**
a. Analgesia/anesthesia without risks of general anesthesia
b. Used in spinal, epidural, regional, and local anesthesia
2. **Dosage considerations**
a. Limit total anesthetic dosage to prevent seizures and arrhythmias or cardiac arrest
b. Add vasoconstrictor to slow vascular absorption
c. Avoid inadvertent vascular injection by preinjection aspiration
d. Impending toxicity—muscle twitching, restlessness, sleepiness
3. **Treatment of toxicity and precautions**
a. Trendelenburg position, $O_2$, IV diazepam (5–10 mg), thiopental (50–100 mg)
b. Never inject solutions containing epinephrine into digits, ear, tip of nose, or penis because may cause local ischemic necrosis.
4. **Commonly used local anesthetics**
a. Lidocaine—dosage maximum: 7 mg/kg with epinephrine, 4.5 mg/kg without epinephrine
b. Mepivacaine—dosage maximum: 7 mg/kg with epinephrine; 4.5 mg/kg without epinephrine
c. Bupivacaine—dosage maximum: 2.5 mg/kg
d. Ropivacaine—dosage maximum: 3 mg/kg

5. Systemic toxicity effects—numbness of the tongue, visual disturbances, unconsciousness, seizures, central nervous system depression, coma, and respiratory arrest

## IV. POSTOPERATIVE MANAGEMENT

### A. POSTOPERATIVE PAIN MANAGEMENT

1. Nonsteroidal antiinflammatory drugs (contraindicated in renal disease and failure, and patients with history of peptic ulcer disease)
a. Ketorolac
b. Ibuprofen
2. Narcotic analgesics
a. Oral narcotics
   (1) Oxycodone +/− acetaminophen
   (2) Hydrocodone +/− acetaminophen
b. IV narcotics
   (1) Intermittent boluses (nurse administered)
   (2) Patient-controlled analgesia

Allows patient to self-administer narcotics (morphine, hydromorphone) with a programmable infusion pump. Attempts to provide optimal pain relief and safety by avoiding peak and trough levels out of the therapeutic range caused by delays in administration, improper dosage, and pharmacokinetic and pharmacodynamic variability. Pumps are programmed to deliver intermittent boluses on demand, a continuous infusion, or a continuous background infusion with intermittent bolus doses. The dose, dose interval, and infusion rate are determined by the physician. Potential complications are respiratory depression, tolerance, nausea, vomiting, and pruritus.

3. Intrathecal analgesia
a. Provides short-term analgesia (24 hours)
b. Morphine is the drug of choice; dosage is 0.5 mg or less.
c. Limited to single-dose administration by risk for spinal headache and nerve damage from multiple punctures
d. Side effects are respiratory depression, nausea, and vomiting.
4. Epidural analgesia

Epidural analgesia attempts to provide pain relief without high systemic levels and side effects of analgesics. Narcotics, local anesthetics, or both can be used.

a. Advantages
   (1) Prevents muscle spasm and splinting, avoiding pulmonary complications
   (2) Allows earlier ambulation
   (3) Possible earlier return of gastrointestinal function after surgery
   (4) Excellent for patients with chest trauma, including rib fractures, pulmonary contusion, and flail chest
b. Adverse side effects
   (1) Local anesthetics—hypotension, motor block, systemic toxicity, urinary retention

   (2) Narcotics—respiratory depression, pruritus, nausea, vomiting, urinary retention
c. Dosing
   (1) Intermittent dosing causes peak systemic levels above those required for analgesia, causing more side effects.
   (2) Continuous infusion prevents peaks and troughs of intermittent dosing.
   (3) Combining infusions of local anesthetics and narcotics reduces the total dose of each, reducing the chance of adverse side effects.

## B. PONV

PONV is a major concern for patients and is a major problem in the postanesthesia recovery unit. Multimodal therapy is best for a patient with a history of PONV.

### 1. Risk factors
a. Female sex
b. Nonsmoker
c. Intraoperative opioid administration
d. History of PONV
e. Type of surgery
   (1) Laparoscopic surgery
   (2) Strabismus surgery
   (3) Inner- or middle-ear surgery

### 2. Treatment
a. Serotonin receptor (5-HT$_3$) antagonists
   (1) Ondansetron
   (2) Tropisetron
   (3) Granisetron
   (4) Dolasetron
b. Metoclopramide
c. Dexamethasone
d. Droperidol
e. Promethazine
f. Scopolamine (usually as transdermal patch)

**17**

**GENERAL ANESTHESIA**

## RECOMMENDED READING

American Society of Anesthesiologists online: Available at: www.asahq.org.
Morgan E, Mikhail M, Murray M: *Clinical Anesthesiology,* 4th ed. United States, McGraw-Hill, 2006.

# PART V

# General Surgery

# Acute Abdomen

*Colin A. Martin, MD*

*There are many who do not appreciate the full significance of the earlier and less flagrant symptoms of acute abdominal disease... or find it hard to believe that a patient with a non-distended abdomen and normal pulse and pressure can be the victim of a perforated gastric ulcer.*

—Zachary Cope, 1921

The acute abdomen is defined as undiagnosed pain that develops suddenly **18** and is less than 7 days in duration.

## I. PHYSIOLOGY OF ABDOMINAL PAIN

### A. VISCERAL PAIN
Visceral or intestinal contraction, spasm, stretching, distension, or chemical irritation results in visceral afferent nerve fiber stimulation

1. **Location—pain experienced in the midline corresponds to the anatomic location of the visceral nerve plexuses and their embryonic relation to the abdominal organs**
   a. Foregut—stomach to second portion of duodenum, pancreas, gallbladder, and liver
      (1) Pain transmitted via celiac plexus.
      (2) Pain experienced in the epigastrium.
   b. Midgut—third part of duodenum to first two thirds of the transverse colon
      (1) Pain transmitted via celiac plexus.
      (2) Pain experienced in the periumbilical region.
   c. Hindgut—last third of transverse colon to rectum
      (1) Pain transmitted via the inferior epigastric plexus.
      (2) Pain experienced in the hypogastrium.

### B. PARIETAL PAIN
Caused by direct parietal peritoneal irritation perceived by segmental somatic nerve fibers

1. **Demonstrative areas**
   a. Anterior abdominal wall
   b. Causes reflex muscle rigidity
2. **Nondemonstrative areas**
   a. Pelvis and central portion of posterior abdominal wall
   b. No reflex muscle rigidity

**Clinical Pearl:** *A pelvic or retrocecal inflamed appendix may cause no somatic or rebound tenderness.*

## C. REFERRED PAIN

Abdominal pain can be referred to distant locations. This is caused by a misinterpretation of visceral afferent impulses that cross the nerve cells to the corresponding somatic dermatome within the central nervous system (Fig. 18-1).

## II. HISTORY

In most cases, a diagnosis can be made from a thorough history and physical examination.

## A. PAIN

1. Location: Location of pain can give information about the cause; however, pain can be referred. Pain can be diffuse or localized. Diffuse pain is associated with visceral pain or uncontained peritonitis.

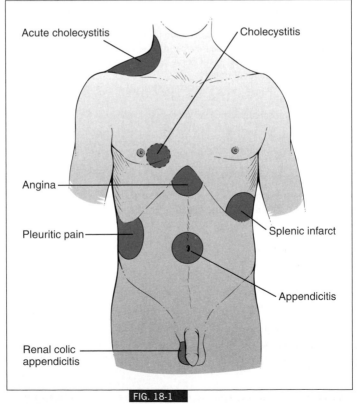

**FIG. 18-1**

Diagram of referred pain.

2. Onset
a. Timing—sudden or gradual
b. Mode—Did the pain develop immediately after an event?
   (1) Trauma can be associated with solid organ injury.
   (2) Fainting and abdominal pain is usually caused by ruptured abdominal aortic aneurysm, perforated duodenal ulcer, acute pancreatitis, or ruptured ectopic pregnancy.
3. Character
a. Burning pain is associated with perforated gastric ulcer or acute pancreatitis.
b. Sharp, constricting pain is associated with biliary colic.
c. Tearing pain is associated with dissecting aneurysm.
d. Gripping pain is associated with intestinal obstruction.
e. Constant, dull, fixed pain is associated with an abscess.
4. Referred pain
5. Exacerbating or ameliorating factors—movement, eating, breathing, vomiting

**Clinical Pearl:** *Abdominal pain associated with driving over bumps is associated with peritonitis.*

## B. VOMITING
Usually caused by irritation of the nerves of the peritoneum or obstruction of an involuntary muscle tube (bile duct, ureter, intestine, or appendix)
1. Relation of pain to vomiting
a. Acute obstruction of the bile duct or ureter causes pain followed shortly by vomiting.
b. Vomiting occurs late in abdominal pain secondary to bowel obstruction.
2. Character
a. Bilious—nonspecific or early obstruction
b. Food particles—proximal obstruction
c. Feculent—caused by bacterial overgrowth in small bowel caused by prolonged distal small-bowel obstruction; rare in colonic obstruction
3. Frequency—increased in proximal bowel obstruction

## C. BOWEL FUNCTION
1. Constipation (absence of bowel movements)/obstipation (absence of bowel movements or gas)—obstruction, paralytic ileus, acute appendicitis
2. Diarrhea—gastroenteritis, early or partial small-bowel obstruction
3. Blood/mucus—intussusception in children, colitis, proctitis in adults

**Clinical Pearl:** *When hypogastric pain and diarrhea are followed by hypogastric tenderness and constipation, suspect pelvic abscess.*

18

ACUTE ABDOMEN

## D. REVIEW OF SYSTEMS
The following causes of acute abdominal pain can be elicited by thorough questioning about each body system.
1. **Cardiopulmonary**
a. Pneumonia
b. Myocardial ischemia
c. Recent upper respiratory infection may precede mesenteric adenitis.
2. **Neuromuscular**
a. Herpes zoster
b. Tabes dorsalis
c. Spine fractures or tumors
3. **Genitourinary**
a. Kidney stones
b. Pneumaturia—frequently seen with a pelvic abscess caused by diverticular disease.
4. **Vascular**
a. Autoimmune vasculitis
b. Abdominal aortic aneurysm
5. **Hematologic**
a. Sickle cell disease
b. Lymphoma
c. Leukemia
6. **Endocrine**
a. Diabetic ketoacidosis
b. Porphyria
c. Addisonian crisis

## E. MEDICAL HISTORY
May give clues about the cause of abdominal pain
1. **Previous abdominal surgery**
2. **History of peptic ulcer disease, gallstones, inflammatory bowel disease, or diverticular disease**

## F. MEDICATION
1. **Steroids**
a. Can decrease symptoms produced by inflammation
b. Can cause atypical perforations of the colon and small intestine
2. **Analgesics, antibiotics, and antipyretics—may mask pain and fever.**

## III. PHYSICAL EXAMINATION
### A. GENERAL APPEARANCE
1. **Facial expression**
2. **Attitude in bed**
a. Restlessness suggests colic.
b. Immobility in patients with peritonitis
c. Knees drawn up to relax abdominal wall tension in peritonitis

3. Dull eyes and ashen countenance in patients with sepsis
4. Pale conjunctiva in patients with anemia

## B.  VITAL SIGNS
1. Temperature
a. 95–96°F—severe shock
b. 99–100°F—early inflammation, usual in acute appendicitis
c. 104–105°F—intraabdominal abscess or urinary source

**Clinical Pearl:** *Oral temperature is likely falsely low if the nasal passages are obstructed or if a nasogastric tube forces the patient to breathe through his or her mouth.*

2. Pulse
a. Tachycardia may be seen in fever, anemia, agitation, dehydration, or pain.
b. Bradycardia can be seen in advanced sepsis or metabolic disturbances (i.e., hypothyroidism).
3. Respiratory rate
a. Kussmaul respirations are present with diabetic ketoacidosis.
b. If respiratory rate is increased to twice the normal rate, the cause is likely thoracic in origin.
4. Blood pressure
a. Hypotension may be associated with anemia, sepsis, or volume depletion.
b. Hypertension may be associated with severe pain.

## C.  ABDOMINAL EXAMINATION
1. Observation, inspection
a. Scaphoid, flat, obese, distended
b. Movement with respiration—note limitation of movement indicating rigidity of the abdominal muscles or diaphragm.
c. Have patient indicate the exact point of maximal pain.
d. Inspect all potential sites for hernias, especially the inguinal and femoral region.
e. Stethoscope is a great tool for palpation in anxious patients.
2. Auscultation
a. Absent or hypoactive bowel sounds—peritonitis or ileus
b. High-pitched bowel sounds with rushes, hyperactive—obstruction
c. Aortic and renal artery bruits—absence of a bruit never excludes the presence of an aortic aneurysm.
3. Palpation/percussion—gentleness is essential.
a. Evaluate presence and extent of muscular rigidity.
b. Palpate four quadrants of abdomen and costovertebral angles to assess tenderness (mild, moderate, or severe). Palpate for abdominal masses, abnormal pulsations, and hernial orifices. Begin away from point of maximal pain. See Table 18-1 for signs and findings in abdominal examination.
c. Rocking the bed can also cause worsening of pain with peritonitis.

18

ACUTE ABDOMEN

## TABLE 18-1

### SIGNS AND FINDINGS ON PHYSICAL EXAMINATION

| Signs/Findings | Description | Associated Clinical Condition(s) |
|---|---|---|
| Balance's sign | Presence of dull percussion noted in both flanks, constant on left side but shifting with change of position on right side | Ruptured spleen |
| Bassler's sign | Sharp pain elicited by pinching appendix between thumb of examiner and iliacus muscle | Chronic appendicitis |
| Charcot's triad | Intermittent right upper quadrant abdominal pain, jaundice, and fever | Choledocholithiasis |
| Claybrook's sign | Transmission of breath and heart sounds through abdominal wall | Ruptured abdominal viscus |
| Courvoisier's sign | Palpable, nontender gallbladder in presence of clinical jaundice | Periampullary neoplasm |
| Cullen's sign | Periumbilical darkening of skin from blood | Hemoperitoneum (especially in ruptured ectopic pregnancy) |
| Cutaneous hyperesthesia | Increased abdominal wall sensation to light touch | Parietal peritoneal inflammation secondary to inflammatory intraabdominal pathology |
| Fothergill's sign | Abdominal wall mass that does not cross midline and remains palpable when rectus muscle is tense | Rectus muscle hematoma |
| Grey Turner's sign | Local areas of discoloration around umbilicus and flanks | Acute hemorrhagic pancreatitis |
| Iliopsoas sign | Elevation and extension of leg against pressure of examiner's hand causes pain | Appendicitis (retrocecal) or an inflammatory mass in contact with psoas |
| Kehr's sign | Left shoulder pain when patient is supine or in the Trendelenburg position (pain may occur spontaneously or after application of pressure to left subcostal region) | Hemoperitoneum (especially ruptured spleen) |
| Murphy's sign | Palpation of right upper abdominal quadrant during deep inspiration results in right upper quadrant abdominal pain and stopping of inspiration | Acute cholecystitis |
| Obturator sign | Flexion of right thigh at right angles to trunk and external rotation of same leg in supine position result in hypogastric pain | Appendicitis (pelvic appendix); pelvic abscess; an inflammatory mass in contact with muscle |
| Ransohoff's sign | Yellow pigmentation in umbilical region | Ruptured common bile duct |

| | | Associated Clinical |
|---|---|---|
| Signs/Findings | Description | Condition(s) |
| Rovsing's sign | Pain referred to McBurney's point on application of pressure to descending colon | Acute appendicitis |
| Summer's sign | Increased abdominal muscle tone on exceedingly gentle palpation of right or left iliac fossa | Early appendicitls; nephrolithiasis; ureterolithiasis; ovarian torsion |

TABLE 18-1—cont'd

SIGNS AND FINDINGS ON PHYSICAL EXAMINATION

4. Muscle rigidity or guarding
a. Involuntary guarding—reflex flexion of abdominal muscles secondary to peritonitis
b. Voluntary guarding—flexion on abdominal muscle in anxious and tender patients; can be relieved by encouraging relaxation and flexing the knees.

## D. EXAMINATION OF PELVIC CAVITY
1. Suprapubic palpation and percussion
2. Rectal examination: A gloved, lubricated finger should be inserted 3 to 4 inches into the rectum. The rectal canal should be palpated in all directions.
a. Pressing forward: In male patients, the examiner can detect a distended bladder, an enlarged prostate, or diseased seminal vesicles. In female patients, pain and swelling in Douglas's pouch or an enlarged uterus can be detected.
b. Passing the finger more proximal can detect a rectal stricture, polyps, or metastatic implants.
c. Pressing laterally: Tender, inflamed appendix or pelvic sidewall abscess can be identified.
d. Pressing anteriorly: Pelvic abscess or a Blumer's shelf (carcinomatous implants).
3. Digital examination of stomas: Assess for strictures, parastomal hernias, or foreign bodies.
4. Bimanual pelvic and speculum examination
a. Palpate bilateral adnexal regions.
b. Examine cervix.
c. Cultures for sexually transmitted diseases

## IV. LABORATORY EXAMINATION
Laboratory tests may be useful; however, they can be misleading, and the clinical evaluation should have the most weight when making the diagnosis. For example, with acute appendicitis, a patient can have a normal white blood cell count, and patients with acute intraabdominal hemorrhage can

18

ACUTE ABDOMEN

have normal hemoglobin. Laboratory tests should be ordered as an adjunct to the history and physical examination. They should also be ordered to evaluate specific organ systems.

## A. WHITE BLOOD CELL COUNT
1. Determines the degree of leukocytosis and the differential.

## B. HEMATOCRIT
1. The hematocrit can indicate anemia, whether chronic (microcytic or macrocytic) or acute.
2. Hemoconcentration may indicate hypovolemia.

## C. PLATELET COUNT
1. Thrombocytopenia is consistent with severe sepsis.

## D. ELECTROLYTES
1. Electrolytes are indicative of volume status and may demonstrate gastrointestinal losses from diarrhea or protracted vomiting (e.g., hypochloremic hypokalemic metabolic alkalosis or "contraction alkalosis").
2. Hyperglycemia can be observed in diabetic ketoacidosis or sepsis-induced glucose intolerance.

## E. ARTERIAL BLOOD GAS
1. Arterial blood gases measure metabolic acidosis or alkalosis. Metabolic acidosis in the presence of generalized abdominal pain in elderly adults is ischemic colitis until proven otherwise.

## F. LIVER FUNCTION TESTS
1. Bilirubin (direct and total) and alkaline phosphatase concentration increases in biliary obstruction and increased transaminase concentration in hepatocellular injury

## G. AMYLASE LEVEL INCREASE
1. Amylase level increases are seen in pancreatitis, although it is relatively nonspecific. It may be increased in mesenteric ischemia, perforated duodenal ulcer, ruptured ovarian cyst, and renal failure. The serum lipase determination is more sensitive.

## V. RADIOGRAPHIC EVALUATION
The radiographic evaluation may be helpful; however, in most patients, the diagnosis can be made from a thorough history and physical examination.

## A. UPRIGHT CHEST RADIOGRAPH
1. Look for pneumonia.
2. Look for free air under the diaphragm suggestive of a perforated viscus.

## B. ABDOMINAL RADIOGRAPH

Look for bowel distension and air–fluid levels consistent with ileus or obstruction, as well as bowel gas cutoff versus air through to rectum.

1. Localized ileus ("sentinel loop") may indicate location of inflammatory process (i.e., pancreatitis).
2. Abnormal calcifications—chronic pancreatitis, 20% of gallstones, 85% of renal calculi.
3. Pneumatosis coli (air in the bowel wall) and air in the biliary tree (pneumobilia) are ominous signs of dead gut.
4. Mass effect from tumor or abscess.

**Clinical Pearl:** *The best opportunity to see free air under the diaphragm is in an upright chest radiograph or in the left lateral decubitus position after the patient has been upright or in the decubitus position for at least 10 minutes before the radiograph.*

## C. ULTRASONOGRAPHY

Ultrasonography is of value in visualizing the hepatobiliary tree, pancreas, vascular structures, kidneys, pelvic organs, and intraabdominal fluid collections. It is inexpensive and noninvasive, but operator-dependent.

## D. CT SCAN

CT scan is beneficial in some cases of acute abdominal pain, but is costly, takes time, and can cause allergic reactions and nephropathy. However, CT is helpful for some causative agents.

1. Acute pancreatitis—helpful in distinguishing among pancreatic necrosis, abscess, or pseudocyst.
2. Blunt trauma—can diagnose solid organ injuries.
3. Ruptured aortic aneurysm
4. Acute appendicitis—usually a clinical diagnosis. In certain cases, CT can be helpful.
a. In course longer than 4 days, CT can demonstrate perforation and abscess that may be amenable to nonoperative percutaneous drainage.
b. CT can used for obese patients where a reliable examination cannot be obtained.
c. Patients with acute appendicitis who get a CT scan as part of their work-up do not have a greater incidence of rupture.
d. There is a lower negative appendectomy rate in female patients.

## VI. DIFFERENTIAL DIAGNOSIS OF ACUTE ABDOMEN

### A. INFLAMMATORY

1. Perforated viscus
a. Stomach, duodenum—ulcer
b. Bowel—diverticulum, appendix, carcinoma, traumatic small-bowel injury
c. Gallbladder

**18**

**ACUTE ABDOMEN**

2. **Primary peritonitis (peritonitis without obvious cause)**
   a. Gram-positive organisms (*Pneumococcus* spp., *Streptococcus* spp.) formerly most common; gram-negative infections increasing, especially in female patients
   b. Tuberculosis—"doughy" abdomen
   c. Patients with cirrhosis with ascites may experience development of spontaneous bacterial peritonitis and have minimal symptoms.
3. **Gastroenteritis, colitis—viral or bacterial**
4. **Inflammatory bowel disease**
5. **Diverticulitis**
6. **Meckel's diverticulitis**
7. **Pancreatitis—alcoholic, biliary, viral, thiazide induced, steroid related, hyperlipidemia, hypercalcemia**
8. **Hepatitis**
9. **Hepatic abscess—look for other primary septic focus.**
10. **Splenic abscess**
11. **Mesenteric lymphadenitis**
12. **Foreign body perforation of bowel**
13. **Gynecologic**
    a. Pelvic inflammatory disease
    b. Fitz–Hugh–Curtis syndrome (gonococcal perihepatitis)
    c. Endometritis
    d. Toxic shock syndrome
    e. Ruptured ovarian cyst
14. **Pyelonephritis**

## B. MECHANICAL

1. **Intestinal obstruction**
   a. Small bowel—adhesions, hernia, neoplasm, volvulus, intussusception, gallstone ileus, Meckel's band, inflammatory mass
   b. Gastric outlet obstruction—peptic ulcer disease (pyloric channel), gastric carcinoma
   c. Colon—neoplasm, hernia, diverticulitis, volvulus
2. **Biliary obstruction**
   a. Cholelithiasis with impacted or "ball-valve" cystic duct stone
   b. Choledocholithiasis
   c. Cholangitis
      (1) Neoplasm
      (2) Choledochal cyst
      (3) Choledocholithiasis
3. **Solid viscera—rare**
   a. Acute splenomegaly—various hematologic disorders
   b. Acute hepatomegaly—pericarditis, hepatitis, congestive heart failure, and Budd–Chiari syndrome
4. **Omental torsion—rare, torsion of appendix epiploic**

5. Gynecologic
a. Torsion of ovarian cyst, uterine fibroid or endometriosis
b. Ectopic pregnancy

## C. VASCULAR
1. Intraperitoneal bleeding
a. Traumatic rupture of liver, spleen, mesentery
b. Delayed splenic rupture
c. Ruptured ectopic pregnancy
d. Ruptured abdominal aortic aneurysm—sudden onset of new back pain in an individual with atherosclerotic risk factors
e. Ruptured splenic or hepatic aneurysm
2. Ischemia
a. Mesenteric thrombosis or embolus
    (1) Usually see other signs of peripheral atherosclerosis
    (2) Atrial fibrillation, valvular heart disease, history of myocardial infarction predispose to embolization.
    (3) Pain out of proportion to examination
    (4) Metabolic acidosis is a late finding and usually indicates intestinal gangrene.
    (5) Short-segment involvement may result in self-limiting episodes and late intestinal stricture formation.
3. Splenic infarction—common in patients with sickle cell disease

## VII. INITIAL TREATMENT AND PREOPERATIVE PREPARATION
### A. ASSESSMENT
1. Prompt work-up and differential diagnosis

### B. DIET
1. Keep the patient NPO (nothing by mouth) until the diagnosis is firm and the treatment plan is formulated.

### C. INTRAVENOUS FLUIDS
1. Intravenous fluid administration should be started early and based on expected fluid losses; large volumes may be required.
2. Correct electrolytes.
3. Central access may be needed.

### D. HEMODYNAMIC MONITORING
1. May be required in cases where fluid status and cardiac status are in question or when septic shock is present.

### E. NASOGASTRIC TUBE
1. Should be inserted for bleeding, vomiting, or signs of obstruction, or when urgent or emergent laparotomy is planned in a patient who has not been NPO.

18

ACUTE ABDOMEN

## F. FOLEY CATHETER
1. Use to monitor fluid resuscitation.

## G. TREATMENT
1. Immediate surgery
a. Consent of patient
b. Use appropriate preoperative antibiotics based on suspected pathology.
c. Develop a primary operative plan.
2. Admit and observe for possible operation.
Serial examinations should be performed every 2 to 4 hours during the first 12 to 24 hours in cases without definite diagnosis and clearly documented in the medical record. Use narcotics and sedatives minimally to avoid masking physical signs and symptoms until treatment plan has been established. Monitor vital signs frequently.

# Appendicitis

*Steven R. Allen, MD*

## I. EPIDEMIOLOGY

### A. GENERAL

1. Appendicitis is the most common cause of acute abdomen requiring surgery, with approximately 300,000 cases per year in the United States affecting 7% of the population.
2. Peak incidence occurs between 10 and 30 years of age, with a slight male predominance.
3. The incidence rate of perforation is 12%.
4. Overall incidence rate of normal appendices after appendectomy is 10% to 15%.

### B. MORBIDITY AND MORTALITY

1. Overall mortality is 0.1% for nonperforated cases and 5% for perforated cases.
2. Infants and elderly adults have much greater morbidity and mortality rates—~85% for infants and ~28% to 60% for elderly adults because of an increase in the perforation rate.
3. The greater morbidity and mortality rates in infants and elderly adults are due to atypical and late presentations.

## II. PATHOPHYSIOLOGY

### A. GENERAL

1. Obstruction of the appendiceal lumen is thought to be the initiating event in two-thirds of cases, most commonly secondary to a fecalith in adults and lymphoid hyperplasia in children.
2. With continued mucosal secretion, luminal pressure increases and eventually exceeds capillary venous and lymphatic pressures, causing venous infarction in watershed areas (middle and proximal antimesenteric regions).
3. Bacterial overgrowth occurs in the inspissated mucus.
4. Polymicrobial infection with anaerobes > aerobes 3:1
5. *Escherichia coli, Bacteroides fragilis, Pseudomonas* spp. present in 80%, 70%, and 40% of cases, respectively

### B. COMPLICATIONS

1. Worsening edema, high luminal pressure, and bacterial proliferation lead to occlusion of arterial blood flow and gangrenous appendicitis.
2. Transmural necrosis and bacterial penetration into the appendiceal wall is associated with perforation, which may either be walled off by omentum or spread throughout the abdomen, inducing diffuse peritonitis.
3. Overall incidence rate is 12% for perforation.

19

## III. PRESENTATION

### A. HISTORY

1. Patient may give history of indigestion lasting hours to 1 day before a painful attack.
2. Pain usually begins as vague midabdominal discomfort caused by appendiceal distention and referred pain along lesser splanchnics.
3. Anorexia and nausea occur almost uniformly after the pain. Almost all adults have anorexia, whereas children with appendicitis may remain hungry.
4. Pain localizes to the right lower quadrant (RLQ) as the parietal peritoneum in that area becomes irritated.
   a. If the appendix lies in the pelvis or retrocecal area, the location of the pain (and tenderness) will be positioned over the area of peritoneal inflammation.
   b. If perforation occurs, diffuse peritonitis may ensue with pain throughout the abdomen, although some may "wall" off the perforation, localizing the symptoms.
5. Patients may have constipation, diarrhea, or no change in bowel habits.
   a. A history of late onset of loose stools may indicate pelvic peritonitis after perforation.

### B. PHYSICAL EXAMINATION

1. Low-grade fever may be present: Temperature is rarely greater than 38°C (101°F), unless perforation, abscess formation, or both have occurred.
2. When appendix lies anteriorly, tenderness is present at McBurney's point (one-third the distance between the anterior superior iliac spine and the umbilicus).
3. Abdominal wall muscular rigidity may be present.
4. With peritoneal irritation, guarding, rebound, and indirect rebound tenderness may occur.
5. Rovsing's sign is pain in RLQ with palpation of the lower left quadrant.
6. Cutaneous hyperesthesia may be present in distribution of T10-T12 in the RLQ and is tested by rolling the skin between the thumb and forefinger, which normally does not cause pain.
7. Rectal examination elicits suprapubic pain if the inflamed appendix tip lies in the pelvis.
8. The psoas sign is pain occurring with extension of the right thigh and indicates an irritative focus overlying that muscle.
9. The obturator sign is pain with passive internal rotation of the flexed right thigh and indicates inflammation overlying that muscle.
10. Male patients may have pain in the right, left, or both testicles, because both are innervated by T10.

## C. LABORATORY AND RADIOLOGIC FINDINGS

1. The diagnosis of appendicitis is largely a clinical one; however, some objective data may be useful.
2. White blood cell (WBC) count increase from 10,000 to 18,000/mm³ is expected, although not always present, with a left shift on differential.
   a. WBC count is normal in approximately 10% of patients.
   b. Patients who are human immunodeficiency virus–positive have the same symptoms, but usually the WBC count is normal.
3. Urinalysis may be normal or reveal few red blood cells or WBCs only, especially in retrocecal or pelvic appendix.
4. Abdominal radiographs are usually nonspecific but may show a fecalith in the RLQ, loss of the right psoas shadow (fat pad), paucity of RLQ gas, and/or a few dilated loops of bowel.
5. Barium enema, though not specific, may rule out appendicitis if normal filling of the appendix occurs.
   a. Mass effect on the cecum or terminal ileum may be seen.
   b. It has a 10% false-negative rate.
6. Computed tomography scan has been shown to be superior to ultrasound in diagnosing acute appendicitis in both pediatric and adult populations.
   a. Both are helpful when pain is associated with an RLQ mass to rule out phlegmon versus abscess.
   b. Computed tomography scan should be used to aid diagnosis in patients with atypical presentation.

## IV. DIFFERENTIAL DIAGNOSIS

1. Gastroenteritis
2. Diverticulitis (adults)
3. Acute mesenteric adenitis (children)
4. Meckel's diverticulitis
5. Intussusception (infants and children)
6. Regional enteritis
7. Perforated peptic ulcer
8. Perforating carcinoma of cecum or sigmoid colon
9. Urinary tract infection
10. Ureteral stone
11. Gynecologic disease (e.g., pelvic inflammatory disease, ectopic pregnancy, ovarian cyst)
12. Male urologic disease (e.g., testicular torsion, epididymitis)
13. Epiploic appendagitis
14. Spontaneous bacterial peritonitis
15. Henoch-Schönlein purpura
16. Yersiniosis

## V. COMPLICATIONS

### A. PERFORATION
1. Occurs more in patients >50 and <10 years of age
2. Associated with more diffuse pain after localized tenderness
   a. Initially, pain may be relieved, followed by peritonitis.
3. Uncommon for perforation to occur within 24 hours of onset of abdominal pain

### B. PERITONITIS
1. Occurs after perforation
2. Localized peritonitis refers to peritonitis that is microscopic and contained by surrounding viscera or omentum, whereas generalized peritonitis refers to gross spillage into the peritoneal cavity.
3. Associated with high fever and may lead to sepsis

### C. ABSCESS
1. May be associated with a RLQ mass on physical examination
2. Computed tomography scan should be performed together with percutaneous drainage.
3. The patient is treated with antibiotics, and an interval appendectomy is performed.
4. If present at the time of operation, the appendix should be removed and drains placed.
5. Recurs in 10% of patients treated with antibiotics and drainage alone

## VI. TREATMENT

### A. GENERAL
1. The treatment of appendicitis is surgical and requires removal of the inflamed appendix, except in cases of appendiceal perforation, in which treatment can vary (drainage and antibiotic treatment).
2. Appendectomy can be performed either open or laparoscopically.
3. Perioperative antibiotics have been shown to be beneficial in decreasing infectious complications, and many authors recommend 3 to 5 days of antibiotics in patients with confirmed appendicitis.

### B. TECHNIQUE
1. With the open technique, use a McBurney (or Rockey–Davis) incision over McBurney's point with a muscle-splitting technique (Fig. 19-1).
2. If there is reasonable doubt about the diagnosis, some surgeons prefer a paramedian or midline incision.
3. After resection of the appendix, the ligated stump may be inverted.
4. In the case of a perforated appendix with phlegmon formation (or significant cecal inflammation), an "interval" (or delayed) appendectomy is usually performed. Drains are brought out to drain discrete collections only, and the fascia is closed while the skin and subcutaneous tissue are left open.

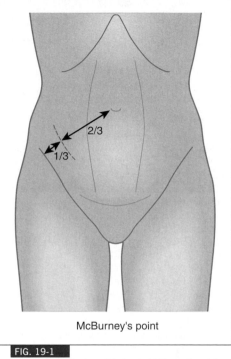

McBurney's point

**FIG. 19-1**

Diagram of method used to locate McBurney's point.

5. Patients with a walled-off abscess may be managed by ultrasound- or computed tomography–guided percutaneous drainage, followed by interval appendectomy 6 to 8 weeks later.
6. If no appendiceal inflammation is present, a careful search for other causes of the symptom should be undertaken.
a. Examination of pelvic organs
b. Gallbladder and gastroduodenal area are inspected.
c. Gram stain of any peritoneal exudate
d. Inspection of the mesentery for lymph nodes
e. Thorough examination of the small bowel to rule out regional enteritis and Meckel's diverticulum
f. Palpation of the colon and kidneys

## C.  LAPAROSCOPY

Laparoscopic appendectomy has no major differences in results when compared with open appendectomy.

1. Advantages
a. Evaluation of the abdomen/pelvic structures when the diagnosis is in question
   (1) Women in childbearing years—can visualize pelvis, fallopian tubes, and ovaries
   (2) Elderly adults—can evaluate for perforated cecal cancer or diverticulitis
b. Postoperative stay is less, and some patients may be discharged the day of surgery.
c. Time of return to normal activity is shorter.
d. The procedure is technically easier in obese patients.
e. In the case of a perforated appendix, there is better visualization of the peritoneum, allowing more adequate drainage.
f. Lower incidence of wound infections
2. **Procedure: Multiple variations exist. In general, the technique at the University of Cincinnati Medical Center is as follows:**
a. It is performed under general anesthesia with bladder and stomach decompression.
b. The appendix is grasped with a forceps to expose its base through the RLQ cannula.
c. Using either a vascular stapler or clips to ligate vessels, the mesoappendix is ligated and divided.
d. The appendix can either be amputated with a linear stapler or excised after endoloops have been placed at its base.
e. The appendix is placed in a bag and removed through the 10- to 12-mm cannula, with care taken not to contact the subcutaneous tissue with the inflamed appendix.

## VII. SPECIAL CIRCUMSTANCES

### A. ELDERLY ADULTS
1. Account for nearly 50% of the deaths from appendicitis
2. Greater mortality rate is due to delay of definitive treatment, uncontrolled infection, and a high incidence of coexistent disease.
3. Constellation of symptoms is usually much more atypical.
a. Abdominal pain may be minimized.
b. Fever and leukocyte count are less reliable signs.
4. Perforation rates reach 75%.
5. Morbidity and mortality rates are much greater because of the delay in accurate diagnosis.

### B. INFANTS
1. Similarly high rates of rupture and secondary complications as in elderly adults because of delayed or atypical presentation.
2. Accurate diagnosis is made more difficult by the fact that infants are unable to give a history, the index of suspicion is usually lower, and progression of disease is usually faster.

3. The ability of the infant to wall off perforated appendicitis is inefficient and results in rapid, diffuse peritonitis and distant abscesses.

## C. PREGNANCY

1. Although appendicitis is the most common extrauterine surgical emergency in pregnant patients, 1 in every 1500 to 2000 pregnancies, it occurs with the same frequency in pregnant women as it does in nonpregnant women.
2. It does occur more frequently in the first two trimesters than in the third trimester.
3. Diagnosis is obscured by the lateral and superior displacement of the appendix by the gravid uterus, with an accompanying change in the point of maximum tenderness.
a. The appendix is in its "normal" position until 12 weeks, when it is displaced upward and laterally.
b. It reaches the umbilicus by 20 weeks and the iliac crest at 24 weeks.
4. Diagnosis is also made more difficult by the fact that abdominal pain, nausea, vomiting, and an increased WBC count are normal findings during pregnancy.
a. An increased neutrophil count is not a normal finding.
b. Ultrasound may be helpful, especially in the first trimester.
5. Laparoscopy is as safe as laparotomy in the first and second trimesters.
6. Although maternal mortality rates are low, early operative intervention is essential because perforation and peritonitis result in fetal mortality rates as high as 20% to 25%.
7. Risk for premature delivery is greatest during the first week after surgery, then returns to baseline.

## VIII. APPENDICEAL TUMORS

Tumors are found in almost 5% of removed appendices.

## A. CARCINOID

1. Carcinoid tumors are most commonly located in the appendix and are usually benign.
2. Appendectomy is the treatment of choice if the tumor is <2 cm, involves the tip of the appendix, and there is no nodal involvement.
3. Right hemicolectomy is the treatment of choice if there is nodal involvement, the tumor is >2 cm, or the mesoappendix or base of cecum is involved.

## B. ADENOCARCINOMA

1. Adenocarcinoma of the colon can arise in the appendix.
2. Most of these cases present as acute appendicitis.
3. A right hemicolectomy should be performed.

## C. PSEUDOMYXOMA

1. Pseudomyxoma arises in the appendix in 50% of patients with pseudomyxoma peritonei.
2. Appendiceal mucocele or fluid-filled cyst can be seen on imaging and may be associated with gelatinous ascites.
3. Both ovaries should be examined for secondary disease in female patients.
4. In a patient with a preoperative diagnosis of pseudomyxoma peritonei, surgical debulking of all gross disease is the treatment, together with adjuvant chemotherapy after tissue diagnosis of pseudomyxoma.
5. Patients with undiagnosed disease should undergo a right hemicolectomy without penetration of the tumor. Once the diagnosis is confirmed, further cancer work-up and treatment are then performed.

## RECOMMENDED READING

Brennan GDG: Pediatric appendicitis: Pathophysiology and appropriate use of diagnostic imaging. *Can J Emerg Med* 8:425–432, 2006.

Maxwell JG, Robinson CL, Maxwell TG, et al: Deriving the indications for laparoscopic appendectomy from a comparison of the outcomes of laparoscopic and open appendectomy. *Am J Surg* 182:687–692, 2001.

Wilson EB, Cole JC, Nipper ML, et al: Computed tomography and ultrasonography in the diagnosis of appendicitis: When are they indicated? *Arch Surg* 136:670–675, 2001.

# Benign Gallbladder

*Ryan A. LeVasseur, MD*

> *I profess to learn and to teach anatomy, not from books but from dissections; not from the positions of philosophers but from the fabric of nature.*
>
> —William Harvey, 1621, *An Anatomical Treatise on the Movement of the Heart and Blood in Animals* **20**

## I. ANATOMY

### A. GENERAL
1. Pear-shaped sac with 30- to 50-ml capacity, >300-ml capacity when obstructed
2. Lies in gallbladder fossa on inferior surface of liver
3. Demarcates anatomic division between left and right hepatic lobes
4. Four anatomic areas: fundus, corpus, infundibulum, and neck
5. Lined by tall columnar epithelium

### B. VASCULAR
1. Supplied by cystic artery
a. More than 90% off right hepatic artery
b. May arise from left hepatic, common hepatic, gastroduodenal, or superior mesenteric arteries
c. Found in triangle of Calot: area bound by the cystic duct, common hepatic duct, and liver edge (modern definition)
2. Venous return
a. Via small veins that drain into liver
b. Rarely by a cystic vein that drains to portal vein

### C. EXTRAHEPATIC BILE DUCTS
1. Right and left hepatic ducts
2. Common hepatic duct
3. Cystic duct
4. Common bile duct (CBD)
a. Approximately 7 to 11 cm in length, 5 to 10 mm in width
b. Blood supply from gastroduodenal artery and right hepatic artery
c. Courses in hepatoduodenal ligament, right of the hepatic artery and anterior to portal vein
d. Joins duodenum at ampulla of Vater (surrounded by sphincter of Oddi) 10 cm distal to pylorus
5. Small ducts of Luschka from liver directly into gallbladder

## II. CHOLELITHIASIS AND CHRONIC CALCULOUS CHOLECYSTITIS

### A. INCIDENCE
1. Gallstones are found in 8% of male and 17% of female adults.
2. Predisposing conditions include obesity, multiparity, diabetes mellitus, cirrhosis, pancreatitis, chronic hemolytic states, malabsorption, inflammatory bowel disease, and certain racial/genetic factors (American Indians).

### B. CAUSATIVE FACTORS
The most important factor is composition of bile, which has three major constituents.
1. Bile salts (primary: cholic and chenodeoxycholic acids; secondary: deoxycholic and lithocholic acids)
2. Phospholipids—90% lecithin
3. Cholesterol—although insoluble, both lecithin and cholesterol are incorporated together with bile salts into more soluble mixed micelles.
a. Conditions that affect the relative concentrations of these components cause lithogenic bile.
b. Bile that contains excess cholesterol relative to bile salts and lecithin is predisposed to gallstone formation.

### C. TYPES OF GALLSTONES
1. Mixed—75%
a. Most common, usually multiple
b. Cholesterol usually predominates—70% of content
c. About 15% to 20% may ultimately calcify and, therefore, become radiopaque.
2. Pure cholesterol—10%
a. Often solitary with large (>2.5 cm), round configuration
b. Usually not calcified
3. Pigment—15%
a. Composed of unconjugated bilirubin, calcium, and variable amounts of organic material
b. About 50% are radiopaque.
c. Black pigment stones are associated with cirrhosis and chronic hemolytic states. Bile is usually sterile, and choledocholithiasis is unusual.
d. Brown pigment stones are found more frequently in the biliary tree than in the gallbladder. Associated with states that predispose to bile stasis (i.e., biliary strictures).

### D. NATURAL HISTORY
1. Eighty percent of gallstones are asymptomatic. Each year, 2% of patients with asymptomatic stones develop symptoms, most commonly (75%) biliary colic.
2. Incidence rate of development of symptoms in patients with asymptomatic stones is 15% to 30% over 15 years.

3. Elective cholecystectomy is recommended for patients with cholelithiasis who develop symptoms.

## E.  BILIARY COLIC
Biliary colic is pain arising from a gallbladder without established infection. It is often difficult to differentiate between colic and intermittent chronic cholecystitis.
1. Cause—thought to be due to transient gallstone obstruction of the cystic duct resulting in gallbladder distention.
2. History—generally presents with moderate intermittent right upper quadrant (RUQ) and epigastric pain usually after a fatty meal.
a. Pain may radiate to back or below right scapula.
b. Pain usually begins abruptly and subsides gradually, lasting from minutes to hours.
c. Pain of biliary colic is usually steady, not undulating like that of renal colic.
3. Physical examination
a. No associated fever
b. May have some mild epigastric or RUQ tenderness, or palpable gallbladder
c. Usually negative Murphy's Sign: Examiner palpates the RUQ and asks the patient to inhale deeply; the diaphragm descends and pushes the inflamed gallbladder against the examiner's fingertips, causing enough pain that patients arrest their inspiration. This can also be done on ultrasound with the tip of the probe.
4. Differential diagnosis—pancreatitis, peptic ulcer disease, hiatal hernia with reflux, gastritis, hepatic flexure carcinoma, hepatobiliary carcinoma, cardiopulmonary disease
5. Complications
a. Prolonged cystic duct obstruction may allow bacterial growth and progress to acute cholecystitis.
b. Stones may pass into the CBD with consequent obstruction or pancreatitis.

## F.  DIAGNOSIS
1. Laboratory findings
a. None is diagnostic.
b. Liver function tests (LFTs), amylase, and white blood cell count should be obtained.
c. Increase of alkaline phosphatase level is common in biliary disease but is nonspecific.
2. Plain films
a. About 30% of gallstones are radiopaque and may be detected.
b. Can exclude other diagnoses
3. Oral cholecystogram (Graham–Cole test)—evaluates presence of gallstones and gallbladder function. It is rarely used today because of use of ultrasound.

4. Ultrasound

a. Ultrasound has become the diagnostic procedure of choice. Identifies stones and determines wall thickness, presence of masses, ductal dilation, and fluid collections. Most sensitive sign for diagnosis is presence of sonographic Murphy's sign.

b. Technical difficulties include obese patients, large amount of bowel gas, and skill required for technician and interpretation.

c. Sensitivity is 95%, with overall specificity of 90%.

5. Radionuclide (hydroxy iminodiacetic acid (HIDA) scan

a. HIDA is radioactive material taken up by the liver and excreted in the biliary system.

b. Diagnosis is acute cholecystitis (up to 95% accuracy) if gallbladder does not visualize within 4 hours of injection and the radioisotope is excreted in the CBD.

c. Reliable with a bilirubin level up to 20 mg/dl

d. Cholecystokinin-HIDA: Cholecystokinin causes contraction of the gallbladder and can be used to measure ejection fraction of GB and aid in the diagnosis of biliary dyskinesia.

## G. TREATMENT

1. Surgery: Cholecystectomy should be performed in most patients with symptoms and demonstrable stones if symptoms cannot be attributed to other causes.

2. Intraoperative cholangiogram (IOC)

a. Small incision on anterior surface of cystic duct. Intubate cystic duct with cholangiogram catheter and inject dye. Make sure there are no air bubbles in tubing because these can appear as stones, or filling defects on the image.

b. Must see filling of the following five structures: right and left hepatic ducts, cystic duct, common duct, and emptying into duodenum.

c. Indications: If unsure of biliary anatomy, or with preoperative increase of LFTs suggesting retained common duct stone or obstruction, some surgeons suggest IOC in every case for experience, documentation of anatomy, and increasing skill for performing IOC.

## H. MANAGEMENT OF ASYMPTOMATIC STONES

1. Truly asymptomatic patients do not require cholecystectomy unless it can be performed safely during laparotomy for another condition ("incidental cholecystectomy"). Postoperative cholecystitis has been reported in up to 20% of patients with cholelithiasis undergoing a second major abdominal procedure.

2. Prophylactic cholecystectomy should be considered in asymptomatic patients in the following situations:

a. Patients with sickle cell disease, on chronic total parenteral nutrition, or undergoing immunosuppression for solid organ transplants

b. The patient with a calcified "porcelain" gallbladder (15–20% associated with carcinoma)

c. Any patient with a history of biliary pancreatitis

d. Roux-en-Y gastric bypass patients

## III. ACUTE CALCULOUS CHOLECYSTITIS

### A. GENERAL CONSIDERATIONS

Approximately 95% of cases of acute cholecystitis are associated with obstruction of the cystic duct by a gallstone. Approximately 30% of patients with biliary colic experience development of acute cholecystitis within 2 years.

### B. SYMPTOMS

Symptoms of acute calculous cholecystitis are constant, severe RUQ or epigastric pain that may radiate to the infrascapular region. Anorexia, nausea, and vomiting are common.

### C. PHYSICAL EXAMINATION

1. RUQ tenderness on palpation and signs of focal peritoneal irritation may be present.
2. Murphy's sign
3. Low-grade fever
4. Palpable gallbladder—uncommon

### D. LABORATORY FINDINGS

1. Moderate leukocytosis—10,000–20,000/mm$^3$
2. Frequent mild increase of bilirubin level: Increase >4 mg/dl is unusual in simple cholecystitis and suggests the presence of choledocholithiasis.
3. Frequent increase of alkaline phosphatase level; transaminases and amylase concentrations may be increased.

### E. IMAGING

Ultrasound shows thickened gallbladder wall, pericholecystic fluid, stones visualized in the gallbladder with echoic shadowing, and positive Murphy's sign with ultrasound probe.

### F. DIFFERENTIAL DIAGNOSIS

The differential diagnosis of acute calculous cholecystitis includes acute peptic ulcer disease with or without perforation, pancreatitis, acute appendicitis, cecal volvulus, right lower lobe pneumonia, myocardial infarction, passive hepatic congestion, acute gonorrheal perihepatitis (Fitz–Hugh–Curtis syndrome), and viral or alcoholic hepatitis.

### G. COMPLICATIONS

1. Hydrops: Cystic duct obstruction leads to a tense gallbladder filled with mucus ("lime bile"). It may lead to gallbladder wall necrosis if pressure exceeds capillary blood pressure. Gallbladder often is palpable.

2. Gangrene and perforation: May be localized, leading to abscess that is confined by the omentum; or free perforation may occur, leading to generalized peritonitis and sepsis. Emergency laparotomy is indicated.

3. Empyema of the gallbladder (suppurative cholecystitis): This is a condition in which the gallbladder contains frank pus. The patient is often toxic, and urgent surgery is indicated.

4. Cholecystenteric fistula
a. Results from repeated attacks of cholecystitis
b. Duodenum, colon, and stomach involved, in decreasing order
c. Pneumobilia: Air is present in the biliary tree in 40% of cases (visible on plain films of the abdomen).
d. May not cause symptoms unless the gallbladder is partially obstructed by stones or scarring
e. Symptomatic cholecystenteric fistulas should be treated with cholecystectomy and fistula closure.

5. Gallstone ileus: Gallstones cause the cholecystenteric fistula to pass into the enteric lumen and cause intermittent bouts of small-bowel obstruction ("tumbling ileus").
a. Symptoms of acute cholecystitis immediately preceding onset of bowel obstruction are uncommon (25–30%).
b. Stones <2 to 3 cm usually pass spontaneously and do not cause bowel obstruction.
c. Terminal ileum is the most common site of obstruction.
d. Overall, responsible for 1% to 2% of bowel obstructions
e. Mortality rate is 10% to 15%—reflects elderly patients, in whom this is more common.
f. Small-bowel enterotomy proximal to the point of obstruction is usually required to remove the stone.
g. Immediate cholecystectomy is not warranted because <4% of patients have further symptoms.

## H. MANAGEMENT OF ACUTE CHOLECYSTITIS

1. Surgery
a. Preferred treatment is cholecystectomy (open procedure or laparoscopic) within 3 days of the onset of symptoms.
b. Conservative management with intravenous fluids and antibiotics (first- or second-generation cephalosporin) may be justified in some high-risk patients to convert an emergency procedure into an elective procedure and in patients with delayed presentation (>72 hours). Lack of noticeable improvement within 1 to 2 days of initiation of conservative treatment suggests possible complicated acute cholecystitis, necessitating more urgent operative intervention.

2. Surgical complications
a. Conservative management is justified after 3 days of symptoms because severe inflammation may increase risk for injury to the CBD, a risk greater

than that of gallbladder perforation. The risk for gangrene and perforation is relatively low during the first 3 days after the onset of symptoms. After this period, the incidence rate increases to 10%. An interval elective cholecystectomy should be performed in the next 4 to 6 weeks.

b. Intraoperative complications—injury to CBD, right or left hepatic ducts or arteries.

c. Postoperative complications—formation of biloma (any patient who presents after cholecystectomy with severe pain must be evaluated for this), abscess formation/infection, prolonged ileus.

### 3. Percutaneous drainage

In extremely high-risk patients (i.e., critically ill patients in an intensive care unit setting), cholecystostomy and percutaneous drainage under radiological guidance may be indicated to decompress the gallbladder, saving formal cholecystectomy until the patient is more stable.

### 4. Microbiology and antibiotics

a. *Escherichia coli, Klebsiella, Enterococcus,* and *Enterobacter* account for >80% of infections.

b. First- or second-generation cephalosporins are first choice of antibiotic coverage, although they do not cover *Enterococcus* sp.

c. Broader-spectrum antibiotics are used depending on the severity of the infection and the patient's response to treatment. Ampicillin, aminoglycoside, and metronidazole (or clindamycin) may be indicated in overtly septic patients.

## IV. ACUTE ACALCULOUS CHOLECYSTITIS

Approximately 5% of cholecystitis occurs in the absence of cholelithiasis; 50% to 80% is present in an advanced state (gangrene, perforation, abscess). This condition is associated with a 40% mortality rate.

### A. ACALCULOUS CHOLECYSTITIS

Primarily seen as a complication of prolonged fasting after an unrelated operation or trauma (e.g., acute burns, multiple organ failure, multiple fractures). Causative factors are believed to include the following:

1. Ischemia of the gallbladder during episodes of relative hypoperfusion

2. Dehydration leads to formation of extremely viscous bile, which may obstruct or irritate the gallbladder.

3. Bacteremia may result in seeding of the stagnant bile.

4. Sepsis with resultant mucosal hypoperfusion may promote gallbladder wall invasion of organisms.

5. Bile stasis results from a lack of cholecystokinin-stimulated gallbladder contraction.

6. May be associated with large amounts of parenterally administered narcotics with resultant spasm of the sphincter of Oddi

7. Acalculous cholecystitis may also be due to cystic duct obstruction by another process, for example, tumor or nodal enlargement.

## B. DIAGNOSIS

1. May be difficult and often delayed because patients often are in the intensive care unit setting with multiple medical problems; requires high degree of suspicion

## C. DIAGNOSIS IS OBTAINED BY HIDA SCAN OR ULTRASOUND; TREATMENT IS EMERGENT CHOLECYSTECTOMY.

## V. CHOLEDOCHOLITHIASIS

### A. GENERAL CONSIDERATIONS

1. Approximately 8% to 16% of patients with cholelithiasis will be found to have stones in the CBD.
2. Most CBD stones arise from the gallbladder and pass into the CBD (secondary stones).
3. Stones forming de novo within the CBD are referred to as primary CBD stones; they are almost always associated with partial duct obstruction.
4. Complications include biliary colic, cholangitis, pancreatitis, late benign biliary stricture, and biliary cirrhosis.

### B. DIAGNOSIS

1. Increases of serum bilirubin, alkaline phosphatase, and 5-nucleotidase are characteristic; amylase level is increased with concomitant biliary pancreatitis. White blood cell count is increased if cholangitis is present; it is normal otherwise.
2. Ultrasound is not useful in detecting CBD stones, but it is highly sensitive in detecting associated intrahepatic and extrahepatic ductal dilation.
3. Endoscopic retrograde cholangiopancreatography (ERCP) is the procedure of choice after ultrasound.
   a. For CBD >9 mm, abnormal LFTs or history of pancreatitis or jaundice
   b. Can define biliary and upper gastrointestinal anatomy
   c. Can be therapeutic and diagnostic (e.g., sphincterotomy or placement of stents as necessary)
4. Intraoperative cystic duct cholangiography or intracorporeal laparoscopic ultrasonography should be performed in all patients at risk for choledocholithiasis or with uncertain anatomy.

### C. TREATMENT

Surgical treatment of stones within the biliary tree requires evacuation of all stones and debris, and establishment of free flow of bile into the gastrointestinal tract. The procedure may be performed before surgery via ERCP; intraoperatively via open, laparoscopic, or endoscopic (ERCP) techniques; or after surgery via ERCP or T tube. Often stones in the biliary tree are diagnosed with IOC as discussed previously.

1. Absolute indications for CBD exploration
   a. Palpable stones in the CBD—90% reliable

b. Jaundice with acute suppurative cholangitis
c. Proven presence of CBD stones on cholangiogram (IOC)

2. **Relative indications for CBD exploration**
a. Dilated CBD >15 mm—35% reliable
b. Bilirubin level >8 mg/dl

3. **Choledochoenteric bypass (choledochoduodenostomy or choledochoje-junostomy) may be performed in the presence of more than five CBD stones, marked CBD dilation, impacted stones that cannot be removed safely, history of previous choledocholithotomy, and primary CBD stones.**

4. **Preoperative ERCP with endoscopic sphincterotomy**
a. For patients with "high likelihood" of having a CBD stone (increased LFTs, bilirubin, or alkaline phosphatase; jaundice; or dilated biliary tree)
b. Cholecystectomy should take place within 48 hours to minimize chance for new stone migration into CBD.
c. Complications of ERCP (6–10%)—hemorrhage, pancreatitis, perforation, cholangitis

5. **Intraoperative CBD exploration**
a. Initial attempt—transcystic approach via a cholangiography catheter. Glucagon may be given to relax the sphincter of Oddi and then saline irrigation to flush the stone from the CBD. If this fails, a balloon catheter may be passed into the duct, inflated, and pulled back to withdraw the stone. For proximal stones, it is possible to "milk" the stone back through the duct and have it exit the incision in the cystic duct. If the above fails, the next attempt can be made with a wire basket catheter passed under fluoroscopy to catch the stones and extract them from the duct.
b. Last attempt—if the cystic duct is well dilated, a choledochoscope may be passed into the biliary tree, and under direct visualization the stones may be caught via a wire basket or pushed into the duodenum.
c. If stone extraction fails by all of the above methods, choledochotomy is required (T tube or antegrade stent necessary).
d. On-table ERCP with endoscopic sphincterotomy has been described, but this is institution and operator dependent.

6. **Postoperative T-tube extraction**
a. About 4 to 6 weeks required for mature tract to form
b. About 80% to 95% successful
c. Management of T tube
   (1) T-tube cholangiogram on postoperative days 5 to 7
   (2) If no evidence of leakage or retained CBD stones, may clamp tube
   (3) Remove tube in 2 to 3 weeks on outpatient basis

7. **Postoperative ERCP with endoscopic sphincterotomy**
a. T tube not required (need not wait 4–6 weeks)
b. Recommended for elderly patients at high risk for complications with CBD exploration

**20**

**BENIGN GALLBLADDER**

## D. RETAINED COMMON DUCT STONES
Retained common duct stones are found in up to 5% of patients undergoing CBD exploration.

1. **Options for the patient with a T tube in place**
   a. Remove stones percutaneously with a basket passed through a mature T-tube tract (4 weeks) using fluoroscopic control (>90% success rate).
   b. Endoscopic sphincterotomy for unstable patients, malfunctioning T tubes, or unsuccessful percutaneous extraction
   c. Chemical dissolution or mechanical lithotripsy rarely indicated or successful
2. **Patients without a T tube**
   a. Endoscopic sphincterotomy and "basket" removal of stones transduodenally
   b. Reoperation
   c. Percutaneous transhepatic approach
   d. Extracorporeal shockwave lithotripsy

## VI. CHOLANGITIS

### A. GENERAL CONSIDERATIONS
1. A life-threatening disease that requires prompt recognition and treatment
2. Caused by obstruction of the biliary tract and biliary stasis, leading to bacterial overgrowth, suppuration, and subsequent biliary sepsis under pressure

### B. CAUSATIVE FACTORS
1. Choledocholithiasis—60%
2. Benign postoperative strictures
3. Pancreatic or biliary neoplasms
4. Miscellaneous—invasive procedures, biliary-enteric anastomoses, foreign bodies, parasitic infections (from the Chinese liver fluke Clonorchis sinensis)

### C. CLINICAL FINDINGS
1. Charcot's triad: (1) RUQ pain, (2) jaundice, (3) fever and chills. The classic Charcot's triad is seen in only 50% to 70% of cases.
2. Reynolds' pentad may be seen: Charcot's triad + shock and mental obtundation.

### D. DIAGNOSIS
1. Leukocytosis, hyperbilirubinemia, increased LFTs (specifically AP)
2. Initial study should be RUQ ultrasound; presence of ductal dilation and gallstones is suggestive. Thickening of bile duct walls, liver abscess, or gas in the biliary tree are strong supportive evidence.

## E. MANAGEMENT

The immediate goal is to decompress the biliary tree. The method by which this is accomplished depends on the particular clinical situation.

1. Initially, provide supportive care with hydration, electrolyte correction, and broad-spectrum antibiotics (successful in up to 85% of patients).
2. The toxic patient is prepared for immediate surgical decompression by CBD exploration.
3. Patients with a protracted course usually have more complicated obstruction and may require percutaneous transhepatic cholangiography or ERCP. Percutaneous transhepatic cholangiography may be therapeutic in the acute situation by decompressing the biliary tree.
4. ERCP may be effective in decompressing the biliary tree by papillotomy or by the endoscopic placement of biliary stents or nasobiliary tube.

# Abdominal Wall Hernias

*Jonathan E. Schoeff, MD*

## I. HISTORICAL PERSPECTIVE

Numerous surgeons and anatomists have participated in the development of the modern-day herniorrhaphy. Several warrant particular interest because of their major contributions to early hernia surgery.

### A. H. O. MARCY (1837–1924)

1. Boston surgeon who described anterior approach to hernia repair with high ligation of the hernia sac in 1871.

### B. EDOARDO BASSINI (1844–1924)

1. In 1887, he wrote "Nuevo Metodo Operativo per la Cura Radicale dell'Ernia Inguinale." In this landmark article, he describes the "triple layer" consisting of the internal oblique muscle, transversus abdominus muscle, and transversalis fascia.

### C. SIR ASTLEY COOPER (1768–1841)

1. Published his description of inguinal anatomy and repair, which included a description of the superior pubic ligament, in 1804. He himself had a right indirect hernia as a teenager and wore a truss for 5 years.

### D. CHESTER MCVAY (1911–1987)

1. Submitted his thesis on groin anatomy in 1939 for a doctorate at Northwestern University, asserting that normal groin anatomy involved Bassini's "triple layer" inserting on Cooper's ligament, not the inguinal ligament. In 1942, while a resident at the University of Michigan, he reported his technique of groin hernia repair, which included the critical "relaxing incision."

### E. EDWARD EARLE SHOULDICE (1890–1965)

1. His interest in treatment of inguinal hernias developed in 1930s. The Shouldice Hospital opened in 1945 and currently has 10 staff surgeons performing 7500 hernia operations per year.

## II. TERMINOLOGY

### A. HERNIA

1. Protrusion of a part or structure through the tissues normally containing it; from the Latin for "rupture"

### B. INCARCERATION

1. Nonreducible hernia sac contents that, in the acute setting, may present with obstructive symptoms and pain, among other symptoms. Also may occur chronically and be essentially asymptomatic.

## C. REDUCIBILITY
1. Contents of the hernia sac can be returned to their normal location.

## D. STRANGULATION
1. Incarcerated hernia with vascular compromise of the sac contents leading to gangrene and perforation of hollow viscus if left untreated. This represents a surgical emergency and is often accompanied by obstructive symptoms (exception is Richter's hernia), pain (potentially focal peritonitis), leukocytosis, fever, and skin changes (e.g. warmth, erythema).

## III. INCIDENCE
### A. GENERAL CONSIDERATIONS
1. Approximately 5% of all people will experience development of a hernia in their lifetime.
2. Hernias of the inguinal region make up ~75% of all abdominal wall hernias.
3. Indirect hernias are the most common type of hernia regardless of sex and outnumber direct hernias 2:1 in male individuals.
a. Right-sided hernias are more common than left because of the slower descent of the right testes and the delay in atrophy of the processus vaginalis.
4. Femoral hernias account for <10% of abdominal wall hernias, yet upward of 40% will present as surgical urgency or emergency in the form of an incarcerated or strangulated hernia.
a. Predominance of right-sided femoral hernias is thought to be due to the tamponading effect of the sigmoid colon on the left femoral canal.

### B. SEX
1. Male-to-female ratio: ~7:1
2. Lifetime risk for development of a hernia reported variably in the literature: male individuals: 5% to 24%; female individuals: 1%

## IV. NATURAL HISTORY
### A. LIKELIHOOD OF STRANGULATION INCREASES WITH AGE; HOWEVER, ONLY ~1% TO 3% OF ALL HERNIAS WILL STRANGULATE.
### B. FEMORAL HERNIAS HAVE A SIGNIFICANTLY GREATER RATE OF STRANGULATION, ~15% TO 20%.

## V. ANATOMIC CONSIDERATIONS
### A. LAYERS OF THE ABDOMINAL WALL
1. The layers of the abdominal wall in order of encounter while performing groin hernia surgery are skin, subcutaneous fat (Camper's), Scarpa's fascia, external oblique muscle laterally and aponeurosis medially, internal oblique muscle, transversus abdominus muscle, transversalis fascia, and peritoneum.

## B.  INGUINAL CANAL

1. A fibrous canal that contains the spermatic cord, the ilioinguinal nerve, the genital branch of the genitofemoral nerve, and hernia sac, if present. The canal is bordered inferiorly by the inguinal ligament, superiorly by the conjoined tendon and the reflections of the transversus abdominus and the internal oblique muscle, anteriorly by the external oblique aponeurosis, and posteriorly by the transversalis fascia.

## C.  SPERMATIC CORD

1. Complex of structures exiting the abdomen, traversing the inguinal canal, and entering the scrotum. Cord is composed of the testicular artery, pampiniform plexus of veins, vas deferens, cremasteric muscle fibers, genital branch of genitofemoral nerve, and hernia sac (if present, often lies anteromedial to the cord structures).

## D.  PROCESSUS VAGINALIS

1. Diverticulum of parietal peritoneum that descends from the abdomen along with the testicle and comes to lie adjacent to the spermatic cord. This structure subsequently obliterates in normal development to remain as the tunica vaginalis.

## E.  DEEP (INTERNAL) INGUINAL RING

1. Composed of fibers of the internal oblique muscle superiorly, and transversalis fascia and inferior epigastric vessels inferomedially.

## F.  SUPERFICIAL (EXTERNAL) INGUINAL RING

1. Composed of a medial and lateral crus of the external oblique aponeurotic fibers through which the spermatic cord in male individuals and round ligament in female individuals together with branches of ilioinguinal and genitofemoral nerve traverse.

## G.  HESSELBACH'S TRIANGLE

1. Site of direct inguinal hernia formed by lateral border of the rectus abdominus muscle medially, inferior epigastric vessels laterally, and the inguinal ligament inferiorly.

## H.  INGUINAL (POUPART'S) LIGAMENT

1. Fibrous band formed by the thickened inferior border of the external oblique aponeurosis that inserts laterally on the anterior superior iliac spine of the ileum and medially on the pubic tubercle; forms the inferior wall of the inguinal canal.

## I.  ILEOPUBIC TRACT

1. Thickening of transversalis fascia inferiorly leading in to inguinal (Poupart's) ligament, only ~7 to 8 mm

## J. LACUNAR (GIMBERNAT) LIGAMENT

1. Medial reflection of the inguinal ligament that reflects inferiorly from the pubic tubercle to the pectineal line of the pubis; acts as the medial border of the femoral canal.

## K. COOPER'S (PECTINEAL) LIGAMENT

1. Fibrous band that joins the lacunar ligament medially and runs laterally along the pectineal line of the pubis.

## L. FEMORAL CANAL

1. Serves as the location for femoral hernias and is defined anatomically by the lacunar ligament medially, the femoral vessels laterally (namely the femoral vein), the inguinal ligament anteriorly, and Cooper's ligament posteriorly.

**Surgical Pearl:** *Femoral canal contents from lateral to medial are NAVEL—nerve (femoral nerve), artery (femoral artery), vein (femoral vein), empty space (site of femoral hernia), and lymphatics.*

## M. INFERIOR LUMBAR (PETIT'S) TRIANGLE

1. Site of Petit's hernia formed by the lateral border of latissimus dorsi medially, posterior/medial margin of the external oblique laterally, and inferiorly by the iliac crest.

## N. SUPERIOR LUMBAR (GRYNFELT'S) TRIANGLE

1. Site of Grynfelt's hernia formed by twelfth rib superiorly, the sacrospinous muscle medially, and the lateral border of the internal oblique muscle inferiorly.

## VI. CLASSIFICATION OF HERNIAS

## A. GROIN HERNIAS (FIG. 21-1)

1. Indirect inguinal hernia—sac exits through internal ring, lateral to the inferior epigastric vessels. Hernia sac is found anteromedial to the spermatic cord in males and the round ligament in female individuals.
2. Direct inguinal hernia—sac exits through Hesselbach's triangle, medial to the inferior epigastric vessels.
3. Pantaloon hernia—inguinal hernia that involves both indirect and direct component straddling the inferior epigastric vessels

**Surgical Pearl:** *Remember, a pantaloon hernia sac is analogous to a pair of pants with the crotch straddling the inferior epigastric vessels.*

4. Femoral hernia—sac exits through the femoral canal, medial to the femoral vein.

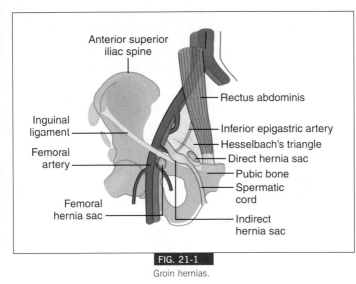

**FIG. 21-1**

Groin hernias.

## B. VENTRAL HERNIAS
1. Umbilical hernia—may be congenital or acquired
2. Epigastric hernia—sac exits in the midline through the linea alba, above the umbilicus.
3. Incisional hernia—defect of the fascia resulting at the site of a previous fascial closure, most commonly after a midline laparotomy; however, it may develop in the setting of any fascial repair, including those from laparoscopic surgical procedures.
4. Rectus diastasis—not a true hernia but is often mistaken for one. Represents a weakening of the linea alba and stretching of the rectus abdominus muscles away from each other. There is no herniation of abdominal contents through this weakened layer.

## C. MISCELLANEOUS HERNIAS
1. Amyand's hernia—inguinal hernia contents include appendix, described first in the setting of acute appendicitis.
2. Grynfeltt's hernia—sac exits through the superior lumbar triangle.
3. Littre's hernia—inguinal hernia contents include Meckel's diverticulum.
4. Obturator hernia—sac exits through the obturator foramen and compresses the obturator nerve and vessels.

**Surgical Pearl:** *Howship–Romberg sign is pain along medial thigh exacerbated by abduction, extension, and medial rotation of the thigh. This is secondary to* *compression on the obturator nerve whose anterior branch supplies sensory fibers to the distal medial thigh. This finding is only present in ~50% of patients.*

5. Parastomal hernia—hernia at ostomy site, more commonly occurring at colostomy sites, in particular, those stomas through the semilunar line
6. Petit's hernia—sac exits through the inferior lumbar triangle.
7. Richter's hernia—condition in which one sidewall of a viscus is incorporated into hernia sac, thus the hernia contents may incarcerate and strangulate without causing bowel obstruction symptoms (Fig. 21-2). Bowel may also reduce after incarceration, leading to intraabdominal perforation with peritonitis.
8. Sciatic hernia—sac exits through the greater or lesser sciatic foramen.
9. Sliding hernia—wall of the hernia sac is composed of a viscus (commonly sigmoid colon or cecum) (Fig. 21-3).
10. Spigelian hernia—abdominal hernia through the semilunar line of Spigelius (lateral to the rectus abdominus) most commonly at the junction of the semilunar line and the semicircular line of Douglas (the point at which the posterior rectus sheath terminates).

## VII. CAUSATIVE FACTORS

### A. INDIRECT INGUINAL HERNIA
1. Persistence of a patent processus vaginalis is primary causative factor in pediatric population; in adults, the cause is likely multifactorial.

### B. DIRECT INGUINAL HERNIA
1. Considered to be an acquired phenomenon related to chronic increases in intraabdominal pressure (see VII.D), placing stress in the area of Hesselbach's triangle, as well as inguinal floor weakness

### C. FEMORAL HERNIA
1. Similar to the causes of direct inguinal hernias involving chronic increases in abdominal pressure together with anatomic variability. Femoral hernias are particularly at risk for incarceration and subsequent strangulation given the relative rigidity of the structures that make up the femoral canal.

### D. CONTRIBUTING FACTORS
1. Contributing factors include obesity, chronic cough (related to smoking/chronic obstructive pulmonary disease), chronic straining from constipation/obstipation, prostatism, pregnancy, and ascites.

## VIII. DIAGNOSIS

### A. HISTORY
1. History of a palpable, soft mass that increases with Valsalva maneuver. This is often a painless mass (in the absence of incarceration or strangulation); a primary complaint of pain should prompt investigation into other sources.

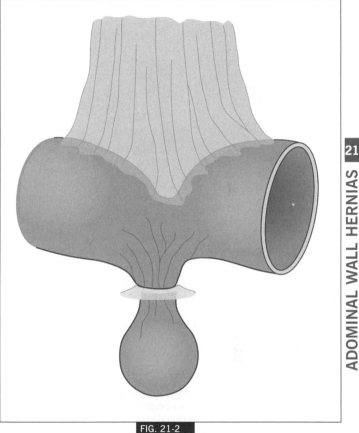

### FIG. 21-2
Richter's hernia.

2. Mass may spontaneously reduce or may require manual reduction.

## B. EXAMINATION
1. Examination reveals a palpable mass that increases in size while the patient performs the Valsalva maneuver. The classic "turn and cough" examination may result in an impulse being appreciated at the external ring that is not a true hernia. It is critical to examine all patients upright (preferably standing) and supine.

**Surgical Pearl:** *In male individuals, a digital inspection should be performed via the scrotum to palpate the external inguinal ring. The finger should parallel*

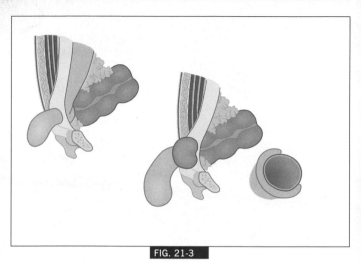

**FIG. 21-3**

Sliding hernia.

*the spermatic cord in the scrotum to follow it up to its exit point at the external ring.*

2. Examination should focus on location of hernia relative to inguinal ligament.
a. Hernias below inguinal ligament may be consistent with a femoral hernia.
   (1) Femoral hernias may reflect above inguinal ligament as well, making it difficult to distinguish between an inguinal and a femoral hernia.
3. Obesity may make it difficult to appreciate small hernias.
4. Obturator, lumbar, sciatic, and small femoral hernias may be easily missed on physical examination.
a. Computed tomography scan may demonstrate hernias not appreciated on physical examination and serve as a useful adjunct to the physical examination.

## C. SMALL-BOWEL OBSTRUCTION
1. May be the first manifestation of a hernia and a thorough examination for any hernias should always be included in the work-up for obstructive symptoms

## D. DIFFERENTIAL DIAGNOSIS OF GROIN MASS
1. Inguinal/femoral hernia, hydrocele, varicocele, inguinal lymphadenitis, ectopic testes, lipoma, epithelial inclusion cyst, neoplasms, arterial aneurysm/pseudoaneurysm

## E. REDUCTION OF INCARCERATED HERNIA

1. Position the patient in steep Trendelenburg position, use adequate sedation, and place ice on hernia. Taxis (process of reducing hernia) requires paradoxical traction on the hernia sac while applying gentle pressure at the neck of the hernia to reduce the contents. This is thought to decrease edema of intestinal contents and also decrease the volume of sac contents being reduced at any one time.
2. Significant tenderness, induration, erythema, or leukocytosis suggest possible strangulation and should prompt urgent surgical exploration; if these signs/symptoms are present, no reduction should be attempted.

## F. REDUCTION EN MASSE

1. Reduction of the hernia sac and contents without exploration of the sac or freeing of the contents within. Patients should be observed after reduction for any signs or symptoms of strangulation.

## IX. REPAIR OF HERNIAS

## A. VENTRAL AND UMBILICAL HERNIAS

1. These hernias can be repaired by suture closure (herniorrhaphy) or closure with mesh, depending on their size and tension.

## B. INGUINAL HERNIAS

1. Multiple repairs have been described. Both laparoscopic and open repairs are used (see section XI for detailed description of laparoscopic procedures). The critical aspect of all hernia surgery is a tension-free repair.
2. Anterior repairs: Uniformly, a transverse/oblique skin incision is made, and the external oblique aponeurosis is incised, revealing the contents of the inguinal canal.

a. Marcy repair: Also known as high ligation of the hernia sac, it is commonly used in pediatric indirect inguinal hernias.

b. Bassini repair: Bassini described an interrupted suture repair of his "triple layer"—the internal oblique muscle, transversus abdominus, and transversalis fascia to ileopubic tract/inguinal ligament. Repair is flawed because of tension.

c. McVay (Cooper ligament) repair: This is the only anterior tissue repair approach that treats all three groin hernia types—indirect, direct, and femoral. This repair is the standard tissue repair that can be used to safely repair groin hernias in which mesh is contraindicated (e.g., strangulated hernia contamination). This repair relies on approximation of the conjoined tendon to Cooper's ligament medially and the inguinal ligament laterally. A "relaxing incision" on the anterior rectus sheath and the "transition" stitch are key elements of the repair.

**Surgical Pearl:** *The "relaxing incision" on the anterior rectus sheath allows this operation to be relatively tension-free.*

**Surgical Pearl:** *The "transition" stitch is critical to this repair and is the suture placed just medial to the femoral vein transitioning from approximation to Cooper's ligament to approximation to the inguinal ligament. If this stitch is placed too far laterally, compression of the femoral vein may occur, which increases the risk for venous thrombosis.*

d. Shouldice repair: This technique expanded on Bassini repair and has essentially replaced it as a tissue repair. The critical difference is the use of a continuous, nonabsorbable suture that sequentially reinforces the inguinal floor. The Shouldice repair will treat inguinal hernias but not femoral hernias.

e. Lichtenstein repair: First described in 1984, this technique has become the standard for inguinal herniorrhaphy because it is a tension-free repair. This involves securing a piece of synthetic mesh (classically polypropylene) medially to the pubic tubercle, inferiorly to the shelving edge of the inguinal ligament (ileopubic tract), and superiorly to the rectus abdominus, internal oblique, and transversus abdominus. This repair recreates the floor of the inguinal canal and the deep (internal) inguinal ring, with the spermatic cord passing through the lateral portion of the mesh.

3. Preperitoneal repairs

a. Nyhus (posterior [preperitoneal] approach) repair: This is a preperitoneal tissue repair advocated for repair of indirect, direct, and femoral hernias. The presence of a satisfactory ileopubic tract is necessary for this repair.

b. Stoppa repair (giant prosthetic reinforcement of the visceral sac): This is a preperitoneal approach to hernia repair that is useful for treating recurrent groin hernias (in particular, incisional hernia), bilateral hernias, or high-risk hernias (those likely to recur). The basic principle is using a large synthetic mesh to either reinforce or replace the transversalis fascia placed in the preperitoneal plane.

c. Total extraperitoneal laparoscopic repair (TEP; see section XI)

## C. PREPERITONEAL APPROACH

1. For groin hernias, this is most commonly a laparoscopic procedure (transabdominal preperitoneal approach [TAPP]; see section XI).

## D. REPAIR OF FEMORAL HERNIAS

Given the high propensity relative to other hernia types for femoral hernias to incarcerate and strangulate, all femoral hernias should be repaired when diagnosed.

1. Tissue-based repair of femoral hernias include McVay (Cooper ligament) repair, Nyhus (preperitoneal) repair, and the infrainguinal repair of the femoral canal.

a. Of note, the Nyhus approach to repair of the femoral hernia involves suturing of the ileopubic tract to Cooper's ligament, thus obliterating the femoral canal.
2. Mesh-based repairs include the Stoppa, TEP, and TAPP.

## X. POSTOPERATIVE COMPLICATIONS

### A. RECURRENT HERNIA

This may be related to missed hernia intraoperatively or failure of repair. Repairs under tension are most likely to recur. Mesh repairs most commonly fail medially.

1. Recurrence rates are reported as ranging from <1% with mesh repairs (e.g., Lichtenstein) to 1.5% with tissue-based repairs (e.g., Shouldice).
a. Recurrence rates are greater in patients with chronic cough, constipation, and obesity. Attempts should be made before surgery to correct these conditions if at all possible.
2. Technical errors
a. Excessive suture line tension
b. Failure to adequately "tighten" internal ring
c. Failure to identify indirect hernia or femoral hernia sac during initial operation
d. Failure to repair "prehernia" laxity in the inguinal floor

### B. INFECTION

1. Infection rates were thought to be greater among mesh repairs; however, this has never been demonstrated in the literature, and the repairs likely share a similar rate of infection when similar elective cohorts are compared.

### C. BLEEDING

1. Bleeding may occur in the preperitoneal space and track retroperitoneally as well as into the scrotum. A significant amount of bleeding may occur before recognition, and a high index of suspicion must be maintained after surgery in any patient with tachycardia, hypotension, or orthostasis.

**Surgical Pearl:** *If worsening scrotal hematoma occurs, reexploration should be performed via inguinal incision to identify and ligate the source of bleeding.*

### D. DYSEJACULATION

1. This is seen in male patients after hernia repair and was initially reported by the Shouldice Clinic, citing an incidence rate in long-term follow-up of ~0.25%. Patients may develop a searing pain with ejaculation and this is thought to be related to constriction of the vas deferens.

21

ADOMINAL WALL HERNIAS

## E. TESTICULAR ATROPHY
1. This is a long-term complication resulting from chronic testicular ischemia. This is seen more commonly in recurrent hernia repairs.

## F. DIFFICULTY VOIDING
1. This is more common in elderly male adults. A thorough history before surgery should focus on symptoms of prostatism, and if the hernia is stable, adequate treatment should be sought before hernia repair.

## G. NEUROMA/NEURITIS
1. Usually results from entrapment of sensory nerve fibers, in particular the ilioinguinal nerve. Symptoms may resolve; however, persistence of symptoms may require reexploration and ligation of the nerve.

## H. PAIN
1. Scrotal swelling may result from inadequate hemostasis intraoperatively or impairment of testicular venous return after surgery.

## XI. LAPAROSCOPIC HERNIA REPAIR

### A. GENERAL
1. Approaches
a. TAPP
b. TEP
c. Additional procedures have been described, including intraperitoneal laparoscopic onlay mesh; however, only TEP and TAPP have remained as mainstays of laparoscopic inguinal hernia repair.
2. Anatomy of the preperitoneal space
a. Both TAPP and TEP require an in-depth understanding of the preperitoneal space (Fig. 21-4).
b. "Triangle of Doom"—bounded medially by the vas deferens and laterally by the gonadal vessels. The external iliac vessels run in triangle.
c. "Triangle of Pain"—bounded by gonadal vessels medially, ileopubic tract superiorly, and the pelvic sidewall inferolaterally. The genitofemoral nerve and lateral femoral cutaneous nerve are at risk for injury if mesh is tacked down in this area.
d. Patient selection—comorbidities as contraindication to general anesthesia, large scrotal component, sliding hernia, recurrent hernia (particularly previously repaired by lap approach), incarcerated or strangulated hernia
3. Details of specific procedures
a. TAPP
(1) Operative procedure
(a) Intraabdominal laparoscopy using three ports: a 10-mm infraumbilical camera port, and bilateral lower quadrant ports for dissection
(b) Hernia contents are reduced into the abdomen.

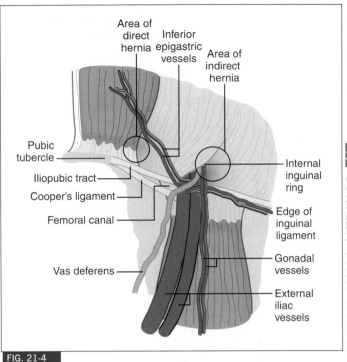

**FIG. 21-4**

Key landmarks of the inguinal anatomy in the preperitoneal space and typical locations of direct, indirect, and femoral hernias. *(From Geis WP, Crafton WB, Novak MJ, Melago M: Laparoscopic herniorrhaphy: Results and technical aspects in 458 consecutive procedures.* Surgery *114:765, 1993.)*

(c) Incision of peritoneum lateral to medial umbilical fold and entry into preperitoneal space

(d) Dissection in preperitoneal space should focus on identification of Cooper's ligament, epigastric vessels, gonadal vessels, vas deferens, and internal inguinal ring.

(e) Reinforcement of posterior abdominal wall with mesh, thereby closing the hernia defect, is critical to secure mesh to Cooper's ligament and pubic symphysis medially, rectus sheath superiorly, and transversalis fascia laterally. Also, all tacks should remain above the ileopubic tract to avoid neurovascular structures.

(f) Peritoneum is then reapproximated over mesh, thereby preventing direct contact between mesh and bowel.

(g) Laparoscopy ports are closed in standard fashion.

      (2) Advantages
         (a) Reduction of hernia sac may be technically easier and hernia sac contents can be directly visualized, particularly if concern for viability exists.
      (3) Disadvantages
         (a) Procedure traverses abdominal cavity, incurring attendant risks for visceral and vascular injury
         (b) If the peritoneum is inadequately closed, there is risk of contact between bowels and mesh, which may increase risk for small-bowel adhesions or fistulization, or both.
  b. TEP
      (1) Operative procedure
         (a) Skin incision in infraumbilical position with incision of the anterior rectus sheath lateral to the midline on the affected side. A dissecting balloon is then inserted in the preperitoneal space and used to dissect this plane.
         (b) Two 5-mm ports are placed in the midline between the pubis and the camera port.
         (c) Dissection and repair of the hernia is the same as TAPP.
      (2) Advantages
         (a) Because the peritoneum is not disrupted, ideally there is no contact between intraabdominal contents and mesh.
         (b) May be performed under regional anesthesia
      (3) Disadvantages
         (a) May be more difficult than TAPP to reduce a large hernia sac
         (b) If peritoneum is unintentionally violated, loss of pneumoperitoneum may make dissection difficult.

**4. Results**
a. In retrospective series, decrease in recovery time and postoperative pain
b. Prospective series have demonstrated similar recurrence rates to open mesh repairs on the order of 1%.

**5. Advantages**
a. Decreased risk for graft infection
b. Ability to diagnose and repair bilateral hernia defects at the time of surgery; data suggest that upward of 50% of patients with a unilateral hernia actually have an asymptomatic hernia on the contralateral side that would be missed with an open repair.
c. Preperitoneal mesh placement offers optimal support for abdominal wall.
d. Improved visualization of neurovascular structures
e. Faster return to full activity

**6. Disadvantages**
a. Increased cost and increased operative time. Authors argue that this is counteracted by shortened recovery time.
b. Learning curve for surgeon requires multiple operations before complication rate is sufficiently low.
c. Requires general anesthesia for TAPP, possible regional anesthesia for TEP

### 7. Complications
a. Mortality—exceedingly low, around 0.1%, most commonly from bleeding complications
b. Morbidity—0% to 6%
   (1) Urinary retention—most common complication, particularly in male patients
   (2) Neuralgias—specific attention must be paid to staying above the ileopubic tract
   (3) Port hernia—specifically in TAPP procedure because TEP should not violate the peritoneum
   (4) Recurrence—long-term follow-up studies demonstrate recurrence rates of ~1% with skilled surgeons.
      (a) Rates higher during learning curve of operation
      (b) Most commonly caused by mesh of inadequate size

# Gastrointestinal Bleeding

*Rajalakshmi R. Nair, MD*

*The only weapon with which the unconscious patient can immediately retaliate upon the incompetent surgeon is hemorrhage.*
—William Stewart Halsted

Gastrointestinal (GI) bleeding can be characterized and managed by its location. Upper GI bleeding is defined as bleeding originating *proximal* to the ligament of Treitz, whereas lower GI bleeding occurs *distal* to the ligament of Treitz. The incidence of GI bleeding increases with advancing age, with a greater than 200-fold increase from the third decade to the ninth decade of life.

**22**

## I. HISTORY

History and physical examination can elucidate the cause of GI bleeding. History should include type, nature, and duration of bleeding; abdominal symptoms; bowel habits; risks and precipitating factors; and medical and surgical history.

### A. INITIAL PRESENTATION
1. Initial assessment should include the type of bleeding and estimated amount of blood loss. This assessment should be conducted simultaneously with resuscitation.
   a. Hematemesis (bright red or coffee-ground emesis)—usually indicates an upper GI source. However, massive pulmonary, upper airway, or nasopharyngeal hemorrhage should not be mistaken for GI bleeding.
   b. Hematochezia (bloody stool)—usually a lower GI source but may also be caused by brisk upper GI bleeding
   c. Melena (black tarry stool)—caused by gradual bleeding, usually from an upper GI source
   d. Occult blood (guaiac positive stool)—may be an upper or a lower GI source
2. Associated abdominal pain
   a. Painless bleeding—varices, angiodysplasia, diverticulosis, or cancer
   b. Epigastric pain—ulcer disease, gastritis, or esophagitis
   c. Cramping abdominal pain—diverticulitis, inflammatory bowel disease, colitis, or partially obstructing cancer
   d. Severe, acute, sudden onset of pain usually indicates perforated viscus.
   e. Pain out of proportion to abdominal pain associated with lower GI bleeding is **hallmark** for bowel ischemia.
3. Risks and precipitating factors
   a. Iatrogenic—GI instrumentation (nasogastric tube, colonoscopy, esophagogastroduodenoscopy)

   b. Ulcerogenic agents—steroids, aspirin, nonsteroidal antiinflammatory drugs, alcohol use, and tobacco use

   c. Severe stress—major trauma or massive burns (Curling's ulcer), intracranial pathology (Cushing's ulcer)

   d. Blunt or penetrating trauma

**4. Medical history**

   a. Bowel habits—constipation, diarrhea, bowel patterns (regular vs. irregular)

   b. Prior episodes of GI bleeding, including severity, frequency, and previous diagnostic and therapeutic interventions

   c. Surgical history

   d. Significant medical history—cardiac, vascular, pulmonary, diabetes, cirrhosis, anticoagulation therapy, blood dyscrasias

**5. Systemic complaints**

   a. Fevers and chills—infectious or inflammatory causative agent

   b. Weight loss, anorexia, and fatigue—malignancy

   c. Dizziness, orthostatic symptoms—indicate large, acute volume loss or severe anemia

**6. Social history**

   a. Note any alcohol or drug use.

## II. PHYSICAL EXAMINATION

### A. GENERAL APPEARANCE

1. Does the patient appear anxious, pale, or diaphoretic? These may reveal the severity of the bleeding.

### B. VITAL SIGNS

1. Blood pressure—check for hypotension or orthostatic changes (decline in systolic blood pressure >20 mm Hg on standing)
2. Pulse—tachycardia (>110 beats/min indicates >15% blood loss)
3. Temperature—may be increased with infection or falsely low or normal with dehydration

### C. SKIN

1. Note the appearance of the patient's skin. Jaundice, palmar erythema, and spider angiomata are associated with cirrhosis and portal hypertension.

### D. HEAD AND NECK

1. Inspection may reveal sclera icterus or an oropharyngeal source.

### E. ABDOMEN

1. Abdominal distention, caput medusae, scars, bruit from abdominal vascular lesion
2. Bowel sounds—usually increased with upper GI bleeding
3. Palpation to localize abdominal tenderness, masses, ascites, hepatosplenomegaly

### F. DIGITAL RECTAL EXAMINATION

1. Include the stool guaiac. Attention should be paid to presence of hemorrhoids, anal fissures, fistula, or rectal mass.

## III. INITIAL MANAGEMENT

### A. ASSESS THE MAGNITUDE OF HEMORRHAGE.

1. Is the patient stable or unstable?

### B. STABILIZE HEMODYNAMIC STATUS.

1. Two large-bore intravenous lines (14–16 gauge)
2. Begin resuscitation with isotonic solution.
3. Place Foley catheter to facilitate monitoring of intravascular volume status.
4. Place nasogastric tube: This may help to differentiate between an upper and lower GI bleeding source. Saline lavage should be continued until the fluid aspirate is clear.

### C. MONITOR FOR CONTINUED BLOOD LOSS.

1. Generally, an intensive care unit setting is required.
2. Continuous monitoring of vital signs with hourly urinary output
3. Frequent laboratory tests to assess the adequacy of transfusion and correction of coagulopathy. The hematocrit should be maintained >30 ml/dl, especially in elderly patients with cardiovascular disease.
4. Central venous pressure or pulmonary artery monitoring in unstable patient
5. If bleeding persists despite transfusion of four to six units of packed red blood cells, further diagnostic testing or surgical intervention is required (see algorithm in Fig. 22-1).

## IV. LABORATORY EVALUATION

### A. TYPE AND CROSS-MATCH

1. Should be done immediately, and four to six units of packed red blood cells should be available at all times.

### B. HEMOGLOBIN/HEMATOCRIT

1. May underestimate the volume in cases of acute blood loss before resuscitation because equilibration has not yet occurred
2. Hypochromia or microcytosis suggest chronic blood loss.
3. Megaloblastosis suggests nutritional abnormalities caused by alcohol abuse.

### C. PLATELET COUNT

1. Thrombocytopenia is present in coagulopathies secondary to massive hemorrhage. This is also seen in patients with cirrhosis secondary to hypersplenism.

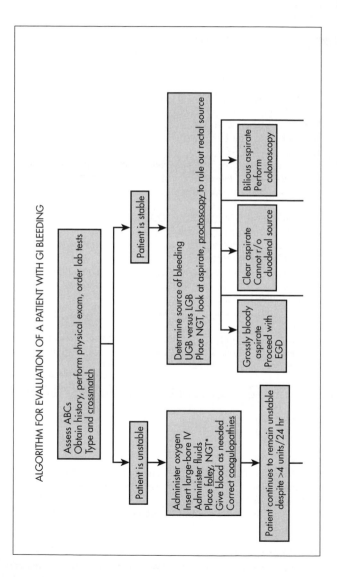

ALGORITHM FOR EVALUATION OF A PATIENT WITH GI BLEEDING

Assess ABCs
Obtain history, perform physical exam, order lab tests
Type and crossmatch

Patient is unstable

Patient is stable

Administer oxygen
Insert large-bore IV
Administer fluids
Place foley, NGT*
Give blood as needed
Correct coagulopathies

Patient continues to remain unstable
despite >4 units/24 hr

Determine source of bleeding
UGB versus LGB
Place NGT, look at aspirate, proctoscopy to rule out rectal source

Grossly bloody
aspirate
Proceed with
EGD

Clear aspirate
Cannot r/o
duodenal source

Bilious aspirate
Perform
colonoscopy

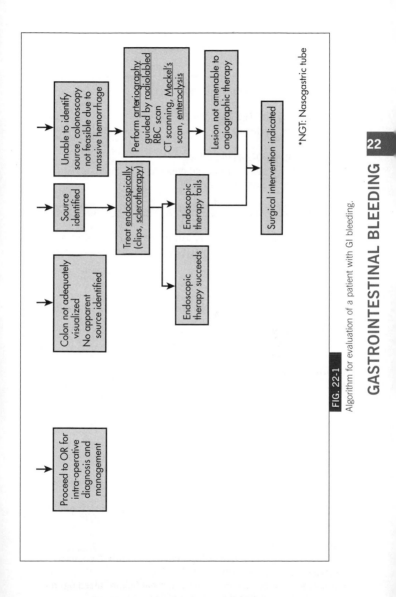

**FIG. 22-1**
Algorithm for evaluation of a patient with GI bleeding.

*NGT: Nasogastric tube

**GASTROINTESTINAL BLEEDING** 22

### D. PROTHROMBIN AND PARTIAL THROMBOPLASTIN TIMES
1. Screen for coagulation defects or abnormalities.

### E. RENAL PROFILE
1. Renal failure and electrolyte disturbance secondary to volume loss or emesis
2. Increased blood urea nitrogen can be caused by the increased protein absorbed from blood in the GI tract as well as a state of dehydration.

### F. LIVER FUNCTION TESTS
1. Assess hepatic dysfunction

### G. CHEST AND ABDOMINAL FILMS
1. Check for the presence of free air, pulmonary infiltrate, abdominal aneurysm, and hepatosplenomegaly.

## V. INVESTIGATIVE AND DIAGNOSTIC PROCEDURES

### A. NASOGASTRIC TUBE
1. A nasogastric tube is inserted as part of the initial management.
2. The character of the aspirate may help differentiate between upper and lower GI source.
a. If the aspirate contains gross blood, esophagogastroduodenoscopy (EGD) is indicated.
b. An aspirate that contains copious amounts of bile is strongly suggestive of lower GI source.
c. The choice is less clear-cut when the aspirate is clear. In the absence of bile, such an aspirate cannot rule out a duodenal source of bleeding.

### B. ENDOSCOPY
1. EGD
a. For upper GI source, it has 95% diagnostic accuracy if used within the first 24 hours.
b. The stomach must first be lavaged clear if possible.
c. EGD can also be used as a therapeutic modality, including sclerotherapy, thermal coagulation, and mechanical occlusion of bleeding sites (clipping or banding of varices).
2. Anoscopy/sigmoidoscopy/colonoscopy
a. Used for lower GI source
b. Overall diagnostic accuracy up to 97%. Lack of adequate bowel prep in the acute setting may render these tests inconclusive.

### C. ANGIOGRAPHY
1. Requires bleeding at a rate >0.5 ml/min to identify the source
2. Overall diagnostic yield from 27% to 67%
3. Complications include contrast allergy, renal failure, bleeding from puncture site, and embolism from a dislodged thrombus.

4. Can be used for therapeutic interventions including vasopressin infusion and embolization of bleeding vessels.

## D. TECHNETIUM-LABELED RED BLOOD CELL SCAN
1. It is sensitive (requires 0.1 ml/min bleeding) and less invasive; however, it is far less specific.
2. May identify the location of the bleed but not the source
3. No therapeutic interventions can be performed.
4. Best used in patients for non–life-threatening lower GI bleeding as a prelude and a guide to angiography after hemorrhage has been confirmed.

## E. COMPUTED TOMOGRAPHY
1. Radiographic contrast studies are rarely useful and may interfere with other diagnostic procedures.

## VI. NONSURGICAL TREATMENT
### A. SCLEROTHERAPY
1. Sclerotherapy can be used for bleeding varices during EGD.

### B. ELECTROCAUTERY
1. Electrocautery of bleeding vessels is used in peptic ulcer disease. This is especially useful in high-risk patients and can be performed at the time of diagnostic study.

### C. VASOPRESSIN INFUSION
1. Can be given systemically or by selective arterial infusion
2. Selective infusion may be started at the time of the diagnostic angiogram and may minimize the systemic effects of the drugs.
3. Recent myocardial infarction or significant coronary artery disease are relative contraindications to this form of therapy. Simultaneous infusion of nitroglycerin may also help reduce risks for infarction.
4. Dosage:
a. Loading dose: 20 units over 20 to 30 minutes
b. Infusion dose: 0.2 to 0.4 units/min

### D. EMBOLIZATION
1. Embolization is reserved for upper GI sources of bleeding because of high risk for ischemia with infarction or perforation with colonic embolization.

## VII. DISEASE-SPECIFIC THERAPY
### A. ACUTE HEMORRHAGIC GASTRITIS
1. Managed medically with $H_2$ receptors blocker, proton-pump inhibitors (PPIs), sucralfate, or antacids alone and with antibiotic if *Helicobacter pylori* is present.
2. Stress ulcer prophylaxis in severely ill or traumatized patients is essential.
3. Prompt resuscitation of shock

22

GASTROINTESTINAL BLEEDING

4. Usually stops after lavage
5. In a patient who remains unstable or continues to have continued blood loss, total or near total gastrectomy is required; however, the mortality rate associated in this setting is high.

## B. PEPTIC ULCER DISEASE
1. Conservative management
2. Nasogastric suctioning and prophylaxis with proton-pump inhibitors, antacids, and cytoprotective agents.
3. Therapeutic EGD
4. For gastric ulcer, biopsy should always be done to rule out malignancy.
5. Giant duodenal ulcer (ulcer >2 cm) will most likely require surgical intervention.
6. Surgery is performed if there is an ongoing need for transfusion or if rebleeding is present on maximal medical therapy.

## C. ESOPHAGOGASTRIC VARICES
1. Lactulose, neomycin for prophylaxis of encephalopathy
2. Endoscopy (banding, sclerotherapy)
3. If the bleeding cannot be controlled endoscopically, balloon tamponade is indicated.
a. Sengstaken–Blakemore tube (rarely used)
b. Four-port Minnesota tube: This tube has gastric balloon, esophageal balloon, and aspiration ports for esophagus and the stomach. The gastric balloon is inflated first and placed on traction. If the bleeding is not controlled, the esophageal balloon is then inflated. Pressure in the balloon is released in 24 to 48 hours to prevent necrosis.
4. Vasopressin infusion should be started with the above-stated measures (beware of use in patients with coronary artery disease).
5. Surgical—determine if the patient is a transplant candidate.
a. If the patient is a candidate for transplant, an operation should be avoided and the bleeding managed by decompressing the portal venous system with transjugular intrahepatic portosystemic shunt.
b. If the patient is not a transplant candidate, either of the following is acceptable:
   (1) Nonshunting (esophagogastric devascularization)
   (2) Shunting
       (a) Nonselective (portocaval)
       (b) Selective (distal splenorenal)
6. Orthotopic liver transplant in select patients with severe hepatic dysfunction

## D. MALLORY–WEISS TEAR
1. A linear mucosal tear at the gastroesophageal junction secondary to violent retching or vomiting
2. Most heal spontaneously with supportive measures alone. In rare cases, the tear will have to be oversewn at the time of operation.

### E. ESOPHAGITIS
1. Medical management or operation for intractable disease may be required.

### F. DIEULAFOY LESION (EXULCERATIO SIMPLEX)
1. Rupturing of a 1- to 3-mm bleeding vessel through the gastric mucosa without any surrounding ulceration. It is usually found high on the lesser curvature of the stomach.
2. No mucosal or vascular abnormalities are noted on histology.
3. Managed endoscopically with either coagulation or mechanical application of clips or rubber bands. Endoscopic therapy has 95% success rate with excellent long-term control.
4. Operative treatment may be required if this fails (resection of lesion vs. ligation of vessel).
5. Embolization may be used in patients too ill to tolerate surgical intervention.

### G. NEOPLASM
1. Benign tumors (leiomyomas, hamartomas) bleed at times. Wedge resection is the procedure of choice.
2. Malignant tumors—bleeding should be controlled initially with endoscopic measures; however, rebleeding rates are high.
3. If lesion is resectable, it should be excised promptly once the patient is stable. If disease is advanced, surgical options are limited.

### H. DIVERTICULOSIS
1. Prevalence of colonic diverticulosis in Western societies can reach 45%.
2. About 17% of patients with colonic diverticulosis will experience bleeding.
3. Up to 80% of hemorrhage stops spontaneously.
4. Surgery indicated for blood loss exceeding 5 units in 24 hours.
5. The risk for the second bleeding episode is approximately 25%. Surgical options should be considered after the second significant bleed. For persistent hemorrhage, resect the involved segment of colon. If question exists, subtotal colectomy with ileoproctostomy is the procedure of choice. Preoperative localization should be attempted to minimize the extent of necessary resection.

### I. ARTERIOVENOUS MALFORMATIONS
(Vascular ectasias, angiomas, and angiodysplasias)
1. Incidence of colonic arteriovenous malformations is 2% to 30% in older patients and approximately 0.8% in healthy, asymptomatic adults.
2. Colonic arteriovenous malformations are believed to arise from chronic colonic wall muscle contraction, which leads to chronic partial obstruction of the submucosal veins. Eventually, the precapillary sphincter becomes incompetent, resulting in direct arterial venous communication.

22

GASTROINTESTINAL BLEEDING

3. Can occur throughout the GI tract, commonly in the right colon.
4. Diagnosis is made at the time of angiography or colonoscopy.
5. Typically, the bleeding is chronic, slow, and intermittent.
6. Bleeding stops spontaneously in 85% to 90% of cases.
7. Surgical treatment for massive acute bleeding or chronic intermittent bleeding
8. Segmental resection of localized segment is preferred.

## J. MECKEL'S DIVERTICULUM
1. Ileal ulceration secondary to Meckel's diverticulum containing gastric mucosa is treated with segmental resection and end-to-end anastomosis or wedge resection.
2. The lesion can be localized before surgery using a nuclear medicine scan.

## K. BENIGN ANORECTAL DISEASE
1. An estimated 11% of lower GI bleeding can be attributed to benign anorectal pathology; however, this does not eliminate the possibility of a more proximal cause for hemorrhage.
2. Portal hypertension, congestive heart failure, and splenic vein thrombosis can cause anorectal varices.
3. In general, patients with hemorrhoids on examination should still undergo thorough endoscopic evaluation of the colon to rule out other pathologic conditions.

## L. AORTOENTERIC FISTULA
(Status post abdominal aortic aneurysm repair)
1. Patients will present with a small herald bleed usually more than 6 months after abdominal aortic aneurysm repair. This is followed a few days later by massive hemorrhage. Triad consists of GI hemorrhage, pulsatile mass, and infection.
2. Usually found in the third or fourth portion of the duodenum at the proximal suture line.
3. Computed tomographic scanning is the procedure of choice for diagnosis. Finding of air around the aorta of the aortic graft is diagnostic.
4. Resection of the graft with extraanatomic bypass is the preferred surgical treatment of choice.

## RECOMMENDED READING

Cameron J: *Current Surgical Therapy,* 8th ed. St. Louis, Elsevier-Mosby, 2004, pp 285–290.
Rosen R, Ponsky J, Harold K, Schlinkert R: *ACS Surgery: Principles and Practice,* WebMD, 2006.
Sabiston DC: *Textbook of Surgery: The Biological Basis of Modern Surgical Practice,* 15th ed. Philadelphia, WB Saunders, 1997.

# Intestinal Obstruction

*Janice A. Taylor, MD*

*Never let the sun set on a bowel obstruction.*

## I. TERMINOLOGY

### A. ILEUS (ALSO KNOWN AS "PARALYTIC ILEUS" OR "ADYNAMIC BOWEL")

1. Mechanical or functional obstruction, usually caused by failure of movement of luminal contents secondary to poor motility

### B. MECHANICAL OBSTRUCTION

1. Partial or complete physical blockage of lumen

### C. SIMPLE OBSTRUCTION

1. Occlusion at one area of the bowel

### D. CLOSED-LOOP OBSTRUCTION

1. Afferent and efferent bowel limb blockage (i.e., volvulus)
2. Occasionally seen with strangulation

### E. STRANGULATION

1. Ischemic damage to obstructed area of bowel
2. Usually secondary to restricted circulation, often seen with closed-loop obstruction, or caused by increased intraluminal pressure

## II. CAUSATIVE FACTORS

### A. SMALL-BOWEL OBSTRUCTION (SBO)

1. Adhesions
   a. Most common cause of SBO (80%)
   b. Occur as a result of prior abdominal surgery
2. Hernia
   a. Second most common cause of SBO overall; most common cause in patients who have not had previous abdominal surgery
3. Intraluminal
   a. Neoplasia
   b. Inflammation
      (1) Enteritis, Crohn's disease
      (2) Radiation enteritis or stricture
   c. Gallstone ileus (elderly)
   d. Foreign bodies
   e. Meconium ileus
   f. Intussusception
   g. Congenital lesions
      (1) Small-bowel atresia, stenosis, webs
      (2) Small-bowel duplications or mesenteric cysts

(3) Meckel's diverticulum

**4. Extraluminal/mass effect**

a. Carcinomatosis/adjacent tumor compressing bowel wall

b. Intraabdominal abscess

c. Hematoma

d. Malrotation/volvulus

e. Annular pancreas (duodenal obstruction)

f. Endometriosis

g. Superior mesenteric artery syndrome

    (1) Superior mesenteric artery compression of third portion of duodenum

    (2) More commonly seen in thin patients who have experienced recent dramatic weight loss

## B. LARGE-BOWEL OBSTRUCTION

**1. Intraluminal**

a. Colon cancer—most common cause (60%) of large-bowel obstruction

b. Inflammation

    (1) Ulcerative colitis, Crohn's disease

    (2) Diverticulitis

    (3) Radiation enteritis

c. Congenital

    (1) Imperforate anus

d. Ischemic colitis

e. Foreign bodies

f. Meconium ileus

g. Intussusception

h. Fecal impaction

**2. Extraluminal/mass effect**

a. Adhesions

b. Hernia (particularly sliding type)

c. Volvulus

    (1) Sigmoid—60% to 80% of cases

    (2) Cecal—20% to 40% of cases

    (3) Transverse colon—<5% of cases

## C. OFTEN MISDIAGNOSED AS SBO OR LARGE-BOWEL OBSTRUCTION

**1. Adynamic ileus (see later)**

**2. Vascular insufficiency**

a. Nonocclusive mesenteric ischemia

b. Mesenteric thrombosis

c. Mesenteric embolism

**3. Hirschsprung's disease**

## D.  ILEUS
### 1.  Metabolic
a.  Hypokalemia, hypomagnesemia, hyponatremia
b.  Ketoacidosis
c.  Uremia
d.  Porphyria
e.  Heavy metal poisoning
### 2.  Medications
a.  Narcotics
b.  Dopaminergics
c.  Antipsychotics
d.  Anticholinergics
e.  Ganglionic blockers
f.  Diuretics
g.  Polypharmacy
### 3.  Infection
a.  Sepsis
b.  Peritonitis
c.  Localized process—appendicitis, cholecystitis, diverticulitis, pyelonephritis, abscess, urinary tract infection
### 4.  Retroperitoneal process
a.  Pancreatitis
b.  Hematoma
c.  Vertebral or pelvic fracture
### 5.  Neuropathic process
a.  Diabetes mellitus
b.  Multiple sclerosis
c.  Scleroderma
d.  Lupus erythematosus
e.  Hirschsprung's disease
### 6.  Bed rest
### 7.  Postoperative (after abdominal surgery)
a.  Forty-eight or fewer hours after surgery: return of small-bowel function (reason physician listens for bowel sounds).
b.  Forty-eight hours after surgery: return of stomach motility (when nasogastric tube is typically removed).
c.  Three to 5 days after surgery: return of colonic motility (why patient is asked whether he/she has passed gas or stool).
### 8.  Ogilvie's syndrome
a.  Pseudoobstruction, colonic
b.  Patient population typically elderly, institutionalized, bedridden, presence of retroperitoneal process, narcotic use, polypharmacy
c.  Cecal dilation—more than 12 cm increases perforation risk.
d.  Treatment—decompression
   (1) Enema first

**23**

INTESTINAL OBSTRUCTION

(2) Colonoscopic decompression if enema unsuccessful or if patient has significant cecal dilation——~40% recurrence.

(3) Intravenous (IV) neostigmine——~20% recurrence. Caution in cardiac patients (bradycardia).

(4) Cecostomy or right hemicolectomy if perforated, ischemic, or colonoscopy unsuccessful

## III. PRESENTATION

### A. HISTORY

**1. Signs and symptoms**

a. Nausea/vomiting, abdominal fullness, *decreased flatus,* constipation/obstipation

(1) Proximal obstruction—bilious emesis early in course, minimal distention. May still have bowel movements, pass gas while moving bowels distal to obstruction.

(2) Distal obstruction—obstipation and distention may occur before feculent emesis. Obstipation is characteristic of complete obstruction.

(3) Bloody emesis—suggests strangulation.

b. Abdominal pain

(1) Proximal obstruction—cramping pain referred to periumbilical region; caused by bowel distention from continued peristalsis against the obstructed point. The pain may decrease after a long time secondary to inhibited bowel motility from distention.

(2) Distal obstruction—cramping pain referred to lower abdomen. When succeeded by continuous severe pain, suspect strangulation and peritonitis. Immediate torsion and vascular compromise of a segment of bowel can cause early obstruction and ischemia.

c. Duration of symptoms, tolerance of oral intake, recent unintentional weight loss

**2. Surgical and medical history**

a. Previous abdominal operations

b. Suspicion of intraabdominal neoplasia or previous radiation for cancer

c. History of ventral/incisional/inguinal hernia

d. Review of medications

e. Atherosclerotic disease, previous myocardial infarction, arrhythmia history

f. History of inflammatory bowel disease or diverticulitis

g. History of chronic biliary colic

**3. Age**

a. Adhesions can be a source of obstruction at any age, given a history of previous intraabdominal surgery.

b. Neonate

(1) Meconium ileus, Hirschsprung's disease, intestinal atresias, *volvulus*/malrotation

c. Two to 24 months

(1) Intussusception, Hirschsprung's disease

d. Young adult
   (1) Inflammatory bowel disease, hernia
e. Adult
   (1) Inflammatory bowel disease, hernia, neoplasm, diverticulitis
f. Elderly
   (1) Hernia, neoplasm, diverticulitis, Ogilvie's syndrome, sigmoid/cecal
       volvulus

## B. PHYSICAL EXAMINATION
1. Fever—rule out infectious/inflammatory process or strangulation.
   May be afebrile if uncomplicated disease.
2. Bowel sounds—initially active with intermittent rushes and
   borborygmus, but decreases with time. Usually have absent
   bowel sounds in adynamic ileus.
3. Hiccups or belching—sign of gastric distention, given the suspicion
   of obstruction.
4. Abdominal tenderness—if localized or if patient is guarding,
   increased probability of strangulation or perforation. Tenderness may
   also be mild.
5. Abdominal distention—tympany on percussion.
6. Note any surgical abdominal scars.
7. Presence of mass/hernia. May be able to palpate fixed distended
   bowel loop, carcinoma, or inflammatory mass.
8. Empty rectal vault.
   a. Can also rule out fecal impaction with rectal examination.
   b. Extrinsic pelvic masses and colonic lesions can be palpated on digital
      rectal examination.
9. Guaiac positive stool—strangulation/cancer/inflammatory
   process
10. Tachycardia—secondary to dehydration and hypovolemia, but it can
    be an early indicator of strangulation if patient has increased WBC
    count and localized tenderness.

## C. LABORATORY TESTS
1. Leukocytosis—may be mild increase in uncomplicated obstruction.
2. Increased hemoglobin, hematocrit, blood urea nitrogen,
   creatinine—implies hemoconcentration, dehydration.
   a. Alternatively, anemia in the setting of SBO or colonic obstruction is
      often characteristic of colon carcinoma.
3. Electrolyte imbalances (particularly hypokalemia)
4. Metabolic alkalosis—usually seen in proximal SBO or pyloric
   obstruction. Emesis causes loss of HCl from the gastric
   secretions.
5. Metabolic acidosis, base deficit—typically seen late in obstruction.
   Normal pH does not rule out bowel infarction. Lactic acid level is
   nonspecific finding suspicious for ischemia.

23

INTESTINAL OBSTRUCTION

6. Urinalysis—rule out urinary tract infection as cause of SBO-like symptoms, especially in elderly adults.
7. Amylase—may or may not be increased in SBO.

## IV. IMAGING

### A. PLAIN FILMS

1. Basic principle of imaging for obstruction
a. Determine the presence of colonic (distal) gas. Gas in the large bowel favors a diagnosis of ileus, not SBO. This is based on the premise that something obstructing passage through the small bowel will not allow anything past that point in the lumen.
2. Abdominal series versus upright and flat versus supine and left lateral decubitus (Fig. 23-1)
a. Abdominal series—upright abdominal, supine abdominal, upright chest films
b. Air-fluid levels, seen best in upright or decubitus positions
   (1) "Stair-step" or "ladder pattern" of air-fluid levels in distended bowel, proximal to an obstruction, can be seen progressing down the abdomen. More pronounced in obstructive disease than in ileus.
c. Distention of bowel with empty rectal vault
d. Identification of closed loops (U-shaped, "bird's beak") can indicate bowel strangulation or volvulus.
e. Bowel gas may be seen distally with partial obstruction, in early complete obstruction, or if air has been introduced during rectal examination or enema.
f. Note diameter of distention. **(Law of Laplace: Tension = pressure × radius)**
   (1) Colonic obstruction or ileus—increased risk for perforation if cecal diameter is larger than 12 cm. Consider emergent decompression.
   (2) When cecal diameter dilates acutely to 12 to 14 cm, wall tension exceeds perfusion pressure and focal areas of necrosis can develop. Necrosis may progress even after decompression.
g. Sigmoid volvulus—"omega" or "bent inner tube" appearance of large, dilated bowel loop. Apex in left lower quadrant and convexity in right upper quadrant.
h. Cecal volvulus—large, dilated, ovoid, air-filled cecum in the upper abdomen. Caused by rotation of hypermobile cecum around the ileocolic vessels. Apex in right lower quadrant.
3. Upright chest radiograph can help rule out free air (look under diaphragm).

### B. CONTRAST STUDIES

1. Contrast enema
a. To identify the site of obstruction, not define mucosal detail. Useful when diagnosis is uncertain.

b. Most commonly used to rule out colonic (distal) obstruction
c. Conduct under low pressure. Free barium in peritoneum has high mortality rate. Use water-soluble contrast, particularly if perforation is suspected.
d. Do not force contrast beyond partial obstruction; can create complete obstruction.
e. Can do before upper gastrointestinal series if distal SBO suspected. Reflux through ileocecal valve can identify a collapsed terminal ileum, confirming SBO.
f. If intussusception is suspected, perform hydrostatic or air contrast barium enema. Functions as diagnosis and treatment (reduction); 60% to 70% of pediatric intussusceptions reduce with enema alone. No hydrostatic reduction in adults: High likelihood of neoplasm as the lead point.
g. In sigmoid or cecal volvulus, see "bird's-beak" pattern at volvulus point.

2. **Upper gastrointestinal series with small-bowel follow-through**
a. Useful if diagnosis is uncertain, or to visualize partially obstructing lesion
b. If suspect colonic obstruction, rule out by performing barium enema first.
   (1) Great care must be taken when administering contrast above an obstruction; additional volume above a fixed obstruction point may exacerbate proximal bowel distention without a means for relief.
c. Study of choice when ruling out malrotation

## C. CT
1. **Sensitivity of 85% and specificity of 80% for identifying SBO; less than 50% sensitivity for identifying partial SBO**
a. If unable to find transition zone on CT, upper gastrointestinal series with small-bowel follow-through will be more sensitive.
2. **Preferably oral and IV contrast**
a. Oral contrast may worsen distention in the setting of a true SBO.
b. Better to give isotonic, not hypertonic, oral contrast solution to minimize osmotic distension of potentially obstructed bowel
3. **Identification of transition point**
a. Dilated proximal bowel, collapsed distal bowel
b. Inability to identify oral contrast past the point of dilation
c. Identification of closed-loop or vascular compromise
d. Identification of intraabdominal or intraluminal mass

## V. MANAGEMENT
### A. EXPECTANT/PREOPERATIVE MANAGEMENT
1. **Early versus late obstruction**
a. Early postoperative SBO typically resolves on its own. If symptoms occur during postoperative days 1 to 14, the obstruction will likely re-solve with bowel rest, nasogastric tube decompression, and IV hydration.

23

INTESTINAL OBSTRUCTION

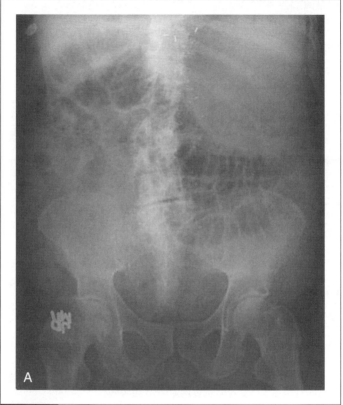

**FIG. 23-1**

*A,* Supine abdominal plain film showing multiple loops of dilated small bowel. The plicae circulares of the small bowel are well-defined secondary to the distention, helping to differentiate it from the haustral markings of the large bowel. Plicae circulares traverse the entire diameter of the small bowel; haustra extend one half to two thirds the diameter of the colon. This patient's small bowel obstruction was secondary to an incarcerated inguinal hernia. *(Courtesy Susan Sharp, MD, and Doan Vu, MD, Department of Radiology, University of Cincinnati.)*

    b. After 14 days from surgery, surgical intervention is more likely required to resolve a fixed point of obstruction.
  2. True bowel obstruction is a surgical emergency; patients should undergo laparotomy with few exceptions.
  a. Exceptions—partial obstruction; patient with history of previous laparotomies for bowel obstruction and now with a hostile abdomen; severely

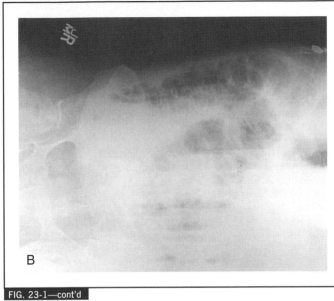

FIG. 23-1—cont'd

*B*, Left lateral decubitus (LLQ) plain film from same patient as in *A*. Note the ability to define air-fluid levels with the patient in this position. *(Courtesy Susan Sharp, MD, and Doan Vu, MD, Department of Radiology, University of Cincinnati.)*

medically debilitated patients who would have high postoperative complications and for whom the team would want to give a short trial of expectant management.

b. Partial or early SBO (patient still passing gas or stool) may also be caused by an exacerbation of inflammatory bowel disease, like Crohn's disease, that may resolve. If partial SBO is the diagnosis, continue to resuscitate and evaluate.

3. **NPO (nothing by mouth)**
a. IV hydration
b. Correct electrolyte imbalances.
c. Potential need for total parenteral nutrition

4. **Nasogastric tube (14 Fr at least) to continuous low suction**
a. Prevents vomiting with aspiration
b. Partially decompresses small bowel
c. Prevents further stomach distention due to swallowed air

5. **Foley catheter to monitor urine output and success of resuscitation**

6. **Small bowel intubation with "long tube" (i.e., Miller–Abbott or Cantor tube)**

a. Generally inappropriate; may delay operation for mechanical obstruction
b. Major indications—resolving partial obstruction, postoperative partial obstruction, obstruction caused by inflammation that will likely resolve and not result in strangulation (carcinomatosis, radiation enteritis)

## B. SURGICAL

1. Indicated when no improvement or when worsening of patient condition during expectant management for initial diagnosis of partial obstruction
2. Antibiotic coverage of gram-negative aerobes and anaerobes
3. Operative treatment of SBO
   a. If patient exhibits signs of peritonitis, leukocytosis, fever, and tachycardia with a diagnosis of SBO, take to operating room when hemodynamically stable. Appropriate to assume that the patient has ischemic or necrotic bowel.
   b. If patient has complete SBO but no ischemic or necrotic bowel, resuscitate and take to operating room as soon as possible when optimal operative resources are available.
   c. Lysis of all adhesions or resection of the involved segment is recommended. Limit manipulation and surgical intervention if obstruction is caused by radiation enteritis; injured bowel may be "revascularized" by the adhesions.
   d. If SBO is due to malignancy, may need to bypass the involved segment.
   e. If SBO is due to hernia, resect any necrotic bowel and repair hernia with autologous tissue (e.g., Bassini repair with relaxing incision; lateral release for large defect). Mesh in this setting is associated with increased infection.
   f. If patient has multiple adhesive SBOs, plication of bowel in an organized fashion has been described in the literature by using fibrin glue or placing seromuscular stitches. The goal is to position adjacent bowel loops to promote adhesion formation in a nonobstructive pattern. These methods are not widely used or accepted as standard of care.
4. Operative treatment of colonic obstruction
   a. Ischemic colon needs to be treated with resection and end colostomy with mucous fistula or rectal (Hartmann's) pouch.
   b. Obstructive right colon carcinoma
      (1) Resection and primary anastomosis if no fecal contamination, massive edema, shock, or long-standing peritonitis. Otherwise, perform decompressive ileostomy and mucous fistula.
   c. Obstructive left colon carcinoma
      (1) Primary resection with colostomy and mucous fistula or Hartmann's pouch
      (2) If patient is debilitated or unstable but has no abscess or perforation, perform diverting colostomy to allow decompression and stabilization. Return later for resection, then colostomy closure.
      (3) Controversial data have been reported regarding success of primary anastomosis with on-table bowel preparation. This is also difficult to perform neatly.

d. Obstructing diverticulitis
   (1) Resect involved segment and perform primary anastomosis or end colostomy with Hartmann's pouch.
   (2) See "Diverticular Disease" chapter for more details.
e. Sigmoid volvulus
   (1) First attempt decompression via sigmoidoscopy, placing rectal tube past obstruction. Immediate reduction in 80% of cases. Inspect mucosa for viability.
   (2) Greater than 50% recurrence rate; therefore, recommend elective sigmoid resection after the first episode if patient is a reasonable surgical candidate.
   (3) If cannot endoscopically reduce (no stool or flatus), suspect strangulation and resect emergently.
f. Cecal volvulus
   (1) Operative treatment. Do not attempt endoscopic reduction.
   (2) Resect for vascular compromise; otherwise, cecopexy or cecostomy.
5. Determining bowel viability: color, motility, arterial pulsation
   (1) Resect anything obviously nonviable.
   (2) If questionable, release adhered segment, place in warm saline-soaked gauze for 15 to 20 minutes, then reexamine. If bowel has normal color and motility, may be returned safely. If any further question of viability, can perform second-look laparotomy at 24 to 48 hours.
   (3) Tools to help determine viability: IV fluorescein dye and Wood's lamp, Doppler examination

## C. POSTOPERATIVE CARE
1. Nasogastric decompression until bowel activity returns
2. Postoperative antibiotic coverage if septic, gross contamination, preoperative long-standing peritonitis
3. If bowel function does not return within 5 days or if the total NPO time (including the preoperative course) is longer than 5 days, consider total parenteral nutrition.

## D. PARALYTIC ILEUS
1. Common in the immediate postoperative period from intraabdominal procedure. Typically resolves after 2 to 3 days.
2. Nasogastric decompression, IV fluids
3. Correct electrolytes.
4. Long-tube or colonoscopic decompression for severe distention
5. Exclude obstructive processes if ileus persists without an obvious cause.

## VI. OUTCOMES
### A. RECURRENCE
1. Ten percent of patients having undergone lysis of adhesions will obstruct in the future.

23

INTESTINAL OBSTRUCTION

2. Incidence of recurrence increases with each subsequent operative intervention.

## B. OPERATIVE MORTALITY

### 1. SBO
a. Occurs in 0% to 5% of cases
b. Occurs in 4.5% to 31% of cases if gangrene develops

### 2. Colonic obstruction
a. Occurs in 1% to 5% when caused by diverticulitis
b. Occurs in 5% to 10% when caused by carcinoma
c. Occurs in 40% to 50% in cases of bowel necrosis secondary to volvulus

## RECOMMENDED READING

Dayton MT: Small bowel obstruction. In Cameron JL (ed): *Current Surgical Therapy.* Philadelphia, Mosby, 2004.

Hayanga AJ, Bass-Wilkins K, Bulkley GB: Current management of small-bowel obstruction. *Adv Surg* 39:1–33, 2005.

Person B, Wexner SD: The management of postoperative ileus. *Curr Probl Surg* 43: 6–65, 2006.

Whang EE, Ashley SW, Zinner MJ: Small intestine. In Brunicardi FC (ed): *Principles of Surgery.* New York, McGraw-Hill, 2005.

# Esophagus Benign Disease

*Prakash K. Pandalai, MD*

## I. ANATOMY

### A. GENERAL DESCRIPTION

1. A muscular tube ~25 cm long that begins 15 cm from incisors, at the cricopharyngeus muscle, and ends at the gastroesophageal (GE) junction along the cardia of the stomach. There are three normal areas of anatomic narrowing: (1) the cricopharyngeal muscle (the narrowest point of the esophagus), (2) the aortic arch and left main stem bronchus, and (3) the diaphragmatic hiatus.
2. The cervical esophagus (5 cm) spans the C6 vertebra to T1–2. Recurrent laryngeal nerves lie in the tracheoesophageal grove on either side.
3. The thoracic esophagus (20 cm) begins at the thoracic inlet and lies between the trachea anteriorly and prevertebral fascia posteriorly. The azygous vein lies to the right and the thoracic aorta on the left of the esophagus.
4. The abdominal esophagus (2 cm) enters the abdomen at the esophageal hiatus at T11. Right and left vagal trunks also enter here.

### B. BLOOD SUPPLY AND NERVES

1. Arterial supply is segmental from superior and inferior thyroid, aortic, bronchial, and esophageal branches, inferior phrenic, and left gastric arteries.
2. Venous drainage is to the hypopharyngeal, azygous, hemiazygous, intercostal, and gastric veins. All are a potential source of varices if portal hypertension is present.
3. Innervation is from both parasympathetic and sympathetic systems. The cervical esophagus receives innervation from the recurrent laryngeal nerves and branches of the vagus. Damage to these nerves interferes with not only the function of the vocal cords but with the function of the cervical esophagus, predisposing to pulmonary aspiration with swallowing.

**Pearl:** *LARP (left vagus lies anteriorly and right vagus lies posteriorly) on the distal esophagus.*

### C. HISTOLOGY

1. Mucosa is lined by squamous epithelium, changing to columnar epithelium at or near the GE junction.

**Pearl:** *Squamous to columnar metaplasia is a hallmark of Barrett's esophagus.*

2. Submucosa contains glands, arteries, Meissner's neural plexus, lymphatics, and veins.
3. Muscularis is composed of two layers, an outer longitudinal and an inner circular layer. Nerves and blood vessels run between the layers. The upper one-third is composed of striated muscle, and the lower two-thirds are smooth muscle.
4. No serosa. The lack of a serosal layer potentially contributes to an increase in anastomotic leaks and early mediastinal invasion by cancer.

## II. PHYSIOLOGY

The esophagus functions to transport swallowed material, in a coordinated fashion, from the pharynx to the stomach. Once initiated, swallowing is entirely a reflex act coordinated by the swallowing center of the medulla and involving cranial nerves 5, 7, 10, 11, and 12 and motor neurons of C1–3.

### A. SWALLOWING MECHANISM

1. Oropharyngeal phase
a. Food is chewed and ready for swallowing.
b. Tongue pushes the food bolus into the hypopharynx.
c. Simultaneously, the soft palate elevates to prevent regurgitation of food into the nasopharynx and the hyoid bone moves anteriorly and superiorly to open the retrolaryngeal space.
d. Epiglottis moves over the larynx to prevent aspiration with the movement of the hyoid bone.
e. Rapid increase in the pressure of the hypopharynx and a subsequent relaxation of the upper esophageal sphincter (cricopharyngeus muscle)
2. Esophageal phase
a. Primary peristalsis—initiated by relaxing the upper esophageal sphincter that propels swallowed material from pharynx to stomach in a progressive and sequential manner; occurs over 9 seconds.
b. Secondary peristalsis—involuntary waves, initiated in the smooth muscle layer, that clear locally distended segments of the esophagus.
c. Tertiary peristalsis—repetitive, nonprogressive, and uncoordinated smooth muscle contractions

### B. SPHINCTERS

1. Upper esophageal sphincter or cricopharyngeal muscle is ~3 cm long with resting pressure of 20 to 60 mm Hg.
2. Lower esophageal sphincter (LES)
a. The LES is not an anatomically defined sphincter in humans; more appropriately referred to as a zone of high pressure that serves to reduce gastric regurgitation and reflux. It is located in distal 3 to 5 cm of esophagus and defined by "pull-back" manometric studies. Its normal resting pressure is 10 to 20 mm Hg.
b. LES pressure increases with inspiration and drug and/or hormone levels.

(1) Pressure is increased by gastrin, caffeine, α-adrenergic drugs, bethanechol, and metoclopramide.

(2) Pressure is decreased by secretin, cholecystokinin, glucagon, progesterone, alcohol, nitroglycerin, nicotine, anticholinergics, and β-adrenergic drugs.

## III. MOTILITY DISORDERS

### A. DEFINITION

Motility disorders are conditions that interfere with swallowing and are not caused by intraluminal obstruction or external compression.

### B. HISTORY

1. A careful, detailed history should be obtained.
2. Dysphagia with liquids more than solids suggests motility disorder.
3. Dysphagia progressive from solids to liquids suggests mechanical obstruction.
4. Odynophagia suggests spasm or esophagitis. Increased pain with cold liquids is suggestive of spasm.
5. Difficulty with swallowing or nasopharyngeal reflux suggests a neurologic or muscular disorder.
6. Symptoms of reflux
7. Duration of symptoms
8. Hematemesis, weight loss, and alcohol/tobacco use should be questioned.
9. Gurgling with swallowing or regurgitation of undigested food suggests a Zenker's diverticulum.

### C. UPPER ESOPHAGEAL SPHINCTER DYSFUNCTION— CRICOPHARYNGEAL ACHALASIA

1. Caused by abnormalities in central and peripheral nervous systems; metabolic, inflammatory myopathy; GE reflux; and others
2. Patients describe a "lump" in the throat, excessive expectoration of saliva, weight loss, and intermittent hoarseness.
3. Diagnosis by barium swallow and manometric studies; however, these may be normal.
4. Treatment depends on the cause—antireflux procedure, bougienage, or cervical esophagotomy.

### D. ESOPHAGEAL BODY DISORDERS

1. Achalasia—failure of relaxation
a. Abnormal peristalsis secondary to absence or destruction of Auerbach's (myenteric) plexus and failure of LES to relax; affects body and distal esophagus
b. Causative factor is unknown, multiple associations.
c. Patients report dysphagia, regurgitation, weight loss, retrosternal chest pain, and recurrent pulmonary infections.

**24**

**ESOPHAGUS BENIGN DISEASE**

d. Barium swallow demonstrates "bird's beak" narrowing of distal esophagus with proximal dilation.
e. Manometric studies show incomplete LES relaxation and lack of progressive peristalsis. Aperistalsis is observed in the esophageal body. An increased LES pressure (>6 mm Hg) is common.
f. About 1% to 10% of patients experience development of squamous cell carcinoma after 15 to 25 years of disease.
g. Treatment options include:
  (1) Medical therapy including sublingual nitroglycerin, calcium channel blockers, botulinum toxin injection, and repeated dilation; 65% of patients improve with pneumatic or hydrostatic dilation.
  (2) Surgical treatment is Heller myotomy; 85% of patients improve. There is a 3% rate of reflux after this procedure. Heller myotomy in combination with an antireflux procedure is commonly performed using robotic assistance and laparoscopic approach today.
  (3) Patients with end-stage achalasia with megaesophagus may require an esophagectomy.

2. **Diffuse esophageal spasm**
a. Repetitive, simultaneous, high-amplitude contractions
b. Pain greater than dysphagia; symptoms increased by emotional stress
c. Diagnosis by motility studies. Barium swallow may show "coiled spring" or "corkscrewing."
d. Medical treatment includes small, soft meals and calcium channel blockers.
e. Surgical treatment is extended esophagomyotomy.

3. **Nutcracker esophagus**
a. Defined as a manometric abnormality with hypertensive contractions with mean pressures in the distal esophagus >180 mm Hg
b. A normal peristaltic sequence occurs in the body of the esophagus.
c. Complaints include chest pain and dysphagia.
d. Medical therapy is indicated for these patients.
e. Most common esophageal motility disorder

4. **Hypertensive LES**
a. Defined as an increased LES pressure >45 mm Hg with normal LES relaxation
b. Main complaints are chest pain and dysphagia.
c. Medical therapy and dilation are the first line of therapy.
d. Myotomy may be indicated in those not responding to medical therapy and dilation.

5. **Scleroderma**
a. Fibrous replacement of esophageal smooth muscle and atrophy
b. LES loses tone and normal response to swallowing; results in GE reflux.
c. Medical/surgical treatment directed at antireflux measures to decrease esophagitis.
d. Operative therapy usually avoided in these patients.

## IV. DIVERTICULA

### A. DEFINITION

Diverticula are epithelial-lined mucosal pouches that protrude from the esophageal lumen.

### B. PHARYNGOESOPHAGEAL (ZENKER'S DIVERTICULUM)

1. Located between oblique fibers of the thyropharyngeus muscle and the horizontal fibers of the cricopharyngeus
2. Most common esophageal diverticulum (pseudodiverticulum) that contains only mucosa and submucosa
3. Pulsion-type diverticula are created by increased intraluminal pressure.
4. Patients are usually 30 to 50 years of age and report cervical dysphagia, effortless regurgitation of undigested food, choking, gurgling in throat, and recurrent aspiration.
5. Diagnosis is made with a barium swallow.
6. Treatment includes diverticulectomy with myotomy of the cricopharyngeus muscle via a neck approach.
a. Exposure of diverticulum using an incision lateral to the sternocleidomastoid muscle
7. Low mortality and recurrence rates of 2% and 4%, respectively

### C. PERIBRONCHIAL

1. Located near tracheal bifurcation
2. Traction diverticulum resulting from inflammatory reaction, typically mediastinal granulomatous disease of adjacent lymph nodes that adhere to the esophagus and pull on wall during healing
3. Rarely symptomatic, tend to be small, and are discovered incidentally

### D. EPIPHRENIC

1. Located in distal 10 cm of esophagus
2. Pulsion type arise from distal obstruction or motor dysfunction.
3. Patients report regurgitation, dysphagia, and retrosternal chest pain.
4. Treatment—usually none. If the diverticulum is large, the appropriate treatment is a long extramucosal thoracic myotomy and diverticulectomy.

## V. GASTROESOPHAGEAL REFLUX

### A. ANATOMY

1. Normally, the distal 2 to 3 cm of esophagus is intraabdominal.
2. Endoabdominal fascia (continuous with transversalis fascia) inserts into the esophageal wall at the esophageal hiatus.
3. No discrete LES in humans

### B. PATHOPHYSIOLOGY

1. Decreased LES tone
2. Delayed gastric emptying

3. Increased intraabdominal pressure because of obesity, tight garments, or large meal
4. Motor failure of esophagus with loss of peristalsis
5. Iatrogenic injury to LES

## C.  ACID-PROTECTING MECHANISMS
1. Distal esophagus prevents reflux through influence of intraabdominal pressure.
2. Peristalsis rapidly clears gastric acid.
3. Bicarbonate-rich saliva (1000–1500 ml/day)

## D.  REFLUX ESOPHAGITIS
1. Gastric acid and pepsin are corrosive to the esophageal mucosa.
2. Complications
a. Pain and spasm
b. Stricture
c. Hemorrhage
d. Shortening of esophagus
e. Ulceration
 f. Barrett's esophagus
   (1) Definition—squamous to columnar metaplasia of the distal esophagus
   (2) Associated with an increased risk for development of adenocarcinoma (10–15%) over 10 years
   (3) Correction of reflux does not prevent malignant transformation, and it requires serial endoscopic surveillance and possible biopsy. Esophageal resection is indicated for severe dysplasia.
g. Dysmotility
h. Schatzki's ring—a constrictive band at the squamocolumnar junction composed of mucosa and submucosa, not esophageal muscle.
 i. Aspiration pneumonia
3. Symptoms
a. Heartburn, retrosternal pyrosis
b. Regurgitation of sour or bitter liquids, aggravated by postural changes
c. Nocturnal aspiration with recurrent pneumonia, lung abscesses, or bronchiectasis
d. Dysphagia secondary to obstruction or motility disorder
4. Diagnosis
a. Upper GI series
   (1) Spontaneous reflux in 40% of patients with true GE reflux
   (2) Able to document stricture or ulcer
b. Esophagoscopy combined with mucosal brushings and biopsy is essential to diagnosis for reflux esophagitis.
c. Esophageal pH probe (aka BRAVO study)
   (1) Accurate for determining magnitude and duration of reflux
   (2) Twenty-four-hour test most precise and quantitative method

(3) Acid reflux test—HCl is placed into the stomach; esophageal pH proximal to LES is monitored as intragastric pressure is increased; pH <4 is a positive test.

d. Manometry

(1) Does not test reflux; however, reflux more common with low LES pressure (<6 mm Hg)

(2) Useful in identifying underlying motility disorder (present in up to 25% of patients)

## 5. Treatment

a. Medical

(1) Dietary

(a) Avoid substances that decrease LES tone, that is, cigarette smoking, chocolate, alcohol, and fatty foods.

(b) Do not eat 2 hours before sleeping.

(c) Avoid excessive eating; eat small meals.

(2) Avoid anticholinergics, tranquilizers, and muscle relaxants.

(3) Reduce weight, if obese.

(4) Elevate head of bed 6 inches on blocks.

(5) Increase LES pressure.

(a) Metoclopramide 10 mg every 8 hours

(b) Bethanechol 10 to 50 mg three or four times daily

(6) Decrease gastric acid.

(a) Antacids

(b) $H_2$ blockers

(c) Proton-pump inhibitors

b. Surgical—antireflux procedures

(1) Goals

(a) Restore segment of intraabdominal esophagus

(b) Maintain distal esophagus as small-diameter tube

(c) Narrow the hiatus

(d) Avoid increasing the resistance of the relaxed sphincter to level that exceeds peristaltic force of esophagus

(2) Indications

(a) Failure of medical therapy

(b) Esophagitis with frank ulceration or stricture

(c) Complications of reflux esophagitis

(d) Severe symptoms or progressive disease

(3) Procedures

(a) Nissen fundoplication—a 360-degree fundoplication. Currently, the accepted first-line procedure is the laparoscopic procedure. Provides symptomatic relief for most patients. The Nissen may also be performed as an open abdominal or thoracic operation.

(b) Partial fundoplications such as the Belsey Mark IV or the Toupet are indicated if esophageal motility is poor. The Belsey is a transthoracic open procedure done with the additional indication of a foreshortened esophagus, whereas the Toupet is a laparoscopic operation. Both feature a 270-degree fundoplication designed to limit reflux but allow transit of esophageal contents.

(c) Other older, rarely indicated, antireflux operations include the following:

(1) Hill gastropexy—features a 180-degree wrap with the phrenoesophageal ligament anchored to the median arcuate ligament of the diaphragm.

(2) Collis gastroplasty—used in patients with an extremely fore-shortened esophagus. The esophagus is lengthened with a gastric tube, allowing a tension-free fundoplication around the new esophagus.

(d) In the morbidly obese patient (body mass index >35) with other comorbid conditions, performing a laparoscopic or open Roux-en-Y gastric bypass is the surgical treatment for reflux disease.

(4) Complications

(a) Perforation of the esophagus—most dreaded complication. Prompt intraoperative recognition is crucial for repair and prevention of potential mediastinitis.

(b) Excessively tight wrap causing dysphagia—decreases with increasing experience and can be prevented with intraoperative manometry.

(c) Excessively loose or short wrap causing reflux

(d) "Slipped-Nissen" occurs when wrap slides down, the GE junction retracts into the chest, and the stomach is partitioned. This is usually due to a foreshortened esophagus unrecognized at the first operation.

(e) "Gas bloat syndrome" is described as difficult eructation because of swallowed air in the stomach of a patient with a restored LES.

## E. HIATAL HERNIA

### 1. Type I—sliding or axial (Fig. 24-1)

a. GE junction migrates above diaphragm; phrenoesophageal membrane intact; no true peritoneal sac.

b. Most common hiatal hernia—90% of cases

c. Significant only if reflux symptoms

d. Causative factors

(1) Chronically increased intraabdominal pressure, including obesity

(2) Weakness of supporting structures at esophageal hiatus

### 2. Type II (paraesophageal)

a. Herniated gastric fundus with GE junction in normal position

b. Peritoneal sac

c. Reflux rare

d. Uncommon type of hernia

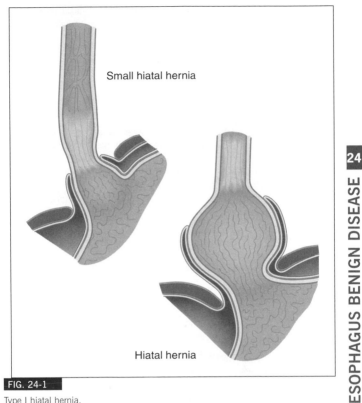

Small hiatal hernia

Hiatal hernia

**FIG. 24-1**

Type I hiatal hernia.

   e. Can result in gastric volvulus or strangulation
   f. All type II hernias should be repaired
  3. Type III—combination of types I and II

## VI. BENIGN TUMORS OF THE ESOPHAGUS

The incidence of benign tumors of the esophagus is rare (<1% of esophageal tumors).

### A. LEIOMYOMA

1. Most common benign tumor of esophagus—75% of cases
2. Less common in esophagus than stomach or small bowel
3. Usually located in distal two thirds of esophagus
4. Lesions <5 cm are usually asymptomatic.
5. Multiple in 3% to 10% of patients

6. Ninety-seven percent are intramural (within the circular muscle layer); histologically appear as interlacing smooth muscle bundles.
7. Symptoms
a. Progressive intermittent dysphagia
b. Vague retrosternal ache
c. Heartburn
d. Odynophagia
e. Regurgitation
8. Diagnosis by chest radiograph, barium swallow, and endoscopy (avoid biopsy if suspected). Endoscopic ultrasound is the gold standard for diagnosis.
a. Five discrete layers exist on ultrasound.
b. Alternating layers of hyperechoic and hypoechoic concentric rings
c. The ultrasonographic layers from intraluminal to periesophageal—superficial mucosa, deep mucosa, submucosa, muscularis propria, and periesophageal tissue
d. Esophageal leiomyoma are found in the fourth layer, the muscularis propria.
e. Ultrasound also allows for fine-needle aspiration of nodes in the periesophageal tissue.
9. Treatment
a. Excision of leiomyoma via thoracotomy, mortality rate <2%
b. Tumors not amenable to enucleation (10%) may require esophageal resection (mortality 10%).

## B. OTHER BENIGN TUMORS
1. Esophageal cysts—20% of cases
2. Polyps
3. Lipomas
4. Hemangiomas

## VII. ESOPHAGEAL RUPTURE AND PERFORATION
## A. CAUSATIVE FACTORS
1. Iatrogenic—most common causative factor
a. Endoscopic injury more common with rigid versus flexible scope and occurs most commonly at pharyngoesophageal junction. Direct injury frequently results from foreign body removal.
b. Dilation (balloon or bougienage)
c. Biopsy
d. Intubation (esophageal or endotracheal)
e. Operative—devascularization or perforation with pulmonary resection, vagotomy, or antireflux procedure
f. Placement of nasoenteric tubes
2. Noniatrogenic
a. Barogenic trauma

(1) Postemetic (Boerhaave's syndrome)—transmural tear after forceful or repeated vomiting. Usually associated with gluttony, bulimia, or alcoholic binge. Esophageal and gastric contents forced into chest under pressure.

(2) Blunt chest or abdominal trauma

(3) Other—labor, convulsions, defecation

b. Penetrating neck, chest, or abdominal trauma

c. Foreign body

d. Postoperative—anastomotic disruption

e. Corrosive injury

f. Erosion by adjacent inflammation

g. Carcinoma

## B. CLINICAL PRESENTATION

1. Can be dramatic and catastrophic with tachycardia, hypotension, and respiratory compromise

2. Others include dyspnea, neck or chest pain, fever, subcutaneous emphysema, and pneumothorax.

## C. DIAGNOSIS

1. Chest radiograph may reveal pneumothorax, pneumomediastinum, pleural effusion, or subdiaphragmatic air.

2. Contrast swallow—controversy whether water-soluble or barium swallow is best. Most would perform water-soluble study first because its effects on mediastinum are less than barium if perforation is present. However, this material is worse if aspirated. Barium study can be obtained if initial study is negative and suspicion remains high.

## D. TREATMENT

1. Early recognition and treatment are essential to survival. The differential diagnosis also must include myocardial infarction, perforated viscus, dissecting aortic aneurysms, and pulmonary embolus.

2. Resuscitation

a. Operative versus chest tube drainage

b. Nothing by mouth

c. Fluid resuscitation

d. Broad-spectrum antibiotics

e. Nutritional support in recovery period; parenteral route is preferred.

f. If perforation occurs in the presence of other pathology, the underlying disease must be treated at the time of surgery or the repair will break down.

3. Nonoperative management of esophageal perforation

a. Controversial; applicable only in patients with the following conditions

(1) Hemodynamic stability

(2) Small perforation

(3) Cervical perforation

(4) A contained leak
(5) No evidence of sepsis
(6) Wide drainage back into esophagus on esophagram
b. Nasogastric suction, antibiotics, and close observation
4. **Operative management depends on the location and extent of the perforation.**
a. Cervical esophagus—cervical incision, repair, drainage, antibiotics
b. Distal thoracic perforation—approach via a left thoracotomy (sixth intercarpal space)
    (1) Stable patient—suture closure, wide drainage, and antibiotics. Bolstering repair with patch is of controversial benefit.
    (2) Unstable patient—operative drainage and antibiotics. Suture closure is unlikely to succeed. Some advocate esophagectomy, oversewing the cardia, and creating a cervical esophagostomy.
c. Midportion of esophagus (rare; can consider right thoracotomy)
d. When in doubt, left thoracotomy
5. Complications of esophageal perforation include sepsis, abscess, fistula, empyema, mediastinitis, and death.

## VIII. CAUSTIC INJURY

### A. BACKGROUND
1. Usually results from ingestion of alkalis, acids, bleach, or detergents
2. Patients usually younger than 5 years or adolescent or adult attempting suicide
3. Alkalis cause liquefactive necrosis that results in greater depth of injury.

### B. CLINICAL PRESENTATION
1. Oral and oropharyngeal burns (pseudomembranes)
2. Signs and symptoms of laryngotracheal edema (hoarseness, stridor, aphonia, and dyspnea)
3. Signs and symptoms of esophageal or gastric perforation
4. In the absence of perforation, acute manifestations resolve in a few days. Clinical improvement may continue for several weeks.
5. Stricture can occur as a late complication.

### C. DIAGNOSIS
1. Upper endoscopy to establish severity of the injury
2. Contrast examination of esophagus can demonstrate injury and suspected perforation.

### D. TREATMENT
1. Initial therapy
a. Induction of emesis should be avoided, as should attempts to dilute the caustic agent (damage is nearly instantaneous, and intake of large volumes of fluid may only cause distention and emesis).

b. Nothing by mouth
c. Intravenous hydration
d. Broad-spectrum antibiotics after diagnosis confirmed
e. Efficacy of corticosteroids in attempt to limit stricture is debatable.

**2. Operative intervention**

a. Patients with evidence of esophageal or gastric perforation require immediate operation.
  (1) Best explored through abdominal incision; prep patient from mandible to pubis to allow for possibility of cervical incision.
  (2) G-tube to drain stomach; feeding J-tube for enteral nutrition
  (3) Restoration of alimentary continuity should await resolution of the acute insult.

b. Stricture formation tends to be the rule.
  (1) Dilation is traditional therapy.
  (2) Stricture that cannot be dilated or remains refractory to dilation after 1 year requires esophageal substitution.
    (a) Stomach is preferred substitute but often is unusable secondary to scarring from original injury.
    (b) Esophagus should be excised.

# Peptic Ulcer Disease

*Rebecca J. McClaine, MD*

## I. OCCURRENCE

A. **LIFETIME RISK—10%**
B. **U.S. PREVALENCE—2%**
C. **AGE**
1. Duodenal ulcers are more common in younger patients.
2. Gastric ulcer incidence peaks at age 55 to 65 years.

D. **MALE PREDOMINANCE FOR BOTH TYPES**

E. **RISK FACTORS**
1. Nonsteroidal antiinflammatory drug (NSAID) use
a. Twenty-five percent prevalence rate of peptic ulcer in chronic users
b. Risk for adverse gastrointestinal events is three times that of healthy control subjects (>60 years, risk increases to five times normal).
2. Cigarette smokers are twice as likely to experience development of peptic ulcer disease as nonsmokers.
3. Stressful life events
a. Burn injury—Curling's ulcer, can be in stomach, duodenum, or jejunum
b. Head injury—Cushing's ulcer

## II. PRESENTATION AND EVALUATION

A. **SYMPTOMS**
1. Abdominal pain (90% of cases)—epigastric, burning, nonradiating
a. Gastric ulcer—with eating
b. Duodenal ulcer—2 to 3 hours postprandial, relieved by food
2. Nausea, bloating
3. Weight loss
4. Complicated disease—worsening abdominal pain, hematemesis, melena

B. **PHYSICAL EXAMINATION**
1. Epigastric tenderness
2. Complicated disease—tachycardia, hypotension, peritonitis

C. **LABORATORY STUDIES**
1. Positive *Helicobacter pylori* tests
2. Complicated disease—decreased hemoglobin, acidosis, or metabolic alkalosis (gastric outlet obstruction with vomiting)

D. **DEFINITIVE DIAGNOSIS**
1. Esophagogastroduodenoscopy (EGD)—95% accurate for diagnosis, direct visualization of ulcer; the gold standard
2. Upper gastrointestinal series (with air and barium contrast)—75% to 80% accurate, filling defect in wall

### E. MODIFIED JOHNSON CLASSIFICATION
1. Type I—lesser curvature
2. Type II—synchronous ulcers in gastric body and duodenum
3. Type III—prepyloric
4. Type IV—near gastroesophageal junction
5. Type V—related to pill, can be located anywhere, but typically greater curvature

### III. PATHOGENESIS
**A. FOCAL DEFECT IN GASTRIC OR DUODENAL MUCOSA, EXTENDING TO SUBMUCOSA OR DEEPER (Fig. 25-1)**
**B. INCREASED GASTRIC ACID PRODUCTION**
1. Acid produced by parietal cells, located mostly in corpus of stomach
   a. Stimulated by acetylcholine from branches of vagus nerve in response to smell, taste, and sight of food (cephalic phase of acid secretory response)
   b. Stimulated by gastrin from G cells in antrum in response to amino acids in lumen (gastric phase)
   c. Gastric distension also stimulates acetylcholine and gastrin release.
   d. Histamine, released from enterochromaffin-like cells (basal acid secretion), mediates large portion of parietal cell stimulation in response to acetylcholine and gastrin release.
   e. Inhibited by somatostatin, released from D cells in response to antral acidification
2. Zollinger–Ellison syndrome—pancreatic, duodenal, or nodal gastrinoma, leading to increased gastrin secretion

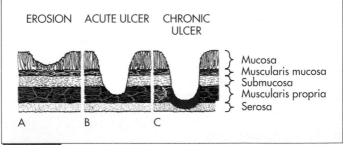

**FIG. 25-1**

Diagram of gastric erosions and ulcers. *(From Dempsey DT: Stomach. In Bruni-cardi FC (ed): Schwartz's Principles of Surgery, 8th ed. New York, McGraw-Hill, p 953.)*

a. Eighty percent sporadic, 20% inherited (most common pancreatic tumor associated with multiple endocrine neoplasia type 1, tend to be multiple tumors; see Chapter 62)
b. Diarrhea is most common symptom.
c. Ninety percent of patients with Zollinger–Ellison syndrome have peptic ulcer disease.
d. Diagnosed by increased gastrin levels (can be falsely increased with proton-pump inhibitor [PPI] use), confirmed by secretin stimulation test (increase of 200 pg/ml serum gastrin after 2 units/kg intravenous secretin bolus)
e. Fifty percent are malignant.
f. Surgical enucleation of gastrinoma is curative in 60% of patients.
g. Most are found in gastrinoma triangle (junction of second and third portions of duodenum, junction of cystic and common bile ducts, junction of head and neck of pancreas).
h. Preoperative localization by computed tomography scan, transabdominal ultrasound, endoscopic ultrasound, or octreotide scan (gastrinoma cells contain type 2 somatostatin receptors, which bind radiolabeled somatostatin analogue with high affinity). In rare situations, angiography with selective venous sampling may be used.
i. Intraoperative localization—exploration of gastrinoma triangle/pancreas, longitudinal duodenotomy, sampling of lymph nodes (portal, peripancreatic, celiac). Intraoperative ultrasound is helpful in identifying the lesion.
3. Duodenal ulcers, concurrent duodenal and gastric ulcers (Johnson type II), and prepyloric gastric ulcers (Johnson type III) associated with increased acid production.

## C. WEAKENED MUCOSAL DEFENSES
1. Defenses consist of mucosal barrier, bicarbonate secretion, and healthy epithelial cell barrier.
2. Mediators of defense system include prostaglandins and nitric oxide.
a. NSAIDs inhibit prostaglandin production.
b. Cigarette smoking inhibits prostaglandin and bicarbonate production.
3. Gastric outlet obstruction causes increased exposure of gastric mucosa to acid and can overwhelm defenses.
4. Gastric ulcers along the lesser curvature (Johnson type I), near the gastroesophageal junction (Johnson type IV), and those associated with pills (Johnson type V) are associated with weakened defenses.

## IV. HELICOBACTER PYLORI
### A. CHARACTERISTICS
1. Oxidase-positive, catalase-positive, microaerophilic gram-negative rod

### B. ASSOCIATED WITH;
1. 90% of duodenal ulcers and 70% to 90% of gastric ulcers

25

PEPTIC ULCER DISEASE

## C. FIFTY PERCENT OF ADULTS WORLDWIDE
And 33% of adults in the United States are infected.

## D. ASSOCIATED, ALTHOUGH NOT CAUSALLY
1. With gastric cancer and mucosa-associated lymphoid tissue lymphoma

## E. PREDISPOSES TO ULCER FORMATION
By both increasing acid production and weakening defenses
1. Local alkalinization of antrum leading to increased acid production
a. To survive in acidic environment, possesses urease, which converts urea to ammonia and bicarbonate
b. Increased bicarbonate → inhibition of D cells → decreased somatostatin production → less inhibition of G cells → hypergastrinemia → increased acid in stomach
2. Colonization of duodenum leading to decreased bicarbonate production
a. After antral epithelial metaplasia of duodenum, because of increased acidity from stomach
b. Leads to further decrease in bicarbonate production
3. Production and release of toxins (vacA, cagA) and cytokines (interleukin-8)

## F. DIAGNOSIS OF INFECTION
1. Endoscopic biopsy, if endoscopy is otherwise indicated
a. Histologic analysis to directly visualize organisms (gold standard)
b. Rapid urease test (CLOtest)—sensitivity of 80% to 95%, specificity of 95% to 100%
2. Serologic test—test of choice when endoscopy not indicated; "scar" remains after eradication following treatment; sensitivity of 80%, specificity of 90%
3. Fecal antigen test—for active infection and to confirm cure
4. Urea breath test—gold standard to confirm cure after 4 weeks of treatment
a. Ingest urea labeled with $^{13}C$, converted to $CO_2$ by urease, exhaled $^{13}CO_2$.
5. Culture only with treatment failure, when antibiotic resistance is suspected.

## G. TREATMENT OF KNOWN INFECTION WITH "TRIPLE THERAPY" (AMOXICILLIN, CLARITHROMYCIN, AND PPI) FOR ERADICATION OF INFECTION
1. May substitute metronidazole for amoxicillin
2. Levofloxacin for resistant strains

## V. TREATMENT OF UNCOMPLICATED DISEASE
## A. PREVENTION
1. High-risk NSAID users (>60 years, before gastrointestinal event, concomitant steroid use or anticoagulation, high NSAID dose) should take a PPI.

## B. EMPIRIC MEDICAL THERAPY

For peptic ulcer if patient younger than 45 years, no alarm symptoms (weight loss, recurrent vomiting, dysphagia, bleeding/anemia)

1. Smoking cessation
2. Avoidance of NSAIDs
3. Acid-reducing medication alone
a. PPIs (omeprazole, pantoprazole), OR
b. Selective histamine H2 receptor blockers (ranitidine, famotidine)
4. Continue treatment for 3 months.
5. Consider testing for *H. pylori* if infection is suspected and change to eradication therapy for positive test.
6. If no improvement in symptoms, change to *H. pylori* eradication therapy, even with no test or with negative results.

## C. CONCERN FOR GASTRIC CANCER

1. If patient older than 45 years, or with alarm symptoms—EGD with test for *H. pylori* and biopsy of edges of gastric ulcer

## D. SURGICAL THERAPY

1. Indicated for bleeding, perforation, obstruction, or intractability

## VI. TREATMENT OF COMPLICATED DISEASE

## A. CONCERN FOR GASTRIC CANCER

With complicated disease:

1. All gastric ulcers visualized during surgical procedure should undergo biopsy (ulcer edges).

## B. BLEEDING PEPTIC ULCER

1. This is the most common complication.
2. A 10% to 20% mortality rate, greater with bleeding gastric ulcers because patients are typically older with more comorbidities
3. Initial treatment—NPO and PPI drip; 75% stop bleeding with this therapy.
4. EGD to control bleeding by cauterization, epinephrine injection, or clipping
5. Early surgical therapy (without prior EGD) indicated for patients presenting in shock, requiring ≥4 units of blood in 24 hours, in patients older than 60 years, or in patients with recurrent bleeding ulcer disease.
6. Surgical therapy after EGD indicated with failure of endoscopic control of bleeding, rebleeding after endoscopy, ulcer location on lesser curvature, or posterior duodenal bulb (because of risk for erosion into large vessels).
7. Surgical options
a. Unstable patient—oversewing to control bleeding
b. Stable patient—vagotomy and drainage or vagotomy and antrectomy depending on patient history, characteristics, and location of ulcer

## C. PERFORATED PEPTIC ULCER

This is the second most common complication.

1. Surgery always indicated, unless patient is stable with radiographic demonstration of sealed perforation.
2. Surgical options
a. Unstable patient or significant peritoneal contamination—omental patch
b. Stable patient (duodenal ulcer)—patch with PPI therapy, highly selective vagotomy, or vagotomy and drainage
c. Stable patient (gastric ulcer)—removal of ulcer by excision and primary repair of stomach; antrectomy is ideal, or patch with PPI and *H. pylori* therapy.

## D. OBSTRUCTION

Acute (caused by inflammation) or chronic (caused by cicatrix)

1. Acute obstruction—can be managed by nasogastric decompression
2. Endoscopic balloon dilation associated with 50% recurrence rate.
3. Surgical options (patients typically stable, or resuscitated from acute obstructive event)—vagotomy and antrectomy, vagotomy and drainage, or highly selective vagotomy, with gastrojejunostomy

## E. INTRACTABILITY—RARE TODAY

1. Differential diagnosis—gastric cancer, noncompliance with PPI therapy, gastric motility disorder, Zollinger–Ellison syndrome
2. Surgical options—highly selective vagotomy; highly selective vagotomy and wedge resection

## VII. DETAILS OF SURGICAL OPTIONS

## A. HIGHLY SELECTIVE VAGOTOMY (HSV; OR PROXIMAL GASTRIC OR PARIETAL CELL)

1. Surgical technique—ligation of vagus nerve branches to proximal two-thirds of stomach
a. Vagal innervation to pylorus controls relaxation of the pyloric sphincter, thus denervation of pylorus may require a drainage procedure.
b. May be performed laparoscopically
2. Mortality rate <0.5%, which is the highest recurrence of procedures discussed.
3. Decreases acid production by 65% to 75% (similar to PPI therapy)

## B. OMENTAL (GRAHAM) PATCH

1. Surgical technique: Patch of greater omentum is loosely placed over perforated portion of duodenum, with or without (true Graham patch) underlying primary closure of duodenum.
2. Low mortality, recurrence rate unchanged unless acid-reducing procedure performed in addition to patch.
3. Historically described for duodenal perforation, but may also be used for perforation of gastric ulcer.

## C. VAGOTOMY AND DRAINAGE

1. Surgical technique—truncal vagotomy (denervates pylorus), plus drainage of stomach by pyloroplasty or gastrojejunostomy
   a. Heineke–Mikulicz pyloroplasty—close longitudinal incision in transverse fashion
   b. Gastrojejunostomy—loop of proximal jejunum sutured to dependent part of greater curvature, antecolic or retrocolic fashion
2. Low mortality, 10% recurrence rate
3. Ten percent of patients experience dumping or diarrhea after pyloroplasty.

## D. VAGOTOMY AND ANTRECTOMY

1. Surgical technique—excision of antrum, leaving 60% to 70% gastric remnant, with reestablishment of continuity with either gastroduodenostomy (Billroth I) or loop gastrojejunostomy (Billroth II)
2. Greater mortality rate; should be avoided in hemodynamically unstable patients
3. Low recurrence rate
4. Gastrojejunostomy side effects possible.

## E. DISTAL GASTRECTOMY

1. Surgical technique—excision of antrum and portion of stomach affected by ulcer, leaving 40% to 50% gastric remnant, with Billroth I or II reconstruction.
2. Similar mortality, recurrence, and side-effect profile as vagotomy and antrectomy

## F. POSTOPERATIVE COMPLICATIONS

1. Early dumping (5–10% of patients)—occurs after pyloroplasty or gastrojejunostomy.
   a. Postprandial diaphoresis, weakness, light-headedness, tachycardia, followed by diarrhea
   b. Caused by abrupt delivery of hyperosmolar load into small bowel, leading to peripheral and splanchnic vasodilatation
   c. Relieved by supine position
   d. Treated initially by dietary modification (small, frequent, low-fat, low-carbohydrate, high-protein, low-liquid meals), octreotide
   e. Most patients improve with time, after months or years.
   f. Reoperation in rare patients—Roux-en-Y gastrojejunostomy to slow gastric emptying
2. Late dumping—occurs after pyloroplasty or gastrojejunostomy.
   a. Similar symptoms to early dumping, occurring 2 to 3 hours postprandial
   b. Due to hypoglycemia from release of large amount of insulin
   c. Treat by eating carbohydrates when symptoms occur, acarbose.
3. Diarrhea (5–10% of patients)—occurs after vagotomy, pyloroplasty, or gastrojejunostomy.

a. Differentiate from dumping by lack of other symptoms.

b. Mechanism caused by accelerated transit, bile acid or fat malabsorption, or blind loop syndrome (see later).

c. Treatment options include loperamide, cholestyramine, pancreatic enzymes, and trial of empiric antibiotics.

**4. Delayed gastric emptying—occurs after gastrojejunostomy.**

a. Characterized by emesis, epigastric distension or pain, and weight loss.

b. Evaluate objectively by gastric emptying scan (nuclear medicine)—liquid transit typically normal, solid transit delayed.

c. Must rule out mechanical obstruction by EGD, upper gastrointestinal series.

d. Treat with promotility agents (erythromycin, metoclopramide).

e. Reoperation in rare patients—more extensive gastrectomy accompanied by Roux-en-Y gastrojejunostomy

**5. Afferent loop syndrome—occurs after gastrojejunostomy.**

a. Characterized by bilious emesis (sometimes 1–2 hours postprandial), epigastric distension or pain, weight loss

b. Caused by obstruction of afferent intestinal limb (containing duodenum and coming toward stomach), either acutely by postoperative edema or chronically by intermittent obstruction

c. Malabsorption caused by bacterial overgrowth in afferent limb, leading to deconjugation of bile salts ("blind loop syndrome").

d. Treat with antibiotics if blind loop syndrome is suspected; reoperation (conversion to Roux-en-Y gastrojejunostomy).

**6. Marginal ulcer—occurs after gastrojejunostomy.**

a. Presents with abdominal pain, bloating, vomiting

b. Diagnose with EGD, usually on intestinal side of anastomosis.

c. Usually responds to medical therapy with PPI; refractory cases require reoperation

**7. Bile reflux gastritis—occurs most often after gastrojejunostomy.**

a. Symptoms include nausea, epigastric pain, bilious vomiting.

b. May occur years after initial operation

c. Treat with PPI or sucralfate, rarely reoperation (Roux-en-Y gastrojejunostomy with long Roux limb).

**8. Cholelithiasis—caused by vagotomy with disruption of vagal branches to gallbladder, leading to bile stasis.**

**9. Nutritional deficiencies after gastrojejunostomy.**

a. Weight loss may be caused by insufficient intake (due to early satiety or dietary modifications to treat dumping or diarrhea) or malabsorption.

b. Iron deficiency: Iron absorption requires acidic environment.

c. Vitamin $B_{12}$ deficiency: Parietal cells synthesize intrinsic factor, which is necessary for vitamin $B_{12}$ absorption.

d. Calcium deficiency: This is caused by poor absorption of calcium (which occurs in duodenum) or vitamin D (fat-soluble vitamin).

## RECOMMENDED READING

Behrman SW: Management of complicated peptic ulcer disease. *Arch Surg* 140: 201–208, 2005.

Dempsey DT: Stomach. In Brunicardi FC (ed): *Schwartz's Principles of Surgery.* 8th ed. New York: McGraw-Hill, pp 933–995.

Marshall BJ, Warren JR: Unidentified curved bacilli in the stomach of patients with gastritis and peptic ulceration. *Lancet* 1(8390):1311–1315, 1984.

# Inflammatory Bowel Disease

*Grace Z. Mak, MD*

## I. INFLAMMATORY BOWEL DISEASE (IBD)

### A. ULCERATIVE COLITIS (UC)
1. Diffuse inflammatory disease limited to mucosa of colon and rectum.
2. Operative therapy is almost always curative.

### B. CROHN'S DISEASE (CD)
1. Chronic, relapsing, transmural, usually segmental, and often granulomatous inflammatory disorder involving any portion of the gastrointestinal (GI) tract from mouth to anus
2. Surgical intervention reserved for treatment of complications or intractable disease.

### C. INDETERMINATE COLITIS
1. Fifteen percent of cases are indistinguishable between UC and CD.

## II. EXTRAINTESTINAL MANIFESTATIONS
Occur in one third of IBD cases

### A. CUTANEOUS
1. Erythema nodosum
   a. Five percent to 15% of IBD patients
   b. Usually coincides with clinical disease activity
   c. Three to four times more frequent in female patients
   d. Characteristic lesions are red, raised, and predominately located on lower legs.
2. Pyoderma gangrenosum
   a. Almost exclusively seen in IBD patients
   b. Begins as erythematous plaque, papule, or bleb generally located on pretibial region of leg or occasionally near a stoma
   c. Progresses to an ulcerated, painful, and necrotic wound
   d. May respond to resection of affected bowel segment
3. Erythema multiforme

### B. OCULAR
1. Occurs in up to 10% of IBD patients
2. Conjunctivitis, iritis, uveitis, episcleritis
3. Usually develops during acute exacerbations

### C. MUSCULOSKELETAL
1. Arthritis
   a. Incidence 20 times greater than in general population
   b. Usually improves with treatment of colonic disease

2. Sacroiliitis, ankylosing spondylitis
a. Unaffected by medicosurgical treatment of colonic disease
3. Associated with human leukocyte antigen-B27 antigen

## D. HEPATOBILIARY

1. Liver common extracolonic disease site
2. Fatty infiltration of liver
a. Occurs in 40% to 50% of patients with IBD
b. May be reversed by medical or surgical treatment of colonic disease
3. Cirrhosis
a. Develops in 2% to 5% of patients with IBD
b. Irreversible
4. Primary sclerosing cholangitis
a. Progressive disease characterized by strictures of intrahepatic and extrahepatic bile ducts
b. Forty percent to 60% of patients with primary sclerosing cholangitis have UC.
c. Only treatment is liver transplantation.
   (1) Colectomy is ineffective
5. Pericholangitis, hepatitis
6. Bile duct carcinoma
a. Rare complication of long-standing primary sclerosing cholangitis.
b. Generally, patients are 20 years younger than average patient with bile duct carcinoma.

## III. ULCERATIVE COLITIS

## A. CAUSATIVE FACTORS

1. Largely unknown—thought to be multifactorial
2. Infectious
a. Viral, bacterial, mycobacterial
3. Immunologic
a. Poorly regulated mucosal inflammatory response to exogenous antigens
4. Autoimmune
5. Genetic
a. Increased in following populations:
   (1) White individuals
   (2) Female individuals
   (3) Individuals of Jewish ancestry
      (a) Two to four times greater risk
b. Familial disposition
c. Associated with certain human leukocyte antigen phenotypes
6. Environmental
a. Increased in urban dwellers
7. Diet

## B. PATHOPHYSIOLOGY

1. Increased production of mucosal immunoglobulins in response to initiating antigens
2. Recruitment of inflammatory cells into colonic mucosa and submucosa
3. Altered mucosal function and permeability

## C. EPIDEMIOLOGY

1. Age at onset
a. Bimodal: 15 to 30 and 50 to 70 years of age
2. Female/male ratio of 1.3:1
3. Family history in 10% to 20% of cases
4. Incidence
a. Eight to 15 per 100,000 people in United States and Northern Europe
b. Significantly lower incidence in Asia, Africa, and South America
5. Smoking—suggested to be protective.

## D. CLINICAL MANIFESTATIONS

1. Signs and symptoms
a. Related to degree and extent of mucosal inflammation
b. Characterized by exacerbations and remissions
c. Clinical spectrum
    (1) Inactive, quiescent phase
    (2) Low-grade active disease
    (3) Fulminant disease
d. Most common—bloody diarrhea, rectal bleeding, tenesmus (proctitis)
e. Less common—cramping abdominal pain, weight loss, fever, malnutrition
f. Rare—vomiting, perianal disease, abdominal mass
g. Onset may be insidious or acute and fulminant.
    (1) Fulminant colitis (toxic megacolon)—15% of cases
        (a) Severe abdominal pain, fever
2. Disease distribution
a. Confined to colon and rectum without skip lesions
b. Almost always involves the rectum (95%), then proceeds proximally
    (1) Involvement of rectum—proctitis
    (2) Involvement of rectum and sigmoid colon—proctosigmoiditis
    (3) Involvement of rectum and left colon—left-sided colitis
    (4) Involvement of rectum and colon proximal to splenic flexure—pancolitis
c. "Backwash" ileitis (10%), resolves after colonic resection.
    (1) Inflammatory changes within terminal ileum

## E. DIAGNOSIS

1. Laboratory findings
a. Anemia, leukocytosis, increased erythrocyte sedimentation rate
b. Negative stool cultures for ova and parasites

c. Severe disease
   (1) Hypoalbuminemia, dehydration, electrolyte/vitamin depletion, steatorrhea
2. **Serologic markers**
a. Perinuclear antineutrophil cytoplasmic antibody
3. **Radiographic findings**
a. Sixty percent to 80% of patients
b. Plain films
   (1) Abdominal radiographs—evaluate colonic distension during acute phase to exclude toxic megacolon.
   (2) Upright chest radiograph—evaluate for free air caused by perforation.
c. Barium enema
   (1) Less sensitive than colonoscopy and may not detect early disease
   (2) Mucosal irregularity, "collar-button" ulcers, and pseudopolyps
   (3) Chronic disease characterized by loss of haustrations and colonic shortening and narrowing ("lead pipe" appearance).
   (4) Ileum typically spared.
   (5) Strictures are highly uncommon, have late manifestations, and imply malignancy.
4. **Endoscopy**
a. Essential for diagnosis and determination of extent of disease
b. Findings
   (1) Early—mucosal edema with loss of normal vascular pattern, confluent erythema, rectal involvement
   (2) Moderate
      (a) Granularity, friable mucosa with contact bleeding, multiple inflammatory pseudopolyps
      (b) Pus and mucus present.
   (3) Late—foreshortened colon, discrete ulcers, mucosa replaced by scar
5. **Pathology**
a. During acute phase, biopsy often shows only nonspecific inflammation.
b. Diagnostic in chronic phase
c. Mucosal depletion of goblet cells
d. Mucosal atrophy
e. Inflammatory polyps in healing stage
f. Crypt abscess

## F. COMPLICATIONS
1. **Rectal or colonic strictures**
a. Highly uncommon because of restriction of inflammation to mucosa
b. Presumed to be malignant until proved otherwise
2. **Toxic colitis with or without megacolon (10% of cases)**
a. May be initial presentation of UC in 30% of cases
b. Greatest risk for perforation with initial attack of toxic megacolon
c. Clinical findings—fever, abrupt onset of bloody diarrhea, abdominal pain, nausea, vomiting, abdominal distention, systemic toxicity

   d. Radiographic findings—transverse colon 8 to 10 cm in diameter on plain abdominal films
   e. Pathology—inflammation extends into muscle layers of bowel wall.
   f. Perforation can lead to localized abscess or generalized peritonitis.
   g. Mortality
      (1) Mortality rate of 40% with perforation
      (2) Mortality rate of 2% to 8% with surgery before perforation
   h. Treatment
      (1) Aggressive intravenous fluid resuscitation
      (2) Electrolyte repletion
      (3) Bowel rest
      (4) Nasogastric tube decompression
      (5) Broad-spectrum intravenous antibiotics
      (6) Consider total parenteral nutrition.
      (7) Avoid colonoscopy, barium enema, and antidiarrheal agents.
      (8) Medical treatment includes high-dose intravenous steroids (hydrocortisone 100 mg every 6 hours, methylprednisolone 16–20 mg every 8 hours, or prednisone 20 mg every 8 hours) and/or immunosuppression (cyclosporine, 6-mercaptopurine).
      (9) Surgery indicated if conservative therapy fails after 24 hours, patient clinically deteriorates, or free perforation, peritonitis, or massive hemorrhage develops.
         (a) Total abdominal colectomy with end ileostomy and closure of rectum
         (b) Proctectomy and ileoanal anastomosis can be performed once patient is stable.
3. **Massive hemorrhage—can occur in toxic colitis, though rare.**
   a. Treatment is total abdominal colectomy, end ileostomy, and closure of rectum.
   b. Sphincter-sparing operation can be performed at a later date.
4. **Carcinoma of colon/rectum**
   a. Five times normal risk, related to severity of disease
   b. Begins to appear after 5 to 10 years of active disease
      (1) 2% risk after 10 years
      (2) 8% risk after 20 years
      (3) 18% risk after 30 years
      (4) 1% to 2% risk per year if disease is present more than 10 years.
   c. More common in patients with initial colitis before 25 years of age
   d. Risk increases with amount of colon involved (greatest with pancolonic disease).
   e. Carcinoma more likely to arise from areas of flat dysplasia (in contrast with sporadic colon cancer)—difficult to diagnose at an early stage.
   f. Presence of stricture—must rule out carcinoma.
   g. Surveillance
      (1) Colonoscopy with 40 to 50 random biopsies as well as biopsies of suspicious lesions to identify dysplasia

26

INFLAMMATORY BOWEL DISEASE

(a) Invasive carcinoma present in up to 20% of patients with low-grade dysplasia.

(b) Any patient with dysplasia should have proctocolectomy.

(2) Annually in patients with pancolitis for 8 years and left-sided colitis for 15 years.

h. Short-term prognosis worse compared with idiopathic colon cancer.

i. Long-term (5-year) survival equivalent

5. **Malnutrition**

a. Decreased oral intake because of abdominal pain and obstructive symptoms

b. Diarrhea can lead to protein losses.

c. Ongoing inflammation can lead to catabolic physiologic state.

d. Can result in growth retardation in children

e. Nutritional status should be assessed before surgical intervention by nutritional parameters such as prealbumin, transferrin, and retinol-binding protein.

## G. MEDICAL MANAGEMENT

1. **Goal is to decrease inflammation and alleviate symptoms.**
2. **Mild-to-moderate flares can be treated as outpatient care.**
3. **More severe flares require hospitalization.**
4. **Aminosalicylates—sulfasalazine, mesalamine, olsalazine, balsalazide**

a. First-line agents for mild-to-moderate disease

b. Decrease inflammation by inhibiting cyclooxygenase and 5-lipoxygenase in gut mucosa

(1) Inhibit prostaglandins and leukotriene production

(2) Inhibit bacterial peptide-induced neutrophil chemotaxis

(3) Scavenge reactive oxygen metabolites

c. Require direct contact with affected mucosa

d. Enemas may be used for proctitis and proctosigmoiditis.

e. Good for sustaining remission

f. Side effects—dose-related toxicity

(1) Oligospermia

(2) Inhibition of folate absorption

(3) Hemolytic anemia

(4) Nausea, vomiting, headaches, abdominal discomfort

(5) Allergic hypersensitivity (10–15%)

g. Sulfasalazine

(1) Conjugated to prevent small-bowel absorption

(2) Metabolized by bacteria to 5-aminosalicylic acid, the active component, and sulfapyridine, which is responsible for major side effects

h. Mesalamine

(1) Fewer side effects than sulfasalazine at comparable doses

(2) Various formulations allow different areas to be targeted.

(a) Rowasa, Canasa—rectal

(b) Asacol, Salofalk—pH dependent, distal ileum and colon

(c) Pentasa—time release, jejunum to colon

5. Antibiotics—used only in setting of fulminant colitis or toxic megacolon.
6. Corticosteroids
   a. Used to control acute exacerbations
      (1) No relapse prevention
      (2) No proven maintenance benefit
   b. Nonspecific inhibitors of the immune system
   c. Seventy-five percent to 90% exhibit improvement after treatment.
   d. Side effects
      (1) Should limit treatment to shortest possible time course
      (2) Potential adverse effect on growth in children
      (3) Failure to wean—relative indication for surgery.
   e. Intravenous steroids
      (1) Severe or fulminant disease
      (2) Hydrocortisone 100 to 300 mg/day
      (3) Prednisolone 20 to 80 mg/day
   f. Oral steroids
      (1) Less severe or improving disease
      (2) Prednisone 20 to 60 mg/day
   g. Enemas or topical preparations for proctitis or proctosigmoiditis—have fewer side effects compared with systemic preparations.
   h. Newer preparations
      (1) Budesonide, beclomethasone dipropionate, tixocortol pivalate
      (2) Rapid hepatic degradation decreases systemic toxicity significantly
7. Immunosuppressives
   a. Azathioprine (6-mercaptopurine, active metabolite)
      (1) Antimetabolite drugs
      (2) Interfere with nucleic acid synthesis, decreasing proliferation of inflammatory cells
      (3) Used for disease refractory to salicylate therapy or corticosteroids and for patients dependent on corticosteroids
         (a) Allows gradual tapering of corticosteroids; may be required up to 6 months
      (4) Onset of action in 6 to 12 weeks
      (5) Possible increased risk for lymphoma
      (6) Adverse side effects—bone marrow suppression, hepatotoxicity, pancreatitis
   b. Cyclosporine
      (1) Interferes with T-cell function
      (2) Used in severe, acute toxic colitis otherwise needing urgent proctocolectomy refractory to high-dose corticosteroids
      (3) Up to 80% of patients with an acute flare will improve after treatment.
         (a) Up to 50% of patients will eventually need proctocolectomy within a year.
      (4) Long-term use limited by toxicity.

c. Methotrexate
  (1) Folate antagonist
  (2) Reports of >50% of patients improving after treatment
d. Infliximab (Remicade)—reports of efficacy, though used more commonly in CD

## H. SURGICAL MANAGEMENT
### 1. Indications
a. Elective
  (1) Chronic, debilitating disease intractable to maximal medical therapy
  (2) High risk for development of major complications from medical therapy—aseptic necrosis of joints caused by chronic steroid use
  (3) Growth failure in children
  (4) Severe extraintestinal complications
  (5) Carcinoma or high risk for carcinoma—biopsy with dysplasia
b. Emergent
  (1) Perforation, toxic megacolon, massive life-threatening hemorrhage, obstruction
  (2) Fulminant colitis that has failed to respond rapidly to medical therapy
  (3) Total abdominal colectomy with end ileostomy
    (a) Total proctocolectomy not recommended because of time required for pelvic dissection and increased risk for massive hemorrhage from pelvis.
    (b) May perform loop ileostomy with decompressing colostomy if patient too unstable to undergo colectomy. Definitive surgery can be performed at later date.
### 2. Surgical procedures
a. Total abdominal colectomy, mucosal proctectomy, ileal reservoir, and ileoanal anastomosis
  (1) Curative procedure
  (2) Procedure of choice for most patients
  (3) Sphincter-sparing procedure preserves continence.
  (4) Minimal bladder and sexual dysfunction
  (5) Disadvantages include pouch fistulas, frequent soiling, nighttime incontinence, pouchitis, anal excoriation, and risk for intestinal obstruction.
  (6) Contraindications include CD, diarrhea, and distal rectal cancer.
  (7) Pouch created from 30 cm of terminal ileum with anastomosis to anus.
    (a) J pouch—simple
    (b) S pouch—can have less tension to anus.
b. Total proctocolectomy with standard (Brooke) end ileostomy
  (1) Until recently it was the gold standard operation; now replaced by sphincter-sparing operations.
  (2) One-step operation

(3) Curative procedure, no contraindications
(4) Disadvantages include permanent ileostomy and impotence (10–15% male patients).
(5) Complications include stoma revisions, perineal wound infections, small bowel obstructions, bladder dysfunction, and sexual dysfunction.
(6) Must empty ostomy bag four to eight times per day.
(7) One percent to 3% elective operative mortality rate

c. Total proctocolectomy with continent (Kock) ileostomy
   (1) Avoids need for conventional ileostomy/appliances
   (2) Major problem—stability of continent nipple valve within ileal reservoir (40–50% require reoperation).
   (3) Use is now limited to patients who strongly desire continence-restoring procedure after total proctocolectomy.

d. Total abdominal colectomy with ileostomy, rectal preservation
   (1) Reserved for emergency procedures (hemorrhage, toxic megacolon) to decrease operative morbidity and mortality rates (3–10%)
   (2) Proctectomy and ileal pouch anal anastomosis can be subsequently performed to control proctitis, reduce cancer risk, and preserve continence.

## I. PROGNOSIS
### 1. Mortality
a. Five percent mortality rate over 10 years (pancolitis)
b. Elective surgery (2%)
c. Emergent surgery (8–15%)

### 2. Left-sided colitis and pancolitis
a. Acute intermittent presentation (60%)—most relapse within first year.
b. Chronic, unremitting presentation (20%)
c. Fulminant presentation (10%)
d. Up to 50% require colectomy in first 10 years.

### 3. Ulcerative proctitis
a. Left-sided colitis develops in 20% of patients.
b. Only 2% to 15% reported to progress to pancolitis.

## IV. CROHN'S DISEASE
### A. CAUSATIVE FACTORS
1. Cause is largely unknown, though many theories exist.
2. Infectious
a. Typical mycobacteria (Mycobacteria paratuberculosis, Mycobacteria avium)
b. Measles virus and paramyxovirus
c. Yersinia enterocolitica
d. Listeria monocytogenes

26

INFLAMMATORY BOWEL DISEASE

3. Genetic
a. NOD2—chromosome 16
b. Fifteen percent to 20% of patients have a positive family history of IBD.
4. Environmental—temperate climates
5. Smoking—two to four times increased risk, increased relapse

## B. EPIDEMIOLOGY
1. Bimodal—peak incidence is 20 to 30 years of age and 50 to 60 years of age.
2. Equal sex distribution
3. Increased in white population
4. Incidence—1 to 5 per 100,000 people
5. Prevalence—400,000 cases
6. Greatest incidence in North America and northern Europe

## C. PATHOPHYSIOLOGY
1. Chronic granulomatous disease that affects any portion of the GI tract from mouth to anus.
2. Early superficial aphthous ulcers can progress to transmural inflammation.
3. Linear ulcers produce transverse clefts and sinuses ("cobblestoning").
4. Submucosal/muscularis inflammation can lead to bowel lumen narrowing.

## D. CLINICAL MANIFESTATIONS
1. Characterized by exacerbations and remissions
2. Signs and symptoms
a. Depend on severity of inflammation or fibrosis, as well as the location of inflammation
b. Diarrhea—90% of cases, usually nonbloody
c. Recurrent abdominal pain—mild colicky pain, often initiated by meals, relieved by defecation
d. Abdominal distention, flatulence
e. Obstructive symptoms caused by strictures
f. Fever, malaise
g. Anorectal lesions
(1) Chronic, recurrent, or nonhealing anal fissures, ulcers, complex anal fistulas, perirectal abscesses
(2) May precede bowel involvement in 4% of cases
(3) Present with pain, swelling, and drainage
h. Malnutrition—protein-losing enteropathy, steatorrhea, mineral and vitamin deficiencies, growth retardation
i. Weight loss caused by protein loss and obstructive symptoms
j. Acute inflammatory presentation

(1) Acute appendicitis-like presentation caused by acute inflammation of distal ileum; only 15% of patients with isolated terminal ileitis experience development of chronic CD.

(2) Acute inflammation can be complicated by fistulas, intraabdominal abscesses, or both.

k. Chronic fibrotic presentation—strictures in any portion of GI tract; chronic strictures generally do not improve with medical therapy.

**3. Extraintestinal manifestations in 30% (see section II)**

**4. Disease distribution**

a. May involve any segment of entire GI tract (from mouth to anus)

b. Skip regions (12–35%)—key in differentiating UC from CD

c. Ileocolic and small-bowel CD

  (1) Distal ileum most frequently involved.

  (2) Terminal ileum and colon (55%)—ileocolic CD

  (3) Small bowel only (30%)

  (4) Most common surgical indications

    (a) Internal fistula or abscess (30–38%)

      (1) Psoas abscess

      (2) Treatment

        (a) Percutaneous abscess drainage

        (b) Antibiotics

    (b) Obstruction (35–37%)

    (c) Risk for recurrence after resection high—>50% of patients have recurrence within 10 years (majority requiring second operation).

d. Colon only (15%)

  (1) May present as fulminant colitis or toxic megacolon

    (a) Management is the same as for UC (resuscitation, bowel rest, broad-spectrum antibiotics, and parenteral corticosteroids).

    (b) If conservative management fails, total abdominal colectomy with end ileostomy recommended.

    (c) Elective proctectomy may be necessary for refractory Crohn's proctitis.

  (2) Surgical indications

    (a) Intractability

    (b) Complications of medical therapy

    (c) Risk for development of malignancy

    (d) Strictures

e. Rectal sparing (40%)

f. Distal rectum and anal canal—perianal CD (35%)

  (1) Isolated anal CD uncommon (3–4%)—detection of anal disease should prompt evaluation of remainder of GI tract.

  (2) Most common perianal lesion—waxy skin tags; minimally symptomatic

(3) Fissures
(a) Common
(b) Tend to occur in unusual locations (lateral rather than anterior or posterior midline)
(c) Often unusually deep or broad
(4) Perianal abscess and fistula—fistulas tend to be complex, often with multiple tracts.

## E. DIAGNOSIS

1. **Diagnosis is more difficult compared with UC because of nonspecific, indolent symptoms.**
a. Mean time from onset to diagnosis—35 months
2. **Laboratory findings**
a. Anemia—caused by iron, vitamin $B_{12}$, or folate deficiency.
b. Hypoalbuminemia
c. Tests of bowel function (D-xylose absorption, bile acid breath test) are abnormal with extensive disease.
3. **Serologic markers—anti–Saccharomyces cerevisiae antibody**
a. Sixty percent of patients with CD compared with 5% of patients with UC
b. Less than 5% in normal population
4. **Radiographic findings**
a. Upper GI with small-bowel follow-through or enteroclysis
(1) Narrowed terminal ileum (Kantor's string sign)
(2) Fistulas
(3) Nodules, sinuses, clefts, linear ulcers
b. Barium enema
(1) Thickened bowel wall, longitudinal ulcers, transverse fissures, cobblestone formation, and rectal sparing
(2) Terminal ileum may contain strictures (string sign).
c. Abdominal computed tomography
(1) Intraabdominal abscesses
(2) Thickened bowel wall
(3) Fistulas—enterovesical or enteroentero
5. **Endoscopy**
a. Esophagogastroduodenoscopy
b. Colonoscopy
(1) Normal rectum (rectal sparing) in 40% to 50% of patients.
(2) Random biopsies required because grossly normal-appearing rectum may have histologic disease.
(3) Characteristic lesions
(a) Aphthous ulcers
(b) Mucosal ulcerations
(c) Anal fissures
(d) Cobblestoning
(4) Chronic inflammation may ultimately lead to fibrosis, strictures, and fistulas in either small or large intestine.

  (5) Segmental (skip) lesions
  (6) Annual surveillance with multiple biopsies recommended for patients with long-standing Crohn's colitis (>7 years in duration)

6. Pathology
a. Inflammation
b. Noncaseating granulomas

## F. COMPLICATIONS
1. Intestinal obstruction
2. Abscess formation
3. Fistulas
a. Internal
  (1) Between segments of bowel
  (2) Between bowel and other viscera (bladder, uterus, vagina)
  (3) Between bowel and retroperitoneal sites
b. External
4. Anorectal lesions—abscess, fistula, fissure
5. Free perforation and hemorrhage
a. Rare because of gradual fibrosis and formation of strictures
b. Adjacent structures generally "wall off" perforation sites—cause formation of internal fistulas.
6. Carcinoma
a. It is less common than UC, but Crohn's colitis (particularly pancolitis) has nearly the same risk for malignancy as UC.
b. Finding of dysplasia on biopsy is indication for total proctocolectomy.
7. Toxic megacolon
a. Occurs in 5% of patients with colonic involvement
b. Responds to medical therapy better than UC
8. Extraintestinal (see section II)
a. More common with colonic involvement
b. Urinary—cystitis, calculi (oxalate), ureteral obstruction
9. Strictures

## G. MEDICAL MANAGEMENT (SEE SECTION III.G)
1. Aminosalicylates—oral agent (mesalamine) used for mild-to-moderate disease.
2. Antibiotics
a. Decrease intraluminal bacterial load
b. Metronidazole—reported to improve Crohn's colitis and perianal disease.
c. Fluoroquinolones—may be effective in some cases.
3. Corticosteroids—acute exacerbations
4. Immunosuppressants
a. Azathioprine, 6-mercaptopurine, cyclosporine
  (1) Useful during remission to decrease steroid requirements, usually added after 7 to 10 days of high-dose intravenous steroids. May be required for 2 to 3 months.

(2) Cyclosporine
    (a) Two thirds of patients will note some improvement with therapy.
    (b) Improvement generally seen within 2 weeks of starting treatment.
b. Methotrexate—used in steroid-dependent active disease and to maintain remission.
c. Infliximab (Remicade)
    (1) Monoclonal antibody against tumor necrosis factor-$\alpha$
    (2) Intravenous administration decreases systemic inflammation.
    (3) More than 50% of patients with moderate-to-severe disease will show improvement.
    (4) Useful with perianal disease—some efficacy in healing chronic fistulas
    (5) Recurrence common—many patients require lifelong infusions.

**5. Supportive measures**
a. Bowel rest and nasogastric decompression
b. Intravenous fluid resuscitation
c. Total parenteral nutrition
    (1) Fistulas
    (2) Malnutrition
d. Low-residue/high-protein diet for mild disease

**6. Acute flare**
a. Antiinflammatory medications as above
b. Bowel rest
c. Antibiotics
d. Total parenteral nutrition if patient is malnourished
e. Drainage of intraabdominal abscess by interventional radiology
f. Surgical resection of diseased bowel likely necessary, though can be performed once patient has been stabilized, nutrition optimized, and inflammation decreased.

**7. Anal and perianal CD**
a. Symptom alleviation
b. Skin tags and hemorrhoids should not be excised unless extremely symptomatic because of risk for creating chronic, nonhealing wounds.
c. Fissures may respond to local or systemic therapy.
    (1) Sphincterotomy is contraindicated because of the possibility of creating chronic, nonhealing wound and the increased risk for incontinence in patients with diarrhea from underlying colitis or small bowel disease.
d. Imperative that all abscesses be drained before initiation of immunosuppressive therapy

**H. SURGICAL MANAGEMENT**
**1. Eventually required in 70% to 75% of cases over lifetime of disease**
**2. Indications for surgery**
a. Reserved for treatment of complications only

b. Surgery not curative because all at-risk intestine cannot be resected as in UC.

c. Small-bowel obstruction
   (1) Caused by strictures
   (2) Indication in 50% of surgical cases

d. Fistula

e. Abscess

f. Hemorrhage

g. Perianal disease unresponsive to medical therapy

h. Disease intractable to medical management

i. Failure to thrive—chronic malnutrition, growth retardation

j. Toxic megacolon

k. Dysplasia seen on biopsy

3. **Intraoperative findings**

a. Creeping of mesenteric fat toward antimesenteric border

b. Serosal and mesenteric inflammation

c. Bowel wall thickening

d. Strictures

e. Shortening of bowel and mesentery

f. Mesenteric lymphadenopathy

g. Inflammatory masses, abscesses, adherent bowel loops

4. **Surgical procedures**

a. Midline incision should be used because of possible need for stoma.

b. Conservative resection of diseased or symptomatic bowel segment
   (1) Only resect grossly diseased bowel with short, "normal-appearing" margins; unnecessary to get histologically free margins for anastomosis.
   (2) Primary end-to-end anastomosis can be safely created if patient is medically stable, nutritionally optimized, and on minimal immunosuppressive medications.
   (3) Stomas should be created in patients who are hemodynamically unstable, septic, malnourished, taking high-dose immunosuppressive medications, or with extensive intraabdominal contamination.
   (4) Distal ileum and cecal resection with ileocolostomy is a common procedure.
   (5) Fistulas
      (a) Generally require resection of only bowel segment with active CD
      (b) Secondary fistula sites often normal and require only repair of fistula site with simple closure rather than resection.
   (6) Sixty percent recurrence rate in long-term follow-up

c. Stricturoplasty
   (1) Relieves obstruction in chronically scarred bowel without resection; especially useful for multiple symptomatic strictures
   (2) Short strictures—bowel opened along antimesenteric surface, then closed transversely (transverse stricturoplasty).

       (3) Long strictures—bowel opened along antimesenteric surface, then folded into an inverted U-shape to create a side-to-side anastomosis.

  d. Total proctocolectomy
     (1) Indicated for dysplasia seen on biopsy
     (2) Ileal pouch—anal reconstruction not recommended because of high risk for CD developing within the pouch and high risk for complications (fistula, abscess, stricture, pouch dysfunction, pouch failure).

  e. Exclusion bypass—has a greater incidence of recurrence and carcinoma; may be indicated in the following:
     (1) Bypass unresectable inflammatory mass
     (2) Gastroduodenal CD
     (3) Multiple, extensive skip lesions

  f. Continent (Kock) ileostomy and mucosal proctectomy procedures are contraindicated.

  g. Recurrent perianal abscesses or complex anal fistulas
     (1) Local drainage of abscesses if possible
     (2) Sphincter preservation
        (a) Endoanal ultrasound or magnetic resonance imaging is useful to delineate complex anatomy and fistulous tracts.
        (b) Liberal use of setons
        (c) Endoanal advancement flaps should be considered for definitive therapy if the rectal mucosa is uninvolved.
        (d) Intractable perianal sepsis may require proctectomy (10–15%).

  h. Rectovaginal fistula: If rectal mucosa appears healthy with minimal rectovaginal septum scarring, rectal or vaginal mucosal advancement flap can be used.

## I. PROGNOSIS
1. Cure is not possible in chronic disease.
2. Medical therapy does not avoid surgery.
3. Recurrence rates 10 years after initial operation
  a. Ileocolic disease (50%)
  b. Small-bowel disease (50%)
  c. Colonic disease (40–50%)
4. Reoperation rates at 5 years
  a. Primary resection (20%)
  b. Bypass (50%)
5. Eighty percent to 85% of patients who require surgery lead normal lives.
6. Mortality rate of 15% at 30 years
See Table 26-1 for a comparison of inflammatory bowel disease.

## V. INDETERMINATE COLITIS
### A. TYPICALLY PRESENT WITH SYMPTOMS SIMILAR TO UC
1. Endoscopic and pathologic findings include features common to both UC and CD.

**TABLE 26-1**

COMPARISON OF INFLAMMATORY BOWEL DISEASE

| Characteristics | Ulcerative Colitis | Crohn's Disease |
|---|---|---|
| Epidemiology | Bimodal: 15–30 and 50–70 years of age | 20–30 and 50–60 years of age |
| | Females > males | Females = males |
| Clinical presentation | Bloody diarrhea | Nonbloody diarrhea |
| | Rectal bleeding | Colicky abdominal pain |
| | Tenesmus | Anorectal lesions |
| | Weight loss | Weight loss |
| | Abdominal pain | Intermittent periods of active disease |
| Gross pathology | Continuous disease | Skip lesions |
| | Friable mucosa | Longitudinal fissures |
| | Pseudopolyps | Focal strictures |
| | Stovepipe narrowing | Bowel wall thickening |
| | Granular irregularity | "Cobblestoning" |
| Microscopic pathology | Confined to mucosa | Transmural |
| | Loss of goblet cells | Granulomas |
| | Crypt abscesses | Mesenteric adenopathy |
| | Plasma cell infiltrate | |
| Gastrointestinal distribution | Continuous from anus proximally | 30% small bowel only |
| | <5% rectal sparing | 55% small bowel and colon |
| | No skip lesions | 15% colon only |
| | 10% terminal ileitis | 30% rectal involvement |
| | | 20% skip lesions |
| | | 50% perianal disease |
| Complications | Toxic megacolon | Abscesses |
| | Perforation | Fistulas |
| | Sclerosing cholangitis | Intestinal obstruction |
| | Extraintestinal less common | Extraintestinal more common |
| | Malnutrition | Strictures |
| | Colon cancer | Colon cancer |
| Surgical intervention | Potential for cure | Reserved for complications, not curative |
| | | Conservative bowel resections |
| Mortality | 2–3% elective surgery | 3–6% elective surgery |
| | 8–25% emergent surgery | |

2. Differential diagnoses—infectious colitis caused by *Campylobacter jejuni*, *Entamoeba histolytica*, *Clostridium difficile*, *Neisseria gonococcus*, *Salmonella* sp, and *Shigella* sp.
3. Indications for surgery
a. Intractability

b. Complications of medical therapy
c. Malignancy or high risk for malignancy
**4. Surgical options**
a. Total abdominal colectomy with end ileostomy may be best initial procedure for patients who prefer sphincter-sparing operation.
    (1) Pathology may provide more accurate diagnosis
        (a) UC—ileal pouch-anal anastomosis
        (b) Still indeterminate—completion proctectomy with end ileostomy
b. Abdominal colectomy with ileorectal anastomosis for patients with rectal sparing

# Benign Colorectal Disease

*Konstantin Umanskiy, MD*

## I. ANATOMY

### A. RECTUM

1. The rectum is 12 to 15 cm in length and extends from the sacral promontory to the levator ani muscles.
2. The three teniae coli spread out at the rectosigmoid junction and fuse into a continuous smooth muscle layer with obliteration of the haustral markings.
3. Three horizontal rectal mucosal folds are visible internally as the valves of Houston.
4. The proximal third of the rectum is covered by peritoneum anteriorly and laterally. The anterior peritoneal reflection extends deep into the pelvis to 7 cm above the anal verge and lies behind the bladder in male individuals and behind the uterus (pouch of Douglas) in female individuals.

### B. ANAL CANAL

1. Anatomic anal canal is 3 cm in length and extends from anal verge to the dentate line.
2. Surgical canal—extends from the anal verge to the top of the anorectal ring.
3. The rectum is lined by colonic columnar epithelium. The transitional zone is lined with cuboidal epithelium that lines the anal canal from the columns of Morgagni to the dentate line. Anal glands located in the intersphincteric plane drain into the anal crypts that are pockets formed between each column. Below the dentate line, the anal canal is lined by squamous epithelium.
4. Internal sphincter (involuntary)—thickened continuation of the circular smooth muscle of the rectum under control of the autonomic nervous system.
5. External sphincter (voluntary)—downward extension of the puborectalis, which is striated muscle with somatic innervation (branch of the internal pudendal nerve S2-S4).

### C. LEVATOR ANI MUSCLE—COMPOSED OF ILIOCOCCYGEUS AND PUBOCOCCYGEUS; CONSTITUTES THE PELVIC FLOOR AND IS INNERVATED BY THE FOURTH SACRAL NERVE.

### D. BLOOD SUPPLY AND LYMPHATIC DRAINAGE

1. Arterial supply—segmental but with rich anastomoses
   a. Superior hemorrhoidal—last branch of the inferior mesentery artery
   b. Middle hemorrhoidal—branch of the internal iliac artery
   c. Inferior hemorrhoidal—branch of the internal pudendal artery

27

2. Venous drainage—parallels the arterial supply.
a. Superior hemorrhoidal—drains the rectum and upper part of anal canal into the portal system.
b. Middle hemorrhoidal—drains rectum and upper anal canal into internal iliac vein (systemic circulation).
c. Inferior hemorrhoidal vein—drains rectum and lower anal canal into the systemic venous return.
d. The superior, middle, and inferior hemorrhoidal veins converge to form the inferior hemorrhoidal plexus in the submucosa of the columns of Morgagni.
3. Lymphatic drainage follows the paths of the arteries.
a. Superior and middle rectum—drains into the inferior mesentery artery nodes.
b. Lower rectum and upper anal canal—drains into the superior rectal lymphatic (leading to the inferior mesentery artery) and to the internal iliac nodes.
c. Anal canal distal to the dentate line—has dual drainage to the inguinal nodes and the internal iliac nodes.

## II. HEMORRHOIDS

### A. TYPES
1. Internal hemorrhoids: Cushions of dilated submucosal veins of the superior rectal plexus that lie proximal to the dentate line and are covered by transitional or columnar epithelium. Typically found in three locations:
a. Left lateral
b. Right posterolateral
c. Right anterolateral
2. Classification of internal hemorrhoids
a. First degree: Painless, bleeding usually associated with defecation.
b. Second degree: Protrude during defecation but spontaneously reduce.
c. Third degree: Protrude during defecation and must be reduced manually.
d. Fourth degree: Permanently prolapsed.
3. External hemorrhoids—dilated veins arising from the inferior hemorrhoidal plexus below the dentate line that are covered with squamous epithelium; generally asymptomatic, unless thrombosed.

### B. SIGNS AND SYMPTOMS
1. Pain, pruritus, rectal bleeding (usually bright red with spotting of the toilet paper) with or without iron deficiency anemia, perianal moistness, or drainage.
2. Symptoms are most commonly caused by prolapsing internal hemorrhoids. Mucoid discharge and soiled undergarments occur when columnar mucosa is prolapsed beyond the anal verge, resulting in irritation and inflammation of the perianal skin.

3. Severe pain is not typically associated with internal hemorrhoids but is commonly seen with thrombosed external hemorrhoids.

## C. DIAGNOSIS

1. Although internal hemorrhoids are the most common cause of rectal bleeding, it is important to exclude other sources such as inflammatory bowel disease, other forms of colitis, neoplasia, diverticular disease, and angiodysplasia. The physical examination should include visual inspection of the anus, digital rectal examination, and anoscopy. Additional endoscopic procedures may include proctoscopy, flexible sigmoidoscopy, or both. More extensive endoscopic evaluation with complete colonoscopy should be considered in all patients with rectal bleeding, but it is mandatory for those who fulfill the following criteria:
   a. Age >50 years if no complete examination within 10 years
   b. Age >40 years with a history of a single first-degree relative with colorectal cancer or adenoma and no complete examination within 10 years
   c. Age >50 years if the history is positive for two or more first-degree relatives with colorectal cancer or adenomas diagnosed at age >60 and no complete examination within 3 to 5 years
   d. Positive fecal occult blood test
   e. Iron-deficiency anemia

## D. TREATMENT

1. Nonoperative treatment for first- and second-degree internal hemorrhoids consists of dietary modification and avoidance of prolonged straining during defecation. Sitz baths provide symptomatic relief and improve hygiene. Increasing dietary fiber, bulk agents (psyllium), and adequate fluid intake minimize constipation and straining. Hydrocortisone acetate (Anusol-HC) suppositories help resolve inflammation.

## E. OFFICE TREATMENT

1. Rubber band ligation—used in the treatment of grade II and sometimes grade III internal hemorrhoids; rubber bands must be placed above the dentate line where somatic pain innervation is absent. Usually only one to two hemorrhoids are ligated per week. Further ligations can be performed every 4 weeks until symptoms have resolved.
2. Infrared coagulation involves direct application of infrared light resulting in protein necrosis. It is most applicable to grades I and II hemorrhoids.
3. Sclerotherapy—submucosal injection of hemorrhoid with sclerosing agent, which obliterates the hemorrhoid by fibrosis.
4. Other therapies—include cryotherapy, bipolar diathermy, and direct current therapy.

**F. SURGICAL HEMORRHOIDECTOMY—INDICATED WHEN OFFICE THERAPIES FAIL OR IN PATIENTS WITH MIXED INTERNAL AND EXTERNAL DISEASE, INCARCERATION, EXTENSIVE EXTERNAL THROMBOSIS AND PAIN, OR PERSISTENT BLEEDING.**

1. We most commonly perform a closed or Ferguson hemorrhoidectomy.
   a. The hemorrhoidal bundle is gathered within the tines of a forceps, and the anoderm is excised.
   b. The hemorrhoid is then elevated off the external and internal sphincter and excised to the proximal anal canal.
   c. The pedicle is then sutured with a chromic gut suture ligature.
   d. The wound is then closed with a running chromic gut suture beginning at the apex and extending to the anoderm. Small bits of internal sphincter are included into suture line to achieve pexy of rectal mucosa. One, two, or three hemorrhoidal bundles may be excised in this fashion.
   e. It is essential that only minimal amounts of anoderm are excised. If large amounts of anoderm are excised, closing the anal wounds can result in significant postoperative pain and even long-term anal stenosis.
2. Circumferential stapled hemorrhoidectomy involves transanal circular stapling of redundant anorectal mucosa with a specialized circular stapling instrument. Redundant mucosa is drawn into the instrument and excised within the "stapled doughnut." No incisions are made in the somatically innervated, highly sensitive anoderm, resulting in significantly less postoperative pain.
3. Thrombosed external hemorrhoids: These can be extremely painful and should be excised if seen within 48 hours. Beyond this time, conservative therapy with analgesics and sitz baths is appropriate.

## III. ANAL FISSURE

**A. ANAL FISSURE IS ONE OF THE MOST FREQUENT CAUSES OF SEVERE ANAL PAIN.**

1. Represents an acute or chronic tear in the anal squamous epithelium, usually in the posterior midline. The fissure extends from the dentate line to the anal verge. The fissure is usually located at posterior midline. Lateral or multiple fissures should raise suspicion of trauma, inflammatory bowel disease, lymphoma, neoplasm, or infection, and require further investigation such as proctosigmoidoscopy.
2. Equal frequency among male and female individuals, and most common in young adults.
3. Typically associated with spasm of the internal sphincter.

**B. SIGNS AND SYMPTOMS**

1. Sharp tearing or burning pain is associated with defecation. Blood may streak the toilet paper.
2. Physical examination may reveal a sentinel tag or hypertrophied papilla. Internal sphincter muscle fibers may be seen at the base of the fissure.

## C. TREATMENT

1. Nonoperative management is usually the first step in treatment of anal fissures.
a. Stool softeners and bulk laxatives relieve straining.
b. Sitz baths offer symptomatic relief and improve hygiene.
c. Anesthetic suppositories and nitroglycerin 0.2% cream may be helpful but may be complicated by headache.
d. Botulinum toxin 20 units can be administered as two injections on each side into the internal anal sphincter.
2. Operative therapy is indicated for unsuccessful response to conservative management. The goal of surgery is to break the cycle of internal anal sphincter spasm and pain. Lateral-internal sphincterotomy is the surgical treatment of choice.

## IV. ANORECTAL ABSCESS

Anorectal abscesses originate from an infection arising from the anal glands that communicate with the anal crypts. The acute phase of the infection causes an anorectal abscess, whereas the chronic stage is referred to as a fistula. An anorectal abscess typically forms in the intersphincteric space. Subsequent spread can occur along various paths (Fig. 27-1). Factors implicated in the development of abscess include constipation, diarrhea, trauma, Crohn's disease, tuberculosis, actinomycosis, anorectal malignancy, leukemia, and lymphoma, although most patients will have no precedent history. The disease is more common in diabetic and immunocompromised patients than in the

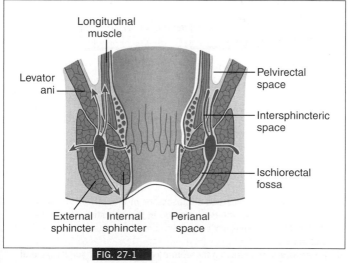

FIG. 27-1

Pathways of infection in perianal spaces.

general public, and the incidence is much greater in men (3:1). Typically, it is polymicrobial (*Escherichia coli, Proteus* spp, *Streptococcus* spp, and *Bacteroides* spp).

## A. CLASSIFICATION

1. Perianal abscess—superficial abscess that lies beneath the skin of the anal canal but does not traverse the external sphincters.
2. Ischiorectal abscess—occupies the ischiorectal fossa below the levators and lateral to the sphincters. The abscess can cross the midline to form bilateral abscess called a *horseshoe abscess.*
3. Intersphincteric abscess—located between the external and internal sphincter muscle; most common in the posterior quadrant. Typically exists without evidence of perianal swelling or induration.
4. Supralevator abscess—occurs above the levators; more difficult to diagnose and drain; can mimic an intraabdominal condition.
5. Postanal space abscess—originates in the posterior midline and causes an abscess in the deep postanal space anatomically bounded by the levators, anococcygeal ligament, and anal canal. Typically, patients present with severe pain without evidence of perianal swelling or induration. A mass can be felt posteriorly by digital rectal examination.

## B. SIGNS AND SYMPTOMS

1. Usually presents with extreme perianal pain
2. A mass is commonly felt on rectal examination. Cellulitis and fluctuance are often seen.
3. Systemic symptoms of fever, chills, and leukocytosis warrant urgent surgical decompression.
4. Vague pain and a high, ill-defined mass may be evidence for a supralevator abscess.

## C. TREATMENT

1. Surgical drainage is always indicated, and drainage alone is usually sufficient therapy.
2. Most small, superficial perianal abscesses can be drained in the emergency department. Packing is left in overnight and removed with the institution of sitz baths or showers. Alternatively, long-term, indwelling, mushroom-tip catheters may be used.
3. Broad-spectrum antibiotics are indicated for diabetic or immunocompromised patients, or patients with valvular heart disease or prosthetic implants.
4. Ischiorectal abscesses and all abscesses in diabetic or immunocompromised patients should be drained in the operating room. Necrotizing fasciitis and Fournier's gangrene are serious complications if left undrained.
5. Supralevator abscesses may require computed tomography–guided drainage or proximal fecal diversion in complex cases.

6. If not previously performed, a proctosigmoidoscopy should always be performed to rule out other proximal causes.

## V. FISTULA IN ANO

### A. GENERAL

1. An abnormal communication between the anal canal (internal opening) at about the level of the dentate line and the perianal skin (external opening).
2. It typically represents the incomplete healing of a drained anorectal abscess and is commonly secondary to a pyogenic process and, less frequently, a granulomatous disease.
3. Those fistulas arising above the dentate line are typically secondary to diverticulitis neoplasm or trauma.

### B. CLASSIFICATION

1. Intersphincteric fistula—located in the intersphincteric space with external opening typically on the perianal skin near the anal verge.
2. Trans-sphincteric fistula—most common type of fistula. Starts in the intersphincteric space and traverses the external sphincter into the ischiorectal fossa, with external opening lateral to the anal verge. Horseshoe fistula falls into this category.
3. Suprasphincteric fistula—starts in the intersphincteric space, passes above the puborectalis muscle, and tracks laterally between the levator and the puborectalis muscle.
4. Extrasphincteric fistula—complicated fistula. Passes from the perianal skin through the ischiorectal fossa and levator ani muscles, and subsequently through the rectal wall.

### C. GOODSALL'S RULE (FIG. 27-2)

1. Relates the position of the internal opening of a fistula to the external opening
2. Fistulas with external openings anterior to a transverse line through the anal opening have a fistula tract that extends directly to the anal canal anteriorly.
3. Refers to those fistulas with an external opening posterior or >3 cm from the verge, have a tract that curves, and have their internal opening in the posterior midline. Fistulas defying this rule should raise the suspicion of inflammatory bowel disease. Anterior midline is the 12-o'clock position by convention.

### D. SIGNS AND SYMPTOMS

1. Chief complaint is typically intermittent or constant drainage. A history of recurrent perianal abscess may be found.
2. The external opening is represented by a red cluster of granulation tissue. A cordlike tract may be palpated on rectal examination.

27

BENIGN COLORECTAL DISEASE

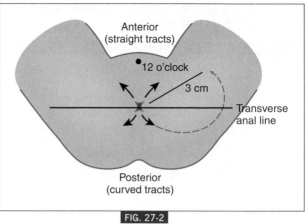

**FIG. 27-2**
Goodsall's rule.

### E. TREATMENT

1. Delineation of the fistula tract must be performed under anesthesia by gentle probing with an anal probe or, if unable to locate an internal opening, with hydrogen peroxide or milk.
2. The entire tract must be unroofed for drainage and curettaged. The wound is then marsupialized and allowed to heal secondarily.
3. Fistulas traversing both internal and external sphincters require placement of a seton to prevent incontinence (Fig. 27-3). A heavy suture or vascular loop is passed through the tract to improve drainage and stimulate fibrosis of the tract. The seton may be sequentially tightened, and after significant fibrosis, the tract is ultimately opened with a greatly reduced risk for incontinence. A more complex procedure may be required to close a high transsphincteric fistula: mucosal advancement flap, fibrin glue, and an anal fistula plug consisting of SIS have all been described.
4. Horseshoe fistulas involve infection of the deep postanal space with extension into the ischiorectal spaces on both sides. These can be treated by opening the postanal space and placing appropriate counterincisions laterally for drainage.

## VI. PILONIDAL DISEASE

### A. GENERAL

1. A common skin lesion of the sacrococcygeal area
2. Most frequently seen in young men after puberty and rarely in men older than 40 years
3. The prevalence in adolescent boys suggests a hormonal relation. However, it is believed to be a result of obstruction of the hair follicles

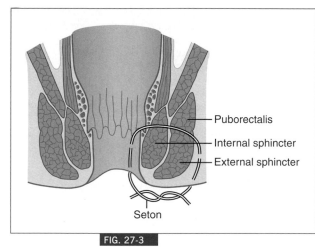

**FIG. 27-3**

Use of a seton in a high fistula.

in this area, which then leads to formation of cysts, sinuses, or abscesses.

4. Sinuses or cysts are typically seen in the midline.
5. Most patients present with pain and swelling resulting from infection.

## B.  TREATMENT

1. Acute abscess—incision and drainage with curettage of the cavity. Impacted hair is removed. The wound is packed open. Up to 40% of patients experience development of chronic draining pilonidal sinuses, which will require further treatment.
2. Chronic pilonidal sinus—many treatment options are available, and their use depends on the severity of disease.
a. Lay open technique—open sinus with incomplete excision and curettage; recurrence rate of 15%; prolonged wound healing is 6 weeks.
b. Excision and marsupialization—recurrence rate of 5% to 15%; accelerated healing.
c. Simple pilonidal cystectomy with primary closure—recurrence rate of 15%; primary healing within 2 weeks.

## VII. ANAL AND PERIANAL INFECTIONS
### A.  CONDYLOMATA ACUMINATA
1. General

Condylomata acuminata (venereal warts) are caused by human papilloma-virus and may occur on perianal skin, anorectal mucosa, or genital region. The incubation period is 1 to 6 months. Presenting symptoms include a lump in the perianal region, pruritus ani, bleeding, or pain. Examination reveals cauliflower-like masses that are typically pink or white and tend to grow in rows. There is a high incidence of dysplasia and an increased risk for cancer.

2. Treatment—combination of local ablation and improved hygiene with concomitant treatment of sexual contacts. Genital lesions should be treated concurrently.

a. Fulguration under anesthesia for extensive involvement.

b. Podophyllin resin—25% solution in mineral oil or tincture of benzoin for small, scattered lesions

c. Imiquimod—applied topically three times a week for up to 6 weeks.

d. Surgical excision of large masses may be necessary.

e. Giant condyloma (Buschke–Löwenstein tumor) may appear to be histologically benign but is locally invasive and malignant. It may require wide local excision or abdominoperineal resection.

### B. ANORECTAL HERPES

1. Usually presents with severe pain

2. Characteristic herpetic lesions are seen on examination and are confirmed by Giemsa (Tzanck prep) stain, viral culture, and biopsy.

3. Treatment: No cure exists for herpes; however, antiviral agents such as valacyclovir shorten the clinical course and the frequency of recurrence.

### C. GONOCOCCAL PROCTITIS

1. Symptoms of gonococcal proctitis include pain and discharge.

2. Anoscopy reveals mucosal erythema and purulence of the anal crypts. Gonococcus is confirmed by Gram stain and culture.

3. Treatment: Because of the increase in prevalence of penicillinase-producing *Neisseria gonorrhoeae,* ceftriaxone 250 mg IM (single dose) followed by doxycycline 100 mg orally twice daily for 7 days is recommended.

### VIII. PRURITUS ANI

Pruritus ani is embarrassing for patients and frustrating for physicians. The condition begins insidiously, but the area of involvement spreads as intensity of itching increases and the patient starts scratching and irritating the skin, creating a vicious cycle.

### A. CAUSES—ANY CONDITION THAT LEADS TO PERIANAL MOISTURE, DRAINAGE, OR SOILING.

1. Hemorrhoids, fissures, fistula

2. Other causes include fungi, pinworms, and other infectious agents.

3. Underlying disease—diabetes, jaundice, Crohn's disease

4. Topical or dietary sensitivities

5. Neoplasm—carcinoma, melanoma, Paget's disease of bone, Bowen disease

6. Approximately 50% ultimately are classified as idiopathic.

## B. DIAGNOSIS

1. A detailed history is important and should include dietary and bowel habits, hygiene practice, menopausal state, systemic diseases, prior anorectal surgeries, and previous radiation.
2. A careful examination of the perianal skin and anorectum is required. Biopsy and specimens for cultures are obtained when necessary.

## C. TREATMENT

1. Therapy is directed at achieving clean, dry, intact skin.
2. Judicious use of an inert skin barrier such as a zinc oxide ointment can help to avoid continued skin irritation.
3. Use of a 1% or 2% hydrocortisone-containing preparation can help in the short term.
4. Careful perianal cleansing seems to be as effective as topical corticosteroids at relieving symptoms of pruritus ani.
5. If symptoms continue in the compliant patient despite aggressive therapy, a second opinion from a dermatologist should be considered.

## IX. ANAL NEOPLASM

Malignancies of the anal canal are relatively uncommon and represent only 2% to 3% of all anorectal carcinomas. The position of the tumor in the anal canal relative to the dentate line is important with regard to the biologic behavior of the tumor. This is based on the lymphatic drainage in these two areas. Most tumors spread by direct extension and lymphatic drainage. Hematologic spread is less common. Anal tumors are classified into two groups based on location: (1) anal canal tumors and (2) anal margin tumors.

## A. TUMORS OF THE ANAL CANAL

1. Anal intraepithelial neoplasia, Bowen disease
a. Squamous carcinoma in situ
b. Precursor to invasive squamous cell carcinoma
c. Associated with infection of human papillomavirus types 16 and 18
d. Treatment—resection or ablation
e. High-risk, immunosuppressed patients should have Pap smears every 3 to 6 months.
f. Abnormal Pap smear should be followed by high-resolution anoscopy, biopsy, and ablation.
2. **Epidermoid carcinomas are referred to as squamous, basaloid, cloacogenic, or transitional carcinomas. Although each has different histologic features, they exhibit similar biologic behavior and are thus grouped together.**
a. Typically seen in patients 50 to 70 years of age, more frequently in women
b. Two cell types—squamous cell (keratinizing) and transitional cell (nonkeratinizing)
c. Rectal pain, bleeding, or mass are common presenting symptoms.

d. About 40% to 50% of patients have pelvic lymph node involvement at diagnosis, whereas 15% to 36% have inguinal nodal involvement and 10% have distant metastasis.

e. Excellent prognosis when discovered before nodal involvement and invasion to adjacent structures; 80% of tumors are cured by chemotherapy/radiation therapy alone (the Nigro protocol).

f. Chemotherapy with mitomycin C and 5-fluorouracil combined with radiation is the treatment of choice. Abdominoperineal resection is indicated for residual disease or recurrence.

**B. MALIGNANT MELANOMA—0.5% TO 1% OF MALIGNANT ANAL TUMORS**

1. Anal canal is the third most common site after skin and eyes.
2. Most typically occur adjacent to the dentate line.
3. Rectal bleeding is the most frequent complaint.
4. Most are not highly pigmented, and diagnosis is difficult.
5. Tumor is aggressive and often widely metastatic. Abdominoperineal resection is indicated in selected patients.
6. Tumors are often radioresistant and unresponsive to chemotherapy.

**C. TUMORS OF THE ANAL MARGIN: THESE TUMORS ARE SIMILAR TO SKIN TUMORS ELSEWHERE AND ARE TREATED LIKEWISE.**

## X. RECTAL PROLAPSE

**A. CLASSIFICATION (FIG. 27-4)**

1. Type I (false prolapsed or mucosal prolapsed)—redundant prolapsed rectal mucosa with radial folds in orientation
2. Type II (incomplete prolapsed)—rectal intussusception without a sliding hernia
3. Type III (true prolapsed or complete prolapsed)—protrusion of the entire rectal wall through the anal orifice with herniation of the pelvic peritoneum or cul-de-sac; circular mucosal folds are seen; most common type

**B. CLINICAL FEATURES**

1. Eighty-five percent of patients are female, with greatest incidence in patients older than 50 years; also seen in children younger than 5 years
2. Many patients have had prior gynecologic surgery.
3. In men, the incidence is more evenly distributed throughout the age range.
4. There is a high incidence rate of associated chronic neurologic or psychiatric disorders (5–50%).
5. Possible pathogenesis includes either sliding-type hernia, where the rectum herniates through a defect in the pelvic fascia, or intussusception of the rectum.

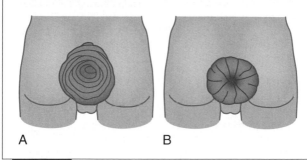

**FIG. 27-4**

Depiction of a true rectal prolapse *(A)* and a type I mucosal prolapse *(B)*.

6. Presenting complaints may be related to the prolapse itself or to the disturbance of anal continence that frequently coexists and includes the following:
a. Extrusion of a mass with defecation, exertion, coughing, sneezing, and so forth
b. Difficulty in bowel regulation—tenesmus, constipation, fecal incontinence
c. Permanently extruded rectum with excoriation, ulceration, and constant soiling
d. Associated urinary incontinence or uterine prolapsed
7. **Physical findings**
a. Demonstrated prolapse during Valsalva maneuver
b. Compromised sphincter tone
c. Excoriation or circumferential inflammation of midrectum on proctosigmoidoscopy

## C.  EVALUATION
1. Reduce the prolapsed segment, if possible, and perform sigmoidoscopy to determine the condition of the bowel and the presence of any associated lesion or carcinoma.
2. Assess sphincter tone and the degree of fecal continence by exam defecography and manometry. Many patients with rectal prolapse have poor sphincter tone.
3. Barium enema or colonoscopy
4. Intravenous pyelogram—the ureters may be pulled with the rectum into the sliding hernia.
5. Radiographs of the lumbar spine and pelvis—look for neurologic disease.
6. Cinedefecography—useful in the evaluation of occult prolapse (type II)
7. Anal manometry and pudendal terminal motor nerve latencies may be indicated to assess sphincter function before surgery. Identification of

a nonrelaxing puborectalis may be useful in planning additional therapy such as biofeedback.

8. Transit time studies document functionally delayed transit (colonic inertia) as a cause of chronic constipation and straining, and assess the need for colon resection.

## D. TREATMENT OPTIONS

1. False prolapse.
a. Common in young children. Conservative therapy is often successful. Gently replace the prolapsed rectum after each defecation or straining. Excision of redundant mucosa is rarely necessary.
b. In adults, hemorrhoidectomy with excision of redundant mucosa is effective. Circumferential stapled hemorrhoidectomy may be used with similar results.
2. True prolapse: Typically a progressive disorder that is not responsive to nonsurgical therapy. Basic features of the repairs include correction of the following anatomic characteristics:
a. Abnormally deep or wide cul-de-sac
b. Weak pelvic floor with diastasis of the levators
c. Patulous anal sphincter
d. Redundant rectosigmoid
e. Lack of fixation of the rectum to the sacral hollow with abnormal mobility and loss of the normal horizontal position of the lower rectum
f. Associated incontinence is not treated initially because it may resolve after treatment of the prolapse.

## E. ABDOMINAL APPROACHES

1. Abdominal proctopexy with sigmoid resection: The lateral rectal stalks are used to anchor the rectum to the presacral fascia and periosteum. This is a treatment option in young, healthy patients and can be performed laparoscopically.
2. Rectal sling (Ripstein procedure): The rectum is fixed to the sacrum using a sling of synthetic mesh. This must be loose enough to prevent obstruction. Foreign material makes concomitant sigmoid resection more hazardous and provides an increased risk for pelvic sepsis.

## F. PERINEAL APPROACH: THE PERINEAL APPROACH IS USEFUL IN DEBILITATED PATIENTS WHO WOULD NOT TOLERATE AN ABDOMINAL INCISION.

1. Perineal rectosigmoidectomy (Altemeier procedure)—involves resection of the redundant prolapsing bowel with primary anastomosis, high ligation of the hernia sac, and approximation of the levator ani muscles. This is well tolerated even in high-risk patients and may be performed under regional anesthesia.
2. Thiersch procedure—of historical note only and is rarely (if ever) done. This technique was used in those patients who were too ill to

tolerate even a perineal resection. The sphincters are encircled with a wire or band of synthetic material.

## XI. ANOSCOPY

### A. GENERAL
1. Examination of the lower rectum and anal canal
2. Patient preparation is not necessary; however, an enema may improve the examination depending on the clinical situation.

### B. TECHNIQUE
1. Position the patient in right or left lateral decubitus position with hips and knees flexed. Alternatively, an examining table providing prone jackknife positioning is ideal.
2. Inspection: Note the presence of fissures, hemorrhoids, skin tags, blood, or pus.
3. Palpation: Digital examination must be done before anoscopy.
   a. Note masses, induration, spasm, tenderness, or discharge.
   b. Palpate normal structures, including prostate.
   c. Inspect examining finger for blood, pus, stool, or mucus. Stool should be analyzed for occult blood.
4. Anoscopy
   a. Lubricate generously and insert obturator.
   b. Introduce anoscope into anus and point in direction of umbilicus. Once the upper end of the anal canal is reached, direct the anoscope posteriorly toward sacral hollow.
   c. Note the character of mucosa, presence of lesions, masses, or foreign body.
   d. Slowly withdraw scope, observing the mucosa as the scope passes.

## XII. RIGID SIGMOIDOSCOPY

### A. GENERAL: RIGID SIGMOIDOSCOPY REACHES TO 25 TO 30 CM.

### B. PATIENT PREPARATION
1. Gentle lavage such as magnesium citrate the evening before procedure
2. Clear liquids after midnight
3. The patient is given an enema in the morning or before the procedure.

### C. TECHNIQUE
1. Position the patient in the lateral decubitus position or in elbow-to-chest position over a sigmoidoscopy table. Alternatively, an examining table providing prone jackknife positioning is ideal.
2. Inspect the perianal area and perform a digital examination, as in anoscopy.
3. Insert the scope into the anus directed toward the umbilicus.
4. As soon as the rectum is entered, remove the obturator and close the window. The scope should be advanced farther only under direct visualization of the lumen. Insufflation is used as needed.

27

BENIGN COLORECTAL DISEASE

5. Slowly advance the scope though the lumen of the bowel. Movements are initially posterior into the sacral hollow, then anterior and left into the sigmoid colon.
6. Once the scope is fully inserted, it is slowly withdrawn in a circular fashion to carefully examine sigmoid and rectal mucosa.
7. Biopsy should be performed last so that blood does not obscure the rest of the examination.
8. Before the scope is removed, insufflated air should be evacuated for the patient's comfort.

## RECOMMENDED READING

Cataldo P, Ellis CN, Gregorcyk S, et al; The Standards Practice Task Force, The American Society of Colon and Rectal Surgeons: Practice parameters for the management of hemorrhoids (revised). *Dis Colon Rectum* 48:189–194, 2005.

Orsay C, Rakinic J, Perry WB, et al; Standards Practice Task Force, American Society of Colon and Rectal Surgeons: Practice parameters for the management of anal fissures (revised). *Dis Colon Rectum* 47:2003–2007, 2004.

Whiteford MH, Kilkenny J, Hyman N, et al; The Standards Practice Task Force, The American Society of Colon and Rectal Surgeons: Practice parameters for the treatment of perianal abscess and fistula-in-ano (revised). *Dis Colon Rectum* 48:1337–1342, 2005.

# Benign Pancreatic Disease

*Ryan M. Thomas, MD*

*"For me, the tiger country is the removal of the pancreas. The anatomy is very complex and one encounters anomalies."*
Sir Andrew Watt Kay, 1978

## I. ANATOMY

### A. EMBRYOLOGY

1. Begins as dorsal (from duodenum) and ventral (from hepatic diverticulum) budding from the foregut endoderm at approximately 5th week of gestation

2. Both the dorsal and ventral portions of the pancreas possess a main duct and fuse when the two pancreatic buds join. However, the portion of the dorsal duct between the anastomosis and the duodenum regresses. The main duct of the ventral pancreas leading to the duodenum is thus the definitive pancreatic duct (duct of Wirsung).
a. If the two ducts do not fuse, the majority of the pancreas will drain via the dorsal bud duct, the duct of Santorini, which is termed pancreas divisum.
b. If the dorsal bud duct (duct of Santorini) fuses with the ventral bud duct (duct of Wirsung) but does not regress, then it will persist as a blind accessory duct or drain via the lesser papilla.
3. Anomalies of pancreatic development include:
a. Annular pancreas: a ring of pancreatic tissue that encircles the duodenum and rarely can cause duodenal obstruction.
b. Heterotopic pancreatic tissue: found most commonly in the duodenum, stomach mucosa, and in approximately 6% of Meckel's diverticulum

### B. HISTOLOGY

1. Endocrine
a. Islets of Langerhans—originate from embryonic ductal epithelium and migrate toward capillaries to form isolated islands of cells within the pancreatic exocrine tissue (acini).
   (1) Alpha-cells—cells within the islets that produce glucagon. First cells to develop (8-9 weeks).
   (2) Beta-cells—cells within the islets that produce insulin.
   (3) Delta-cells—cells within the islets that produce somatostatin.
   (4) PP-cells—secrete pancreatic polypeptide.
2. Exocrine
a. Acini—develop in three stages from pancreatic "founder" cells to become differentiated cells that store inactive digestive enzymes as zymogen granules.
   (1) Endopeptidases (trypsinogen, chymotrypsinogen, proelastase)
   (2) Exopeptidases (procarboxypeptidase A and B)
   (3) Others (amylase, lipase, phospholipase, colipase)

b. Ductal—develops from the same pancreatic cellular cords as acinar cells. Originates from the centroacinar cells of each acinus and terminates in the main pancreatic excretory duct.

## C. GROSS ANATOMY
### 1. Basics
a. Retroperitoneal location posterior to the stomach at the level of L1-2 that is nested in the C-loop of the duodenum and lies obliquely to meet the splenic hilum
b. Access gained via separating the gastrocolic omentum from the transverse mesocolon to enter the lesser sac. The body and tail of the pancreas will be visible on the floor of the lesser sac.
### 2. Regions
a. Head—positioned within the C-loop of the duodenum and posterior to the transverse colon. The head is anterior to the inferior vena cava, right renal artery, and bilateral renal veins.
b. Uncinate process—portion of the pancreatic head that projects to the right and posterior to the superior mesenteric vein. It terminates posterior to the superior mesenteric artery and vein but anterior to the inferior vena cava and aorta. The tissue connecting the uncinate to the superior mesenteric artery is what is termed the retroperitoneal margin and is an important margin during pancreatectomy for pancreatic cancer.
c. Neck—divides the pancreas into near equal halves and is adjacent to the L1-2 vertebral bodies, making it susceptible to injury during blunt trauma. At the inferior edge of the neck, the splenic vein and superior mesenteric vein join to form the portal vein, which travels directly posterior to the neck of the pancreas on its way to the porta hepatis.
d. Body—lies directly anterior to the splenic artery and vein, with the artery running superior to the vein. Lies directly anterior to the aorta at the takeoff of the superior mesenteric artery, a good landmark to note on abdominal CTs.
e. Tail—extends to the left from the pancreatic body to lie near the splenic hilum anterior to the splenic artery and vein.

## D. VASCULAR/LYMPHATIC ANATOMY
### 1. Arterial (Figure 28-1)
a. Celiac trunk
   (1) The celiac trunk gives rise to the common hepatic artery, the left gastric artery and the splenic artery. The hepatic artery gives off the gastroduodenal artery (GDA). The GDA divides into the anterior and posterior superior pancreaticoduodenal artery as it passes posterior to the first portion of the duodenum.
   (2) The splenic artery supplies the body and tail of the pancreas as it courses along the superior posterior surface of the pancreas toward the spleen.
b. Superior mesenteric artery (SMA)

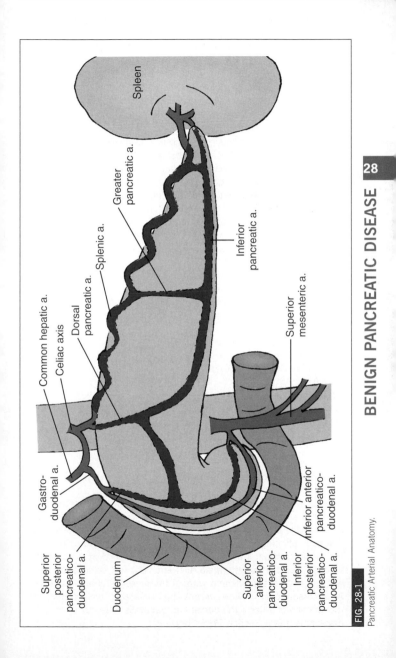

FIG. 28-1

Pancreatic Arterial Anatomy.

(1) The SMA gives off the inferior pancreaticoduodenal artery. This divides into anterior and posterior branches and forms an anastomosis with the anterior and posterior branches of the superior pancreaticoduodenal artery within the pancreatic parenchyma. This anastomosis not only supplies the head of the pancreas but also the medial aspect of the duodenal C-loop. Therefore, any resection of the pancreatic head involves resection of this portion of the duodenum; otherwise it will be devascularized.

(2) The dorsal pancreatic artery is a branch of the splenic artery that becomes the inferior pancreatic artery and travels parallel to the splenic artery but at the inferior border of the pancreas. Two main arteries run perpendicular to the pancreatic body and create an anastomosis between the splenic and inferior pancreatic arteries. They are the dorsal and greater pancreatic arteries (medial to lateral).

2. **Venous**

a. Drainage follows similar routes as the arteries, but veins are more superficially located.

b. The head of the pancreas is drained via veins located anterior and posterior to it.

   (1) The anterior and posterior superior pancreaticoduodenal veins drain directly into the portal vein.

   (2) The anterior inferior pancreaticoduodenal vein drains via the right gastroepiploic and right colic veins into the superior mesenteric vein.

   (3) The posterior inferior pancreaticoduodenal vein drains into the inferior mesenteric vein.

c. The body and tail of the pancreas drain into the splenic vein.

3. **Lymphatics**

a. Diffuse drainage, which likely accounts for early and aggressive metastatic spread of tumor cells.

b. Communication exists between pancreatic lymphatics and the transverse mesocolon and proximal jejunum mesentery.

## E.  DUCT SYSTEM

1. Main pancreatic duct (duct of Wirsung) is approximately 2-3 mm in diameter.

2. Runs between the superior and inferior borders of the pancreas (one-third of the way up from the caudal margin), closer to the posterior aspect of the organ (two-thirds of the way in from the ventral surface).

3. The main pancreatic duct joins the common bile duct to empty into the second portion of the duodenum (medial aspect) at the ampulla of Vater (9% of the time the main duct and CBD will be separate and will drain into the duodenum without the presence of an ampulla).

4. An accessory duct may be present approximately 2 cm proximal to the ampulla of Vater if the dorsal bud duct fails to regress during development (see Section IA: Embryology).

## II. ACUTE PANCREATITIS

### A.  BASICS

1. Many factors may play a role in the pathogenesis (see Section IIB).
2. Disease spectrum ranges from mild peripancreatic edema, to intraparenchymal hemorrhage, systemic inflammatory response syndrome (SIRS), and multi-system organ failure.
3. Self-limited in the vast majority of cases (90%)
4. Responsible for approximately 220,000 hospital admissions and over 3,000 deaths annually

### B.  PATHOGENESIS

1. Not mutually exclusive hypotheses, but at the same time may be mutually contradictory. Hypotheses apply to both acute and, over time, chronic pancreatitis.
2. Toxic-metabolic hypothesis
a. Alcohol may be directly toxic to acinar cells through alterations in cellular metabolism.
b. Alcohol has been shown to induce lipid accumulation within acinar cells leading to fatty degeneration and necrosis as well as induce fibrosis.
3. Oxidative stress hypothesis
a. Hepatocytes with overactive mixed-function oxidases lead to the secretion of free radical byproducts into the bile which can reflux into the pancreatic duct and induce damage in susceptible acinar and ductal cells.
b. Fibrosis results after repeat exposure.
c. Overactivity of mixed-function oxidases may be due to high substrates (i.e., fats) or enzyme inducers (i.e., ethanol).
4. Stone and ductal obstruction hypothesis
a. Long-standing alcohol exposure has been shown to increase the incidence of protein plugs and eventually stones within the pancreatic ducts.
b. Pressure from lodged stones within the ducts leads to ulceration, obstruction, stasis, and further stone formation, which leads to atrophy and fibrosis.
5. Necrosis-fibrosis hypothesis
a. Periductal scarring and chronic disruption of the glandular architecture leads to repeated inflammation and tissue necrosis.
b. Represents a step-wise progression of fibrosis leading to chronic pancreatitis as a result of repeated episodes of acute or subacute pancreatitis
6. Primary duct hypothesis
a. Immune-mediated destruction of the ductal epithelium leading to inflammation and fibrosis (similar to primary sclerosing cholangitis)
b. Helps to explain large duct pancreatitis when alcohol is not a factor
7. Sentinel acute pancreatitis event (SAPE) hypothesis
a. Attempts to combine several of the above hypotheses into one coherent explanation
b. Long-term alcohol ingestion leads to metabolic/oxidative stress that, once a "sentinel" event is reached, leads to acinar cell injury and an acute pro-

28

BENIGN PANCREATIC DISEASE

inflammatory response. Later, with recurrent metabolic stress, the pancreas has already been "primed" by the sentinel event and an antiinflammatory response predominates, leading to fibrosis and chronic pancreatitis.

## C. ETIOLOGY/RISK FACTORS

### 1. Cholelithiasis
a. Most common cause of acute pancreatitis (40%) worldwide
b. Although mechanical obstruction may lead to pancreatic ductal hypertension with rupture of smaller ductules and leakage of pancreatic enzymes, the exact mechanism is unclear.

### 2. Alcohol
a. 10-15% of people who ingest 100-150 g of ethanol daily will develop pancreatitis. Alcohol is responsible for ~40% of cases of acute pancreatitis in the United States.
b. Enzymes may precipitate out with calcium resulting in ductal obstruction, and continued enzyme release results in ductal hypertension.
c. Finally, ethanol has been shown to decrease pancreatic blood flow which may perpetuate pancreatic cellular necrosis.

### 3. Obstruction
a. Gallstones (as discussed above)
b. Periampullary tumors
c. Duodenal ulcers or diverticulum
d. Parasites (*Ascaris* and *Clonorchis*) which can block the pancreatic duct.
e. Pancreas divisum (rare)

### 4. Hypercalcemia
a. May be the cause of pancreatitis in a patient with hyperparathyroidism or multiple myeloma
b. Likely involves pancreatic hypersecretion with the formation of calcium stones intraductally resulting in obstruction

### 5. Trauma
a. Blunt
b. Penetrating

### 6. Hereditary
a. Hyperlipoproteinemia syndromes (Types I, IV, and V)
b. *CFTR* (cystic fibrosis transmembrane regulator gene) gene mutation
c. *PRSS1* (cationic trypsinogen gene) gene mutation
d. *SPINK1* gene mutation

### 7. Iatrogenic
a. Endoscopic retrograde cholangiopancreatography (ERCP)-related pancreatitis occurs in 2-10% of patients as a result of intraductal hypertension or trauma.
b. Various surgical procedures near the pancreas (biopsy, ductal cannulation/exploration, gastrectomy, splenectomy)
c. Cardiopulmonary bypass may result in a pancreatic low-flow state resulting in ischemia and injury.

d. Billroth II may allow the reflux of activated pancreatic enzymes into the pancreatic duct owing to afferent limb obstruction.

**8. Drugs**

a. Antibiotics (sulfonamides, tetracycline, nitrofurantoin)

b. Azathioprine

c. Diuretics (thiazide and furosemide)

d. Estrogens

e. Methyldopa

f. Valproic acid

**9. Idiopathic**

a. Responsible for 15% of cases

b. Third largest group after biliary and alcoholic causes

## D. DIAGNOSIS

**1. History**

a. First episode is usually the most severe.

b. A history of alcohol ingestion or cholelithiasis may be elicited.

c. Onset of epigastric pain (50% with radiation to the back) usually occurs several hours after a meal, is constant in nature, is described as sharp or knife-like, and may be relieved by sitting up and aggravated by lying flat or movement.

d. Nausea/vomiting usually accompany the abdominal pain.

**2. Physical exam**

a. Fever, tachycardia, possible hypotension secondary to fluid sequestration (3rd spacing)

b. Abdominal pain can range from epigastric to diffuse abdominal tenderness with possible peritoneal signs.

c. A paralytic ileus can develop, resulting in abdominal distension. Grey Turner's sign (left flank ecchymosis) or Cullen's sign (periumbilical ecchymosis) may develop in cases of hemorrhagic pancreatitis. This is due to blood-stained peritoneal fluid dissecting through the planes of the abdominal wall to the flank or along the falciform ligament to the umbilicus (very uncommon).

**3. Labs**

a. CBC—evaluate for possible infectious etiology (inc. white blood cell count), baseline hematocrit (hemoconcentration may be present because of 3rd spacing in the retroperitoneum).

b. Basic metabolic profile—evaluate electrolyte status, renal function, and acid/base status.

c. Prothrombin time/partial thromboplastin time—especially important in cases of hemorrhagic pancreatitis in order to correct any coagulopathies.

d. Amylase

(1) Elevated in 90% of cases

(2) Levels >1000 IU/dl are suggestive of gallstone pancreatitis.

(3) Rises soon after the onset of symptoms and returns to normal in 3-5 days, a good marker to follow disease progression

(4) Sensitive but not specific for pancreatitis; serves a diagnostic and not a prognostic role

e. Lipase
   (1) Specific but not sensitive for pancreatitis; especially useful 24 hours after presentation
   (2) Remains elevated longer than serum amylase
   (3) Serves a diagnostic and not a prognostic role

f. EKG—exclude myocardial infarction.

4. **Imaging**

a. Chest X-ray
   (1) Findings may include left pleural effusion, elevated hemidiaphragm, or basilar atelectasis.
   (2) Helps to rule out perforated viscus (air under the diaphragm)

b. Abdominal X-ray
   (1) "Sentinel loop" may be visualized, which represents a loop of distended bowel lying next to an inflamed pancreas.
   (2) Air in the duodenal sweep (C-loop) may be evident.
   (3) The "Colon Cutoff" sign represents dilation from the proximal colon to the transverse colon with a paucity of gas distal to the splenic flexure.

c. Ultrasound
   (1) Evaluate for cholelithiasis if gallstone pancreatitis is suspected.
   (2) Can determine extra-pancreatic ductal dilatation, pancreatic edema, or peri-pancreatic fluid
   (3) Not used often because bowel gas can prevent an adequate assessment of the pancreas

d. CT scan with IV contrast (Figure 28-2)
   (1) Most common diagnostic imaging modality
   (2) Can detail pancreatic anatomy, fluid collections, extrapancreatic ductal dilatation
   (3) Findings include enlargement of the pancreas with loss of peri-pancreatic fat planes, fat stranding, and areas of decreased density.
   (4) In non-contrast studies, pancreatic parenchyma has CT attenuation of 30-50 Hounsfield units, which should increase by at least 50 with IV contrast. A decrease or lack of enhancement is consistent with necrosis.
   (5) Non-enhancement of the pancreas on CT indicates necrosis and, in the face of patient instability, it must undergo fine-needle aspiration (FNA) to rule out infected necrosis.
   (6) Approximately 4 days after presentation, the sensitivity of CT to diagnose necrosis approaches 100%.

e. ERCP/magnetic resonance cholangio-pancreatography (MRCP)
   (1) ERCP is not warranted in cases of acute pancreatitis unless the diagnosis is obstructive gallstone pancreatitis or biliary sepsis, in which case early ERCP has been shown to reduce morbidity when compared with delayed ERCP for severe gallstone pancreatitis (but no difference in mortality).

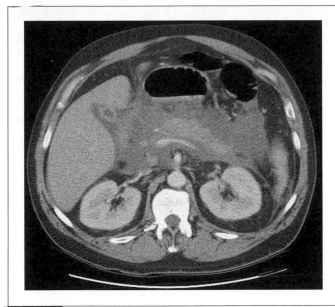

**FIG. 28-2**

**CT Scan of Acute Pancreatitis**

CT imaging of acute pancreatitis demonstrating an edematous pancreas with peripancreatic fluid and fat stranding. CT is useful in evaluation of potential complications including hemorrhage, pseudocyst formation, abscess formation, and necrotizing pancreatitis.

    (2) ERCP is indicated for recurrent disease after the resolution of an acute attack.
    (3) MRCP may be useful to diagnose gallstone pancreatitis without subjecting the patient to the complications of ERCP, such as worsening pancreatitis, but cannot treat retained stones.

## E. TREATMENT

1. If patient is unstable or at high risk, ICU monitoring is essential.
2. Restriction of oral intake (food and fluids) with the administration of parenteral fluids and electrolyte replacement is the initial mainstay of treatment.
3. Nasogastric decompression in those patients with nausea/vomiting
4. Foley catheter to monitor urine output
5. In cases of necrotizing pancreatitis, broad-spectrum antibiotics are recommended (imipenem is the drug of choice).
6. Serial labs (electrolytes, amylase) to guide therapy and response
7. Pain management; meperidine is favored over morphine because it is thought to have less sphincter of Oddi contraction.

8. Alcohol withdrawal prophylaxis in selected patients with the use of benzodiazepine as well as thiamine (100 mg IV x1 followed by 50-100 mg IV once daily to prevent Wernicke's encephalopathy), folate (400 $\mu$g PO once daily), and multivitamin (1 tab PO once daily) replacement

9. After stabilization, nasojejunal tube feeds can be instituted to avoid stimulating pancreatic exocrine function while maintaining nutrition and normal intestinal bacterial flora. If a patient cannot tolerate feeds (ileus, nausea/vomiting), then total parenteral nutrition should be started.

10. Surgical management varies depending on the presentation, condition, and complications the patient may possess:

a. Infected pancreatic necrosis based on FNA demands debridement/necrosectomy. Because FNA has a 10% false negative rate, patients with sterile necrosis (i.e., a negative FNA) who continue to deteriorate must be explored for fear of missing an infection.

b. Warranted if a definitive diagnosis cannot be made such that intraabdominal catastrophe cannot be ruled out.

c. In patients whose condition deteriorates despite maximal supportive care

d. Acute gallstone pancreatitis is best managed by either early cholecystectomy (within 48-72 hours of presentation) or delayed cholecystectomy (after 72 hours but during the same hospitalization) to allow the pancreatitis to resolve.

e. Pancreatitis secondary to trauma may require surgical intervention to treat a pancreatic ductal injury or hemorrhagic complications.

## F. PROGNOSIS

1. Mortality based on severity of disease:

a. Acute (edematous) pancreatitis (<2%)

b. Pancreatitis with sterile necrosis (<10%)

c. Pancreatitis with infected necrosis (50%)

2. Approximately 10-30% of patients will develop severe pancreatitis that will progress to pancreatic necrosis.

3. Ranson's criteria (Table 28-1)

a. 11 criteria that predict survival, not used very often.

b. Estimated mortality based on total criteria found at initial presentation and 48 hours after admission.

4. APACHE II score (Table 28-2)

a. "Acute Physiology and Chronic Health Evaluation II"

b. Severity of disease classification system based on physiologic parameters; higher scores predict higher death rates.

c. More accurate than Ranson's criteria

d. Special weight can be given to organ system involvement.

## G. COMPLICATIONS

1. Necrotizing pancreatitis

a. Sterile

**TABLE 28-1**

RANSON'S CRITERIA

| Initial Presentation | 48 Hours after Admission | Calculated Mortality Rate* |
|---|---|---|
| Age >55 years | Decline in hematocrit >10% | 0–2 criteria = 2% mortality rate |
| White blood cell count >16,000/$\mu$L | Fluid sequestration >6 L | 3–4 criteria = 15% mortality rate |
| Glucose level >11 mmol/L (>200 mg/dl) | Hypocalcemia (Ca <8 mg/dl, <2 mmol/L) | 5–6 criteria = 40% mortality rate |
| Lactate dehydrogenase level >350 IU/L | Hypoxemia ($P_{O_2}$ <60 mm Hg) | 7–8 criteria = 100% mortality rate |
| Aspartate aminotransferase concentration >250 IU/L | Blood urea nitrogen increase of >5 mg/dl (>1.98 mmol/L) even after intravenous fluid resuscitation | |
| | Base deficit of >4 mmol/L | |

*Sum of the number of criteria at initial presentation and 48 hours after admission yields the estimated mortality rate.

(1) Far better prognosis than infected necrosis, with a mortality of near 0% without any other systemic complications

(2) It may develop into infected necrosis, chronic pseudocyst, or it may resolve spontaneously.

(3) Some studies suggest the use of prophylactic antibiotics even with sterile pancreatic necrosis as this has been shown to limit the number of cases that convert to infected pancreatic necrosis. However, the results of a recent double-blind placebo study do not concur with these earlier unblinded studies.

b. Infected

(1) Develops in 30-50% of patients with pancreatic necrosis

(2) Incidence peaks in the 3rd week of the disease

(3) High mortality when other systemic complications are present

(4) Fine-needle aspiration of the necrosis to confirm the diagnosis and determine bacterial antibiotic sensitivities

(5) Most common organisms are enteric; *Enterococcus* (most common), *E. coli, Klebsiella, S. aureus, Proteus, Pseudomonas, Enterobacter,* and *Candida.*

(6) Surgical debridement is necessary for those patients with infected necrosis and thus hemodynamic instability.

2. **Pseudocyst (Figure 28-3)**

a. Cyst-like space within or near the pancreas that is *not* lined by epithelium but instead granulated and fibrotic tissue.

b. Accounts for the majority of cystic masses of the pancreas and the most common complication of pancreatitis (10% of acute pancreatitis, 20-40% of chronic pancreatitis).

c. Frequently found in the lesser sac, posterior to the stomach

# TABLE 28-2
## APACHE II SCORING SYSTEM

| | Low Abnormal Values | | | | Normal | High Abnormal Values | | | |
|---|---|---|---|---|---|---|---|---|---|
| | +4 | +3 | +2 | +1 | 0 | +1 | +2 | +3 | +4 |
| Temperature (°C) | <29.9 | 30–31.9 | 32–33.9 | 34–35.9 | 36–38.4 | 38.5–38.9 | | 39–40.9 | >41 |
| MAP (mm Hg) | <49 | | 50–69 | | 70–109 | | 110–129 | 130–159 | >160 |
| HR | <39 | 40–54 | 55–69 | | 70–109 | | 110–139 | 140–179 | >180 |
| RR | <5 | | 6–9 | 10–11 | 12–24 | 25–34 | | 35–49 | >50 |
| (A-a)O$_2$, Pao$_2$ | <55 | 55–60 | | 61–70 | >70 or <200 | | 200–349 | 350–499 | >500 |
| pH | <7.15 | 7.15–7.24 | 7.25–7.32 | | 7.33–7.49 | 7.5–7.59 | | 7.6–7.69 | >7.7 |
| Na (mmol/L) | <110 | 111–119 | 120–129 | | 130–149 | 150–154 | 155–159 | 160–179 | >180 |
| K (mmol/L) | <2.5 | 2.5–2.9 | | 3–3.4 | 3.5–5.4 | 5.5–5.9 | | 6–6.9 | >7 |
| Cr (mg/dl, no renal failure) | | | <0.6 (+4 if renal failure) | | 0.6–1.4 | | 1.5–1.9 (+4 if renal failure) | 2–3.4 (+6 if renal failure) | >3.5 (+8 if renal failure) |
| Hematocrit (%) | <20 | | 20–29.9 | | 30–45.9 | 46–49.9 | 50–59.9 | | >60 |
| White blood cell count (per liter) | <1 | | 1–2.9 | | 3–14.9 | 15–19.9 | 20–39.9 | | >40 |

## APACHE II SCORING SYSTEM

| | Low Abnormal Values | | | | Normal | High Abnormal Values | | | |
| | +4 | +3 | +2 | +1 | 0 | +1 | +2 | +3 | +4 |
|---|---|---|---|---|---|---|---|---|---|
| $HCO_3$ (bicarbonate; mmol/L, use if no arterial blood gases) | <15 | 15–17.9 | 18–21.1 | | 22–31.9 | 32–40.9 | | 41–51.9 | >52 |
| Score | +0 | +2 | +3 | +5 | +6 | | | | |
| Age (yr) | <44 | 45–54 | 55–64 | 65–74 | >75 | | | | |
| Chronic organ insufficiency?* | | Elective after surgery | | Nonoperative or emergent after surgery | | | | | |

Tabulate total number of points based on criteria from each row.

*Chronic organ insufficiency involves liver (biopsy-proved cirrhosis, portal HTN, past upper gastrointestinal bleed, prior encephalopathy/coma), cardiovascular (New York Health Association Class IV), pulmonary (chronic obstructive pulmonary disease, exercise restriction, chronic hypoxia, hypercapnia, pulmonary hypertension >40 mm Hg, or respirator dependency), renal (chronic dialysis), or immunosuppression (chemotherapy, radiation, long-term or recent high-dose steroid therapy, disease that suppresses resistance to infection such as leukemia, lymphoma, or acquired immune deficiency syndrome). Predicted death rate calculated as follows: X = [−3.517 + (Acute Physiology and Chronic Health Evaluation [APACHE] II)] * 0.146. Predicted Death Rate = $e^X/(1 + e^X)$ * 100.

MAP = mean arterial pressure; HR = heart rate; RR = respiratory rate.

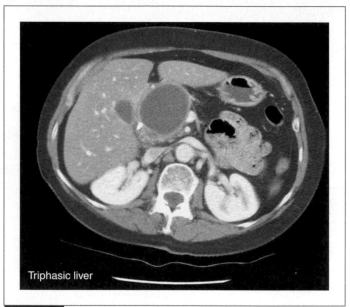

**FIG. 28-3**

**CT Scan of Pancreatic Pseudocyst**
Complications of pancreatitis include pseudocyst formation. By CT the pseudocyst is water density with a thin wall.

d. Communicates with the pancreatic ductal system and contains a watery fluid rich in pancreatic enzymes
e. Many pseudocysts will resolve spontaneously without complications, but further intervention may be required if the pseudocyst:
  (1) Enlarged—pseudocysts >6 cm are more likely to cause symptoms and less likely to resolve spontaneously.
  (2) Causes symptoms (mainly due to size)
    (a) Abdominal pain
    (b) Early satiety (compressed stomach)
    (c) Nausea/vomiting
    (d) Obstructive jaundice (compression of bile duct)
  (3) Creates complications
    (a) Hemosuccus pancreaticus (erosion of the pseudocyst into a neighboring vessel)
    (b) Gastric outlet obstruction (compression of the stomach and/ or duodenum)
    (c) Perforation with peritonitis
  (4) Becomes infected and forms an abscess

    f. Pseudocysts are ideally treated 4-6 weeks after appearance so that a thick, fibrous wall can mature around the cavity and a drainage procedure is then performed:
- (1) Pseudocysts are treated only if symptomatic or associated with a complication (infection, obstruction, bleeding), otherwise they are left alone.
- (2) First modality of treatment is endoscopic drainage, either transgastric, transduodenal, or transpapillary.
- (3) Surgical drainage is the next best option and involves internal drainage (cystogastrostomy, cystojejunostomy, or cystoduodenostomy) or percutaneous external drainage (for infected pseudocysts or those with immature walls, reserved for patients who cannot tolerate the endoscopic or surgical drainage).

## 3. Hemorrhage
a. Due to erosion of a pseudoaneurysm from a pseudocyst, abscess, or necrotizing pancreatitis
b. Bleeding may be gastrointestinal, intraperitoneal, or retroperitoneal.
c. Angiography is used to localize the site of bleeding and possibly embolize the bleeding vessel in an unstable patient. Otherwise, surgical management is necessary when bleeding cannot be controlled by interventional radiology.

## 4. Splenic vein thrombosis
a. Because the splenic vein runs posterior to the pancreas, in cases of severe pancreatitis thrombosis is not unusual.
b. Gastroesophageal varices can form, with a mortality rate of ~20% if they bleed.
c. Splenectomy can be performed to prevent possible or recurrent gastroesophageal bleeding due to splenic vein thrombosis.

## 5. Pancreatic ascites
a. Leakage of pancreatic fluid directly into the peritoneum caused by rupture of a pancreatic pseudocyst or a leaking pancreatic duct that was never able to form a pseudocyst.
b. ERCP can be used to identify the area of leak and possibly place a stent across that area.
c. Octreotide and bowel rest has been shown to be successful in stopping a leak in >50% of patients.
d. If medical management fails, the site of the pancreatic duct leak dictates the surgical management:
- (1) Body—Roux-en-Y pancreaticojejunostomy
- (2) Tail—distal pancreatectomy or internal drainage procedure

## 6. Pancreaticoenteric fistula
a. A pseudocyst can erode into various areas of the GI tract, including the stomach, duodenum, small intestine, bile duct, or splenic flexure of the colon.
b. In some cases, the pseudocyst will decompress via this fistula and no further management is required.

28

BENIGN PANCREATIC DISEASE

c. If the fistula does not resolve spontaneously, ERCP is performed to detail the communication and operative management is dictated by the organ(s) involved.

## III. CHRONIC PANCREATITIS

### A. BASICS
1. Incidence is approximately 10 cases per 100,000 (similar to pancreatic cancer).
2. Characterized by recurrent or persistent chronic abdominal pain with endocrine and exocrine insufficiency
3. Irreversible destruction of the pancreatic parenchyma
4. Patients with chronic pancreatitis may have attacks of acute pancreatitis superimposed on their chronic pain.

### B. ETIOLOGY
1. Alcohol
a. Most common cause
b. Usually manifests in middle age (~40 years of age)
2. Cholelithiasis—recurrent episodes of gallstone pancreatitis can lead to chronic pancreatitis.
3. Autoimmune
a. Associated with primary sclerosing cholangitis and Sjögren's syndrome
b. Responsive to steroid treatment
4. Hypercalcemia
5. Hereditary
a. Onset is usually during the teenage years.
b. *PRSS1* (cationic trypsinogen gene) gene mutation (66% of hereditary cases)
c. *CFTR* (cystic fibrosis transmembrane regulator gene) gene mutation
d. *SPINK1* gene mutation
6. Pancreas divisum
7. Idiopathic

### C. DIAGNOSIS
1. History
a. Recurrent or chronic abdominal pain with characteristics similar to acute pancreatitis but a more "aching" pain
b. Weight loss/anorexia is present in 75% of patients.
c. Steatorrhea
   (1) Pale, bulky, malodorous stool that floats
   (2) Exocrine and endocrine insufficiency result in the inability to digest lipids. However, 90% of exocrine function must be lost before steatorrhea develops.
d. Signs/symptoms of endocrine and exocrine insufficiency

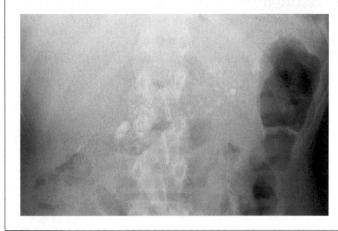

FIG. 28-4

**Abdominal X-Ray of Chronic Pancreatitis**

Plain film finding characteristic of chronic pancreatitis includes coarse calcification crossing the midline of the upper abdomen. Also present in the right upper quadrant are surgical clips from prior cholecystectomy.

28

BENIGN PANCREATIC DISEASE

2. Physical exam
a. Cachectic appearance
b. Pain may be out of proportion to abdominal exam but is usually epigastric in nature.

3. Labs
a. Usually not very helpful
b. Amylase may be normal or only slightly elevated, because of destruction of the pancreatic parenchyma.

4. Imaging
a. Abdominal X-ray may demonstrate calcifications (calcium carbonate) in the pancreas (95% specific, Figure 28-4).
b. CT scan typically demonstrates an atrophic pancreas with calcifications and a dilated duct. The presence of calcifications indicates advanced disease.
c. Endoscopic ultrasound (EUS) demonstrates duct dilation, calcifications, parenchymal fibrosis, and possible pseudocyst with chronic pancreatitis.
d. ERCP delineates the ductal system and is necessary before any surgical procedure, although EUS, CT, and MRCP may provide as accurate information of the duct system.
e. The "chain of lakes" is present due to areas of alternating ductal strictures and dilations.

## D. TREATMENT

1. Medical—first line treatment.
   a. Pain control
   b. Counseling (alcohol abstinence, low-fat meals)
   c. Acid suppression (to prevent orally administered lipase from being inactivated)
   d. Oral pancreatic enzyme supplementation (coated enzymes for insufficiency, uncoated for pain)
   e. Treatment of diabetes
   f. Steroids (for autoimmune pancreatitis)
2. Surgical—nearly 50% of patients with chronic pancreatitis will require some form of surgical intervention. Indications include intractable pain not controlled by medical management (most common indication), recurrent flare-ups requiring repeat hospitalization, sequelae of progressive fibrosis (duodenal, CBD, colonic obstructions), effects of ductal rupture (pseudocyst, pancreatic ascites, etc.), and suspected pancreatic cancer. Surgical treatment includes either a drainage procedure (DP) or resective procedure (RP).
   a. Beger procedure (RP)
      (1) Duodenal-sparing pancreatic head resection
      (2) GI continuity is restored with two pancreaticojejunostomies (one connected to the remaining pancreatic body and another to remnant pancreatic tissue at the duodenal C-loop) and a jejunojejunostomy.
      (3) Indicated for small duct, head-dominant chronic pancreatitis, but contraindicated if pancreatic cancer is suspected.
      (4) Pancreatic tissue should be sent for freezing regardless because of a 5% incidence of occult pancreatic cancer.
   b. Duval procedure (DP)
      (1) Based on the presumption that a single ductal stricture is responsible for the obstructive symptoms
      (2) Involves a distal pancreatectomy with splenectomy and retrograde drainage of the distal pancreatic duct via a pancreaticojejunostomy
   c. Frey procedure (DP)
      (1) Subtotal pancreatic head resection ("coring out") with longitudinal decompression of the pancreatic duct in the body and tail
      (2) Originally described for patients with "head dominant" disease
   d. Puestow procedure (DP)
      (1) Longitudinal pancreaticojejunostomy allows for decompression of the entire pancreatic duct.
      (2) The entire pancreatic duct is longitudinally opened from the duodenum to the tail, which allows for pain relief in 65-85% of patients.
      (3) Patients with a pancreatic duct >10 mm, a length of anastomosis >6 cm, and pancreatic calcifications usually respond well to the Puestow procedure.
   e. Whipple procedure (RP)

    (1) Pancreaticoduodenectomy
    (2) Three anastomoses involved—pancreaticojejunostomy, choledocho-jejunostomy, and duodeno/gastrojejunostomy (pylorus preserving vs. non-preserving).
    (3) Indicated for small duct, head-dominant chronic pancreatitis
 f. Partial/total pancreatectomy (RP)
    (1) Indicated for intractable pain, prior failed operations, and is usually a last resort procedure that is very rarely used for fear of uncontrolled hypoglycemic attacks.
    (2) May be reserved for patients with "small duct" disease in which a decompressive procedure cannot be performed
    (3) Total pancreatectomy can be "near-total," in which a rim of pancreatic tissue is preserved along the duodenal C-loop in addition to preservation of the common bile duct and pancreaticoduodenal vessels. Total pancreatectomy involves removal of the pylorus with reconstruction via a gastrojejunostomy/hepaticojejunostomy. Alternatively, a "pylorus-preserving" procedure is performed with GI continuity restored via duodenojejunostomy.
    (4) Complicated by several endocrine and exocrine insufficiencies. In a few select institutions, autologous islet cell transplantation is carried out at the time of the total pancreatectomy.
 g. Autologous islet cell transplant
    (1) A distal pancreatectomy is performed up to the level of the superior mesenteric vein and it is this portion that is typically used to harvest the islet cells to limit warm ischemia time.
    (2) Once the islet cells have been harvested via continuous cold enzymatic perfusion/digestion of the pancreas, 1-2 ml of packed islet cells are injected into a tributary of the middle colic vein or directly into the portal vein.
    (3) Postoperative care requires stringent glucose control (levels between 100-120 mg/dl) to prevent islet cell "burn-out."
    (4) In one study, 41% of patients were insulin-free, 27% required minimal or sliding scale insulin, and 82% were pain-free and off narcotics after pancreatectomy with autologous islet cell transplantation.
 h. Celiac plexus blockade
    (1) Celiac ganglion innervates the upper abdominal viscera via pre- and post-synaptic sympathetics, pre-synaptic parasympathetics, and pain fibers.
    (2) Blockade is used in cases of continued pain after resection or drainage procedure for chronic pancreatitis that is not due to an anatomic problem (biliary stricture, fluid collection, etc.).
    (3) The celiac plexus is identified after incising the avascular hepatogastric ligament and palpating for a thrill arising from the aorta behind the stomach near the diaphragmatic crura.

**28**

BENIGN PANCREATIC DISEASE

(4) The index finger is placed on the splenic artery, the middle finger on the common hepatic artery (the two most anatomically consistent celiac axis branches) and a neurolytic agent is injected into the soft tissue just lateral to the aorta above and below the operator's fingers (this represents the four quadrants where the plexus lies).

(5) A 50% ethanol solution is used with a 22-gauge spinal needle to inject 10 ml into four quadrants around the celiac plexus.

## E. COMPLICATIONS

1. Diabetes mellitus (Type I) due to endocrine insufficiency (up to 30% of patients)
2. Malabsorption due to exocrine insufficiency
3. Narcotics abuse
4. Increased risk for pancreatic cancer

## RECOMMENDED READING

Ahmad SA, Lowy AM, Wray CJ, et al. Factors associated with insulin and narcotic independence after islet autotransplantation in patients with severe chronic pancreatitis. *J Am Coll Surg* 2005 Nov;201(5):680-7.

Ahmad SA, Wray CJ, Rilo HR, et al. Chronic pancreatitis: Advances and ongoing challenges. *Curr Probl Surg* 2006 Mar;43(3):135-238.

Bell RH. Current surgical management of chronic pancreatitis. *J Gastrointest Surg* 2005;9(1):144-54.

Clancy TE, Benoit EP, Ashley SW. Current management of acute pancreatitis. *J Gastrointest Surg* 2005;9(3):440-52.

Isenmann R, Rünzi M, Kron M, et al. Prophylactic antibiotic treatment in patients with severe acute pancreatitis – A placebo-controlled, double-blind trial. *Gastroenterology* 2004;126:997–1004.

Nathens AB, Curtis JR, Beale RJ, et al. Management of the critically ill patient with severe acute pancreatitis. *Crit Care Med* 2004;32(12):2524-36.

# Spleen

*Amy T. Makley, MD*

The spleen is the largest organ of the reticuloendothelial system, responsible for many filtration and host defense mechanisms; however, it is not well understood. It plays a role in many childhood and adulthood hematologic and immunologic disorders, and can cause significant morbidity and mortality in blunt and penetrating trauma. Previous management included simple and straightforward guidelines for splenectomy; recently, the indications for surgical management of splenic disease have drastically changed, with more conservative treatment dominating.

## 29

## I. ANATOMY

**A. AVERAGE ADULT SPLEEN**
1. 150 g, 7 to 11 cm in length

**B. SURROUNDED BY CAPSULE**
1. Approximately 1 to 2 mm in thickness

**C. SPLENOMEGALY DEFINITION**
1. >500 g
2. >15 cm in length

**D. BLOOD SUPPLY**
1. Arterial
a. Splenic artery off of the celiac trunk
b. Short gastrics contained in gastrosplenic ligament
2. Venous drainage via splenic vein, which joins superior mesenteric vein to form the portal vein

**E. STRUCTURAL SUPPORT**
1. Suspended via four ligaments
2. Splenocolic, gastrosplenic, phrenosplenic, and splenorenal ligaments

**F. MICROANATOMY**
1. Red pulp
a. Comprises 75% of splenic volume
b. Venous sinuses surrounded by reticulum
c. Site of splenic macrophages responsible for filtration system
2. Marginal zone—narrow interface between red and white pulp
3. White pulp
a. Comprises 25% of splenic volume
b. Consists of lymphoid follicles

**G. ACCESSORY SPLEENS**
1. Present in 20% of the population

2. Most common locations
a. Approximately 80% in splenic hilum/vascular pedicle
b. Remainder dispersed in gastrocolic ligament, pancreatic tail, greater omentum, greater curve of the stomach, and mesentery.

## II. FUNCTION
### A. FILTRATION
1. Clearance of damaged/aged red blood cells (RBCs), white blood cells (WBCs), and platelets

### B. HOST DEFENSE/IMMUNOLOGIC FUNCTION
1. Cell mediated and humoral immunity

### C. STORAGE ORGAN FOR HEMATOPOIETIC ELEMENTS
### D. CYTOPOIETIC ORGAN IN EARLY DEVELOPMENT

## III. GENERAL INDICATIONS FOR SPLENECTOMY
### A. TRAUMA
1. Treatment is increasingly more conservative (observation vs. embolization) (see Chapter 63 for details).

### B. RBC DISORDERS
1. Autoimmune hemolytic anemia—warm IgG antibodies
a. Autoantibodies to RBCs causing hemolysis
b. Symptoms of anemia and jaundice
c. Splenomegaly present in one third to one half of cases.
d. Diagnose via direct Coombs' test.
e. Treat first with steroids.
f. Splenectomy if steroids fail—80% success
2. Hereditary spherocytosis
a. Abnormality in spectrin—RBC membrane protein
b. Symptoms of splenomegaly, anemia, jaundice
c. Diagnosis of spherocytes on peripheral blood smear and increased mean corpuscular hemoglobin concentration
d. Treat with splenectomy; perform ideally at age 4 to 6 to minimize postoperative infection (see V.A.).
e. Prophylactic cholecystectomy recommended given associated symptomatic cholelithiasis in 50% of patients secondary to bilirubin stones.
3. Sickle cell disease
a. Deoxygenated hemoglobin sickles and polymerizes, resulting in splenic sequestration and splenomegaly.
b. Often results in autosplenectomy
c. Splenectomy indicated for acute sequestration crisis or abscesses.
d. Approximately 3% of children with sickle cell disease undergo splenectomy.

4. **Thalassemias**
a. Disorder of hemoglobin synthesis
b. Treat first with transfusions and appropriate chelation therapy.
c. Splenectomy indicated if excessive transfusion requirements, painful splenomegaly, or painful splenic infarction.

## C. MYELOPROLIFERATIVE DISORDERS
1. **Chronic myelogenous leukemia**
a. Associated splenomegaly in 50% of cases
b. Splenectomy indicated for symptomatic splenomegaly or refractory anemia.
2. **Polycythemia vera**
a. Treat first with phlebotomy, aspirin, and chemotherapeutic agents.
b. Splenectomy only for late-stage, symptomatic splenomegaly
c. Splenectomy may improve quality of life, not survival.
3. **Essential thrombocytopenia**
a. Reserve splenectomy for late disease only.
b. Bleeding risks make elective splenectomy prohibitive.

## D. WBC DISORDERS
1. **Chronic lymphocytic leukemia**
a. Progressive accumulation of dysfunctional lymphocytes.
b. Symptoms include weakness, fatigue, fevers, night sweats, lymphadenopathy, and frequent infections.
c. Splenectomy to improve cytopenia—allows for the administration of chemotherapy if previously prohibited by cytopenia.
d. May significantly improve survival in patients with advanced stages of chronic lymphocytic leukemia with hemoglobin levels <10 g/dl and platelet counts <50 × $10^9$ per liter.
e. Palliative splenectomy indicated for symptomatic splenomegaly.
2. **Hairy cell leukemia**
a. Rare form of leukemia—2% of cases
b. Chemotherapy is first-line therapy.
c. Splenectomy indicated for symptomatic pancytopenia or splenomegaly.
3. **Non–Hodgkin's lymphoma**
a. Monoclonal lymphocytic proliferation; 80% B-cell type
b. Palliative splenectomy for splenomegaly and pancytopenia
4. **Hodgkin's disease**
a. Four types—lymphocyte predominant, nodular sclerosis, mixed cellularity, and lymphocyte depleted
b. Staging by anatomic distribution of lymphadenopathy.
c. Previously staged by laparotomy; now mainly staged by imaging techniques.
d. Treatment varies with staging; if splenic involvement, chemotherapy and radiation therapy are both indicated.

### E. PLATELET DISORDERS.
1. Immune thrombocytopenic purpura.
a. Incidence 1 in 10,000 people.
b. Clinically presents with low platelet counts and petechial bleeding.
c. Premature removal of platelets with IgG autoantibodies from spleen.
d. Symptom severity correlates with level of thrombocytopenia.
   (1) >50,000 per liter—incidental findings
   (2) 30–50,000 per liter—easy ecchymosis
   (3) 10–30,000 per liter—spontaneous petechial bleeding
   (4) <10,000 per liter—increased risk for internal and intracranial bleeding
e. Diagnosis by platelet counts, megathrombocytes on peripheral blood smears, and exclusion of secondary causes.
f. Adult disease—insidious onset; treat with splenectomy if medical therapy fails (prednisone and intravenous immunoglobulin). Splenectomy achieves 75% to 80% cure rate with no further need for steroid therapy after surgery.
g. Childhood course—generally self-limited disease, with 70% achieving complete remission. Manage conservatively with intermittent steroids/intravenous immunoglobulin and observation; splenectomy is rarely indicated.
2. Thrombotic thrombocytopenic purpura
a. Decreased platelet count, hemolytic anemia, and neurologic complications
b. Abnormal platelet clumping/thrombosis causing deformation of vessel lumen size with resultant RBC hemolysis and splenic sequestration
c. Treat with plasma exchange.
d. Splenectomy is indicated if multiple relapses or excessive plasmapheresis.

### F. OTHER SPLENIC DISORDERS
1. Splenic abscesses
a. Rare (<1% incidence rate)
b. Arise from hematogenous infection, contiguous infection, hemoglobinopathies, immunosuppression, or trauma
c. Clinical picture of fevers, leukocytosis, left upper quadrant pain, and splenomegaly
d. Treat with broad-spectrum antibiotics and splenectomy. Option of percutaneous drainage should be considered if single abscess or patient is unable to tolerate general anesthesia.
2. Splenic cysts
a. Infectious causative agents most commonly parasitic; treat with splenectomy.
b. Noninfectious causative factor most commonly is traumatic "pseudocysts." Treatment is observation if asymptomatic; if symptomatic, may excise if small or unroof if larger.

3. Felty syndrome
a. Triad of splenomegaly, rheumatoid arthritis, and neutropenia
b. Immune complexes coat and sequester WBCs in spleen
c. Occurs in 3% of patients with rheumatoid arthritis; female predominance
d. Splenectomy results in increased WBC counts in 80% of cases.

4. Splenic artery aneurysm
a. Most common visceral aneurysm
b. Female predominance
c. Most commonly found in the mid-to-distal artery
d. Rupture rate averages 3% to 9%.
e. Risk for rupture is much greater in pregnancy.
f. Mortality rate with rupture approaches 50%.
g. Most are diagnosed incidentally.
h. If symptomatic or enlarging, recommend treatment with resection or ligation. If pregnant or of childbearing age, recommend treatment. If >2 cm and asymptomatic, consider elective resection. If located in the distal segment, splenectomy is recommended.

5. Splenic vein thrombosis
a. Associated with chronic pancreatitis
b. Gastric varices and left-sided portal hypertension are complications.
c. If found with accompanying varices, recommended treatment is splenectomy.

## IV. SURGICAL TECHNIQUES
### A. OPEN SPLENECTOMY
1. Position supinely, place nasogastrically before surgery.
2. Exposure
a. Midline incision—massive splenomegaly or trauma
b. Left subcostal incision—most elective splenectomies
3. Division of splenocolic ligament
4. Incision of lateral peritoneal attachments (splenophrenic ligament)
5. Division of short gastrics
6. Dissection of splenic hilum (artery, then vein)
7. Irrigation and evaluation for hemostasis

### B. LAPAROSCOPIC SPLENECTOMY
First successful procedure performed in 1991 by Delaitre and Maignien.
1. Placement of Foley catheter, nasogastrically before surgery
2. Position in right lateral decubitus at 60 degrees, 15-degree reverse Trendelenburg position.
3. Insertion of three 10-mm port sites
4. Dissection as with open technique, using endovascular staples, clips, or cautery
5. Removal of spleen via retrieval bag; may require morcellation of spleen to achieve removal

## C. HAND-ASSISTED TECHNIQUE
1. Allows identification, retraction, and direct palpation, as well as removal of large spleens via hand port.

## V. POSTSPLENECTOMY CONSIDERATIONS
### A. OVERWHELMING POSTSPLENECTOMY INFECTION
1. Increased susceptibility to infection by encapsulated organisms and parasites
2. Incidence rate 1% to 5% over lifetime, typically within 2 years of splenectomy
3. Mortality increased in children, immunocompromised patients, and those with associated hematologic conditions.
4. Responsible organisms include:
a. *Streptococcus pneumoniae* (50–90% of cases)
b. *Haemophilus influenzae*
c. *Meningococcus* sp
5. Prodrome of fever, malaise, headache, vomiting, diarrhea, and abdominal pain
6. Rapid progression into fulminant septic shock
7. Treatment/prevention
a. Pneumococcal vaccine
b. Meningococcal vaccine
c. *H. influenzae* vaccine
d. Administer vaccines 1 to 2 weeks before surgery in elective cases and as soon as possible in emergent splenectomies, usually 2 to 3 days after surgery.
e. Children are candidates for prophylactic antibiotics for 2 years after surgery.

### B. POSTSPLENECTOMY HEMATOLOGIC CHANGES
1. Expect leukocytosis and thrombocytosis after surgery.
2. WBC count increases on postoperative day 1 and remains increased for months.
3. Platelet count increases over several days, peaking 2 to 3 weeks after surgery.
4. Some recommend acetylsalicylic acid for platelet count $>10^6$ per liter.

### C. PULMONARY COMPLICATIONS
1. Left lower lobe atelectasis—16% of open splenectomy cases
2. Pulmonary effusions
3. Pneumonia—up to 10% of cases

### D. HEMORRHAGE
1. Subphrenic hematoma—presents after surgery
2. Usual source—short gastrics
3. Average transfusion rate—3% to 5% of all splenectomies

### E. INFECTION
1. Subphrenic abscesses—increased incidence with left upper quadrant drain placement
2. Wound infection

### F. THROMBOEMBOLIC PHENOMENA
1. Portal vein thrombosis
a. Incidence rate of 5% to 10%
b. Up to 40% with associated myeloproliferative disorders
c. Clinical presentation of anorexia, abdominal pain, leukocytosis, and thrombocytosis after surgery
d. Diagnose with computed tomography imaging.
e. Immediate anticoagulation
2. Preoperative administration of heparin and use of sequential compression devices decreases incidence.

### G. PANCREATITIS, PSEUDOCYST, FISTULA
1. Secondary to pancreatic irritation/injury during dissection of splenic hilum

# PART VI

# Bariatric Surgery

# Bariatric Surgery

*John D. Scott, MD*

Bariatric surgery has become a popular option for the treatment of morbid obesity and its associated comorbidities. Because of the increasing volume of procedures performed across the country, surgery residents should become familiar with the indications, benefits, and complications associated common bariatric operations.

## I. EPIDEMIOLOGY OF MORBID OBESITY

### A. DEFINITIONS
1. Overweight—body mass index [(BMI) = weight in kg/height in m$^2$] between 25 and 29.9
2. Obese (Class I)—BMI between 30 and 34.9
3. Severe obesity (Class II)—BMI between 35 and 39.9
4. Morbid obesity (Class III)—BMI ≥40

### B. CAUSES OF OBESITY
1. Genetic predisposition
2. Environmental conditions
   a. Easy access to food sources
   b. High-calorie, large-portion food choices
3. Sedentary behavior
   a. Lack of leisure-time physical activity
   b. Labor-saving technology
4. Increased caloric intake + reduced energy expenditure = obesity

### C. EPIDEMIOLOGY
1. Worldwide, obesity affects 1.7 billion people.
2. The number of people in the United States with a BMI >40 has tripled in the last decade.
3. In 2000, more than 300,000 deaths were attributed to obesity.
4. Obesity presents a significant economic burden, accounting for 9.4% ($50–70 billion) of all direct U.S. healthcare costs.
5. In 2004, 140,000 bariatric surgeries were performed in the United States.

## II. COMORBIDITY ASSOCIATED WITH MORBID OBESITY

### A. NEOPLASIA
1. Seven-fold increased risk for endometrial cancer in obese women
2. Fifty percent greater risk for breast cancer for the morbidly obese female individual
3. Forty percent greater risk for colon cancer for the morbidly obese female individual

## B. CARDIOVASCULAR DISEASE
1. Seventy-eight percent of all patients with hypertension are obese.
2. Morbidly obese patients have a doubled risk for myocardial infarction.

## C. PULMONARY DISEASE
1. Approximately 98% of obese subjects have increased apnea scores, and 33% of obese subjects have severe sleep apnea.
2. Obese patients have high rates of obesity-hypoventilation syndrome.

## D. ENDOCRINE DISEASE
1. Relative risk for development of type II diabetes mellitus for patients with a BMI >35 versus patients with normal weight is 38.
2. Obese patients are at greater risk for hypoparathyroidism.

## E. GASTROINTESTINAL DISEASE
1. Morbid obesity can increase risks for the following conditions:
a. Nonalcoholic steatohepatitis
b. Gastroesophageal reflux disease
c. Cholelithiasis and choledocholithiasis
d. Acute pancreatitis

## F. OTHER COMORBIDITIES ASSOCIATED WITH MORBID OBESITY
1. Pregnancy-related complications such as preeclampsia, early neonatal death, and meconium aspiration
2. Musculoskeletal pain in hip and knee joints
3. Prothrombic state caused by high intraabdominal pressures, decreased activity, and venous compression by fatty tissues
4. Altered immunologic state
5. Intertriginous dermatitis
6. Psychological complaints
a. Depression
b. Social isolation
c. Decreased libido

## III. MEDICAL THERAPY FOR MORBID OBESITY
### A. DIET MODIFICATION—LOW IN CALORIES, FAT, AND CARBOHYDRATES
### B. INCREASED PHYSICAL ACTIVITY
### C. BEHAVIORAL MODIFICATION—AVOID SNACKING
### D. MEDICATIONS
1. Sibutramine, an appetite suppressant
2. Orlistat, binds to lipases in the stomach and prevents their absorption.

## E. ADVANTAGES/DISADVANTAGES
1. Lower cost to initiate medical therapy.
2. Long-term results are poor: Most medical weight-loss programs have a high attrition rate.
3. Medical treatment is associated with greater rate of rebound weight gain versus surgical treatment.

## IV. TYPES OF PROCEDURES

### A. MALABSORPTIVE OPERATIONS
1. Decrease the intestinal surface area used for nutrient absorption by shortening or rearranging the digestive tract.

### B. RESTRICTIVE OPERATIONS
1. Reduce gastric volume and cause satiety with low food volumes.

### C. COMBINED OPERATIONS ARE RESTRICTIVE AND MALABSORPTIVE.

## V. PREOPERATIVE WORKUP

### A. PATIENT SELECTION CRITERIA
1. BMI ≥40
2. BMI ≥35 with associated comorbidity
3. Failure of nonsurgical weight-loss efforts
4. Well-informed, compliant, motivated patients

### B. PREOPERATIVE ASSESSMENT
1. Bariatric nutritional assessment
2. Psychological assessment
3. Sleep apnea study and pulmonary assessment
4. Cardiovascular assessment

### C. PREOPERATIVE INFERIOR VENA CAVA FILTER IF PATIENT HAS HISTORY OF THROMBOTIC EVENTS

## VI. SURGICAL PROCEDURES FOR THE BARIATRIC PATIENT

### A. LAPAROSCOPIC ROUX-EN-Y GASTRIC BYPASS
1. Most common bariatric operation performed in the United States.
2. Restrictive and malabsorptive
3. A 30-ml gastric pouch is created by dividing stomach, and an approximately 150-cm roux limb is created to anastomose to the gastric pouch.
4. Requires two anastomoses
   a. Gastrojejunostomy
   b. Jejujejunostomy
5. Excellent excess weight loss (60–70%) and resolution of comorbidity
6. Advantages

a. Rapid weight loss
b. Largest U.S. experience of any bariatric procedure
c. Minimal dietary restrictions
**7. Disadvantages**
a. Anatomic rearrangement
b. Increased morbidity and mortality rates (0.2–1%) as compared with laparoscopic adjustable gastric banding
c. Dumping syndrome associated with high carbohydrate intake
d. Nutritional deficiencies such as vitamin $B_{12}$ and iron are common.
**8. Complications**
a. Leaks
   (1) Most dreaded complication
   (2) Incidence rate of 1% to 5.6%
   (3) Mortality rate of 10%
   (4) Clinical characteristics—fever, tachycardia, hypotension, abdominal pain
   (5) Types
      (a) Gastric pouch leaks (49%)
      (b) Staple line leaks (9%)
      (c) Gastric remnant leaks (25%), not seen on postoperative swallow studies
      (d) Jejujejunostomy leaks (13%)
   (6) Treatment
      (a) Percutaneous drainage
      (b) Operative exploration
b. Internal hernias
   (1) More common with laparoscopic procedures than open procedures because of decreased adhesion formation
   (2) Incidence rate: 3% lifetime risk
   (3) Clinical characteristics—obstructive symptoms
   (4) Types
      (a) Transmesocolic (for retrocolic Roux limbs)
      (b) Mesenteric-mesocolic (Petersen's hernia)
      (c) Mesenteric (at jejujejunostomy)
   (5) Treatment: Early operative intervention for any bypass patient with obstructive symptoms can prevent intestinal strangulation and necrosis.
c. Other complications
   (1) Thrombotic events—pulmonary embolism rate between 0.3% and 2.4%
      (a) Prevent with early ambulation
      (b) Subcutaneous heparin before and after surgery
   (2) Bleeding at the staple lines

(3) Marginal ulceration

(4) Gastric-gastric fistula can lead to weight regain.

(5) Stricture formation

## B.   LAPAROSCOPIC ADJUSTABLE GASTRIC BANDING

1. Silicone band lined with inflatable balloon
2. The band is connected to a subcutaneous reservoir, which controls the balloon tightness.
3. The band is wrapped around gastric cardia, forming a 30-ml gastric pouch.
4. Inflation of the balloon tightens the band and promotes early satiety.
5. Advantages
a. Adjustable
b. Reversible
c. Least invasive bariatric surgical procedure
d. No anatomic rearrangement
e. Low morbidity and mortality rates
6. Disadvantages
a. More frequent and intense follow-up with patients
b. Slower rate of weight loss
c. Less overall excess weight loss
7. Complications
a. Band slippage
   (1) Anterior or posterior gastric prolapse through band
   (2) Clinically, causes pouch distention and obstructive symptoms
   (3) Treatment—deflate band, nasogastric tube drainage of pouch, operative band repositioning or removal to prevent strangulation and necrosis
b. Band erosion
   (1) Incidence rate of 0.2% to 1.2%
   (2) Diagnosis—usually endoscopy
   (3) Treatment—band removal and gastric repair

## C.   JEJUNOILEAL BYPASS

1. Developed in the 1950s
2. Malabsorptive
3. Stomach was left intact and the jejunum was connected to the terminal ileum.
4. Operation left a long, blind intestinal limb.
5. Excellent weight loss, but patients suffered many long-term complications.
6. This procedure has been abandoned in the United States.

## D.   VERTICAL BANDED GASTROPLASTY

1. Purely restrictive operation with a stapled 30-ml pouch based off the lesser curvature.

30

BARIATRIC SURGERY

2. No anastomosis required.
3. Polypropylene mesh or silastic ring used to create gastric outlet.
4. Once popular, it is now rarely performed because of weight regain and severe heartburn.
5. Laparoscopic Roux-en-Y gastric bypass has proved to have superior results to the vertical banded gastroplasty.

### E. BILIOPANCREATIC DIVERSION
1. Seventy percent gastrectomy and biliopancreatic diversion with a 100-cm common alimentary channel
2. Restrictive and malabsorptive
3. Usually a two-stage procedure
4. Complex operation that yields excellent weight-loss results (70% excess body weight loss) that is sustainable more than 10 years after surgery.
5. Most common variant performed today is the duodenal switch where the duodenum is transected proximal to the ampulla of Vater and an enteric limb is anastomosed postpylorically.

## VII. RESULTS OF BARIATRIC SURGERY
### A. SURGICAL THERAPY
1. Decreases mortality risk versus nonintervention or medical therapy.

### B. RISK REDUCTION
1. Reduction is 31.6% for death in surgical versus medical treatment for morbid obesity, according to the recent Swedish Obese Subjects study.

### C. LAPAROSCOPIC ROUX-EN-Y GASTRIC BYPASS AND LAPAROSCOPIC ADJUSTABLE GASTRIC BANDING
Demonstrate excellent and near-complete resolution of comorbidity associated with morbid obesity, including the following conditions·
1. Type II diabetes mellitus
2. Hypertension
3. Gastroesophageal reflux disease
4. Sleep apnea
5. Joint pain

### D. EXCESS WEIGHT LOSS
1. Weight loss usually reaches a maximum between 18 and 24 months after surgery.
2. Weight loss is dependent on several factors:
a. Preoperative weight
b. Overall patient health
c. Procedure performed
    (1) Bypass surgery (55–66% excessive weight loss)
    (2) Gastric banding (40–54% excessive weight loss)
d. Commitment to maintaining dietary guidelines

e. Follow-up care
f. Patient motivation

## RECOMMENDED READING

Buchwald H: Consensus conference statement, bariatric surgery for the morbidly obese. *Surg Obes Relat Dis* 1:371–381, 2005.

Buchwald H, Avidor Y, Braunwald E, et al: Bariatric surgery, a systematic review. *JAMA* 292:1724–1737, 2004.

Manson JE, Skerrett PJ, Greenland P, VanItallie TB: The escalating pandemics of obesity and sedentary lifestyle. *Arch Intern Med* 164:249–258, 2004.

Surgerman HJ, Nguyen NT (eds): *Management of Morbid Obesity.* New York, Taylor & Francis Group, 2006.

BARIATRIC SURGERY

# PART VII

# Vascular Surgery

# Thromboembolic Prophylaxis and Management of Deep Vein Thrombosis

*Brian S. Pan, MD*

## I. INTRODUCTION

### A. EPIDEMIOLOGY

1. Deep vein thrombosis (DVT) is a common problem after surgery, and its sequelae, pulmonary embolism (PE), is the leading cause of preventable in-hospital mortality in the United States.

2. DVT must be considered in the postoperative period given the multifactorial insults that surgery inflicts.

a. Prevention begins before surgery by considering the surgical procedure, its risks, and the patient's comorbidities.

b. The physician must consider the length of hospitalization, the normal postoperative course, and the patient's rehabilitation status.

3. Estimates of DVT after surgical procedures without appropriate prophylaxis are as follows:

a. General surgery (intraabdominal procedures): 22% to 33%

b. Orthopedic procedures: 45% to 66%

c. Prostatectomy: 50%

d. Trauma: 20%

e. Postpartum: 3%

### B. CAUSATIVE FACTORS

1. Multiple predisposing factors contribute to development of DVTs; however, they all hold in common the characteristics found in *Virchow's triad:*

a. Venous stasis—inactivity, cardiac factors (congestive heart failure), anesthesia induction

b. Endothelial injury—all operative procedures in which blood flow is interrupted

c. Hypercoagulability—medical conditions/states not limited to cancer, pregnancy, hematologic conditions (factor V Leiden deficiency)

### C. OTHER RISK FACTORS FOR THE DEVELOPMENT OF DVT

1. Age >60 years

2. Malignancy

3. History of DVT, PE, or varicose veins

4. Obesity

5. Major surgery—pelvic surgery

6. Trauma

7. Pregnancy

8. Oral contraceptives
9. Travel

## D. CLINICAL PRESENTATION
Nonspecific and often detected only after PE has occurred.
1. Signs include swelling, tenderness, calf pain elicited on passive dorsiflexion of the ankle (Homan's sign), and fever.
2. *Less than 50% of patients with DVTs will exhibit the above signs.*

## E. DIFFERENTIAL DIAGNOSES
1. Achilles tendonitis, arterial insufficiency, arthritis, cellulitis, lymphangitis, varicose veins, superficial thrombophlebitis, ruptured Baker cyst

## F. DIAGNOSIS
1. Best made by doppler ultrasonography. Other methods include venography, impedance plethysmography, and radiolabeled iodine fibrinogen studies.

## G. SEQUELAE
1. PE is the third most common cause of death in the hospitalized patient. One in every 200 patients undergoing a major operation dies of a massive PE, accounting for 50,000 deaths/year. Ten percent of the deaths occur within 60 minutes of the first symptoms.
a. Thrombosis that occurs below the knees rarely leads to pulmonary embolization unless the thrombus extends into the femoral vein.
b. DVTs from the iliofemoral, pelvic, ovarian, axillary, subclavian, and internal jugular veins, as well as the inferior vena cava and cavernous sinuses of the skull, can lead to PE.
   (1) About 60% to 80% of patients with a DVT will have a PE.
   (2) *More than half of these patients are asymptomatic.*
c. Clinical presentation is inconsistent but can include dyspnea, chest pain, hemoptysis, tachycardia, fever, rales, increased central venous pressures, electrocardiographic changes (arrhythmias, enlarged P waves, ST depression, T-wave inversions notably in leads III, AVF, V1, V3 and V4), and possibly arterial blood gas changes (unlikely acutely).
   (1) Physical examination is inconsistent and often nondiagnostic.
   (2) Most common symptoms according to Prospective Investigation of Pulmonary Embolism Diagnosis (PIOPED) study were dyspnea (73%), pleuritic chest pain (66%), cough (37%), and hemoptysis (13%).
d. Diagnosis is established by radiographic imaging studies.
   (1) The gold standard test—pulmonary angiography
       (a) Highly invasive, technically difficult to perform
   (2) Computed tomographic angiography is less invasive and offers nearly the same specificity and sensitivity as pulmonary angiography.
       (a) Has become the imaging modality of choice

(3) High-probability ventilation/perfusion (V/Q) scans coupled with a high clinical suspicion to PE is also diagnostic.
  (a) V/Q scans are not as frequently used given the accuracy of computed tomographic angiography.
(4) Chest radiographs initially are normal.
  (a) Rare findings include:
    (1) Westermark's sign—dilatation of the pulmonary vessels proximal to an embolism with collapse of distal vessels
    (2) Hampton hump—triangular, pleural-based infiltrate with the apex pointed toward the hilum, a rare late finding of pulmonary infarction

2. Postthrombotic syndrome—occurs in 50% of patients with acute DVT and signifies chronic venous insufficiency. Classic findings include brawny, nonpitting edema and ulcer formation.
3. Upper extremity DVT—presents with upper extremity swelling and/or pain, and less commonly with superior vena cava syndrome and loss of upper extremity vascular access.
a. Classification of upper extremity DVTs
  (1) Primary thrombosis—rare disorder occurring in the dominant arm of a healthy individual (Paget-Schroetter syndrome)
  (2) Heavy exertion or *effort thrombosis* is thought to cause microtrauma to the venous intima, leading to initiation and propagation of the coagulation cascade.
  (3) Secondary thrombosis—axillary or subclavian vein thrombosis caused by indwelling catheters for total parenteral nutrition, chemotherapy, and central cardiovascular monitoring
4. Other DVTs
a. Superior vena cava obstruction—related to tumor invasion, primary thrombosis, chronic fibrosing mediastinitis, or granulomatous disease.
b. Inferior vena cava thrombosis is generally related to the extension of thrombi from the pelvic or thigh veins.
c. Tumor thrombus is a consequence of tumor invasion (e.g., renal, hepatic, adrenal, soft tissue) into the vena cava.

## II. METHODS OF PROPHYLAXIS AND TREATMENT OF DEEP VENOUS THROMBOSES AND PULMONARY EMBOLI

### A.  DVT PROPHYLAXIS
1. Mechanical
a. Leg elevation—no substantial evidence to improve clinical outcomes
b. Graduated compression stockings (thromboembolism deterrent "TED" hose)—must be well fitted, with only a small effect.
c. Early ambulation—simple and extremely effective
d. Pneumatic compression boots or sequential compression devices
  (1) Promote venous return and activate the fibrinolytic system
  (2) Inexpensive and useful in patients who cannot be systemically anticoagulated
2. Pharmacologic agents (see the following section)

31

PE AND DT PROPHYLAXIS

## B. TREATMENT OF DVTS AND PULMONARY EMBOLI

### 1. Warfarin

a. Generally not used for prophylaxis

b. Disrupts the hepatic synthesis of vitamin K–dependent coagulation factors (II, VII, IX, and X, and proteins C and S)

c. Therapeutic levels vary depending on the reason for anticoagulation; however, the goal international normalized ratio is 2 to 3 for DVT.

   (1) Dosing must be individualized.

   (2) Multiple drug interactions

   (3) Effects reversed with the administration of vitamin K and fresh frozen plasma.

d. *Patients should be systemically anticoagulated with heparin before initiation given the prothrombotic state that occurs with depletion of proteins C and S.*

e. Contraindicated in pregnancy and in patients at risk for recurrent hemorrhage (recent CVA or head trauma)

f. Therapy is maintained for 3 to 6 months.

### 2. Unfractionated heparin

a. Used for prophylaxis and treatment

b. Increases the activity of antithrombin III and prevents conversion of fibrinogen to fibrin

c. Does not produce clot lysis but does inhibit active thrombogenesis

d. Therapeutic levels are dependent on the institution's laboratory.

e. Partial thromboplastin time must be monitored every 6 hours.

f. Dosing for systemic anticoagulation is based on weight with an 80-unit/kg intravenous bolus, followed by 18-unit/kg/hr maintenance infusion, and titrated to maintain therapeutic partial thromboplastic time.

   (1) Subtherapeutic dosing is used for prophylaxis and is administered subcutaneously in two or three times daily doses of between 5000 and 8000 units depending on the weight of the patient.

   (2) Reversed with the administration of protamine and fresh frozen plasma

g. Safe to use during pregnancy but contraindicated in patients with a history of HIT (heparin-induced thrombocytopenia)

### 3. Low-molecular-weight heparin (enoxaparin, dalteparin, tinzaparin)

a. Administered in once-daily dosing for prophylaxis and twice-daily dosing for systemic anticoagulation

   (1) Does not require systemic monitoring

   (2) Cannot be reversed with fresh frozen plasma; however, protamine can be given.

b. Primarily enhances the inhibition of factor Xa, but also thrombin, by increasing antithrombin III activity

c. More expensive than unfractionated heparin

d. Contraindicated in patients with HIT

e. Dosing is dependent on weight and is individualized depending on the manufacturer.

4. Thrombolytics (tissue plasminogen activator)
a. Used therapeutically only
b. Promote rapid clot lysis leading to prompt resolution of symptoms, restoration of normal venous circulation, and preservation of venous valvular function
   (1) Does not prevent clot propagation, rethrombosis, or subsequent embolization
   (2) Not effective if the thrombus is organized; will work only on the surface of the clot
   (3) Administered transvenously via a catheter-directed system to allow injection of the agent at the site of the clot
c. Patients must be systemically anticoagulated after administration of thrombolytics.
d. Multiple contraindications exist, including active internal hemorrhage, recent history of intracranial or intraspinal surgery or trauma, intracranial neoplasm, arteriovenous malformation or aneurysm, history of stroke in last 2 months, and bleeding diathesis.
5. Special circumstances—HIT
a. Prothrombotic disorder associated with a decrease in platelets, the administration of unfractionated heparin, and occasionally with low-molecular-weight heparin
b. Occurs typically within 2 weeks of heparin administration
c. Subdivided into HIT types I and II
   (1) HIT I—transient decrease in platelet count that corrects even if heparin treatment continues.
      (a) Platelet counts rarely decline to less than 100/L.
      (b) Not attributed to an immune reaction
   (2) HIT II—autoimmune reaction with antibodies (mainly IgG) reactive to platelet factor 4, neutrophil-activating peptide 2, and interleukin-8, which form complexes with heparin.
      (a) Most common antigen is heparin/platelet factor 4 complex caused by a conformational change in the protein.
d. Clinical diagnosis confirmed with HIT antibody panel; all heparin products should be stopped if suspected.
e. Alternatives for anticoagulation are lepirudin, danaparoid sodium, and argatroban (synthetic thrombin inhibitor).

## C. PROPHYLACTIC INFERIOR VENA CAVA FILTER PLACEMENT

1. Indicated for high-risk patients (quadriplegics, severe closed head injury, recurrent DVTs despite therapy) who have contraindications to other forms of prophylaxis or cannot be anticoagulated, or both
2. *The filter is designed to prevent embolization of a potentially fatal thrombus to the pulmonary circulation, not to prevent DVT.*
3. Technical considerations
a. Prevents embolism of thrombi >3 mm

b. Vena cava should be <30 mm (measured by venography) to deter migration.

c. Can be placed from either an internal jugular or femoral approach

4. Complications include malpositioning, persistent vena caval leak, filter thrombosis, filter migration, and caval thrombosis.

## III. AN APPROACH TO PROPHYLAXIS

### A. DETERMINE THE PATIENT'S RISK FACTORS

1. Low risk—age <40 years; ambulatory or minor surgery
2. Moderate risk—age >40 years; abdominal, pelvic, or thoracic surgery
3. High risk—age >40 years; prior DVT or PE, malignancy, hip and other orthopedic surgery, immobility, hypercoagulable states

### B. PROPHYLAXIS OF CHOICE

1. Encourage early ambulation in all patients and get physical/occupational therapist involved early if indicated.
2. Low-risk patients probably do not need prophylaxis.
3. Moderate-risk patients should have pneumatic compression boots, low-dose heparin prophylaxis, or low-molecular-weight heparin.
4. High-risk patients should have a combination of treatment consisting of pneumatic compression boots plus low-dose heparin or low-molecular-weight heparin. Full anticoagulation with warfarin or inferior vena cava filter placement can be considered in this population.
5. *Prophylaxis should be started before the initiation of anesthesia.*
a. *Vasodilatation associated with induction predisposes to formation of DVT.*
6. Ophthalmologic and neurosurgical patients with intracranial or spinal lesions are not candidates for prophylaxis with anticoagulants.
7. High-risk patients should be watched closely for clinical signs and symptoms of DVT in addition to frequent (every 3–4 days) objective testing. Duplex scanning is the least invasive of these methods, and its sensitivity is 88% in the lower extremity.

## IV. APPROACH TO THE PATIENT WITH PULMONARY EMBOLUS

### A. CONSIDERATIONS

1. Respiratory consequences: Increased physiologic alveolar dead space secondary to V/Q mismatch leads to pneumoconstriction, hypoxemia, and hyperventilation.
a. Hypoxemia is not a consistent finding in the acute presentation, and chest radiograph is normal in the majority of cases.
2. Hemodynamic consequences: PE leads to vascular congestion secondary to a decreased pulmonary vascular bed, leading to increased resistance (pulmonary hypertension). In the cardiac compromised patient, this can lead to cardiac collapse secondary to increased right ventricular afterload.

**B. THE PREVIOUS CONSIDERATIONS MAY NECESSITATE TRANSFER OF THE PATIENT TO A MONITORED CARE SETTING OR THE INTENSIVE CARE UNIT**

1. Aggressive respiratory care and monitoring often are obtainable only in an intensive care unit setting.
2. The patient can be intubated and given mechanical ventilatory support if necessary.

**C. CONSIDER ANTICOAGULATION VERSUS THROMBOLYTIC THERAPY**

1. Anticoagulation is mandatory for all patients suspected to have a PE, and diagnostic investigations should not delay empiric therapy.
2. Thrombolytics should be reserved for patients who are hemodynamically unstable and in patients with poor underlying cardiopulmonary reserve.
3. Refer to section II for a description of treatment modalities.

**D. SURGICAL TREATMENT OPTIONS**

1. Pulmonary embolectomy
   a. Open embolectomy—performed through median sternotomy with cardiopulmonary bypass; associated with >50% mortality and high morbidity.
   b. Transvenous embolectomy with a suction cap–tipped catheter passed via jugular or femoral vein
      (1) Especially useful in massive PE in which there is a contraindication to fibrinolytic therapy

31

PE AND DT PROPHYLAXIS

# The Diabetic Patient

*Rebecca J. McClaine, MD*

Diabetes mellitus currently affects about 10% of the U.S. population, with prevalence rates expected to increase over the next several decades. Although not typically a surgical disease, surgeons must be familiar with the complications and therapies associated with diabetes to appropriately care for this growing segment of their surgical population. This chapter focuses on the care of patients with diabetes before, during, and after surgery; glycemic control during critical illness; wound healing in patients with diabetes; and the one true surgically treated diabetic complication, the diabetic foot ulcer.

**32**

## I. DEFINITIONS

### A. DIABETES

1. Diagnosis of diabetes made by any two of the following tests performed on two different occasions:
a. Fasting blood glucose level (after 8-hour fast) ≥126 mg/dl
b. Oral glucose tolerance test (most sensitive test for diabetes)—8-hour fast, followed by drinking 75 g glucose; check blood glucose 2 hours later, glucose level ≥200 mg/dl
c. Random blood glucose level ≥200 mg/dl, with symptoms of thirst, polyuria, or weight loss
2. Prediabetes diagnosed by fasting blood glucose ≥100 mg/dl, or oral glucose tolerance test ≥140 mg/dl.
3. Type I diabetes (5–10% of total) is caused by autoimmune destruction of islet cells; insulin supplementation required.
4. Type II diabetes (90–95% of total) is caused by peripheral insulin resistance; treated by weight loss, diet modification, oral agents, or insulin.

## II. MEDICAL THERAPIES

### A. ORAL ANTIHYPERGLYCEMICS

1. Sulfonylureas (glipizide [Glucotrol], chlorpropamide, glimepiride, glyburide, tolazamide, tolbutamide)—stimulate insulin release from beta cells.
a. Can cause hypoglycemia for days after last dose
2. Short-acting insulin secretagogues (repaglinide [Prandin], nateglinide)—similar mechanism to sulfonylureas, less risk for hypoglycemia
3. Thiazolidinediones (pioglitazone [Actos], rosiglitazone)—increase peripheral insulin sensitivity.
a. Can cause volume expansion and induce heart failure
4. Biguanides (metformin [Glucophage])—decrease hepatic glucose production and intestinal glucose absorption, increase peripheral insulin sensitivity.

a. Cause lactic acidosis, contraindicated in dehydration and renal failure
b. Hold before administration of intravenous (IV) contrast.
5. α-Glucosidase inhibitors (acarbose [Precose], miglitol)—delay glucose absorption from intestine.

## B. INSULIN

1. **Rapid-acting**—lispro (Humalog), aspart (NovoLog)
a. Onset 15 to 30 minutes, peak 30 to 90 minutes, duration 3 to 4 hours
b. Used in continuous subcutaneous insulin pumps, can be given intravenously
2. **Fast-acting**—regular (Humulin R, Novolin R)
a. Onset 30 to 60 minutes, peak 2 to 4 hours, duration 6 to 10 hours
b. Used in continuous IV infusions
3. **Intermediate-acting**—NPH (Humulin N, Novolin N)
a. Onset 1 to 4 hours, peak 4 to 12 hours, duration 12 to 24 hours
b. Subcutaneously, cannot be given intravenously
4. **Long-acting**—glargine (Lantus)/lente (Humulin L), detemir (Levemir pen)
a. Onset 1 to 2 hours, peak 3 to 20 hours, duration 24 to 30 hours
b. Subcutaneously, cannot be given intravenously
c. Glargine cannot be mixed with other insulins for injection.

## C. ORDERING AN INSULIN REGIMEN IN A PATIENT WITH HYPERGLYCEMIA

1. Goal blood glucose varies, usually 80 to 130 mg/dl before meal and 90 to 140 mg/dl at bedtime.
2. Weight-based estimation of insulin need
a. Type 1 diabetic will require 0.4 to 0.7 unit/kg/day.
b. Type 2 diabetic will require 0.3 to 1 unit/kg/day.
3. Traditional subcutaneous sliding scale insulin
a. Fast- or rapid-acting insulin is dosed before every meal and at bedtime, or on every 4 to 6 hours schedule for patients not eating, based on blood glucose level checked at that time.
b. When 24-hour insulin requirement is known, either after conversion from continuous IV infusion or after doses of subcutaneous sliding scale given for 1 day, may add long-acting insulin to regimen totaling 50% of daily requirement.
c. Advantages include it is commonly used and relatively easy to order and administer.
d. Disadvantages include it is nonphysiologic and reactive in treating hyperglycemia instead of proactive in avoiding it.
4. Basal-bolus-correction subcutaneous dosing.
a. Goal is to administer 50% of daily insulin in a long-acting form to mimic physiologic continuous *basal* insulin secretion and 50% as 3 subcutaneous *boluses* of fast- or rapid-acting insulin to mimic physiologic prandial insulin peaks.

b. Based on premeal blood glucose levels, subcutaneous "correction" dose of fast- or rapid-acting insulin may be given with scheduled bolus. Basal and bolus doses are then adjusted for the next day's orders to try to eliminate need for correction doses.

c. Bolus doses are given on every 6 hours schedule for patient who is not eating and receiving continuous tube feeds.

d. Advantages include being more physiologic and easy to convert to this protocol from continuous insulin infusion (when 24-hour insulin requirement is known).

e. Disadvantages include being a more confusing regimen to order and administer.

5. **Continuous IV insulin infusion (insulin drip)**

a. In most hospitals, used only in intensive care unit (ICU) setting.

b. Usually, regular insulin is used.

c. Blood glucose levels checked every hour for 4 hours, then may be decreased gradually to every 4 hours if blood glucose levels stabilize on set rate of insulin infusion.

d. Blood glucose levels checked hourly for 3 hours after patient starts eating.

e. If nutritional therapy (total parenteral nutrition or continuous tube feeds) is discontinued, decrease infusion rate by 50%.

f. Patient should receive 5 to 10 g glucose/hr as food, tube feeds, total parenteral nutrition, or IV fluids (D5 at 100–200 ml/hr).

g. When converting to subcutaneous therapy, give 40% of daily insulin requirement as intermediate- or long-acting insulin. If ordering basal-bolus-correction regimen, give 40% of daily requirement divided by 3 and given as bolus doses before meals.

6. **Persistent hyperglycemia**

a. Review amount of carbohydrate patient is receiving (should be 5–10 g glucose/hr). Adjust maintenance IV fluids or tube feeds to keep carbohydrates at, but not above, this infusion goal.

b. Other IV medications should be mixed in solution without dextrose when possible.

## D. ADJUSTING MEDICATIONS FOR SURGERY

1. **Preoperative adjustments**

a. Hold chlorpropamide, glyburide, glipizide 48 to 72 hours before surgery (long half-life).

b. All other oral agents may be taken until the day before or day of surgery.

c. One-half usual dose of intermediate- or long-acting insulin given the morning of surgery.

2. **Intraoperative adjustments**

a. Patients with type II diabetes undergoing short procedure with preoperative glucose level <140 mg/dl will likely not need insulin during surgery.

32

THE DIABETIC PATIENT

b. Patients with type II diabetes undergoing short procedure can be managed with glucose checks and doses of subcutaneous rapid- or short-acting insulin.

c. For other patients with type II and all with type I diabetes, use continuous IV infusion (together with infusion of dextrose) intraoperatively; goal blood glucose level is 100–150 mg/dl.

d. Monitor blood glucose levels every 1 to 2 hours intraoperatively.

e. Subcutaneous insulin pumps should be turned off and IV infusion substituted.

**3. Postoperative adjustments**

a. Hold metformin after surgery for 48 hours until normal diet is resumed and until normal renal function has been documented.

b. Other oral agents may be restarted after surgery when patient resumes normal diet.

c. Ideally, can maintain continuous IV insulin infusion until patient starts regular (not liquid) diet.

d. Give normal subcutaneous intermediate- or long-acting dose before meal, then stop insulin infusion 2 hours after meal.

e. If not feasible to maintain continuous infusion after surgery, give patient one-half usual doses of intermediate- or long-acting insulin as part of sliding-scale or basal-bolus-correction orders until normal diet is resumed.

**4. Discharge adjustments**

a. Any patient requiring insulin while hospitalized should have follow-up with primary care physician to be evaluated or treated for diabetes.

b. Patients requiring less than 20 units/day insulin may be discharged without insulin or oral therapy.

c. Patients requiring 20 to 35 units/day insulin should be discharged on an oral antihyperglycemic medication, with glucometer, diabetes teaching, and appropriate follow-up.

d. Patients requiring more than 35 units/day insulin should be discharged on their in-hospital insulin regimen, with glucometer, diabetes teaching, and appropriate follow-up.

## E. HYPOGLYCEMIA (BLOOD GLUCOSE LEVEL <70 MG/DL)

**1. Therapies that increase risk for hypoglycemia**

a. Discontinuation of glucose source without adjustment of dose

b. Administration of regular insulin every 4 hours (half-life is 6 hours, leads to "stacking")

c. Continuous venovenous hemodialysis with bicarbonate substitution fluid

d. Inotropic support

e. Octreotide therapy

**2. Initial therapy**

a. If patient is awake and able to swallow, give 15 g oral glucose (as glucose tablets, 4 oz juice or soda, or 8 oz milk).

b. If patient is unconscious or unable to swallow, give 15 g IV glucose (30 ml dextrose 50%).

c. Recheck blood glucose in 15 minutes.

d. Repeat process until blood sugar level >70 mg/dl.

**3. Prevent recurrence.**

a. If more than 1 hour until next meal, give snack with 15 g carbohydrate and protein/fat.

b. In unconscious patient, give additional 15 g glucose if blood glucose level is <90 mg/dl.

c. Do NOT hold dose of intermediate- or long-acting insulin for single episode of hypoglycemia. If multiple episodes occur, decrease dose as appropriate.

### F. DIABETIC KETOACIDOSIS

1. Usually occurs in patients with type I diabetes and is caused by inappropriate insulin dosing or infection

2. Hyperglycemia (250–800 mg/dl) with anion-gap acidosis and ketotic diuresis

3. Treatment

a. Insulin at 0.1 unit/kg/hr IV infusion, decrease to 50% of rate when bicarbonate increases to greater than 16 mEq/L.

b. Fluids (normal saline) at 1 L/hr for 2 hours, then change to half-normal saline at 250 to 500 ml/hr. Add dextrose to fluids when serum glucose level <250 mg/dl and decrease rate to 100 to 250 ml/hr.

c. Expect profound potassium and phosphate deficits with correction of acidosis and hyperglycemia.

### G. NONKETOTIC HYPEROSMOLAR HYPERGLYCEMIA

1. Usually occurs in patients with type II diabetes and is caused by infection

2. Hyperglycemia (>1000 mg/dl) with hypertonic serum and osmotic diuresis

3. Treatment similar to that for hypovolemic hypernatremia

a. Fluids (normal saline) to replace calculated free water deficit (with correction of plasma sodium level, which will be falsely reduced by hyperglycemia)

b. Insulin therapy only after hypovolemia is corrected

### III. GLYCEMIC CONTROL IN THE CRITICALLY ILL PATIENT

### A. HYPERGLYCEMIC RESPONSE TO SURGERY AND ANESTHESIA

1. Up-regulation of sympathomimetic and hypothalamopituitary-adrenal axis leads to high levels of catecholamines and glucocorticoids, resulting in hyperglycemia.

2. Counterregulatory hormones (glucagons, corticotrophin, growth hormone), up-regulated in response to stress, promote hepatic gluconeogenesis and peripheral lipolysis and glycolysis (insulin resistance).

3. Proinflammatory cytokines (tumor necrosis factor-$\alpha$ and interleukin-6) induce peripheral insulin resistance by blocking expression of insulin-dependent (GLUT 4) membrane glucose transporters.

### B. IATROGENIC HYPERGLYCEMIA
1. Can be exacerbated by IV dextrose infusions, parenteral or enteral nutrition, or steroid administration. Immobility alone also leads to insulin resistance in skeletal muscles.

### C. GLYCEMIC CONTROL
1. Blood glucose between 70 and 110 mg/dl demonstrated to significantly reduce mortality and length of ICU stay in surgical ICU setting.
2. All ICU patients should have blood sugar levels monitored and continuous IV insulin therapy initiated in individuals with hyperglycemia, regardless of personal history of diabetes.
3. Many ICUs have established insulin protocols based on this evidence.

### IV. COMPLICATIONS OF DIABETES
### A. TISSUE HYPOXIA CAUSED BY MICROVASCULAR DISEASE.
1. Endothelial cell dysfunction
a. Hyperglycemia encourages intracellular conversion of glucose to sorbitol, which cannot diffuse across cell membrane.
b. Leads to metabolic alterations and production of abnormal basement membrane proteins
2. Thickening of capillary basement membrane
a. In early diabetes, hyperglycemia leads to increased microvascular blood flow.
b. Capillary hypertension leads to shear stress on vascular wall, leading to accumulation of fibronectin in basement membrane.
c. Leads to changes in capillary permeability
3. Dysregulation of microvascular circulation
a. Rigid basement membrane prevents local vasodilatation in response to tissue damage, leading to hypoxia and tissue breakdown.
4. The process is responsible for retinopathy and nephropathy, and contributes to poor wound healing associated with diabetes.
5. Can be delayed, but not completely prevented, by good glycemic control

### B. INCREASED RISK FOR INFECTION AND SLOW WOUND HEALING BECAUSE OF IMPAIRED IMMUNE FUNCTION
1. Chemotaxis of leukocytes and macrophages impaired by hyperglycemia
2. Leads to prolonged inflammatory phase of wound healing
3. Delay leads to slower rate of collagen synthesis in wound and decreased granulation tissue in wound as healing continues, compared with wounds of patients without diabetes.

4. Patients with diabetes are at increased risk for perioperative infections, including wound infections.
5. Patients with diabetes, compared with those without, are also at increased risk for Staphylococcal infections, Fournier's gangrene, and candidiasis.
6. Risk for infection can be decreased with good glycemic control, but poor healing occurs even in patients with well-controlled disease.

### C. INCREASED RATE OF ATHEROSCLEROSIS LEADS TO MACROVASCULAR DISEASE.

1. Enhanced thrombotic potential in patients with diabetes because of endothelial dysfunction (leading to decreased production of nitric oxide, a vasodilator) and up-regulation of platelet aggregation.
2. Peripheral vascular disease (PVD) and diabetes
a. Patients with diabetes with PVD are at greater risk for amputation than patients without diabetes with PVD.
b. Cardiovascular and cerebrovascular event rates are greater in patients with diabetes with PVD than in patients without diabetes with PVD.
c. Patients with diabetes with PVD may not suffer from claudication, due to peripheral neuropathy, leading to delayed diagnosis.
d. Pattern of occlusive disease typically involves medium-sized arteries (popliteal trifurcation) and spares distal (small) vessels.
e. Diagnostic studies—ankle/brachial indices (often falsely increased because of tibial artery calcification), exercise ankle/brachial indices, segmental pressure and pulse volume recordings, toe pressures
3. Rate of disease progression may be slowed, but not normalized, by good glycemic control.

### D. NEUROPATHIES OCCUR IN MOTOR, SENSORY, AND AUTONOMIC NERVES.

1. Charcot's neuroarthropathy (Charcot's foot)
a. Motor neuropathy leads to muscle weakness, atrophy, and paresis.
b. Sensory neuropathy leads to loss of protective sensations and development of deformities.
c. Autonomic neuropathy leads to vasodilatation and decreased sweating, causing warm feet and dry skin.
2. Gastroparesis, resulting in need for nasogastric decompression or promotility agent (metoclopramide) perioperatively

### V. DIABETIC FOOT ULCERS

### A. OCCURRENCE

1. Risk for patients with diabetes experiencing development of an ulcer is 12% to 25% over lifetime.
2. Amputations are 15 times more common in patients with versus without diabetes.
3. Ulcer precedes amputation in 84% of patients.

32

THE DIABETIC PATIENT

4. Can differentiate from arterial and venous ulcers by location and symptoms.
a. Diabetic ulcers are located on high-weight-bearing areas (metatarsal heads), dry or weeping, and painless unless infected.
b. Arterial ulcers (10% of foot ulcers) are located on distal toes, dry, painful, and surrounded by shiny skin; pain is relieved with dependent positioning.
c. Venous ulcers (70% of foot ulcers) are located superior to medial (or lateral) malleolus, weeping, painless unless infected, surrounded by dry, discolored skin with lower extremity edema.

## B. PATHOPHYSIOLOGY
1. Neuropathy (Charcot's foot, as described earlier)
2. Ischemia—secondary to both microvascular and macrovascular dysfunction
a. Majority of diabetic foot ulcers are not caused by PVD.
b. Ulcers occurring in patients with diabetes with PVD are more likely to lead to amputation.

## C. PREVENTION
1. Routine foot care
a. Daily inspection for skin breakdown
b. Prompt removal (debridement) of any callus
c. Treatment of onychomycosis (nail fungus) with topical or oral agents. Brittle diseased nails present less of a barrier to bacterial infection.
d. Fitting with orthotic shoes to minimize daily trauma to feet
2. Somatosensory (monofilament) testing annually to detect diminished sensation
3. Early detection of PVD (annual ankle/brachial indices in individual with diabetes older than 50 years, with follow-up studies for falsely increased results) and early revascularization procedures
4. Smoking cessation

## D. MANAGEMENT
1. Surgical debridement of hyperkeratotic (callused), necrotic, and infected tissue (including bone) to healthy bleeding wound bed, regardless of depth of wound
2. Assessment for infection—purulent or foul-smelling drainage, warmth, erythema, tenderness
a. Failure of wound to heal after proper debridement may also indicate infection.
b. Deep tissue cultures (not superficial wound swabs) should be obtained at time of debridement or in nonhealing wounds after debridement.
c. Infections are often polymicrobial, with gram-positive cocci, gram-negative rods, and anaerobes, usually NOT *Pseudomonas.*

d. IV antibiotic therapy is often required for optimal tissue penetration. Patients undergoing therapy with oral antibiotics should have close outpatient follow-up to ensure healing of wound or resolution of symptoms/signs of infection.

e. Antibiotic regimen should be tailored to culture results. Empiric regimens include ampicillin/sulbactam (Unasyn), piperacillin/tazobactam (Zosyn), and clindamycin plus ciprofloxacin or levofloxacin.

3. **Osteomyelitis treated by surgical removal of infected bone, followed by IV antibiotics for remaining infection in surrounding soft tissue (usually 6 weeks).**

a. Classic radiographic findings (demineralization, periosteal reaction, bony destruction) take up to 2 weeks to appear, when 30% to 50% of bone has been destroyed.

b. Other imaging modalities include magnetic resonance imaging (most sensitive and specific), bone scan, and bone probe.

c. Often a clinical diagnosis at time of debridement, with appearance of purulent material around bone and spongy texture of bone when removed. During debridement, any bone removed (for biopsy) should be cultured.

4. **Dressings should be designed to keep wound bed moist to promote migration of fibroblasts and epithelialization of wound.**

a. Wet-to-dry dressings also allow for mechanical debridement of fibrinous exudate and devitalized tissue with dressing changes.

b. Packing of deeper tracts with moist packing gauze allows for healing by secondary intention.

c. Wounds with large amounts of exudate usually require dry dressings and frequent changes.

d. Recombinant platelet-derived growth factor-B applied as gel directly to wound under wet-to-dry dressings has demonstrated mixed results in accelerating wound healing.

e. Cultured skin products (biologic dressings) have been used on dry wound with granulation tissue bed with mixed results. Product is usually changed or replaced about every 6 weeks, with frequent wound checks and topical dressing consisting of Adaptic (nonadherent gauze dressing) and Bacitracin or petroleum jelly.

f. Negative pressure wound therapy (vacuum-assisted closure device, V.A.C.) dressings have gained popularity in treating many wounds. For foot ulcers, offer continuous wound drainage, mechanical debridement (when sponge is changed), less frequent dressing changes (every 48–72 hours).

5. **Off-loading of pressure from wound is necessary for healing of ulcer.**

a. Elevate foot above level of heart when sitting or in bed.

b. Previously, total contact casting (Luna-boots), which is molded carefully to shape of foot and distributes weight to all parts of foot during ambulation, often was used. Application performed by specialized technicians, and wound cannot be visualized easily.

**32**

**THE DIABETIC PATIENT**

   c. Current techniques include cast-walkers and half shoes, which are tailored specifically for the involved foot to keep weight distributed to all parts of foot except ulcer.

6. Weekly measurements of wound size to objectively document healing (shrinking).

## E. ALL DIABETIC FOOT WOUNDS WITHOUT ISCHEMIA OR INFECTION (INCLUDING OSTEOMYELITIS) SHOULD HEAL.

## RECOMMENDED READING

Brem H, Sheehan P, Rosenberg HJ: Evidence-based protocol for diabetic foot ulcers. *Plast Reconstr Surg* 117(7 suppl):193S–211S, 2006.

Marso SP, Hiatt WR: Peripheral arterial disease in patients with diabetes. *J Am Coll Cardiol* 47:921–929, 2006.

Van den Berghe G, Wouters P, Weekers F, et al: Intensive insulin therapy in the critically ill patients. *N Engl J Med* 345:1359–1367, 2001.

# Peripheral Vascular Disease

*Alexander J. Bondoc, MD*

This chapter encompasses disease of the renal arteries and the arterial system of the lower extremities.

## I. DEFINITIONS

1. Refers to a constellation of disorders that result from stenotic, occlusive, and aneurysmal diseases of the aorta and its branch arteries, exclusive of the coronary arteries

2. American Heart Association guidelines define peripheral artery disease (PAD) as a vascular disease caused primarily by atherosclerosis and thromboembolic pathophysiology processes that alter the normal structure and function of the aorta, its visceral arterial branches, and the arteries of the lower extremity.

## II. EPIDEMIOLOGY

### A. PREVALENCE
2 million individuals are symptomatic, millions more asymptomatic.

### B. NATURAL HISTORY
Slow progression over time
1. Twenty to 25 percent of symptomatic patients will require revascularization.
2. Five percent of symptomatic patients will progress to critical limb ischemia.
3. Severity of disease often depends on the presence of multilevel disease and concurrent diabetes.

### C. QUALITY OF LIFE, MORBIDITY, AND MORTALITY IMPLICATIONS ARE SIGNIFICANT.
1. Compromised ambulation → impaired exercise tolerance
2. Lower extremity ulceration
3. Need for surgery
4. Predictor for other vascular disease
a. Coronary artery disease occurs in upward of 90% of patients with PAD.
b. Cerebrovascular disease of more than 70% of region is found in 30% of patients with PAD.
c. Furthermore, PAD as demonstrated by decreased ankle/brachial index (ABI) predicts increased rates of overall mortality and mortality related to coronary artery disease and cerebrovascular disease.

## III. PATHOPHYSIOLOGY

### A. ATHEROSCLEROSIS—MOST COMMON CAUSE

1. Risk factors—similar to those related to other atheroembolic disease
a. Advanced age—>70 or those >50 with other atherosclerotic risk factors
b. Sex
c. Smoking—most important modifiable risk factor
d. Diabetes mellitus—increases risk by two- to four-fold.
e. Hyperlipidemia
f. Hypertension
g. Hyperhomocystinemia
h. Increased C-reactive protein level
2. Anatomy influences hemodynamics—formation of plaque on lateral walls.
3. Modified response to injury hypothesis
a. Endothelial injury caused by hyperlipidemia, smoking, shear, and hypertension.
b. Monocytes attach to endothelium because they secrete platelet-derived growth factor.
c. Plaque increases in size.
d. Increased platelet activity leads to more endothelial injury.
e. Smooth muscle cells secrete extracellular matrix and accumulate lipids.
4. Inciting events such as plaque ulceration or rupture can induce thrombosis.

### B. IN SITU THROMBOSIS/THROMBOEMBOLISM

1. Prothrombotic conditions
a. Hypercoagulability disorders—most common is factor V Leiden.
b. Associated prothrombotic state associated with malignancy
2. Thromboembolic disease
a. Macroembolic—often from a cardiac source
b. Microembolic—cardiac or arterial source

### C. DEGENERATIVE DISEASES

Loss of structural integrity of the arterial wall with subsequent dilation
1. Collagen disorders (e.g., Marfan's and Ehlers–Danlos syndromes)
2. Others are less well understood (e.g., cystic medial necrosis, neurofibromatosis).

### D. DYSPLASTIC DISORDERS (E.G., FIBROMUSCULAR DYSPLASIA)

### E. ARTERITIDES

Can affect any vascular bed.
1. Small vessels—often related to autoimmune or connective tissue diseases.
2. Medium vessels (e.g., polyarteritis nodosa, temporal arteritis)
3. Large vessels (e.g., Takayasu's arteritis)

## F. VASOSPASTIC DISEASE

The pathologic vasoconstriction that affects any muscular vessel in the body.

1. Examples in the periphery—Raynaud's phenomenon

**Case:** *A 70-year-old man with a history of previous stroke and insulin-dependent diabetes presents to your clinic with a history of bilateral foot cramping after walking about two to three blocks.*

## IV. DIAGNOSIS

### A. HISTORY

1. Comprehensive cardiovascular evaluation
2. *Claudication*—reports of cramping, tightness, or aching in the lower extremities brought on by exertion and relieved by rest
   a. Note which muscle groups are affected to correlate which vascular beds are affected.
       (1) Iliac occlusive disease often produces hip, buttock, and thigh pain.
       (2) Femoral and popliteal disease causes calf pain.
       (3) Tibial disease often causes calf pain but also foot numbness and pain.
   b. *Leriche syndrome*—aortoiliac disease that causes the triad of buttock claudication, impotence, and muscular atrophy.
   c. Distinguish claudication from "pseudoclaudication," which can be caused by severe venous occlusive disease, chronic compartment syndrome, spinal stenosis, or radiculopathies.
3. Noticeable skin changes, temperature abnormalities, and hair loss of the lower extremities
4. *Critical limb ischemia*—limb pain that occurs at rest or impending limb loss.
   a. Often indicative of chronic, multilevel disease
   b. Pain may sometimes be absent because of concomitant neuropathic disorders.
   c. Ulcers—most often arterial (on the toes and feet, extremely painful) and often become infected with polymicrobial organisms, especially in individuals with diabetes.
       (1) Venous ulcers—located on the malleoli
       (2) Neurotrophic—often deep and infected and found on the foot sole
5. *Acute limb ischemia*—rapid or sudden loss in limb perfusion that threatens tissue viability.
   a. Causes
       (1) Embolism
           (a) Sudden onset without previous symptoms
           (b) Known embolic source—atrial fibrillation, dilated cardiomyopathy
           (c) Usually lodge at arterial branch points where arterial lumina narrow

(2) Thrombosis
  (a) Often superimposed on an ulcerated mural thrombus
  (b) Thrombus also often propagates distally.
  (c) Most commonly occurs at the superficial femoral artery
b. Severity of ischemia depends on:
  (1) Location of occlusion
  (2) Extent of occlusion
  (3) Capacity of collateralization
c. Often characterized by the 6 *P*s—often found in the first webspace
  (1) Pain out of proportion to stimuli
  (2) Paralysis
  (3) Paresthesias
  (4) Pulselessness
  (5) Pallor
  (6) Polar or cold limb
6. Importantly, many patients may have asymptomatic PAD. Claudication questionnaires may detect subtle but clinically significant functional impairments.
a. Slower walking velocity
b. Poor standing balance
c. Slower time to rise from a standing position

## B. PHYSICAL EXAMINATION
1. Blood pressure in bilateral upper extremities
2. Lower extremity inspection
a. Ulcers/gangrene
b. Edema
c. Nail thickness
d. Absence of hair
e. Skin dryness
f. Cool temperature
3. Pulse examination
a. Femoral, popliteal, dorsalis pedis, and posterior tibial
b. Graded as absent, diminished, or normal (scale of 0–2) and compared bilaterally
c. Palpation of the abdomen for aneurysmal disease
d. In acute limb ischemia, pulses are often present in one limb but absent in the contralateral one.
4. Bruit auscultation—carotids, abdomen, and flank

## C. DIAGNOSTIC STUDIES
1. ABI—should be performed in any patients with claudication symptoms.
a. Lower extremity systolic blood pressure divided by the higher of two upper extremity systolic blood pressures
b. Value
  (1) Reference: 1 to 1.3
  (2) Claudication: 0.8 to 0.5

(3) Rest pain: 0.5 to 0.3
(4) Tissue loss: <0.3

c. Advantages
   (1) Inexpensive
   (2) Can monitor disease progression, predict limb survival
   (3) Predictor of cardiovascular morbidity/mortality

d. Limitations
   (1) Calcified distal arteries, specifically in individuals with diabetes, may be noncompressible, producing artificially high ABIs. Instead, toe/brachial index measurements can be performed.
   (2) Inability to localize arterial lesions

e. Exercise testing with ABI
   (1) Can unmask PAD in patients with normal resting ABIs
   (2) Can differentiate between claudication and "pseudoclaudication"

2. **Segmental pressures and pulse volume recordings**
a. Compares bilateral systolic blood pressures at sequential arterial levels, as well as the magnitude and contour of pulse volumes

b. Advantages
   (1) Can provide localization of anatomic lesions
   (2) Good to use as a postoperative monitor of recurrent disease/graft patency

c. Limitations
   (1) Qualitative, not quantitative evaluation of disease
   (2) May not be accurate in more distal arterial beds

3. **Doppler waveform analysis**
a. Measures arterial velocities, which should increase going from proximal to distal, and velocity waveforms

b. Advantages
   (1) Able to assess patients with diabetes with calcified vessels
   (2) Able to assess PAD severity and progression

c. Limitations
   (1) Highly operator dependent
   (2) Inability to pinpoint arterial lesion
   (3) Low accuracy in tortuous or overlapping segments

4. **Duplex ultrasound**
a. Able to diagnose anatomic location and degree of stenosis
b. Can be used for preinterventional decision making
c. Also can evaluate the following conditions:
   (1) Aneurysms
   (2) Arterial dissection
   (3) Popliteal entrapment syndrome
   (4) Soft-tissue masses
d. Advantages
   (1) High specificity
   (2) Delineates flow turbulence, vessel characteristics, and changes in velocity

     (3) Important for postrevascularization surveillance, specifically venous conduits

e. Disadvantages

     (1) High cost relative to other noninvasive tests

     (2) Decreased sensitivity for detecting stenoses downstream from more proximal disease

## 5. Computed tomographic angiography

a. An angiographic image is created from multiple cross-sectional images that can then be rotated to any oblique view.

b. Advantages

     (1) Delineates anatomy and significant stenoses

     (2) Evaluates associated soft-tissue and arterial wall defects

     (3) *Can be a helpful adjunct for operative planning*

c. Limitations

     (1) Spatial resolution improving with multidetector scanners but still limited compared with angiography.

     (2) Arterial phase may be obscured by venous filling or asymmetric contrast boluses.

     (3) Not as reliable and accurate as magnetic resonance angiography

     (4) Iodinated contrast risks

## 6. Magnetic resonance angiography

a. Advantages

     (1) Delineates anatomy and significant stenoses

     (2) Diagnostic accuracy similar to angiography

     (3) *Can also be a helpful adjunct for operative planning*

b. Limitations

     (1) Often overestimates the degree of stenosis caused by flow turbulence

     (2) Cannot be used in patients with magnetic resonance–incompatible metal prostheses

## 7. Contrast angiography

a. Most common diagnostic study to stratify patients before intervention

b. Advantages

     (1) Gold standard—able to delineate inflow and outflow vasculature and to characterize lesion

     (2) Able to preoperatively treat selected lesions with endoluminal therapies

     (3) Able to perform superselective angiography and oblique views

c. Disadvantages

     (1) Contrast load—contrast nephropathy, allergic reaction

     (2) Vascular access complications—atrioventricular fistula, dissection

     (3) Limited views of tibial-pedal circulation, eccentric lesions

## V. MANAGEMENT OF ATHEROSCLEROTIC PAD

### A. MEDICAL MANAGEMENT

It is important to minimize progression of PAD and risk for concurrent coronary or cerebrovascular events.

1. Risk factor modification
   a. Lipid lowering with a statin and/or fibric acid derivative for hypertriglyceridemia
   b. Antihypertensive therapy—beta-blockers and angiotensin-converting enzyme inhibitors have been demonstrated to reduce cardiovascular risks in patients with PAD.
   c. Maintain normoglycemia in patients with diabetes mellitus—goal is hemoglobin $A_{1c}$ <7%.
   d. Smoking cessation
2. **Antiplatelet therapy—important for both asymptomatic and symptomatic patients**
   a. Low-dose acetylsalicylic acid (81 or 325 mg/day) decreases cardiovascular events in patients with PAD.
   b. Clopidogrel is an effective alternative to acetylsalicylic acid therapy.
3. *Exercise rehabilitation is extremely effective with regard to risk factor modification and, more importantly, the improvement of claudication symptoms.*
4. Pharmacologic agents
   a. Cilostazol—a phosphodiesterase inhibitor. Not for use in patients with arrhythmias or heart failure.
   b. Pentoxifylline—modifies platelet shape and has weak antithrombotic properties. Not much difference from placebo and second line to cilostazol.
5. **Proper foot care, especially in patients with diabetes**

## B. REVASCULARIZATION THERAPY
1. Endovascular therapy
   a. Include a variety of therapies:
      (1) Angioplasty with balloon dilation
      (2) Stents
      (3) Atherectomy
      (4) Thrombolysis/thrombectomy
   b. Choosing endovascular therapy versus surgery
      (1) Anatomy of the lesion
      (2) Severity of patient symptoms
      (3) Comorbid conditions
      (4) Risks of surgical intervention
   c. Angioplasty
      (1) Better for more proximal vessels, that is, common iliac lesions
      (2) Patency decreases with the following conditions:
         (a) Long segment disease
         (b) Multiple lesions
         (c) Poor runoff
         (d) Multiple comorbid conditions
   d. Stenting
      (1) Most effective in:

33

PERIPHERAL VASCULAR DISEASE

      (a) A single stenosis of the common or external iliac arteries less than 3 cm (unilateral or bilateral)

      (b) A single stenosis of the superficial femoral or popliteal arteries less than 3 cm

    (2) Can be used as salvage therapy for failed angioplasty in the femoral, popliteal, and tibial arteries

## 2. Surgical bypass therapy

a. Reserved for disabling claudication and critical limb ischemia because the natural history of claudication is relatively benign.

    (1) Lack of response to exercise and pharmacotherapy

    (2) Severe impairment in activities of daily living

    (3) Absence of other significant comorbid conditions

    (4) Suitable vascular anatomy

b. Preoperative assessment

    (1) History and physical examination

    (2) Cardiovascular risk assessment must be performed to stratify patients.

      (a) Identify major, intermediate, and minor clinical predictors of increased perioperative cardiovascular risk.

      (b) Further testing such as electrocardiogram, chemical stress test, or coronary angiography may be necessary.

      (c) Coronary revascularization whether bypass grafting or percutaneous intervention may be necessary before elective intermediate- or high-risk surgery.

    (3) Patients with significant PAD often have significant coronary artery disease.

      (a) *Preoperative beta-blockade* should be used if there are no contraindications.

      (b) Clonidine may have similar cardioprotective properties.

    (4) Patients younger than 50 years with significant claudication often have a more virulent form of PAD and, as a result, have poorer outcomes after surgery.

c. General principles

    (1) Identification of patterns of arterial obstruction

      (a) Inflow disease—stenosis or occlusion of the suprainguinal vessels, most often the infrarenal aorta and iliac arteries

      (b) Outflow disease—stenosis or occlusion of the infrainguinal lower extremity arterial tree

      (c) Runoff disease—stenosis or occlusion in the trifurcation vessels (anterior tibial, posterior tibial, and peroneal arteries)

    (2) Choice of bypass conduit

      (a) Autogenous vein

        (1) Regarded as best, specifically for below knee bypass

        (2) Will restenose at the midpoint and anastomotic sites

      (b) Synthetic material (Dacron, Gore-Tex)

        (1) Best for above knee bypass when vein is not available

          (2) Fail more frequently because of native arterial inflow and vessel outflow

d. Specific procedures

  (1) Inflow disease

    (a) Aortobifemoral bypass—for patients with aortoiliac disease

    (b) Adequate aortic inflow with iliac disease

      (1) Endovascular therapy is a strong consideration.

      (2) Subsequent iliac endarterectomy with iliofemoral or fem-femoral bypass

    (c) Patients with severe comorbidities

      (1) Axillofemoral bypass with subsequent fem-femoral bypass

      (2) Reserved for patients with no other options for revascularization

  (2) Outflow disease—most commonly bypassing superficial femoral artery and proximal popliteal disease

    (a) Popliteal artery bypass

      (1) Vein conduit is preferred whether bypassing to the above or below knee popliteal artery.

      (2) Use of synthetic material should be reserved for bypassing to the below-knee popliteal artery when no autogenous vein is available.

    (b) Distal artery bypass (e.g., femoral-tibial)

      (1) Prosthetic material should be avoided because of high failure rates.

      (2) The least diseased tibial or pedal artery should be used as outflow.

## C. CRITICAL LIMB ISCHEMIA

**1. More aggressive natural history as compared with intermittent claudication**

a. One-year mortality rate for patients with chronic critical limb ischemia is 20%.

b. Approximately 50% of patients will require revascularization.

c. Forty percent of patients who have lesions that cannot be revascularized/reconstructed will require amputation in 6 months.

d. Pharmacotherapy considerations

  (1) Cilostazol and pentoxifylline are not useful.

  (2) Angiogenic growth factors need further investigation.

e. Endovascular therapy—may be used as an adjunct for multilevel disease common in critical limb ischemia. Inflow should be addressed first.

**2. Surgical therapy**

a. As described earlier, but more often, multilevel disease is present.

b. Inflow lesions should be addressed first.

c. Sequential composite grafts (combination vein and prosthetic grafts, jump grafts) may be necessary.

d. If tissue loss or persistent infection is present, limb amputation may be the only surgical option.

3. **Postoperative care**

a. Important to evaluate for recurrent disease and new arterial lesions

b. Infrainguinal revascularization is less durable than aortoiliac revascularization.

c. History and physical examination as described earlier including palpation of the graft pulse

d. Imaging

   (1) ABIs are mandatory.

   (2) Duplex ultrasound of the graft

e. Antiplatelet therapy is essential.

**Case:** *A 66-year-old woman with a history of rate-controlled atrial fibrillation and 1.5 packs/day smoking history presents with severe pain in her left ankle with walking.*

## D. ACUTE LIMB ISCHEMIA
Rapid or sudden loss in limb perfusion that threatens tissue viability.

1. **Causes**

a. Embolism

   (1) Sudden onset without previous symptoms

   (2) Known embolic source—atrial fibrillation, dilated cardiomyopathy

   (3) Usually lodge at arterial branch points where arterial lumen narrows

b. Thrombosis

   (1) Often superimposed on an ulcerated mural thrombus

   (2) Thrombus also often propagates distally.

   (3) Most commonly occurs at the superficial femoral artery

2. **Severity of ischemia depends on the following factors:**

a. Location of occlusion.

b. Extent of occlusion.

c. Capacity of collateralization.

3. **Often characterized by the 6 *P*s—often found in the first webspace**

a. Pain out of proportion to stimuli

b. Paralysis

c. Paresthesias

d. Pulselessness

e. Pallor

f. Polar or cold limb

4. **Diagnosis**

a. Often diagnosed by history and acute onset of symptoms

b. Clinical categories of acute limb ischemia (Table 33-1)

5. **Therapy—determined by limb viability**

**TABLE 33-1**

CLINICAL CATEGORIES OF ACUTE LIMB ISCHEMIA

| Category | Description/Prognosis | Sensory Loss | Muscle Weakness | Arterial Doppler Signal | Venous Doppler Signal |
|---|---|---|---|---|---|
| Viable | Not immediately threatened | None | None | Audible | Audible |
| Marginally threatened | Salvageable if promptly treated | Minimal or none | None | Often inaudible | Audible |
| Immediately threatened | Salvageable with immediate revascularization | More than toes, associated with rest pain | Mild, moderate | Usually inaudible | Audible |
| Irreversible | Major tissue loss or permanent nerve damage | Profound, anesthetic | Profound paralysis | Inaudible | Inaudible |

From Katzen BT: Clinical diagnosis and prognosis of acute limb ischemia. *Rev Cardiovasc Med* 3(suppl 2):S2–S6, 2002.

33

PERIPHERAL VASCULAR DISEASE

a. Local catheter-based thrombolysis for symptoms <14 days in duration
b. Thrombectomy may be a useful adjunct.
c. *Decompressive fasciotomies* may be required distal to the occlusion if compartment pressures (>30 mm Hg) are increased because of muscle and soft-tissue swelling.

**Case:** *A 72-year-old woman with hypertension uncontrolled by beta-blocker, calcium-channel blocker, and angiotensin-converting enzyme inhibitor therapy presents to your office in referral from her primary care physician after being found to have an unexplained increase in her creatinine level to 1.7 mg/dl. One year ago at the time of her yearly physical, her creatinine level was normal.*

## VI. RENAL ARTERY DISEASE

### A. EPIDEMIOLOGY
1. Estimated prevalence of ~7% in the general population
2. However, in patients with known PAD, prevalence rate of hemodynamically significant stenosis (>50%) is as high as 60%.

### B. NATURAL HISTORY
A progressive disease. Progress to occlusion occurs more often in patients with the following conditions:
1. High-grade stenosis (>60% at the time of diagnosis)
2. Diabetes
3. Severe hypertension

### C. CLINICAL CONSEQUENCE
1. Impaired kidney function and renal atrophy
2. Rates of progression to end-stage renal disease are unknown, but patients requiring dialysis secondary to renal artery stenosis have higher rates of mortality and worse prognoses.

### D. PATHOPHYSIOLOGY
1. Type of disease
a. Unilateral stenosis—impaired blood flow activates the renin-angiotensin-aldosterone system (RAS), and serum renin levels remain high.
b. Bilateral stenosis or unilateral solitary stenosis—increases in extracellular fluid lead to hypertension, and increased serum renin levels are transient.
2. Causative factors
a. Renal artery atherosclerosis—90% of renal artery stenosis cases
b. Fibromuscular dysplasia
   (1) Noninflammatory, nonatherosclerotic
   (2) String-of-beads appearance on angiography
c. Renal artery aneurysms
d. Multiple other causes

## E. DIAGNOSIS

1. History
   a. Complete cardiovascular evaluation as described earlier with evidence of systemic cardiovascular disease
   b. Onset of hypertension before the age of 30 years
   c. Presence of resistant (requiring more than three agents to control blood pressure) or malignant (evidence of end-organ damage) hypertension
   d. Unexplained atrophic kidney or discrepancy in size of kidneys >1.5 cm
   e. Sudden onset pulmonary edema (caused by azotemia)
2. **Physical examination—cardiovascular examination as described earlier**
3. **Laboratory evaluation—increased blood urea nitrogen/creatinine, especially after initiation of angiotensin-converting enzyme or angiotensin receptor blocker therapy**
4. Imaging
   a. Noninvasive imaging
      (1) Duplex ultrasound—high sensitivity but operator dependent and can be limited by patient's body habitus and bowel gas
      (2) Computed tomographic angiography—provides three-dimensional angiographic images of renal arteries.
      (3) Magnetic resonance angiography—may be less effective in detecting subtle arterial wall deformities.
      (4) Captopril scintigraphy—provides information about renal size, perfusion, and excretory capacity, but has limited value in patients with azotemia, bilateral RAS, and unilateral solitary RAS.
   b. Catheter angiography—still considered the gold standard, but not used as a first-line study. Contrast risks are similar to aortography.
   c. Studies sampling serum renin (e.g., renal vein sampling and the captopril test) are not used routinely.
5. Treatment
   a. Medical therapy
      (1) Angiotensin-converting enzyme inhibitors, angiotensin receptor blockers, and calcium-channel blockers are useful in the treatment of hypertension related to unilateral RAS.
      (2) Beta-blockers are also effective in the treatment of hypertension related to RAS.
   b. Interventional therapy
      (1) Percutaneous revascularization may be appropriate for the following conditions:
         (a) Asymptomatic bilateral or hemodynamically significant unilateral RAS
         (b) Accelerated, resistant, or malignant hypertension
         (c) Worsening renal insufficiency
      (2) Catheter-based intervention
         (a) Stent placement—indicated in atherosclerotic, ostial lesions.
         (b) Balloon angioplasty—recommended for FMD lesions.

33

PERIPHERAL VASCULAR DISEASE

c. Surgical therapy
   (1) Endarterectomy can be used for ostial atherosclerotic disease.
   (2) Surgical reconstruction indicated for the following conditions:
       (a) FMD
       (b) Atherosclerotic RAS
       (c) RAS in conjunction with aortic aneurysmal or aortoiliac occlusive disease
   (3) Nephrectomy may be necessary if operative intervention fails.

**Case:** *A 64-year-old man with a history of previously diagnosed 4.6-cm abdominal aortic aneurysm (AAA) currently managed with yearly computed tomography scans presents to the emergency department with numbness and tingling of his left lower leg for approximately 5 to 6 days and now has a cool, painful left foot and ankle.*

## VII. LOWER EXTREMITY ANEURYSM DISEASE
### A. EPIDEMIOLOGY
1. The diameters of lower extremity arteries usually increase by 20% to 25% between the ages of 20 and 70.
2. Femoral artery aneurysm
a. Incidence—relatively uncommon
b. Concurrent AAA in 85% of cases
3. Popliteal aneurysm
a. Incidence rate of ~2%
b. Comprise ~70% of all lower extremity arterial aneurysms
c. Concurrent AAA in 62% of cases
4. However, when AAAs are diagnosed, femoral and/or popliteal aneurysms are present in only 3% to 7% of cases.

### B. NATURAL HISTORY
1. Unlike AAAs, peripheral aneurysms do not often rupture; instead, they cause flow disturbances that lead to thrombosis and thromboembolism.

### C. PATHOPHYSIOLOGY
1. Possibly indicative of generalized arterial disease given coexistence of peripheral arteries and the abdominal aorta
2. As compared with the aorta, however, the lower extremity arteries have a histologically different medial layer, consisting mostly of smooth muscle cells.
3. As a result, secretion of matrix metalloproteases and the resultant changes in the elastin and collagen of the artery is not the primary pathologic process.
4. Changes in the smooth muscle layer lead to changes in arterial wall mechanics, thereby altering laminar flow.

## D. DIAGNOSIS

### 1. Femoral artery aneurysm

a. Occurs more often in men

b. Common femoral aneurysm is most prevalent.

c. Presents as a thigh mass with compression of neighboring structures or with thromboembolic complaints

d. Should be evaluated with Duplex ultrasound, computed tomographic angiography, or both

### 2. Popliteal artery aneurysm

a. Majority occur in men.

b. Often patients present with local ischemic or distal embolic complaints.

c. Often found on Duplex ultrasound and differentiated from other popliteal masses, specifically a synovial (Baker's) cyst.

## E. MANAGEMENT

### 1. Femoral artery aneurysm

a. No definitive size at which the aneurysm should be repaired, although these often become symptomatic at 3 cm.

b. Both elective surgical repair and conservative monitoring have pros and cons.

### 2. Popliteal artery aneurysm

a. Routine surveillance with Duplex until size approaches 2 cm

b. If aneurysm is symptomatic as described earlier, angiogram or computed tomographic angiography is necessary to evaluate distal vessel runoff.

c. Elective repair is often performed using bypass grafting, preferably with autogenous vein.

d. Acute limb ischemia because of acute thrombosis

   (1) Catheter-directed thrombolysis/thrombectomy can be used.

   (2) Fasciotomies may be necessary for the lower leg.

## F. FEMORAL ARTERY PSEUDOANEURYSM

### 1. A well-recognized complication of arterial puncture

a. Incidence rate of 0.1% to 0.2% after arterial catheterization

b. Approximately 5% after interventional procedures

### 2. Pathophysiology—incomplete dilation of some but not all layers of the arterial wall

### 3. Diagnosis

a. Frequently present as a pulsatile mass

b. Should be evaluated by Duplex ultrasonography

### 4. Management

a. Pseudoaneurysms <2 cm usually heal spontaneously.

b. Larger, symptomatic pseudoaneurysms can be managed with ultrasound-guided compression or thrombin injection.

c. Pseudoaneurysms complicated by bleeding or acute compression of surrounding structures often need operative management.

**33**

**PERIPHERAL VASCULAR DISEASE**

# Venous Disease

*Janice A. Taylor, MD*

*Varicose veins are the result of an improper selection of grandparents.*
—William Osler

*The detachment of larger or smaller fragments from the end of the softening thrombus which are driven into remote vessels. This gives rise to the very frequent process on which I have bestowed the name of Embolia.*
—Rudolf Virchow

**34**

## I. ANATOMY PEARLS
### A. MAIN LOWER EXTREMITY VEINS
1. Superficial: greater saphenous, lesser saphenous
2. Deep: femoral, popliteal, tibial

### B. MAIN UPPER EXTREMITY VEINS
1. Superficial: cephalic, basilic
2. Deep: brachial, axillary
3. Ten percent of deep venous thromboses (DVTs), but typically not clinically significant

### C. NO VALVES IN INFERIOR VENA CAVA, COMMON ILIAC VEINS, PORTAL SYSTEM, CRANIAL SINUSES
### D. COAGULATION CASCADE (SEE CHAPTER 13)

## II. CAUSATIVE FACTORS
### A. RISK FACTORS FOR DVT (SEE CHAPTER 31)
### B. RISK FACTORS FOR CHRONIC VENOUS INSUFFICIENCY (CVI)
1. Valvular destruction or incompetence resulting in venous reflux
2. Venous obstruction

### C. RISK FACTORS FOR VARICOSE VEINS
1. CVI
2. Obesity
3. Family history
4. Long-term inactivity
5. Female sex
6. Inherent defect of vein

## III. PRESENTATION

### A. HISTORY

1. Presence of risk factors as stated in section II
2. Heaviness, aching, burning of lower extremities after prolonged standing/sitting
3. Recurrent lower extremity ulceration

### B PHYSICAL EXAMINATION

1. DVT
   a. Homans' sign—calf pain on passive ankle dorsiflexion (only positive in 50% of cases)
   b. Swelling in affected extremity
2. Phlegmasia alba dolens ("milk leg syndrome")
   a. Pain, pallor, pitting (edema)
   b. Large DVT of major veins with sparing of venous collaterals
3. Phlegmasia cerulean dolens ("copper leg")
   a. Cyanosis (pathognomonic), pain, edema
   b. Large DVT of major veins and collaterals
   c. If not treated, results in limb threat and high likelihood of amputation
4. CVI
   a. Hyperemic lower extremities
   b. Hyperpigmentation *from hemosiderin deposits*
   c. Lipodermatosclerosis
   d. Venous stasis ulcers
   e. Erythema and pain
   f. Induration, eczema
   g. Lower extremity edema
5. Varicose veins
   a. Dilated, tortuous veins
   b. Aching, "heavy" feeling to leg with varicosities
   c. Relief with elevation
   d. Similar physical findings as with CVI

## IV. DIAGNOSIS

### A. HYPERCOAGULABLE WORKUP

1. Indications for workup after diagnosis of DVT
   a. No obvious trauma and not immediately after surgery
   b. Clot recurrence or occurring in artery
   c. Upper extremity location; no history of recent instrumentation
   d. Abdominal vasculature clots
2. Laboratory tests
   a. Antithrombin III level
   b. Protein C and S levels
   c. Lupus anticoagulant level
   d. Activated protein C resistance

e. Factor V Leiden mutation
f. Homocysteine level

## B. IMAGING
1. Duplex ultrasound of vasculature in question
a. (+) Diagnostic criteria *for DVT:* noncompressible vein, no respiratory flow variation (augmentation), no flow, venous distention
b. *When ordering for CVI, evaluate for reflux and flow velocity with time, and listen for flow sound in the imaged area.*
c. Sensitivity of 50% to 93%; specificity of ~100%
2. Venography
a. Invasive; considered gold standard. *Performed via intravenous contrast dye*
b. Used primarily when intervention being considered
c. (+) Diagnostic criteria: contrast filling defect
3. Magnetic resonance venography
a. Noninvasive
b. Gadolinium contrast used to enhance visibility

## V. DEEP VENOUS THROMBOSIS PROPHYLAXIS
### A. MEDICAL
1. Low-dose unfractionated heparin versus low-molecular-weight heparin
2. Warfarin (Coumadin)
3. Aspirin may be given, but it is not enough on its own.
4. Contraindications
a. Hemorrhage, including intracranial
b. Coagulopathy
c. Spinal hematoma

### B. MECHANICAL (SEE CHAPTER 31 FOR FURTHER DETAILS)
1. Early activity if patient is in postoperative state.
2. Compression stockings
3. Pneumatic compression boots/sequential compression devices
4. Inferior vena cava filter

## VI. TREATMENT
### A. DVT
1. Medical
a. Start patient on unfractionated heparin drip or low-molecular-weight heparin. Convert to warfarin when patient is therapeutic on heparin.
b. Thrombolysis (streptokinase, tissue plasminogen activator)
   (1) Activates plasminogen
   (2) Degrades factors V, VIII, XII, prekallikrein
   (3) Contraindicated if actively bleeding, stroke within 2 months, cranial hemorrhage, major trauma, uncontrolled hypertension, gastrointestinal bleed

34

VENOUS DISEASE

(4) Urokinase is no longer available as an option for treatment.

2. Surgical

a. Inferior vena cava filter (permanent or retrievable)

b. Percutaneous mechanical thrombectomy, venoplasty, possible venous stenting

c. Open thrombectomy

    (1) If limb threat or patient condition worsens even with medical treatment

    (2) Longitudinal incision in vein to remove clot with balloon catheter

    (3) Perform fasciotomy when operating for phlegmasia

3. For further details, see Chapter 31.

## B. CVI

1. Venous stasis ulcer treatment

a. Debridement, wound care, Unna boot, stockings, nonelastic compression

2. Compression garments

a. Gold standard of care

b. Venous stasis ulcer recurrence rate is 100% without compression after healing versus 30% with long-term compression therapy.

3. Surgical options

a. Radiofrequency ablation, laser, stripping, or ligation to treat superficial venous reflux in saphenous system

b. Endoscopic perforator vein ligation for perforator incompetence

c. Venous valve transposition

## C. VARICOSE VEINS

1. Nonsurgical

a. Compression stockings

b. Sclerotherapy (injection of sclerosing agents such as hypertonic saline) of small side branches and spider veins

2. Surgical

a. Radiofrequency ablation, laser, stripping, ligation of saphenous veins

b. Stab phlebectomy of symptomatic large side branches; *also known as ambulatory phlebectomy*

## D. PULMONARY EMBOLISM (SEE CHAPTER 31 FOR FURTHER DETAILS)

## VII. HEPARIN-INDUCED THROMBOCYTOPENIC THROMBOSIS

## A. *PARADOXICAL THROMBOCYTOPENIA* WITH VEIN AND ARTERY THROMBOSIS

1. Results from IgG antibodies forming against heparin-platelet factor 4 complex; *causes platelet destruction.*

2. The heparin-platelet factor 4 complex is a microthrombotic event secondary to consumptive thrombocytopenia.
3. Typically seen about 2 to 3 weeks after starting heparin. Platelet level will decline to less than 100,000/L. Diagnose via enzyme-linked immunosorbent assay.
4. Remove all sources of heparin (remember intravenous tubing, central lines, *flushes*).
5. Start thrombin inhibitor, then convert to warfarin when platelet levels return to normal.

## B. THROMBIN INHIBITOR OPTIONS

1. Hirudin—leech product. Inhibits fibrinogen by binding with thrombin. Good for patients with hepatic failure.
2. Argatroban—binds to thrombin. Good for patients with renal failure.

**34**

### RECOMMENDED READING

Bergan JJ, Schmid-Schonbein GW, Smith PD, et al: Chronic venous disease. *N Engl J Med* 355:488–498, 2006.

Gloviczki P (ed): Section XXI: the management of venous disorders. In Rutherford RB (ed): *Vascular Surgery*. Philadelphia, Elsevier Saunders, 2005.

Lam EY, Giswold ME, Moneta GL: Venous and lymphatic disease. In Brunicardi FC (ed): *Principles of Surgery*. New York, McGraw-Hill, 2005.

van Gent WB, Hop WC, van Praag MC, et al: Conservative versus surgical treatment of venous leg ulcers: A prospective, randomized, multicenter trial. *J Vasc Surg* 44: 563–571, 2006.

**VENOUS DISEASE**

# Abdominal Aortic Aneurysm

*Michael D. Goodman, MD*

## I. EPIDEMIOLOGY

### A. GENERAL

1. Aneurysm—dilation of an artery to at least 1.5 times the normal diameter
   a. Arterial dilation less than 50% increase in diameter—ectasia
2. Abdominal aortic aneurysm (AAA) is the most common type of aneurysm for which patients present for treatment.
3. Found in up to 14% of men and 4% of women 65 to 74 years old
4. Male predominance: male/female ratio of 3:1.
5. Familial tendency (sex-linked and autosomal recessive)—relative risk for first-degree relatives of affected individuals is 11.6 times greater than general population.
6. Fifteenth leading cause of death in the United States

### B. CASE REPORT

A 60-year-old man with a history of hypertension and a 50 pack-a-year smoking history presents to the emergency with an acute onset of back and left flank pain 2 hours before presentation. His initial set of vital signs is as follows: heart rate 128, blood pressure 95/52 mm Hg, respiratory rate 26. Abdominal examination reveals a tender pulsatile mass. He exhibits the classic triad of ruptured AAA—abdominal/back/flank pain, pulsatile mass, and hypotension.

### C. RISK FACTORS

1. Acquired factors—cigarette smoking (90% of AAA cases), hypertension, use of antihypertensive medications, total cholesterol, high plasma fibrinogen
2. Inheritable factors—connective tissue disorders, such as Marfan's and type IV Ehlers–Danlos syndromes, can predispose to aneurysm formation.

### D. CAUSATIVE FACTORS

1. Arterial wall degeneration from atherosclerosis with concurrent loss of elastin caused by proteolysis and inflammation leads to a *fusiform (spindle-shaped) aneurysm.*
2. Infectious process in the arterial wall leads to a *mycotic aneurysm.*
   a. Most commonly caused by *Salmonella* or *Staphylococcal* infection

## II. ANATOMY

### A. AORTIC

1. Abdominal portion of the aorta—from diaphragmatic hiatus at T12 to the aortic bifurcation at L4
2. Normal mean diameter—2 cm

## B. ASSOCIATED BRANCHES AND THEIR LOCATIONS
1. Celiac axis—upper portion of L1
2. Superior mesenteric artery—lower third of L1
3. Renal arteries—upper portion of L2
4. Inferior mesenteric artery (IMA) —L3

## III. PATHOLOGY
### A. LOCATION
1. Infrarenal—95% of cases
a. Distribution factors include elastin/collagen ratio, reflected pulsatility from the aortic bifurcation, diminished vasa vasorum, possible localized autoimmune reaction, and increased metalloproteinase activity.

### B. CHARACTERISTICS
1. Size—ranges 3 to 15 cm in diameter
2. Shape—usually fusiform; mycotic aneurysms tend to be saccular
3. Composition—AAAs are true aneurysms; the entire arterial wall is involved.
4. Extension—25% of AAAs also involve the iliac arteries.

### C. ASSOCIATED MANIFESTATIONS OF DIFFUSE ATHEROSCLEROSIS
1. Hypertension—40%
2. Coronary artery disease—30%
3. Associated occlusive arterial disease
a. Iliac arteries—16%
b. Carotid arteries—7%
c. Renal arteries—2%
4. Other associated aneurysms
a. Thoracic aorta—4%
b. Femoral artery—3%; up to 92% with common femoral artery aneurysm have an AAA
c. Popliteal artery—2%; up to 64% with popliteal artery aneurysm have an AAA
d. Visceral arteries—0.5%

## IV. NATURAL HISTORY
### A. GENERAL CONSIDERATIONS
1. Diameter is the strongest predictor of rupture.
2. *Increased size = increased rate of rupture*
a. Laplace's law: A larger radius increases wall tension, which, in turn, increases the risk for rupture of the aneurysmal wall.
3. Average growth is 0.4 cm/year.

### B. STATISTICS
1. Annual rates of rupture for untreated AAA (from VA Cooperative Study #417 and UK Small Aneurysm Trial):

a. 4.0 to 5.5 cm—1% to 3%
b. 5.5 to 5.9 cm—9.4%
c. 6.0 to 6.9 cm—10.2%; subset 6.5 to 6.9 cm—19.1%
d. >7.0 cm—32.5%
2. Five-year survival rate of untreated AAA:
a. <6 cm—48%
b. >6 cm—6%
3. UK Small Aneurysm Trial suggested that women may rupture at smaller diameters.
4. Renal artery involvement, chronic obstructive pulmonary disease, and diastolic hypertension may also increase the rate of rupture.

## V. CLINICAL PRESENTATION
### A. SYMPTOMS
1. Most AAAs are asymptomatic.
2. Two thirds of AAAs are incidental findings on imaging studies done for other reasons.
3. Most common symptoms include new-onset abdominal pain and low back pain.
4. Symptoms may be caused by compression of surrounding structures—inferior vena cava, ureter, duodenum.

### B. PHYSICAL EXAMINATION
1. Palpation
a. Presence of pulsatile mass on deep palpation—larger than 5-cm aneurysm palpable in up to 75% of patients.
b. Tortuous aorta may mimic AAA, presenting as pulsating, expansile abdominal mass different from other abdominal masses that merely transmit aortic pulsations (e.g., pseudocyst, pancreatic carcinoma).
c. In thin individuals, aortic pulsations may be unusually prominent; careful bimanual palpation should confirm normal diameter.
d. In larger patients, it may be impossible to detect AAAs regardless of diameter.
2. Other pulses: It is important to evaluate peripheral arteries for associated occlusive disease (pulses and bruits) or additional aneurysmal disease.

## VI. DIAGNOSTIC STUDIES
### A. PLAIN FILMS
1. Calcific rim ("egg shell") or large soft-tissue shadow is often visible projecting anterior to the spine.

### B. B-MODE ULTRASOUND
1. Simplest, most cost-effective method of confirming and following AAAs
2. Can also evaluate blood flow in renal and visceral arteries
3. Difficult to evaluate the suprarenal aorta because of bowel gas or obesity

35

ABDOMINAL AORTIC ANEURYSM

## C. COMPUTED TOMOGRAPHY (CT) SCAN

1. Can provide accurate characterization of entire aorta—gold standard for preoperative planning
2. Permits assessment of diameter, length, wall thickness, and thrombus
3. Three-dimensional reconstruction used for endograft evaluation and planning

## D. MAGNETIC RESONANCE IMAGING

1. Comparable in accuracy with CT scan but more expensive and less readily available
2. May have a role in patients in whom intravenous contrast is contraindicated

## E. AORTOGRAPHY

1. Poor study for diagnosis or assessment of size because mural thrombus within AAA can obscure actual aneurysm sac size; expensive and invasive.
2. Being replaced by CT and magnetic resonance angiograms that provide noninvasive three-dimensional images
3. Provides information regarding associated vascular lesions for renals and distal runoff
4. Indications for aortography: evidence of accessory renal arteries, horseshoe kidneys, mesenteric ischemia, and peripheral arterial occlusive disease.

## VII. OPERATIVE INDICATIONS

### A. PRINCIPLES

1. Decision for repair is individualized: There is not a single threshold size.
2. Patients with AAAs larger than 4 to 5 cm are candidates for elective operation unless medical comorbidities significantly increase the operative risk.
3. Surveillance is safe up to 5.5 cm unless symptomatic or rapidly expanding more than 1 cm/year.
4. A region of 5.5 cm is likely appropriate for the average patient, but patient preference for those who are younger, with low operative risk, or female patients with high rupture risk may consider repair at 4.5 to 5.5 cm.

## VIII. ELECTIVE MANAGEMENT OF ABDOMINAL AORTIC ANEURYSM

### A. HISTORY

1. First successful repair of AAA was performed by Dubost in 1951 with a human homograft.
2. DeBakey subsequently developed the Dacron graft in 1953, which remains the current gold standard.

## B. CARDIAC WORKUP

1. Clearance should follow American College of Cardiology/American Heart Association 2006 guidelines (see Chapter 4), according to low-, intermediate-, or high-risk patient categorizations.
2. Consider preoperative β-blockade to decrease myocardial oxygen demand.

## C. PREOPERATIVE PREPARATION

1. Severity of coronary artery disease, creatinine, and chronic obstructive pulmonary disease are independent predictors of mortality.
2. Bowel prep optional
3. Selective Swan-Ganz catheter use may be helpful during preoperative hydration and perioperative maintenance of adequate filling pressures and cardiac output.
4. Epidural anesthesia may be a useful adjunct for postoperative pain management and compromised pulmonary status.

## D. APPROACH

1. Midline incision for transabdominal approach
2. Left flank incision for retroperitoneal approach

## E. ARTERIAL CONTROL

1. Patient is systemically heparinized, and control is obtained proximal to and distal to the aneurysm sac.

## F. IMA

1. Ligated from within the aneurysm to avoid injury to collateral vessels of the left colon, such as the marginal artery of Drummond and meandering mesenteric artery
2. Prevent ischemia and ensure adequate perfusion by several intraoperative maneuvers:
a. Palpate the root of the superior mesenteric artery for pulsatility.
b. Examine the IMA orifice.
c. Doppler ultrasound—audible flow decreases the risk for postoperative ischemic colitis.
d. IMA back-pressure >40 mm Hg indicates adequate collateral retrograde flow.
e. Fluorescein—Ultraviolet luminescence should show bowel viability.
3. In patients with decreased visceral blood supply and patent IMA with back-pressure <40 mm Hg, it may be necessary to reimplant artery into graft.

## G. ANTERIOR WALL

1. Incised longitudinally to open the sac and remove thrombus.

## H. POSTERIOR WALL
1. Back-bleeding lumbar vessels are suture ligated.

## I. PROSTHETIC GRAFT
1. Tube graft if iliac arteries are normal; bifurcated graft if iliacs are aneurysmal

## J. POSTOPERATIVE COURSE
1. Admitted to ICU initially; typical hospitalization of 5 to 7 days
2. CT scan performed at 3 years after surgery for pseudoaneurysm surveillance.

## K. NONOPERATIVE AND ADJUNCTIVE MANAGEMENT
1. Reduce expansion rate and risk for rupture—smoking cessation and blood pressure control.

## IX. COMPLICATIONS

## A. ATHEROEMBOLISM ("TRASH FOOT")
1. Occlusion of small distal lower extremity arteries from embolization of aneurysmal sac fragments or from thrombosis caused by extended aortic clamp time.
2. Large emboli above the ankle can be removed with embolectomy catheter.

## B. LOWER EXTREMITY ISCHEMIA
1. Acute graft occlusion usually from technical error

## C. CARDIAC EVENTS
1. Arrhythmias are common
2. Myocardial infarction occurs in 3% to 16% of repaired patients.

## D. RENAL INSUFFICIENCY
1. Causes
a. Hypovolemia—preoperative dehydration, blood loss, removal of cross clamp
b. Atheromatous debris or thrombus embolizing to the kidney
c. Renal artery occlusion from aortic cross-clamping

## E. STROKE
1. Stroke associated with AAA repair can be embolic or secondary to hypotension.

## F. COLONIC ISCHEMIA
1. Suspect ischemia if patient has bowel movement during the first 24 to 72 hours after surgery. Stool is usually positive for blood (grossly or by Heme test).

a. Mucosal ischemia most common and usually manifested by mucosal sloughing; resolves spontaneously in most cases.

b. *Requires immediate flexible sigmoidoscopy* (or abdominal CT) to diagnose

c. Transmural involvement requires reexploration and colonic resection.

## G. SPINAL CORD ISCHEMIA

1. Anterior spinal artery syndrome—paraplegia with loss of light touch and pain sensation, and loss of sphincter control. Proprioception and temperature sensation are spared.

## H. CHYLOUS ASCITES

1. Results from inadequate ligation of lymphatics.

## I. LATE COMPLICATIONS

1. Aortoenteric fistula

a. Distal portion of duodenum is most common location.

b. Presentation—gastrointestinal bleeding with associated abdominal and back pain; may have "herald bleed" of small amount of hematemesis, followed by exsanguinating hemorrhage per rectum.

c. Diagnosis—perform endoscopy to rule out other sources.

d. Treatment—remove graft, oversew aorta, repair enteric defect; drain retroperitoneum, extraanatomic bypass (axillary-bifemoral).

2. Late infection of prosthetic graft material requires extraanatomic bypass.

3. Sexual dysfunction—retrograde ejaculation and/or inability to maintain erection caused by injury to sympathetic plexus around aorta or inadequate hypogastric perfusion.

## X. ENDOVASCULAR ABDOMINAL AORTIC ANEURYSM REPAIR (EVAR)

### A. HISTORY

1. First transfemoral intraluminal graft placement reported by Parodi in 1991.

2. Approved for use by the U.S. Food and Drug Administration in 1999

3. Thirty to 50% of all AAA repairs are currently endovascular.

### B. INDICATIONS

1. Currently, most appropriate for patients at increased risk for conventional open repair.

2. May be the preferred treatment method if vascular anatomy is appropriate, in older or higher risk patients, or in those with multiple prior abdominal surgeries

a. Current literature demonstrates that EVAR is increasingly being used for patients of older age and greater number of associated comorbidities (coronary artery disease, congenital heart failure, renal failure, peripheral artery disease) compared with those undergoing open AAA repair.

**35**

**ABDOMINAL AORTIC ANEURYSM**

3. EVAR does not currently justify changing the accepted threshold measurements for intervention.
4. Patient preference is of great importance.
5. May not be eligible because of anatomic variability of the aneurysm, such as size and angulation of the proximal neck and extent of iliac aneurysmal or atherosclerotic disease
6. New protocols are being established for use of EVAR in the emergent setting of a ruptured AAA; currently, protocols are institution dependent.

## C. PROCEDURE
1. Preoperative anatomical evaluation is essential. CT angiography with three-dimensional reconstruction is a valuable tool to tailor grafts to the individual anatomy.
2. Endografts are inserted through bilateral cutdowns on the common femoral arteries via the Seldinger technique. Transluminal catheters are used to mark graft placement and ensure appropriate deployment into the aneurysm sac with angiographic confirmation.
3. Aortic endograft with unilateral iliac gate is placed, followed by cannulation of this graft via the contralateral femoral artery to deploy the contralateral iliac gate.

## D. COMPLICATIONS
1. Endoleaks—principal concern of EVAR
a. Type I—persistent perigraft attachment site leak; must be treated
b. Type II—retrograde lumbar or IMA flow; most common type
c. Type III—junctional leak between overlapping graft segments
d. Type IV—transgraft
2. Iliac artery injuries from device insertion—rupture, dissection, limb occlusion
3. Renal failure as a result of embolization, dye toxicity, deployment inadvertently occluding the renal arteries

## E. OUTCOMES
1. Long-term durability and effectiveness remain uncertain; current randomized, controlled trials are evaluating EVAR versus open AAA repair.
2. Most recent retrospective studies demonstrate comparable mortality rates between EVAR and open repair, with EVAR patients having lower 30-day and 1-year mortality rates, shorter ICU and inpatient stays, and earlier functional recovery.
3. Current postoperative surveillance protocols include abdominal CT annually for life to evaluate for endoleaks, graft migration, and aortic morphology.

## XI. PROGNOSIS
Surgical repair has been shown to double the survival time of patients with AAA.

## A. OPERATIVE MORTALITY

1. Rate for elective repair is 1% to 2%, approximately equal to repair of a <5.5-cm AAA.

## B. MORTALITY RATES

1. For emergent repair of ruptured AAA range from 20% to 80% (mean, 50%), depending on the condition of the patient at presentation.

## XII. RUPTURED ABDOMINAL AORTIC ANEURYSM

## A. PRINCIPLES OF MANAGEMENT

1. Clinical examination is most important. Hemodynamically unstable patients go directly to operating room. Stable patients with questionable presence of AAA may undergo emergent abdominal CT scan or ultrasound.
2. Prep and drape before induction of anesthesia. Be prepared for incision on induction because of further hypotension with anesthetic agent.
3. Mortality rate of those who reach the hospital is 50%.
4. Overall mortality rate for AAA rupture is 80% to 90%.

35

ABDOMINAL AORTIC ANEURYSM

# Carotid Disease

*Alexander J. Bondoc, MD*

## I. CASE REPORT

A 68-year-old woman with a history of coronary artery disease and non–insulin-dependent diabetes mellitus is referred to your clinic by her neurologist with a 1-month history of transient ischemic attacks.

## II. STROKE

**A. THIRD MOST COMMON CAUSE OF DEATH IN THE UNITED STATES**

1. 164,000/year

**B. ONE MILLION HOSPITAL ADMISSIONS/YEAR**

**C. SIGNIFICANT NEUROLOGIC MORBIDITY**

**D. RISK FACTORS**

1. Nonmodifiable

a. Sex (male)

b. Age (>55 years)

c. Race (black or Asian American)

2. Modifiable

a. Hypertension—preeminent risk factor

b. Smoking

c. Hyperlipidemia

d. Diabetes mellitus

e. Obesity

**E. CAUSATIVE FACTORS**

1. Ischemic—insufficient blood supply

a. Embolic (two thirds of ischemic strokes)—clot or plaque formation outside of the cerebral vasculature
   (1) *Carotid embolization*—cholesterol or fibrin/platelet matter
   (2) Cardiogenic embolization—valvular disease, atrial fibrillation
   (3) Hematologic causes—hypercoagulability disorders

b. Thrombotic
   (1) Local in situ occlusion of cerebral vessels, *or*
   (2) *Carotid thrombosis* → flow impairment
   (3) Circle of Willis collateralizes in response.
   (4) Chronicity and extent of thrombosis may determine symptoms.
   (5) Acute flow impairment may occur (e.g., a hypotensive event).

2. Hemorrhagic—10% to 15% of strokes

a. Intracranial hemorrhage caused by trauma, among other factors

b. Rupture of cerebral aneurysm

## III. DIAGNOSIS

### A. HISTORY

1. Characteristics of neurologic symptoms—can localize a circulatory impairment (see Table 36-1 for a more complete review)
   a. Onset—two episodes over the last month of left hand and arm weakness with associated difficulty speaking.
   b. Provoking factors—none, onset is sudden and unexplained.
   c. Palliative factors—none, resolves with time.
   d. Timing differentiates between transient ischemic attack and stroke—both episodes have lasted about 4 to 5 hours.
2. Other possible associated symptoms
   a. Nausea/vomiting
   b. Headache
   c. Severity of neurologic impairment may require:
      (1) Emergent admission
      (2) Therapeutic anticoagulation
      (3) Semiemergent operative intervention
3. Medical history—risk factor assessment including diabetes and coronary disease
4. Surgical history
   a. Three-vessel coronary artery bypass grafting 2 years ago
   b. Some authors advocate carotid evaluation in the preoperative workup of potential coronary bypass patients, but this remains controversial.
5. Allergies/medications—no known drug allergies; currently taking atenolol, metformin, lisinopril, and aspirin

### TABLE 36-1

RELATION OF NEUROLOGIC IMPAIRMENT WITH VASCULAR LESION

| Symptoms | Vascular Distribution | Neurologic Distribution |
|---|---|---|
| Transient monocular blindness (amaurosis fugax) | | |
| Visual field disturbances | Retinal artery | Limited to the ipsilateral retina/eye |
| Altered mental status | | |
| Impaired judgment | | |
| Contralateral motor weakness | Anterior cerebral artery | Cerebral hemisphere |
| Contralateral motor weakness | | |
| Loss of sensation | | |
| Speech/language deficits | | |
| Visual field deficits | Middle cerebral artery | Cerebral hemisphere |
| Hemianopsia | | |
| Impaired memory | Posterior cerebral artery | Cerebral hemisphere |
| Dysarthria, dysphagia, diplopia | | |
| Limb or gait ataxia | | |
| Simultaneous motor, sensory, and visual loss | Vertebrobasilar | Brainstem, cerebellum, cerebrum |

6. Social history—nonsmoker, quit 10 years ago; drinks alcohol socially; no recent travel

## B. PHYSICAL EXAMINATION
1. HEENT (head, eyes, ears, nose and throat)
a. No carotid bruits bilaterally
b. *The presence of a carotid bruit has low sensitivity for detecting more than 70% stenosis.*
2. Cardiovascular
a. Regular rate and rhythm, no murmurs
b. *Evaluate pulse and murmurs for possible cardiac sources of emboli.*
3. Pulmonary—clear bilaterally
4. Abdomen—no palpable masses or audible periumbilical bruits
5. Vascular
a. Two plus carotid, radial, femoral, popliteal, and dorsalis pedis pulses bilaterally
b. *A full vascular examination is important to diagnose other possible pathologic conditions including aneurysms.*
6. Neurologic
a. Cranial nerves II-XII intact. Five of 5 strength in all upper and lower extremity muscle groups. No evidence of hyperreflexia.
b. *A full neurologic examination may help identify symptoms in active stroke and localize a lesion.*

## C. IMAGING
1. Angiography—gold standard but not used often anymore.
a. Advantages
   (1) Evaluation of entire carotid system including collaterals and the aortic arch
   (2) Necessary for patients undergoing carotid artery stenting (CAS)
b. Disadvantages
   (1) Invasiveness and cost
   (2) Neurologic and vascular morbidity
   (3) Limited views
2. Carotid duplex ultrasound (Fig. 36-1)
a. Uses gray scale, color flow, and B-mode images
b. Advantages
   (1) Noninvasive
   (2) Can give information on velocities, anatomy, and plaque morphology
   (3) Can achieve high sensitivity and specificity if combinations of parameters are measured together (e.g., peak systolic velocity, spectral broadening, flow reversal)
c. Disadvantages: Ultrasound is limited by the following factors:
   (1) Arterial calcification.
   (2) Patient body habitus.
   (3) Anatomic distortion/normal variant.
   (4) Operator dependence.

36

CAROTID DISEASE

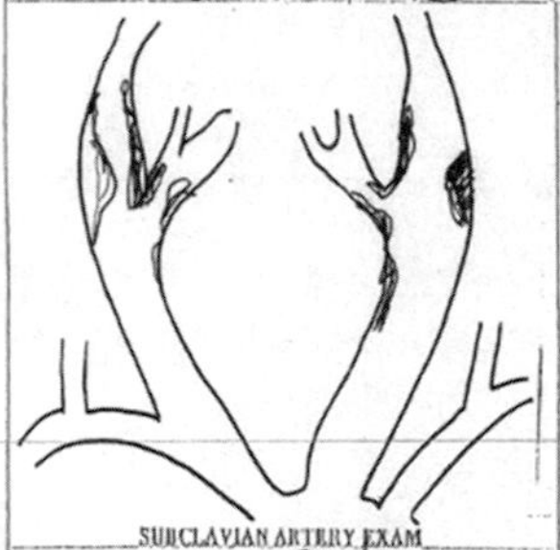

**FIG. 36-1**

Report of carotid duplex ultrasound.

3. Computed tomographic angiography
   a. Advantages.
      (1) For patients who cannot undergo magnetic resonance angiography
      (2) Demonstrates relative position of calcifications and stenosis near the carotid bifurcation
      (3) Provides an estimate of the residual lumen and less likely to over-estimate stenosis

b. Disadvantage—requires a contrast bolus comparable to that of angiography

4. **Magnetic resonance angiography**

a. Advantages
   (1) Not operator dependent
   (2) Avoids nephrotoxic contrast agents
   (3) May allow characterization of plaque morphology
b. Disadvantages
   (1) Can overestimate stenosis
   (2) Incompatible with implanted metallic devices
   (3) Claustrophobia

## IV. DIFFERENTIAL DIAGNOSIS OF CAROTID OCCLUSIVE DISEASE

**A. ATHEROSCLEROTIC DISEASE**

1. Comprise 90% of carotid occlusive disease cases
2. Anatomy influences hemodynamics—formation of plaque on lateral walls.
3. Pathophysiology—modified response to injury hypothesis
a. Endothelial injury (hyperlipidemia, smoking, shear, hypertension)
b. Monocytes attach to endothelium and low-density lipoproteins and then secrete growth factors.
c. Plaque size increase
d. Increased platelet activity furthers endothelial damage.
e. Platelets stimulate intimal smooth muscle cells to secrete extracellular matrix.
f. Muscle cells accumulate lipids, and the plaque center becomes necrotic.
4. **Inciting events**
a. Ulceration of plaque
b. Rupture—similar to acute coronary syndrome
c. Intraplaque hemorrhage

**B. FIBROMUSCULAR DYSPLASIA**

1. Replacement of normal tissue, most often the media, by extracellular matrix leading to a stenosis or aneurysms, or both.

**C. COILS/KINKS BECAUSE OF ANATOMIC VARIATION**

**D. CAROTID ANEURYSMS**

1. False—blunt trauma, iatrogenic injury
2. True—as with other anatomic arterial sites

**E. CAROTID DISSECTION**

1. Intimal tear followed by intimal dissection.

**F. RADIATION ARTERITIS**

**G. TAKAYASU'S ARTERITIS**

1. More common in Asia and in adolescent female individuals. Affects all three vascular layers.

**36**

**CAROTID DISEASE**

## H. CAROTID TRAUMA

1. Often causes stretch or compression injuries

## V. MANAGEMENT

### A. MEDICAL

1. Risk factor modification

a. Hypertension therapy
  (1) Systolic/diastolic goals based on presence of concomitant diabetes and chronic kidney disease
  (2) Angiotensin-converting enzyme inhibitors and angiotensin receptor blockers may be particularly useful because of mechanism of action, decreased smooth muscle cell proliferation, and improvement of endothelial cell function.

b. Smoking cessation

c. Treatment of hyperlipidemia
  (1) Statins
    (a) Lower cholesterol
    (b) Antiinflammatory—decrease cell/endothelial interaction and decrease number of inflammatory cells

d. Treatment of diabetes

e. Obesity—weight loss and physical activity

2. Antiplatelet therapy

a. Acetylsalicylic acid
  (1) May be beneficial as prevention therapy in women but not necessarily in men
  (2) Beneficial as secondary prevention in patients with a history of transient ischemic attack and stroke at low dose (81 or 325 mg daily)

b. Dipyridamole—useful in secondary prevention after transient ischemic attack or stroke

c. Clopidogrel
  (1) Also effective in secondary prevention
  (2) Acetylsalicylic acid plus clopidogrel—increased risk for bleeding without improved benefit as compared with acetylsalicylic acid alone

### B. SURGICAL—CAROTID ENDARTERECTOMY

1. Indications

a. Symptomatic disease with >70% stenosis and in some subgroups with >50% stenosis (e.g., men older than 75 years, history of stroke)

b. Asymptomatic disease with >80% stenosis

c. The clinical trials that drive these recommendations may now be outdated given new "best" medical therapies (e.g., statins, angiotensin-converting enzyme inhibitors).

2. Contraindications

a. Severe neurologic manifestations after stroke may lead to high rates of mortality.

b. Completely occluded carotid
c. Concurrent morbid illness
3. **Timing:** There is no difference in performing an operation during the "subacute period" (<3–6 weeks after onset of symptoms) versus the "stable" period.
4. Cerebral perfusion monitoring
a. Options
   (1) General anesthesia with electroencephalographic monitoring
   (2) Local nerve block with conscious monitoring
     (a) Effective postoperative pain control
     (b) Increased rates of patient satisfaction with lower amounts of narcotic consumption
   (3) Cerebral oximetry—noninvasive method that can approximate electroencephalographic/neurologic evaluation.
b. Anesthetic choice governed by surgeon's choice and patient comorbidity

## C.  ENDOVASCULAR—CAROTID ARTERY STENTING (CAS)
1. Steep learning curve given difficulty of negotiating aortic arch and common carotid system
2. Indications
a. Recurrent stenosis
b. Severe comorbidities
   (1) Advanced age—worse in those older than 80 years
   (2) Severe cardiopulmonary disease
   (3) Contralateral carotid occlusion
   (4) Severe renal disease
c. Surgically hostile neck status post prior radiation therapy
3. Plaque morphology graded on duplex ultrasonography may predict the likelihood of embolic stroke during the procedure.
4. Use of an embolization protection device reduces risk for embolization of dislodged plaque if necessary.
5. Intraoperative complications—often related to prolonged stretch of the baroreceptors in the carotid bulb
a. Bradycardia—premedication with atropine
b. Hypotension—volume replacement, phenylephrine, or both
c. Randomized, controlled trials comparing carotid endarterectomy and CAS are ongoing. However, a recent European study demonstrates greater rates of death and stroke at 1 and 6 months in a CAS group for symptomatic patients with >60% stenosis.

## VI. POSTOPERATIVE COMPLICATIONS
Similar between the carotid endarterectomy and CAS

## A.  CARDIOVASCULAR
1. Myocardial infarction
2. Hemodynamic instability

a. Hypotension—use of phenylephrine (Neo-Synephrine)
b. Hypertension—use of nitroprusside

## B.  NEUROLOGIC
1. Stroke
a. Temporary internal carotid artery occlusion
b. Embolization—platelet
c. Thrombosis—flap dislodgement
2. Intracerebral hemorrhage
3. Seizures

## C.  CAROTID ARTERY
1. Dissection
2. Thrombosis
3. Recurrent carotid stenosis—30% occurrence, 3% symptomatic

## D.  COMPLICATIONS UNIQUE TO CAROTID ENDARTERECTOMY
1. Cranial nerve dysfunction—2% to 7%, most often cranial nerves X and XII
2. Wound infections

## VII. POSTOPERATIVE CARE
1. Lifetime aspirin
2. Clopidogrel for 4 weeks after procedure
3. Screening carotid duplex ultrasound at 1 month, 6 months, and annually after procedure
4. Continued risk factor modification

# Mesenteric Ischemia

*Grace Z. Mak, MD*

Mesenteric ischemia is an uncommon entity with an unfortunately high mortality rate ranging from 50% to 75%, usually because of a delay in diagnosis and treatment. It is defined by insufficient perfusion to meet the metabolic needs of the end organs supplied by the mesenteric vasculature. These organs include the stomach, small intestine, colon, liver, gallbladder, and spleen. Successful treatment requires a high index of suspicion, early recognition of both acute and chronic presentations, and prompt treatment before the onset of irreversible intestinal ischemia and infarction.

## I. ANATOMY AND PHYSIOLOGY

### A. VASCULAR SUPPLY

Circulation deficits in the gastrointestinal tract are uncommon because of abundant collateral circulation among the following:

1. Celiac axis
a. Supplies foregut (stomach to second portion of duodenum)
2. Superior mesenteric artery (SMA)
a. Supplies midgut (second portion of duodenum to proximal two thirds of transverse colon)
3. Inferior mesenteric artery (IMA)
a. Supplies hindgut (distal third of transverse colon to rectum)

### B. COLLATERAL VESSELS

1. Pancreaticoduodenal arcade (celiac artery and SMA)
2. Branch of left colic artery (SMA and IMA)
3. Marginal artery of Drummond—often small, not continuous, especially at splenic flexure (SMA and IMA)
4. Arc of Riolan (SMA and IMA)

### C. PHYSIOLOGY

1. Occlusive
a. Macrovascular acute or chronic interruption of segmental blood flow
b. Usually occurs in patients with generalized atherosclerosis
c. Acute—thrombotic and embolic
  (1) SMA most commonly involved vessel
  (2) Thrombotic ischemia occurs in patients with mesenteric atherosclerosis involving mesenteric arterial origins sparing collateral branches.
    (a) Development of collateral circulation more likely with gradual occlusion rather than a sudden event
  (3) Embolic ischemia results from emboli typically originating from a cardiac source (atrial fibrillation or after myocardial infarction).
d. Chronic

      (1) Progressive luminal plaque narrowing caused by atherosclerotic progression

      (2) Typically involves at least two of the three main visceral arteries

**2. Nonocclusive**

a. Low-flow state caused by microvascular vasospasm in response to systemic physiologic stress in otherwise normal vasculature

b. Sympathetic stimulation

c. Decreased blood flow

d. Drugs—digitalis and others

**3. Less common syndromes**

a. Median arcuate ligament syndrome

      (1) Chronic intermittent ischemia symptoms

      (2) External compression of celiac artery by the diaphragm; often seen in healthy individuals as well

b. IMA ligation during aortic surgery

      (1) Acute symptoms

      (2) Absence of adequate collateral circulation

c. Aortic dissection involving mesenteric arteries

      (1) Acute symptoms

d. Mesenteric arteritis, polyarteritis nodosa, lupus erythematosus, Kawasaki's disease, fibromuscular dysplasia

e. Radiation arteritis

f. Cholesterol emboli

g. Intimal hyperplasia of visceral arteries

      (1) Patients who smoke heavily or young women taking oral contraceptives

h. Mesenteric venous thrombosis

## II. EPIDEMIOLOGY

1. One in every 1000 hospital admissions in the United States
2. Increasing prevalence because of increased awareness and advancing age of population with multiple comorbidities

## III. ACUTE MESENTERIC ISCHEMIA

**A. RISK FACTORS**

1. Cardiac arrhythmias, advanced age, low cardiac output states, valvular heart disease, myocardial infarction, and malignancy

**B. CLINICAL PRESENTATION**

1. Hallmark of mesenteric ischemia is severe, acute midabdominal pain out of proportion to examination.
2. Early

a. Prominent symptoms of gastrointestinal emptying (i.e., nausea, vomiting, diarrhea); sudden onset of abdominal cramps; diffuse abdominal tenderness without peritoneal signs; active bowel sounds may be present.

**3. Late**

a. Symptoms of intestinal infarction

b. Bloody diarrhea caused by mucosal sloughing and intestinal spasm from ischemia

c. Fever and peritonitis develop late and are ominous findings indicative of bowel infarction.

d. Hypotension and acidosis eventually lead to shock.

e. Eighty to 85% mortality rate at this point despite intervention

**4. Early diagnosis improves survival.**

## C. CAUSATIVE FACTORS

**1. Embolization of SMA**

a. Occurs in 40% of cases

b. Occurs in one third of patients with antecedent embolic episodes (lower extremity embolus, cerebrovascular accident)

c. SMA usually otherwise normal

d. Most emboli lodge 3 to 10 cm distal to SMA origin, proximal to middle colic artery origin.

   (1) "Meniscus sign" with abrupt cutoff of normal proximal SMA seen on mesenteric angiography.

**2. Thrombosis of SMA**

a. Occurs in 40% of cases

b. Thrombus formation on atherosclerotic plaque or stenotic lesion often caused by low-flow state (dehydration).

   (1) Collateral vasculature usually well developed because of chronicity of mesenteric atherosclerosis.

c. More insidious presentation compared with embolic ischemia

d. Often preceded by symptoms of chronic mesenteric ischemia (abdominal angina), for example, postprandial pain, weight loss, bloating, diarrhea

e. Mesenteric angiogram shows occlusion at most proximal SMA with tapering seen 1 to 2 cm from origin with collateral circulation.

**3. Nonocclusive ischemia**

a. Occurs in 20% of cases

b. Vasoconstriction of mesenteric vasculature caused by low cardiac output (low-flow state).

c. Common predisposing conditions include myocardial infarction, congestive heart failure, renal or hepatic disease, medications (e.g., digoxin, epinephrine), trauma, sepsis, and hypovolemia or hypotension.

d. Abdominal pain (70%) usually severe.

e. Mesenteric angiogram shows segmental vasospasm with relatively normal-appearing main SMA trunk.

## D. DIAGNOSIS

1. Biplanar mesenteric angiography (with lateral views of aorta) is the definitive diagnostic test.

a. Typically demonstrates occlusion or near occlusion of celiac artery or SMA at or near aortic origins

b. IMA often occluded because of diffuse infrarenal aortic atherosclerotic disease.

2. Laboratory derangements nonspecific.

a. Increased hematocrit consistent with hemoconcentration.

b. Leukocytosis with left shift

c. Increase in amylase, lactate dehydrogenase, creatine phosphokinase, or alkaline phosphatase

d. Evidence of marked metabolic acidosis with persistent base deficit

3. Radiographs nonspecific.

a. Can exclude pneumoperitoneum, obstruction, or volvulus

b. Commonly see adynamic ileus with gasless abdomen

## E. MANAGEMENT

1. Expeditious evaluation
2. Aggressive fluid resuscitation
3. Nasogastric tube, Foley catheter
4. Hemodynamic status monitoring (central venous catheter, arterial line)
5. Parenteral antibiotics
6. With peritonitis or evidence of intestinal infarction, immediate abdominal exploration warranted.
7. Systemic anticoagulation with heparin to prevent further thrombus propagation
8. Embolus

a. Arteriography shows SMA occlusion with embolus lodged proximal to middle colic artery (meniscus sign).

b. Angiography catheter may be used to infuse papaverine both before and after surgery.

c. Immediate exploration after adequate resuscitation

   (1) Primary goal—restore arterial perfusion with embolectomy

d. SMA exposure

   (1) Reflection of transverse colon superiorly and retraction of small bowel into right upper quadrant

      (a) SMA located at root of small bowel mesentery passing over third/fourth portion of duodenum as it emerges beneath pancreas.

   (2) Retraction of duodenum medially after incision of retroperitoneum lateral to fourth portion of duodenum

e. Embolectomy performed via transverse arteriotomy in proximal SMA using standard balloon embolectomy catheters.

   (1) Arteriotomy may be closed with or without a vein patch.

f. For more distal SMA emboli, individual jejunal and ileal branches can be isolated at root of small-bowel mesentery.

g. Once SMA blood flow restored, assess bowel viability by direct inspection, fluorescein examination, or Doppler assessment.
   (1) Assess bowel supplied by SMA from midjejunum to ascending/ transverse colon.
   (2) Administer intravenous sodium fluorescein (1 g) and inspect bowel under ultraviolet (Wood's) lamp. Viable bowel has smooth, uniform fluorescence.
   (3) Doppler assessment of antimesenteric intestinal arterial flow
   (4) All nonviable bowel should be resected.
h. Consider second-look operation 24 to 48 hours after embolectomy to reinspect bowel with questionable viability with resection of all nonviable bowel.

**9. Thrombosis**
a. Arteriogram shows severe atherosclerosis involving proximal celiac artery and SMA with complete occlusion of SMA at origin, with infrequent collateralization.
b. Extensive bowel necrosis often presents with gray and often pulseless bowel appearance
c. Revascularization required with aortomesenteric bypass graft (prosthetic or saphenous vein) to distal SMA bypassing proximal SMA lesion.
   (1) Saphenous vein is graft material of choice.
   (2) Prosthetic grafts should be avoided in presence of nonviable bowel.
   (3) Origin of graft
      (a) Aorta
         (1) Supraceliac infradiaphragmatic aorta often has no atherosclerotic disease, decreasing risk for embolic complications with cross-clamping of aorta compared with more atherosclerotic infrarenal aorta.
         (2) Allows antegrade graft placement—less prone to kinking
      (b) Iliac artery
d. Resect nonviable bowel after revascularization.
e. Consider a second-look operation.

**10. Nonocclusive**
a. Arteriography shows marked narrowing and "pruning" of distal mesenteric vessels sparing large vessels.
b. Treatment is primarily nonoperative because patients are often extremely ill and poor surgical candidates.
c. Optimize cardiac output.
d. Minimize or stop all vasoconstricting agents.
e. Angiographic catheter at SMA orifice with infusion of vasodilating agents (i.e., papaverine, tolazoline)
   (1) Papaverine 30 to 60 mg/hr with hemodynamic monitoring
      (a) If catheter migrates into aorta, allowing systemic papaverine infusion, patient can experience significant hypotension.
   (2) If abdominal symptoms improve, repeat angiography after 24 hours to document resolution of vasospasm.

f. Systemic anticoagulation via heparin to prevent thrombosis of cannulated vessels

g. Laparotomy if peritoneal signs develop
   (1) Continue papaverine infusion during and after surgery.
   (2) Be sure to maintain adequate body temperature in operating room with use of warm irrigation fluid and laparotomy pads to prevent further intestinal vasoconstriction.

## IV. CHRONIC MESENTERIC ISCHEMIA

### A. CAUSATIVE FACTORS

1. Chronic atherosclerosis of two of the three main visceral arteries (celiac artery, SMA, IMA) supported by a large number of collaterals
2. Often precipitated by illness resulting in dehydration (i.e., nausea, vomiting, diarrhea)

### B. DIAGNOSIS

1. Symptoms often attributable to multiple causative factors, for example, gallbladder disease and occult gastrointestinal cancer.
2. Often present with chronic epigastric abdominal pain—colicky in nature, occurring 30 to 60 minutes after meal.
3. Seventy percent of cases have history of abdominal angina.
4. Involuntary weight loss because of "food fear"
5. Presence of abdominal bruit
6. Computed tomographic angiography or magnetic resonance angiography
7. Angiography (less common)
a. Used after other disease entities ruled out
b. Should include lateral view of aorta and take-off vessels

### C. TREATMENT

1. Surgical revascularization with prevention of bowel infarction
a. Transaortic endarterectomy
   (1) Indicated for ostial lesions of patent celiac artery and SMA
   (2) Approach via left medial visceral rotation exposing aorta with mesenteric branches
   (3) Lateral aortotomy encompassing both celiac artery and SMA
   (4) Careful not to create intimal flap—must visualize termination site of endarterectomy
b. Mesenteric artery bypass
   (1) Indicated for occlusive lesions 1 to 2 cm distal to mesenteric origin
   (2) Antegrade from supraceliac aorta
   (3) Retrograde from infrarenal aorta or iliac artery
   (4) Can use autologous saphenous vein grafts or prosthetic material
2. Percutaneous angioplasty and stenting of SMA

**D. PROGNOSIS**
1. Relief of pain in 90% of cases
2. Best long-term results with multivessel revascularization
3. Recurrence
a. Ten to 30% with multivessel revascularization versus 50% with single-vessel revascularization

## V. MEDIAN ARCUATE LIGAMENT SYNDROME (CELIAC ARTERY COMPRESSION SYNDROME)

**A. CAUSATIVE FACTORS**
1. Narrowed celiac artery origin caused by extrinsic compression or impingement by median arcuate ligament

**B. PRESENTATION**
1. Nonspecific abdominal pain usually located in upper abdomen and precipitated by meals
2. Often in young women between 20 and 40 years of age

**C. DIAGNOSIS**
1. Computed tomographic angiography or magnetic resonance angiography
2. Mesenteric duplex of celiac artery and SMA with inspiration and expiration
3. Aortogram
a. Lateral views show significant celiac artery compression.
b. Imaging with inspiration and expiration

**D. TREATMENT**
1. Based on combination of appropriate symptom complex with celiac artery compression without other pathology identified
2. Patient must be counseled that relief of celiac compression may not relieve symptoms
3. Release of ligament compressing proximal celiac artery with bypass graft to correct any persistent stricture

## VI. MESENTERIC VENOUS THROMBOSIS

**A. CAUSATIVE FACTORS**
1. Associated with other pathologic processes
a. Malignancy, visceral infection, pancreatitis, portal hypertension, trauma
2. Hypercoagulable states
3. Idiopathic

**B. CLINICAL PRESENTATION**
1. Five to 15 percent of acute mesenteric ischemia cases
2. Insidious onset of symptoms

37

MESENTERIC ISCHEMIA

a. Nonspecific abdominal pain followed by diarrhea, nausea, and vomiting
3. **Peritoneal signs in less than 50% of patients**
a. Bowel wall edema, systemic hypovolemia, and hemoconcentration can lead to compromised arterial inflow leading to life-threatening complications.

## C. DIAGNOSIS
1. **Leukocytosis**
2. **Radiographs**
a. Generally nondiagnostic showing nonspecific bowel gas pattern
b. May show distended small bowel loops, portal venous gas, or gas in bowel wall
3. **Barium enema**
a. Thumbprinting and luminal narrowing; may limit angiographic evaluation
4. **Angiography**
a. Prolonged arterial phase; nonvisualization of the venous phase, reflux of contrast into the aorta
5. **Computed tomography scan**
a. Study of choice
b. Visualization of intraluminal thrombus, enlargement of thrombosed vein, focal or segmental bowel wall thickening
c. Also can detect portal and ovarian vein thrombosis
6. **Duplex ultrasound scan of mesenteric and portal veins**
a. Often limited by distended bowel gas pattern

## D. TREATMENT
1. **Fluid resuscitation**
2. **Early heparinization for suspected thrombosis**
3. **Nasogastric tube with bowel rest**
4. **Foley catheter**
5. **Broad spectrum antibiotics**
6. **Laparotomy for peritonitis or suspected infarction**
a. Often find edema and cyanotic discoloration of mesentery and bowel wall with thrombus of distal mesenteric veins
b. Complete SMV thrombosis rare (12%)
c. Arterial supply usually intact
d. Wide resection of nonviable bowel followed by reanastomosis
e. Thrombectomy considered for large segments of compromised bowel.
f. Consider second-look operation.
7. **Postoperative care**
a. Continue anticoagulation, possibly for life
8. **Evaluate cause of thrombosis including workup for hypercoagulable state**

## E. PROGNOSIS
1. **Mortality rate as high as 50%**

# Renovascular Hypertension

*Sha-Ron Jackson, MD*

Renovascular hypertension is systemic hypertension resulting from decreased renal blood flow and subsequent activation of the renin-angiotensin system.

**Case Scenario:** *A 65-year-old man with a medical history of hypertension, peripheral vascular disease, and three-vessel coronary artery bypass graft presents with hypertension newly refractory to triple-drug antihypertensive therapy. Physical examination is positive for left upper quadrant bruit.*

## I. BACKGROUND

Renovascular hypertension was originally described by Goldblatt in 1934. He demonstrated that hypertension could be produced by 70% narrowing of the renal artery—renal artery stenosis (RAS).

1. Found in less than 5% of individuals with hypertension
2. Activation of the renin-angiotensin system is protective to prevent renal parenchymal injury during times of inadequate perfusion.
3. Most common cause of surgically correctable hypertension
4. Other surgical causes—primary aldosteronism, pheochromocytoma, coarctation of the aorta, abdominal coarctation, Takayasu disease, Cushing syndrome, renal parenchymal disease

## II. SPECIFIC FUNCTIONS

### A. RENIN

1. Released from the juxtaglomerular apparatus at the afferent arteriole in response to sympathetic stimulation, decrease in sodium and chloride ion concentrations in the adjacent distal tubule, or decreased perfusion pressure (hypotension)
2. Proteolytically cleaves angiotensinogen to angiotensin I in the liver

### B. ANGIOTENSIN-CONVERTING ENZYME (ACE)

1. Causes cleavage of angiotensin I (a decapeptide) to angiotensin II (an octapeptide) in the lung

**Pearl:** *Patient newly prescribed an ACE inhibitor for essential hypertension (HTN) describes persistent cough. You recognize that this is a not uncommon adverse effect of ACE inhibitors and make appropriate changes to the patient's antihypertensive medications.*

### C. ANGIOTENSIN II IS THE MOST POTENT VASOCONSTRICTOR KNOWN.

1. Acts directly on smooth muscle in nearly all vascular beds, increasing systemic vascular resistance

2. Stimulates posterior pituitary to release antidiuretic hormone and stimulation of aldosterone secretion from the adrenal cortex
3. Is cleaved to form angiotensin III, which also causes aldosterone release
4. Increased adrenergic function by increased norepinephrine release and decreased reuptake

### D. ALDOSTERONE
1. Produced by the zona glomerulosa of the adrenal gland
2. It contributes to hypertension by stimulating active absorption of sodium and water at the distal tubules of the kidney, leading to increased intravascular volume.

## III. ADDITIONAL FEATURES

**A. RENOVASCULAR HYPERTENSION CAN BE EITHER RENIN- OR VOLUME-DEPENDENT.**

**B. RENIN-DEPENDENT DISEASE**
1. Occurs with unilateral RAS. Activation of the renin-angiotensin system results in a compensatory natriuresis by the unaffected kidney. The patient remains euvolemic; thus, the hypertension is caused only by vasoconstriction. (Angiotensin II inhibitors are effective in the treatment of unilateral RAS.)

**C. VOLUME-DEPENDENT DISEASE**
1. Occurs with bilateral RAS. Compensatory diuresis is lost, so the hypertension is driven primarily by volume expansion. (Angiotensin II inhibitors are ineffective in the treatment of bilateral RAS and for patients with solitary kidney.)

## IV. ATHEROSCLEROSIS

1. Atherosclerosis represents 75% of renovascular hypertension cases.
2. Eighty-five percent of atheromatous plaques occur at the renal artery ostia.
a. Most are contiguous with aortic lesions
3. Atherosclerosis primarily occurs in elderly men (in their sixth decade of life).
4. The proximal third of left renal artery is more commonly affected.
5. Thirty percent to 50% of cases are bilateral.

## V. FIBROMUSCULAR DYSPLASIA

Fibromuscular dysplasia is an idiopathic disorder with several different histologic subtypes; it accounts for 20% of renovascular hypertension.

## A. MEDIAL FIBROPLASIA

1. Accounts for 85% of dysplastic lesions
2. Occurs primarily in young (30–50 years of age) multiparous women
3. Forms focal stenosis surrounded by microaneurysms in the midrenal artery and distal renal artery, which resemble a "string of beads" on angiogram
4. About 85% of cases involve the distal third of right renal artery; 50% are bilateral.
5. Causative factors may be related to changes in smooth muscle cells under the influence of estrogens or damage caused by stretching during pregnancy.
6. Other arteries, such as the internal carotids and iliacs, can be affected.
7. Excellent cure results (2/3) with balloon angioplasty

## B. INTIMAL FIBRODYSPLASIA

1. Accounts for 5% of dysplastic disease cases
2. Occurs primarily in children and adolescents, with no sex predominance
3. Most common cause of renovascular hypertension in the pediatric population
4. Results in smooth focal or tubular stenosis of the renal artery
5. Causative factor is thought to be related to persistence of embryonic myointimal cushions, trauma, or abnormal flow patterns.

## C. PERIMEDIAL FIBRODYSPLASIA

1. Accounts for 10% of dysplastic lesions; usually affects young women
2. More progressive than medial fibrodysplasia
3. Solitary or multiple areas of stenosis without dilations in the distal renal artery

## VI. DEVELOPMENTAL RENAL ARTERY DISEASE

1. Rare cause of renovascular hypertension
2. Found equally among the sexes
3. Accounts for 40% of renovascular hypertension cases in children
4. Arteries are hypoplastic at their origin from the aorta, with an hourglass shape.
5. Causative factors
a. May stem from abnormal fusion of the dorsal aorta during development. Can be associated with coarctation of the abdominal aorta or aortic hypoplasia.

## VII. OTHER CAUSES OF RENOVASCULAR HYPERTENSION

Other causes of renovascular hypertension include aneurysms, arteriovenous malformations, dissections, traumatic disruptions, renal artery thrombosis, and emboli from arterial plaques.

38

RENOVASCULAR HYPERTENSION

## VIII. CLINICAL FINDINGS

### A. ABDOMINAL BRUIT (50–80% OF PATIENTS)

### B. HYPERTENSION

1. New onset before 35 or after 50 years of age
2. Hypertension refractory to triple-drug therapy
3. Sudden worsening of stable hypertension, especially in patients with known atherosclerosis
4. Malignant hypertension presenting with signs of end-organ damage

### C. DECREASED RENAL FUNCTION

1. There is decreased renal function after starting an ACE inhibitor or angiotensin receptor blocker.

### D. UNILATERAL SMALL KIDNEY ≤9 CM, ASYMMETRY IN KIDNEY SIZE >1.5 CM

1. 75% correlation with large-vessel occlusive disease

## IX. SCREENING STUDIES

The 2005 American College of Cardiology/American Heart Association Guidelines on Peripheral Artery Disease recommend screening for RAS only if a corrective procedure for RAS would be considered.

### A. LABORATORY STUDIES

1. Captopril challenge test—plasma renin levels measured before and after administration of captopril accurately discriminate between renovascular and essential hypertension.
2. Plasma renin activity profile—plasma renin plotted against 24-hour urine sodium excretion can identify right ventricular hypertrophy; however, plasma renin levels can be normal in up to 50% of patients with the disease.
3. Obtain necessary serum and urine chemistries to rule out other potential causes of hypertension, for example, primary hyperaldosteronism (sodium, potassium), pheochromocytoma (urine catecholamines), hyperthyroidism (thyroid-stimulating hormone, thyroxine), and hyperparathyroidism (calcium).

### B. DUPLEX ULTRASOUND

1. Reliable, noninvasive method to detect RAS
2. Peak systolic velocity is measured in the pararenal aorta and in each renal artery.
3. A ratio of renal-to-aortic peak systolic velocities greater than 3.5 correlates with a significant (>60%) stenosis.
4. Obesity, bowel gas, or recent surgery often prevents a technically adequate study.
5. Often used for surveillance after angioplasty or surgery

## C. INTRAVENOUS PYELOGRAM
1. Widely used but highly inaccurate screening test
2. Renovascular hypertension is suspected if there is a difference of $\geq 1.5$ cm in renal length or if there is a delay in the appearance of contrast material on one side.
3. Up to 30% of patients with renovascular hypertension demonstrate no abnormal findings.

## X. FUNCTIONAL STUDIES
### A. CAPTOPRIL RENAL SCAN
1. Baseline radionuclide scintigraphy is performed, after which 25 to 50 mg captopril is administered orally. The scan is then repeated after 1 hour.
2. A decline in glomerular filtration rate after the administration of captopril is specific for hemodynamically significant RAS.
3. Asymmetry of appearance and excretion of the radioisotope are also suggestive of renal artery disease.
4. Less accurate study when bilateral RAS is present.
5. ACE inhibitors must be withheld 1 week before the study for accurate results. Other antihypertensive agents may be continued.
6. The 2005 American College of Cardiology/American Heart Association Guidelines recommend not using as a screening tool for RAS—false-negative rate of 20% to 25%.

### B. SELECTIVE RENAL VEIN RENIN ASSAY
1. The test is performed by cannulating each renal vein and sampling blood renin levels.
2. A positive test is indicated by an increase in renin from the affected kidney by a ratio of $\geq 1.5$ compared with the normal kidney.
3. Test has limited value in patients with bilateral RAS.
4. Patients should be fluid and salt restricted, and not taking any antihypertensive medications for accurate results, further limiting its usefulness.

## XI. ARTERIAL STUDIES
### A. CONTRAST ANGIOGRAPHY
Intraarterial digital subtraction angiogram
1. The gold standard in the diagnosis of RAS
2. If functional studies are positive, angiography is performed to confirm anatomic stenosis and to plan appropriate interventions.
3. $CO_2$ angiography can be used to reduce the contrast load for patients with impaired renal function.

### B. MAGNETIC RESONANCE ANGIOGRAPHY
1. A high-quality, noninvasive imaging modality that may eventually replace conventional angiography

38

RENOVASCULAR HYPERTENSION

2. Ideal for patients with impaired renal function or contrast agent allergies
3. Sensitivity of 100%, specificity of 70% to 90%
4. Limited to centers with appropriate equipment and experienced radiologists

### C. SPIRAL COMPUTED TOMOGRAPHY WITH ANGIOGRAPHY
1. Highly accurate noninvasive screening tool
2. Sensitivity of 98% and specificity of 94% in those patients with plasma creatine levels less than 1.7 mg/dl
3. Lower sensitivity in fibromuscular disease

## XII. MEDICAL THERAPY

### A. MEDICAL THERAPY
1. Requires close follow-up, compliant patients, and lifelong medications—even with control of hypertension, renal mass and function can be lost in up to 40% of patients.

### B. PHARMACOLOGIC MANAGEMENT OF RENOVASCULAR HYPERTENSION
1. Restricted to patients not amenable to interventional therapies
2. Operative therapy has proved to be safer than long-term medical management.
3. Reported mortality rates from surgical and medical therapies are 30% and 70%, respectively.

### C. ACE INHIBITORS ARE THE MOST EFFECTIVE THERAPY.
1. Can be associated with a substantial decrease in renal excretory function, especially in patients with atherosclerotic disease
2. Not recommended if bilateral RAS is present

### D. CALCIUM CHANNEL BLOCKERS ARE SECOND-LINE AGENTS

## XIII. ENDOVASCULAR THERAPY

### A. PERCUTANEOUS TRANSLUMINAL RENAL ANGIOPLASTY
1. Involves a controlled disruption of the vessel wall via balloon dilation
2. Treatment of choice for medial fibromuscular dysplasia, short segments of stenosis in the main renal artery, and nonostial atherosclerotic lesions
3. Plaque lesions, especially ones involving the ostia and aorta, have a high rate of technical failure and restenosis.
4. More than 90% of patients improve, but long-term results are still unclear; restenosis occurs in 12% to 25% of patients over 6 months with 2-year follow-up.

### B. PERCUTANEOUS TRANSLUMINAL RENAL ANGIOPLASTY WITH STENT PLACEMENT

1. Intraluminal stents have improved patency rates of ostial lesions and other renal lesions refractory to traditional balloon angioplasty.
2. Treatment of choice for patients at high risk for surgical intervention with ostial lesions

## XIV. SURGICAL THERAPY

Ideal candidates are younger patients with recent-onset HTN less likely to have atherosclerotic disease, those who have not responded successfully to multidrug regimens, medically noncompliant or intolerant individuals, and those with ischemic nephropathy associated with RAS.

### A. RENAL ARTERY REVASCULARIZATION

1. An aortorenal bypass using autogenous saphenous vein is the procedure of choice when the aorta is relatively spared of atherosclerotic change.
2. Prosthetic grafts with polytetrafluoroethylene Gore-Tex or Dacron are acceptable alternatives with similar patency rates.
3. Saphenous vein should be avoided in children because it is prone to aneurysmal degeneration. Autogenous hypogastric artery is the conduit of choice in the pediatric population.
4. Initial revascularization is critical; reoperation is associated with a high nephrectomy rate (50%).
5. Renal artery bypass often accompanies aortic repairs for occlusive or aneurysmal disease.
6. It is effective only if initiated before irreversible parenchymal loss.

### B. RENAL ENDARTERECTOMY

1. Appropriate for atherosclerotic disease and the treatment of choice for bilateral ostial lesions
2. Can be performed either through a longitudinal aortotomy with primary closure or through a transverse aortotomy extending into each renal artery with patch closure

### C. HEPATORENAL/SPLENORENAL BYPASS

1. Extraanatomic bypass is a useful alternative in high-risk patients or patients who have had prior aortic surgery.
2. Bypass procedures avoid cross-clamping of the aorta and are associated with less cardiac and pulmonary morbidity.
3. Hepatorenal bypass using the gastroduodenal artery or saphenous graft is used for right renal revascularization.
4. Splenorenal bypass is used for revascularization of the left kidney.
5. Angiography of visceral arteries must precede revascularization to exclude atherosclerotic disease.

38

RENOVASCULAR HYPERTENSION

## D. NEPHRECTOMY (<10% OF PATIENTS)

1. Indicated in unilateral renovascular disease in a small (<8-cm) kidney with minimal excretory function and persistent hypertension
2. Atrophic kidneys do not contribute to creatinine clearance, but do continue to produce renin and hypertension.
3. Also indicated for patients who have not responded successfully to revascularization
4. Traumatic disruption

## E. SURGICAL OUTCOMES

1. Mortality rate of 3% to 6%
2. Overall, 80% to 90% of patients are better or cured in carefully selected patient groups.
   a. Pediatric fibrodysplasia—97% improve
   b. Adult fibrodysplasia—94% improve
   c. Adult focal atherosclerosis—91% improve
   d. Adult diffuse atherosclerosis—72% improve, but only 24% cured
3. Patients with fibrodysplastic disease respond better. Older patients with atherosclerosis have poorer outcomes.
4. Nephrectomy is uniformly successful.

# Endovascular Surgery

*Karen Lissette Huezo, MD*

The specialty of endovascular surgery currently encompasses the use of angiography, intravascular ultrasound, and/or angioscopy via catheter-based systems through a remote vascular site to remove, remodel, stent, or bypass vascular stenoses, blockages, dissections, aneurysms, and injuries. This chapter outlines angiography and endovascular interventions such as endoluminal angioplasty and stenting/grafting. Endovascular surgery is invasive and, therefore, has inherent risks. The indications, risks, and benefits have to be clear, as with any other invasive procedure.

## I. ANGIOGRAPHY

### A. DEFINITION

1. Angiography is the evaluation of arteries and veins through imaging that allows characterization of disease by looking at intraluminal anatomy and flow.
2. This usually includes the infusion of a contrast agent that passes intraluminally, allowing blood vessels to stand out against the background of other soft tissues, and the use of serial film or digital systems.
3. In general, angiography is indicated in patients for whom an intervention is planned that requires information that cannot be obtained by noninvasive means.
4. The angiographer is usually prepared to proceed with an endovascular intervention, depending on the diagnostic findings during angiography.

### B. COMMON INDICATIONS FOR DIAGNOSTIC ANGIOGRAPHY

1. Evaluation of mesenteric vessels for visceral ischemia or before surgery for cancer resection (pancreatic cancer)
2. Evaluation of renal arteries for renovascular hypertension or renal donor anatomy
3. Evaluation of extremities for acute or chronic ischemia
4. Evaluation of cerebral vasculature for cause of neurologic symptoms
5. Evaluation of traumatic arterial injuries
6. Evaluation and treatment of pulmonary embolus

### C. THE RISKS OF ANGIOGRAPHY

Depend on the vascular bed to be imaged, the contrast agent being used, and the preprocedural diagnosis. These risks are related to the following:

1. **Access site**
   a. Bleeding/hematomas at access site
   b. Arteriovenous fistulas
   c. Pseudoaneurysms
   d. Retroperitoneal hematomas

e. Perforation of a vessel by catheters or balloons (increased in arterial tortuosity)

2. **Embolization or occlusion of the vascular bed distal to the access or catheterization site (i.e., stroke for carotid or kidney infarct for renal catheterization)**

3. **Contrast induced**

a. Allergic reactions

   (1) Urticaria

   (2) Anaphylactic reactions

   (3) May be ameliorated by diphenhydramine and steroids administered before contrast agent

b. Renal failure

   (1) May be dose related

   (2) Increased risk in prior renal failure/insufficiency, proteinuria, diabetes, advanced age, gout, hypertension, and dehydration

   (3) Prehydration with normal saline is recommended.

      (a) Usually begins 3 to 12 hours before contrast and continues 6 to 24 hours after contrast

      (b) Use caution in those with left ventricular dysfunction, cirrhosis, or acute respiratory distress syndrome.

   (4) Mannitol and furosemide have potentially detrimental effects (secondary to hypovolemia).

   (5) Theophylline has demonstrated beneficial effects in prevention of contrast-induced nephropathy. It needs to be studied further. It is not yet recommended as standard prophylaxis.

   (6) Acetylcysteine may reduce the incidence of contrast-induced nephropathy, but trials are inconsistent.

   (7) Sodium bicarbonate may be beneficial but needs to be studied further.

   (8) Usually transient and resolves spontaneously in 7 days but can be progressive

c. Cardiac

   (1) Congestive heart failure

      (a) Usually occurs in patients with renal failure

      (b) Increased risk during pulmonary artery injections and in patients with preexisting cardiac dysfunction

   (2) Can affect intracardiac conduction, myocardial function, or coronary artery tone induced by hyperosmolarity of the contrast agents (decreased by use of low-osmolality agents)

d. Nausea and vomiting

e. Burning in distribution of the vascular bed being infused with contrast agent (secondary to extravasation of the contrast)

## D. PREOPERATIVE EVALUATION

1. **Complete history**

a. Reactions to seafood, iodine, anesthetics, contrast agents, or sedatives/narcotics

(1) Contrast is iodinated.
(2) Seafood usually contains iodine.
(3) Lidocaine or similar drugs are used for local anesthesia.
(4) Sedation with narcotics or other sedatives is common.
b. Documented evidence or review of systems that suggests renal, cardiac, pulmonary, diabetic, or bleeding diseases
c. Family history of any of the above
d. Medications
   (1) Diuretics
       (a) Suggest chronic dehydration
       (b) May need preoperative hydration
   (2) Metformin
       (a) Can increase renal failure
       (b) Should be avoided 24 hours before and 48 hours after procedure

**2. Complete physical examination**
a. Preoperative vascular and neurologic exam is *extremely* important.
   (1) Any neurologic deficit needs to be documented.
   (2) Pulse/Doppler status needs to be documented for all extremities.
   (3) Preoperative blood pressure measurements in both arms should be recorded.

**3. Laboratory data**
a. Complete blood cell count
b. Renal panel
c. Prothrombin time/partial prothrombin time

**4. All patients are potential candidates for an intervention such as thrombolytics and should fulfill the following criteria:**
a. Eighteen-gauge intravenous catheter—at least one, preferably two
b. No arterial punctures just before procedures
c. No attempted central venous access just before procedure unless there is no other access and it is approved by the surgeon.
d. No intramuscular injections
e. Type and screen
f. Foley catheter
g. NPO (nothing by mouth)

## II. ENDOVASCULAR INTERVENTION

Endovascular interventions include angioplasty, stenting, endoluminal grafting, thrombectomy, and catheter-directed thrombolysis. The details of these procedures are beyond the scope of this handbook, but the risks, benefits, and preoperative evaluations are important to understand while caring for these patients.

### A. PREOPERATIVE CONSIDERATIONS

1. Preoperative evaluations and preparation are the same as for diagnostic angiography.

39

ENDOVASCULAR SURGERY

a. All patients undergoing angiography should also consent to possible percutaneous transluminal angioplasty and stenting to avoid having to come back for another procedure that could have been completed at the time of the initial angiogram.

b. Preoperative imaging: Which modality is used depends on the vascular bed to be studied—spiral computed tomography (CT), CT angiography, and intravascular ultrasound.

   (1) Intravascular ultrasound

      (a) This is an invasive procedure.

      (b) It can be used as an adjunct to other procedures, such as contrast angiography and balloon angioplasty.

      (c) It can be used for prediagnostic evaluation in patients when contrast agents are contraindicated or CT scans are inconclusive.

c. Special historical facts are important to risk analysis, especially for thrombolytic therapy. The following are not all absolute contraindications, but they may increase patient risks:

   (1) Recent fall, trauma, or both

   (2) Recent surgery or recent obstetric delivery

   (3) History of intracranial pathology—recent stroke, subdural hematoma, or aneurysm

   (4) History of metastatic cancer

   (5) Active bleeding from any source

   (6) Recent cardiopulmonary resuscitation

   (7) Hemorrhagic retinopathy

   (8) Pregnancy

   (9) Peptic ulcer disease

   (10) Uncontrolled hypertension

   (11) Left-sided heart thrombus

   (12) Bacterial endocarditis

   (13) Atrial fibrillation with mitral valve disease

**2. Postprocedural care includes assessment of the following conditions:**

a. End-organ ischemia after stenting or angioplasty secondary to dissection, thrombosis, or embolus

b. Renal function, especially in high-risk patients

c. Inspection of access site for bleeding

## B. CATHETER-DIRECTED THROMBOLYSIS

**1. All thrombolytic agents currently used are plasminogen activators (recombinant tissue-type plasminogen activator).**

**2. Goals**

a. Dissolve the occluding thrombus.

b. Restore perfusion.

c. Identify underlying cause of arterial or graft thrombus.

**3. Good candidates for lytic therapy**

a. Acute embolic or thrombotic occlusion of inaccessible arteries that would require involved surgical exposure for operative thromboembolectomy

b. Wound complications in a new surgical wound
c. Acute thrombosis of a popliteal aneurysm causing limb-threatening foot ischemia
d. Acute arterial thrombosis
e. Thrombosed saphenous vein grafts that have been functioning for 1 year or longer
4. **Patients undergoing continuous thrombolytic infusions should have the following evaluations:**
a. Serial complete blood cell count, prothrombin and partial thromboplastin times, and fibrinogen levels checked no less than every 8 hours, usually every 6 hours
b. Serial evaluations for local or remote site bleeding such as hematuria, gastrointestinal bleeding, strokes, pericatheter bleeding, or retroperitoneal hematomas
   (1) Medical adjuncts to thrombolytic therapy that increase the risk for bleeding complications include:
      (a) Aspirin
      (b) Heparin
      (c) Clopidogrel (Plavix)
      (d) Glycoprotein IIb/IIIa antagonist
   (2) Bleeding risk can last for up to 36 hours with current agents.

## C. GENERAL RISKS AND BENEFITS
Of intervention or diagnostics in specific vascular beds
1. **AAA endovascular repair (also refer to Chapter 35)**
a. Anatomic considerations
   (1) The infrarenal aneurysm neck must be smaller than the expanded graft diameter (less than 30 mm with newer Cook grafts) and 10 to 15 mm in length.
   (2) Infrarenal neck angulation less than 45 to 60 degrees
   (3) Common iliac artery landing zone of ≈2 cm
b. Patient follow-up
   (1) CT scan at 1 month
   (2) Additional CT scans: Timing is dependent on presence or absence of endoleak.
   (3) Secondary endoleaks require angiographic evaluation.
c. Complications (in addition to angiography complications)
   (1) Endoleak—presence of blood outside of the lumen of the endovascular graft but within the aneurysm sac (maintenance of some degree of pressurization of the aneurysm sac)
      (a) Type I—perigraft blood flow at the attachment sites. Persistent type I endoleaks should be treated.
      (b) Type II—retrograde blood flow from patent lumbar arteries/inferior mesenteric artery
         (1) Most common type
         (2) Can be followed if decrease in size of sac

        (3) Treatment of enlarging aneurysm sac is controversial. Can perform superselective coil embolization.

     (c) Type III—leakage through detached or inadequately sealed modular segments or through structural defects in the graft

        (1) Requires reintervention

     (d) Type IV—diffusion of blood through needle holes or interstices of graft material

        (1) Self-limited

        (2) Usually resolves within 24 hours

  (2) Graft migration

  (3) AAA rupture

d. Results

  (1) Decreased 30-day mortality after endovascular repair. This decrease is not present 1 year after repair.

  (2) One percent per year risk for rupture after endovascular repair

  (3) Endovascular repair is associated with fewer postoperative complications.

  (4) Stabilization or shrinkage of aneurysm sac is seen in 80% to 90% of patients.

  (5) Reintervention is required in $\approx$10% of patients.

## 2. Carotid stenting

a. Carotid endarterectomy (CEA) remains the gold standard.

b. Alternative to CEA in high-risk patients—remains under investigation

  (1) Severe cardiac disease, chronic obstructive pulmonary disease, chronic renal insufficiency (CRI)

  (2) Prior CEA

  (3) Surgically inaccessible lesions

  (4) Prior radiation therapy to neck

  (5) Prior ipsilateral radical neck dissection

c. Incidence of restenosis most commonly reported between 5% and 10% at 12 to 24 months

d. Reported stroke and mortality rate between 0% and 27%

e. Embolic stroke is most common complication.

  (1) Incidence may be affected by use of embolic protection devices.

## 3. Cerebral angiography

a. Angiogram carries 1% to 2% risk for stroke.

## 4. Renal (also refer to Chapter 38)

a. Overall complication rate: 17%, including puncture site (4.5%)

b. Complication related to catheterization of renal artery

  (1) Direct injury, spasm, occlusion, or infarction: $\approx$10%

  (2) Decrease in renal function: $\approx$3%

  (3) New dialysis requirement: <0.5%

  (4) Requiring surgery: $\approx$2%

  (5) Thirty-day mortality rate: $\approx$1.3%

c. Percutaneous transluminal angioplasty alone

  (1) Restenosis rate: $\approx$18% at 1 to 2 years

    d. Percutaneous transluminal angioplasty and stent
      (1) Renal function benefit: reported between 0% and 55%
      (2) Hypertension benefit: ≈51%
      (3) Restenosis rate: ≈18% at 1-2 years
      (4) Major complications (requiring additional therapy or change in treatment plan): ≈9%

**5. Lower extremity interventions (also refer to Chapter 33)**
a. Iliac arteries
    (1) Primary patency: 81% at 2 year and 72% at 5 years
    (2) Major complications: ≈10%
b. Femoropopliteal vessels
    (1) Primary patency: 48% at 5 years
    (2) Major complications: ≈10%

**6. Vena cava interruption (also refer to Chapter 31)**
a. Specific complications
    (1) Inferior vena cava occlusion
    (2) Vena caval penetration
    (3) Filter migration
    (4) Filter maldeployment

**7. General follow-up**
a. Close monitoring after endovascular intervention is important
b. Duplex ultrasound is most frequently used.
c. Clinically significant stenosis is usually defined as greater than 50% stenosis as identified by duplex ultrasound.
d. Suggested follow-up—1, 3, and 6 months, and every 6 months thereafter
e. Suspected restenotic lesions should be confirmed with angiography and addressed quickly.

## RECOMMENDED READING

Brunicardi F (ed): *Schwartz's Principles of Surgery,* 8th ed. New York, McGraw Hill, 2005.

Narins C, Illig K: Patient selection for carotid stenting versus endarterectomy: A systematic review. *J Vasc Surg* 44:661–672, 2006.

Rutherford RB: *Vascular Surgery,* 6th ed. New York, Elsevier-Saunders, 2005.

39

ENDOVASCULAR SURGERY

# PART VIII

# Cardiothoracic Surgery

# Cardiac Surgery

*Jefferson M. Lyons, MD*

## I. PREOPERATIVE EVALUATION

### A. HISTORY

1. History of present illness—detailed account of symptom chronology: acute versus chronic
   a. Angina, arrhythmia, congestive heart failure
   b. Timing of recent intervention
2. Medical and surgical history—detailed
3. Medications and allergies—detailed list and dosages
4. Social history including tobacco, ethyl alcohol, and drug use
5. Family history
6. Review of symptoms

### B. PHYSICAL EXAMINATION—COMPLETE AND SYSTEMS BASED

1. Neurologic—cranial nerves, strength, and motor bilaterally
2. Pulmonary—rales, rhonchi, wheezing (pneumonia, congestive heart failure, chronic obstructive pulmonary disease)
3. Cardiovascular
   a. Signs or symptoms of congestive heart failure—jugular venous distention, rales, S3 gallop
   b. Arrhythmias, presence of a pacemaker, and/or defibrillator
   c. Previous sternotomy/thoracotomy incisions, chest tubes
   d. Vascular examination
      (1) Documentation of peripheral pulses—radial, ulnar, femoral, dorsalis pedis
      (2) Evidence of tissue loss or ischemic extremities
      (3) Evaluation of carotid disease, bruits
      (4) Evaluation of neck/groin for potential internal jugular/femoral cannulation
4. Gastrointestinal—old incisions, hernia
5. Musculoskeletal—strength, sensation, gait, among others

### C. PREOPERATIVE TESTING

1. Electrocardiogram—arrhythmias, ischemic changes, conduction delays, chamber enlargement
2. Laboratory—complete blood cell count, electrolytes, coagulation profile, type and cross-match for 2 units of packed red blood cells
3. Posteroanterior and lateral chest radiograph—visualize plane between sternum and heart on lateral.
4. Nuclear perfusion testing
   a. Myocardial reserve—hibernating myocardium that may benefit from revascularization.
   b. Functional significance of coronary lesion

5. Cardiac catheterization and echocardiogram
a. Distribution of coronary artery disease
b. Evaluation of ventricular wall motion and ejection fraction
c. Presence of valvular dysfunction

## D. PREOPERATIVE ORDERS
1. Accurate height and weight recorded in chart to calculate body surface area
2. Twelve-lead electrocardiogram
3. Posteroanterior and lateral chest radiograph (recent)
4. Hibiclens scrub and clipper prep to chest the night before surgery
5. Nothing by mouth (NPO) after midnight
6. Antibiotics on call—cefuroxime 1.5 g intravenous on call or use vancomycin 1 g intravenous for reoperative/valve patients.
7. Medications
a. In general, medications are continued until surgery, especially antianginal agents, antihypertensive agents, nitroglycerin, and heparin drips.
b. Continue all antiarrhythmic agents.
c. Perioperative steroid and insulin coverage is per routine.
8. Perioperative monitors are generally placed in preop immediately before operation.
a. Right radial/brachial arterial line (femoral line as well as dissection)
b. Swan–Ganz catheter (some institutions omit this step for straightforward procedures)

## II. OPERATIVE PROCEDURES
### A. CORONARY ARTERY BYPASS GRAFTING (CABG)
1. Indications
a. Chronic stable angina unrelieved by medication
b. Unstable angina despite treatment
c. Acute myocardial infarction—if significant coronary disease exists beyond the area of infarction, ongoing angina after infarction, or unstable hemodynamic status. Controversy exists on the timing of surgical intervention.
d. Ventricular arrhythmias with coronary disease
e. Failed percutaneous transluminal coronary angioplasty
2. CABG has been shown to be superior to medical treatment of coronary disease in the following situations:
a. In patients with asymptomatic or mild angina and the following conditions:
   (1) Significant left main disease (Veterans Affairs Cooperative Study 1972–1974)
   (2) Three-vessel coronary artery disease with proximal left anterior descending disease or double-vessel disease in conjunction with left main disease (European Coronary Surgery Study Group 1973–1976)

(3) Three-vessel disease and ventricular dysfunction (Coronary Artery Surgery Study 1975–1979)
b. In patients with chronic moderate-to-severe angina
c. Unstable angina despite full medical therapy
d. Failed percutaneous transluminal coronary angioplasty with reasonable targets
e. Persistent ventricular arrhythmias in patients with coronary artery disease
f. Patients with diabetes with double-vessel disease
3. No difference in rates of myocardial infarction in CABG and medically treated patients.
4. Internal mammary artery grafts are the conduit of choice because of superior patency rates compared with saphenous vein grafts (in situ and free grafts) (90–95% vs. 50–60% at 10 years).

## B. VALVE REPLACEMENT OR REPAIR
1. Aortic stenosis
a. Commonly caused by bicuspid valve, rheumatic disease, or calcific aortic stenosis
b. Symptoms include triad of dyspnea, angina, and syncope.
c. Indications for surgery
   (1) Symptomatic patients with valve gradient of >50 mm Hg or valve area <0.8 cm$^2$/m$^2$
   (2) Asymptomatic patients with significant stenosis and left ventricular hypertrophy should be considered.
   (3) Asymptomatic patients with evidence of decreased systolic function should also be considered.
d. Coronary angiography is performed before surgery because of high rate of concomitant coronary artery disease.
2. Aortic insufficiency
a. Causative factors include rheumatic disease, annular ectasia, endocarditis, and aortitis.
b. Frequently asymptomatic, but symptoms of congestive heart failure may be present
c. Indications for surgery
   (1) Symptomatic patients
   (2) Patients with cardiomegaly or deteriorating systolic function as assessed by echocardiography
3. Mitral stenosis
a. Primarily rheumatic
b. Symptoms—dyspnea, orthopnea, and paroxysmal nocturnal dyspnea. Radiographs may demonstrate left atrial enlargement and pulmonary venous hypertension.
c. Indications for surgery—presence of chronic symptoms or acute episodes of pulmonary venous hypertension.
d. Chronic atrial fibrillation—a complication of progressive left atrial enlargement.

4. Mitral regurgitation
  a. Causative factors—rheumatic disease, myxomatous valve structure, endocarditis, ischemia or papillary muscle dysfunction, and congenital structural defects
  b. Severity and development of symptoms—varies with causative factor; rheumatic disease is more insidious in onset, whereas ischemic mitral regurgitation is often acute in onset.
  c. As with mitral stenosis, indications for surgery depend on the severity of symptoms.
  d. Ischemic mitral regurgitation is usually corrected at the time of coronary bypass, with either valve replacement or annuloplasty. Often mild ischemic mitral regurgitation may improve by coronary bypass only.
  e. Rheumatic or myxomatous valve disease may be corrected by valve repair or replacement. The advantages of repair versus replacement are the low rate of endocarditis and lack of need for long-term anticoagulation.

## C. AORTIC DISSECTION
1. Causative factors—hypertension, atherosclerosis, cystic medial necrosis (e.g., Marfan's syndrome), infections, trauma, pregnancy
2. Clinical considerations
  a. Dissections diagnosed within 2 weeks from onset of symptoms are acute.
  b. Mortality secondary to acute dissection ranges from 57% to 89%.
3. DeBakey classification
  a. Type I—intimal disruption of ascending aorta that extends to involve the entire descending thoracic aorta and abdominal aorta.
  b. Type II—involves the ascending aorta only (stops at the innominate artery).
  c. Type III—involves the descending thoracic and abdominal aorta only (distal to left subclavian artery).
4. Stanford classification
  a. Type A—any dissection that involves the ascending aorta.
  b. Type B—any dissection that involves only the descending aorta, distal to the left subclavian artery.
5. Diagnosis is usually made by aortogram or chest computed tomography scan. Preoperative control of hypertension with nitroprusside and beta-blockers is an essential part of management.
  a. Start beta-blockade first to decrease heart rate and aortic wall dP/dt.
  b. Nitroprusside can then decrease the blood pressure (if sodium nitroprusside [SNP] given first, it actually increases cardiac work and the dP/dt; this theoretically can increase propagation of the dissection).
6. Dissection may advance proximally, disrupting coronary blood flow or inducing aortic valve incompetence, or distally, causing stroke, renal failure, paraplegia, or intestinal ischemia.
7. Indications for emergent operative repair

a. Acute type A dissection
  (1) Operative repair involves replacement of the affected aorta with a prosthetic graft.
  (2) Cardiopulmonary bypass is required, and hypothermic circulatory arrest is often used for transverse arch dissections.
  (3) Aortic valve replacement and coronary reimplantation may be required for type A aneurysms that involve the aortic root.
b. Type B dissection with failed medical therapy such as hypertension, inadequate pain control, progressive dissection by radiographic studies, impaired organ perfusion, or impending aortic rupture
  (1) Type B dissections can be medically managed unless expansion, rupture, or compromise of branch arteries develops or hypertension becomes refractory.
8. Postoperative complications include renal failure, intestinal ischemia, stroke, and paraplegia.

## D. TRAUMATIC AORTIC DISRUPTION
1. This injury results from deceleration injury and usually occurs just distal to the left subclavian artery, at the level of the ligamentum arteriosum.
2. Chest radiograph findings include widened mediastinum, pleural capping, associated first and second rib fractures, loss of the aortic knob, hemothorax, deviation of the trachea or nasogastric tube, and associated thoracic injuries (scapular and clavicular fractures).
3. Definitive diagnosis is made by aortogram, but chest computed tomography and transesophageal echocardiography also aid in the diagnosis.
4. Imperative that immediate life-threatening injuries (e.g., positive diagnostic peritoneal lavage) be treated before repair.

## E. CONGENITAL HEART SURGERY
Numerous congenital anomalies have been described, but in general, most congenital heart diseases can be broken down according to the physiologic disturbances.
1. Obstructive lesions: Lesions include valvular stenoses and coarctation of the aorta. Long-term sequelae include concentric cardiac hypertrophy and subsequent failure because of ventricular pressure overload. Repair or replacement of the involved valve or segment is the mainstay of operative treatment.
2. Left-to-right shunts (acyanotic): Atrial and ventricular septal defects make up most patients in this group. Also included are patent ductus arteriosus and truncus arteriosus. Symptoms are due to chronic volume overload of the pulmonary circulation, which eventually leads to pulmonary hypertension. Cyanosis is a late finding in these anomalies because of right-sided heart pressures exceeding left-sided heart pressures (Eisenmenger syndrome). Operative repair involves patch closure of the septal defect or ductal ligation.

3. Right-to-left shunts (cyanotic): These defects include tetralogy of Fallot, transposition of the great arteries, tricuspid atresia, total anomalous pulmonary venous drainage, and Ebstein's anomaly. These defects involve complex repairs that are usually performed during infancy. Palliative procedures include Blalock–Taussig shunts (subclavian artery to pulmonary artery) and aortopulmonary artery shunts.

## III. POSTOPERATIVE CARE

### A. HEMODYNAMICS

1. Invasive monitors include arterial lines, pulmonary artery catheters, and occasionally left atrial catheters.
2. Every effort should be made to optimize ventricular filling pressures and systemic blood pressures. In general, up to 2 L of crystalloid is used; after that, blood or colloid is used to increase filling pressures. Hypertension aggravates bleeding along suture lines and is controlled by a nitroprusside drip. Lower blood pressures are preferred as long as a mean blood pressure >60 mm Hg is maintained. There are numerous causes for hypotension after surgery; before beginning specific treatment, know the filling pressures, cardiac rhythm, cardiac index, and systemic vascular resistance.

### B. ANTIARRHYTHMICS

1. Digoxin is not routinely used unless patient has been taking it previously.
2. Once patient has been weaned from postoperative drips, metoprolol is started and titrated to effect.
3. Atrial fibrillation may be treated with intravenous (IV) beta-blockade, calcium-channel blockade, or amiodarone, depending on surgeon preference.
a. Amiodarone is often loaded as a 150-mg bolus and started on a gtt (drops/min) of 1 mg/min for 6 hours. The gtt is then decreased to 0.5 mg/min for the next 18 hours.
b. Conversion to oral dosing (200 mg orally twice daily) is usually done when gtt is finished, continued for 6 weeks, and then weaned off.
4. Ventricular arrhythmias are often treated with amiodarone.

### C. ANTICOAGULATION

1. Aspirin is given to all CABG patients.
2. Clopidogrel (Plavix) is restarted in all patients with recent stents.
a. Patients with fresh stents may need to undergo intervention.
b. Sometimes Plavix is continued intraoperatively.
3. Patients with bioprosthetic valves are started on warfarin therapy and kept therapeutic (international normalized ratio, 2–3) for 3 months.
4. Patients with mechanical valve replacements are given warfarin starting postoperative day 1, and the dosage is adjusted to maintain international normalized ratio (INR) between 2.5 and 3.5 for life.

## D. HARDWARE

1. Mediastinal tubes are discontinued when drainage is <200 ml/ 8 hours and no air leak is present.
2. Antibiotics are discontinued after the mediastinal tubes are removed or at 24 hours (depending on surgeon preference).
3. Pacing wires are (by convention) atrial on right side and ventricular on left side. They are removed at 3 days or the day before discharge.

## IV. POSTOPERATIVE COMPLICATIONS

### A. ARRHYTHMIAS

1. Ventricular ectopy is the most common complication.
   a. For frequent (>6–10/min) or multifocal premature ventricular complexes, treat with lidocaine bolus of 1 mg/kg, followed by drip at 2 to 4 mg/min.
   b. Cardioversion needed if it progresses to symptomatic ventricular tachycardia or if ventricular fibrillation develops.
   c. Atrial or atrioventricular pacing at a slightly greater rate may suppress ectopy.

2. Nodal or junctional rhythm
   a. May not need treatment for asymptomatic, normotensive patient
   b. Rule out digoxin toxicity; make certain serum $K^+$ level >4.5; rule out hypomagnesemia.
   c. May require atrioventricular sequential pacing if loss of atrial kick has significant hemodynamic sequelae

3. Supraventricular tachycardia—includes atrial fibrillation and flutter.
   a. Onset may be preceded by multiple premature atrial contractions.
   b. Atrial electrocardiogram using atrial pacing leads is often helpful in distinguishing fibrillation from flutter during rapid rates.
   c. Atrial fibrillation—may consider IV beta-blockade, calcium-channel blockade, or amiodarone.
   d. Atrial flutter may be treated by the following:
      (1) Rapid atrial pacing >400 beats/min
      (2) IV beta-blocker or calcium-channel blocker. Calcium-channel blockers must be given judiciously because wide complex supraventricular tachycardia can mimic ventricular tachycardia.
      (3) IV amiodarone
   e. In both instances, if any significant decline in blood pressure or cardiac output occurs, the arrhythmia should be treated with synchronous direct current cardioversion at 50 to 100 joules. This may be repeated with increasing energy levels (100-200-360 joules).
   f. Adenosine can be used initially as a diagnostic and therapeutic intervention. Transient bradycardia/asystole allows interpretation of rhythm and may be therapeutic.

CARDIAC SURGERY

40

## B. BLEEDING

1. Causative factors—include medications, clotting deficits, reoperation, prolonged operation, technical factors, hypothermia, and transfusion reactions.
2. Treatment
a. Ensure normothermia.
b. Measurement of clotting factors—prothrombin time, partial thromboplastin time, fibrinogen, platelet count, activated clotting time
c. Correction
   (1) Fresh frozen plasma, cryoprecipitate, platelets
   (2) Protamine for prolonged heparinization
d. Transfusion reaction protocol if suspected
3. Exploration for postoperative hemorrhage—indications include mediastinal tube output of >200 ml/hr despite correction of clotting factors. Technical factors found as cause >50% of the time.

## C. RENAL FAILURE

1. Incidence rate of 1% to 30%
2. Diagnosis—renal versus prerenal azotemia
3. Management
a. Optimize volume status and cardiac output.
b. Discontinue nephrotoxic drugs.
c. Maintain urine output >30 ml/hr (low-dose dopamine, furosemide, ethacrynic acid as indicated; furosemide (Lasix) or furosemide/chlorothiazide (Diuril) drips for persistent oliguria.
d. Dialysis—either continuous venovenous or hemodialysis may be used.
e. Outcome—mortality rate of 0.3% to 23% depending on the degree of azotemia; if dialysis is required, mortality rate ranges from 27% to 53%.

## D. RESPIRATORY FAILURE

1. Mechanical—mucus plugging, malpositioned endotracheal tube, pneumothorax
2. Intrinsic—volume overload, pulmonary edema, atelectasis, pneumonia, pulmonary embolus (uncommon)

## E. LOW CARDIAC OUTPUT SYNDROME

Cardiac index <2.0 L/min/m$^2$
1. Signs—decreased urine output, acidosis, hypothermia, altered sensorium
2. Assessment—heart rate and rhythm (electrocardiogram: possible acute myocardial infarction), preload and afterload states (pulmonary artery catheter readings), measurement of cardiac output
3. Treatment
a. Stabilize rate and rhythm.
b. Optimize volume status and systemic vascular resistance.

c. Correct acidosis, hypoxemia if present (chest radiograph for pneumothorax).
d. Inotropic agents (e.g., dobutamine or milrinone drips).
e. Persistent low cardiac output despite inotropic support requires placement of intraaortic balloon pump.

## F. CARDIAC TAMPONADE

1. Onset—suggested by increasing filling pressures with decreased cardiac output; decreasing urine output, and hypotension; quiet, distant heart sounds, and eventual equalization of right- and left-sided atrial pressures.
2. High degree of suspicion that coincides with excessive postoperative bleeding
3. Chest radiograph may demonstrate wide mediastinum; echocardiogram if readily available or diagnosis uncertain.
4. Treatment—emergent reexploration is treatment of choice and may be needed at bedside for sudden hemodynamic decompensation. Transfusion to optimize volume status and inotropic support; avoid increased positive end-expiratory pressure.

## G. PERIOPERATIVE MYOCARDIAL INFARCTION

1. Incidence rate of 5% to 20%
2. Diagnosis—new-onset Q waves after surgery; serial isoenzymes, increased myoglobine (MB) fractions; segmental wall motion abnormalities by transthoracic or transesophageal echocardiogram
3. Treatment—vasodilation (IV nitroglycerin is preferred to nitroprusside). Continued hemodynamic deterioration should be treated with immediate intraaortic balloon counterpulsation. This "unloads" the ventricle and may preserve nonischemic adjacent myocardium.
4. Outcome—associated with increased morbidity and mortality, as well as poorer long-term results.

## H. POSTOPERATIVE FEVER

1. Common in the first 24 hours after surgery; most commonly cytokine storm; however, may be associated with pyrogens introduced during cardiopulmonary bypass. Treat pyrexia with acetaminophen and cooling blankets because associated hypermetabolism and vasodilation can be detrimental to hemodynamic status and increase myocardial work.
2. Postoperative fevers in valve patients should be followed closely with cultures. CABG patients should have full fever workup on 5th postoperative day if still febrile.
3. Special attention should be paid to invasive monitors, and should be changed if infection is suspected.
4. Sternal wound—daily inspection for drainage and stability. Sternal infections are disastrous in the cardiac patient, and early evidence of postoperative infection should be treated with operative debridement.

5. Postpericardiotomy syndrome—characterized by low-grade fever, leukocytosis, chest pain, malaise, and pericardial rub on auscultation. Usually occurs 2 to 3 weeks after surgery and is treated with nonsteroidal antiinflammatory agents. Steroids are necessary for some cases.

## I. CENTRAL NERVOUS SYSTEM COMPLICATIONS

1. Causative factors—preexisting cerebrovascular disease, prolonged cardiopulmonary bypass, intraoperative hypotension, and emboli (either air or particulate matter)
2. Transient neurologic deficit—occurs in up to 12% of patients. Improvement usually occurs within several days.
3. Permanent deficit—suspect in patients with delayed awakening postoperatively; may have pathologic reflexes present.
4. Postcardiotomy psychosis syndrome—incidence rate of 10% to 24%. Starts around postoperative day 2 with anxiety and confusion; may progress to disorientation and hallucinations. Treat with rest and quiet environment; antipsychotics may be given as necessary. It is essential to rule out organic cause of delirium, for example, substance withdrawal, hypoxemia, hypoglycemia, and electrolyte abnormality.
5. Computed tomography scan early for suspected localized lesions; electroencephalogram in patients with extensive dysfunction
6. Treatment—optimize cerebral blood flow and avoid hypercapnia.
a. Postoperative seizures are treated with lorazepam and phenytoin.
b. Mannitol may be needed in presence of increased intracranial pressure, depending on hemodynamic status.

## RECOMMENDED READING

Booth DC, Deupree RH, Hultgren HN, et al: Quality of life after bypass surgery for unstable angina: Five-year follow up results of a Veterans Affairs Cooperative Study. *Circulation* 83:87, 1991.

DeBakey ME, McCollum CH, Crawford ES, et al: Dissection and dissecting aneurysm of the aorta: Twenty-year follow up of five hundred twenty-seven patients treated surgically. *Surgery* 92:1118, 1982.

Emergency Cardiac Care Committee and Subcommittees, American Heart Association: Guidelines for resuscitation and emergency cardiac care. *JAMA* 268:2171, 1992.

Gersh BJ, Califf RM, Loop FD, et al: Coronary bypass surgery in chronic stable angina. *Circulation* 79(suppl I):46, 1989.

# Benign Tumors of the Lung

*Lynn C. Huffman, MD*

## I. OVERVIEW

1. Account for <1% of all lung tumors
2. May be derived from epithelial, mesodermal, or endodermal cell lines
3. Infectious granulomas account for 70% to 80% of typical pulmonary nodules.
4. Hamartomas are the next most common single cause, accounting for about 10% of cases.
5. Endobronchial tumors present with signs and symptoms related to airway obstruction and bleeding.
6. Peripheral airway and parenchymal tumors usually present as undiagnosed asymptomatic solitary pulmonary nodules.

41

## II. HISTORY

1. In patients younger than 30 years, probability of malignancy is low.
2. In individuals older than 50 years, there is a significantly greater chance of lesion being malignant.
3. Only 5% of all lung nodules prove to be malignant.
4. Tobacco use is associated with more than 85% of all lung cancers.
5. Chemical exposure, asbestos, or coal mining are risk factors.

## III. PHYSICAL EXAMINATION

1. Lymph node assessment—cervical, supraclavicular, and axillary
2. SOB (shortness of breath)
3. Chest pain
4. Cough
5. Weight loss
6. Hemoptysis

## IV. INITIAL EVALUATION

1. Characterize the mass.
2. Establish a histologic diagnosis.

## V. IMAGING

### A. OLD RADIOGRAPHS ARE ESSENTIAL.

### B. TUMOR DOUBLING TIME

1. Malignant tumors double in weeks to months.
2. Benign tumors double over years or remain unchanged.

### C. COMPUTED TOMOGRAPHY

1. Computed tomography scanning provides information on the following features:

a. Location
b. Morphology

c. Invasive nature
d. Mediastinal adenopathy
e. Presence of adrenal or liver lesions

## VI. TISSUE OBTAINED

1. Sputum cytology
2. Fiberoptic bronchoscopy
3. Transbronchial needle aspiration
4. Transthoracic needle aspiration

## VII. EPITHELIAL TUMORS

### A. POLYPS

1. Can be solitary or multiple
2. Polypoid areas of bronchial mucosa with a fibrous stalk
3. Covered by ciliated columnar epithelium with possible areas of squamous metaplasia
4. Polyps are thought to be secondary to a chronic inflammatory process.
5. They are always benign but may cause bronchial obstruction.

### B. PAPILLOMA

1. Classified as squamous or multiple
2. Multiple papillomatosis is usually a childhood disease with multiple papillomas of the vocal cords and trachea.
3. Thought to be caused by the human papillomavirus
4. Squamous papillomas are a benign neoplasm of squamous epithelium.
5. Thin central fibrovascular core covered by stratified squamous epithelium
6. Occur as solitary lesions in adults and multiple in children
7. Papillomas are usually located in segmental or more proximal bronchi.
8. Human papillomavirus types 6 and 11 are associated with benign lesions, whereas types 16 and 18 have been found in patients with squamous cell carcinoma.
9. Treatment is usually conservative with laser ablation.
10. May require endoscopic removal or even bronchotomy or sleeve resection

### C. MUCOUS GLAND ADENOMA

1. Also known as mucous gland cystadenoma, adenomatous polyp, and adenoma of mucous gland type
2. Benign tumor of the bronchus derived from bronchial mucous glands
3. The tumor must be composed of cystic glands, be superficial to the cartilaginous plate, be in the bronchus, and have some normal bronchial seromucous glands.

4. Patient age ranges from 25 to 67 in reported cases.
5. Symptoms are cough, fever, recurrent pneumonia, and hemoptysis.
6. Chest radiograph often demonstrates obstructive pneumonitis and postobstructive atelectasis.
7. Most often found in the major bronchi of the middle and lower lobes
8. Grossly, tumors vary in size from 0.8 to 6.8 cm and project into the bronchial lumen.
9. Usually encapsulated by a thin membrane and easily removed from the bronchus
10. Composed of small, mucous-filled cysts lined with well-differentiated mucous epithelium
11. The differential diagnosis is low-grade mucoepidermoid carcinoma.
12. Rarely have a stalk but can be completely removed endoscopically
13. Surgical resection is indicated when the distal lung has been destroyed or if endoscopic removal is contraindicated or incomplete.
14. Complete surgical resection results in cure.

## VIII. MESENCHYMAL TUMORS

### A. VESSEL

1. Sclerosing hemangioma

a. Rare, benign tumor of undetermined histogenesis
b. Most patients are asymptomatic with a solitary nodule usually in a lower lobe.
c. Histologically of two cell types—cuboidal surface cells and round cells within the surface layer
d. Calcifications present in one third of tumors.
e. Architecture is a combination of papillary, sclerotic, solid, and hemorrhagic patterns.
f. May be derived from type 2 alveolar pneumocytes
g. Others have found that there is no good evidence of pneumocyte origin.
h. Magnetic resonance for imaging
i. Surgical excision is the treatment of choice for bleeding or obstruction.

2. Lymphangioma

a. Four basic types:
   (1) Lymphangioma
   (2) Lymphangiectasis
   (3) Lymphangiomatosis
   (4) Lymphatic dysplasia
b. Usually small and peripheral
c. High-resolution computed tomography shows the lesion to have a smooth border.
d. May be associated with dyspnea or hemoptysis
e. Surgical resection has excellent outcomes.

**41**

BENIGN TUMORS OF THE LUNG

### 3. Nerve
a. Granular cell tumor
   (1) Were called *granular cell myoblastomas* because thought to be derived from skeletal muscle. Now thought to be derived from Schwann cells.
   (2) Patients are 20 to 60 years of age, and cases are evenly distributed among men and women.
   (3) Found incidentally for >50% of cases; otherwise, usually present with symptoms of obstruction.
   (4) Chest radiograph shows lobar infiltration, coin lesions, and lobar atelectasis.
   (5) Solitary lesions are present in 75% of cases, <10% are multiple; remainder are solitary lesions with multiple skin lesions.
   (6) Gross tumors vary from 0.5 to 5 cm.
   (7) Commonly present as an endobronchial lesion
   (8) Microscopically composed of large cells with abundant pink granular cytoplasm
   (9) Conservative treatment except with a malignant association
   (10) Complete resection is curative, but tumors may recur.
   (11) Laser treatment may be appropriate in certain cases.
   (12) With associated damaged lung, surgical resection is indicated.
b. Neurilemoma
   (1) Equal sex distribution
   (2) May occur in a major bronchus, but majority are seen in the lung parenchyma
   (3) May be difficult to classify because of degenerative changes
c. Neurofibroma
   (1) Most occur in an endobronchial location.
   (2) Seen in young to middle-aged adults
   (3) Surgical resection or endobronchial ablation is indicated as dictated by the extent and location of the tumor.

### 4. Muscle
a. Leiomyoma
   (1) These tumors account for 2% of benign tumors.
   (2) May occur in the trachea, bronchus, or parenchyma. Usually equally distributed.
   (3) Seen in young to middle-aged adults
   (4) More common in women than men
   (5) In women who have had a uterine leiomyoma removed in the past, it is difficult to differentiate a true pulmonary leiomyoma from a benign metastasizing leiomyoma from the original uterine tumor.
   (6) These tumors may be managed by laser resection and close monitoring.

## IX. MISCELLANEOUS TUMORS

### A. FIBROMA

1. Most commonly found arising from visceral pleura
2. Found in the mediastinum, retroperitoneum, external surface of the stomach, and small intestine
3. Tumors are composed of spindle cells with dense bundles of collagen.
4. Adequate resection is curative.
5. Commonly presents as an endobronchial lesion

### B. HAMARTOMA

1. Most common benign tumor of the lung. Comprises about 75% of all benign lesions.
2. Hamartomas consist of abnormal arrangements of normal cells.
3. Slow growth pattern
4. Present as solitary pulmonary nodule 90% of time
5. Radiographically well-circumscribed nodule that may contain popcorn calcifications
6. Needle biopsy is frequently diagnostic of a cartilaginous benign lesion.
7. Surgical excision if symptomatic or when located more proximally with endobronchial compression; also when carcinoma cannot be ruled out
8. Most often, hamartomas consist of cartilage with fatty tissue being a frequent component.
9. The tumor is sometimes referred to as a *fibrolipochondroma.*
10. Most common in middle-aged adults, but no age group is exempt.
11. It has been reported that they present twice as often in male as in female individuals.
12. When symptomatic, patients may present with hemoptysis, cough, phlegm, or chest pain.
13. Usually 1 to 2 cm
14. Calcifications on computed tomographic scanning are usually 30% or less.
15. Occurs most often in a diffuse or popcorn distribution
16. It is now accepted that a fat density identified by high-resolution computed tomography in a peripheral solitary lesion is strong presumptive evidence that the lesion is a benign hamartoma.
17. Endobronchial lesions are not detectable radiographically except when distal lung changes are observed.
18. Biopsy is indicated in any patient with symptoms.
19. Transthoracic needle biopsy is diagnostic in 85% of lesions.
20. There is a 50% incidence rate of postaspiration pneumothorax that is twice the incidence of biopsy of other peripheral lesions.
21. When the diagnosis is made by needle biopsy, observation is safe.

22. Endobronchial lesions are best treated by laser ablation.
23. Rare reports of malignancy in a hamartoma; however, no real evidence exists that these tumors arise from the underlying hamartoma.

### C. TERATOMA
1. Occur rarely as primary lung tumors
2. Most that are found in the lung have an anterior segment of the left upper lobe.
a. Clear cell (sugar) tumor
3. Unknown histogenesis
4. Equally distributed among the sexes
5. Most patients are asymptomatic.
6. The lesions are solitary, peripheral, and 1.5 to 3 cm.
7. Excision is curative.

## X. OTHER TUMORS
### A. LIPOMA
1. These tumors arise from the wall of the bronchus in 80% of cases.
2. More common in male than in female individuals
3. May cause obstruction with pulmonary complications
4. Computed tomographic examination is used to determine pulmonary extension.
5. Commonly presents as an endobronchial lesion
6. Bronchial laser vaporization is the treatment of choice when possible.

### B. CHONDROMA
1. These are true pulmonary mesenchymal tumors.
2. Often confused with hamartomas
3. Most chondromas are endobronchial in location and most often occur in men.
4. Extension requires surgical resection, which is curative.
5. There is a subgroup of these tumors that occur in women that are associated with gastric sarcomas or an extraadrenal paraganglioma (located in the neck, thorax, or abdomen—association is known as Carney's triad).
6. The location of these tumors is primarily parenchymal.
7. They have a tendency to become multiple.
8. In more than half of cases they contain areas that are calcified and need to be differentiated from hamartomas.
9. Microscopically mature bone and cartilage are seen peripherally with degenerative changes centrally.
10. The triad is a chronic persistent indolent disease. Treatment consists of repeated resections of respective tumors. (*Note:* Refers

to Carney syndrome, inherited autosomal disorder, melanotic schwannoma, multiple myomas, multiple areas of skin pigmentation, and one or more endocrine disorders; this is not the same as Carney's triad.)

## XI. INFLAMMATORY PSEUDOTUMORS

### A. PLASMA CELL GRANULOMA

1. This tumor has been called a variety of names, including fibrous histiocytoma, inflammatory pseudotumors, and fibroxanthoma.
2. Because of the low-grade malignant potential of these tumors, wide local excision is recommended (lobectomy or bronchial sleeve lobectomy).

### B. PULMONARY HYALINIZING GRANULOMA

1. A tumor of dense hyalinized connective tissue that occurs as the result of inflammatory or postinflammatory changes.
2. Patients are asymptomatic or present with cough, shortness of breath, chest pain, and weight loss.
3. Lesions are nodular and vary from a few millimeters to 15 cm.
4. Many patients have multiple lesions with most being bilateral.
5. Half of the patients have a history of an autoimmune disorder or past fungal or mycobacterial disease.

## XII. OTHER BENIGN TUMORS

### A. MUCINOUS CYSTADENOMA

1. Defined as a unilocular cystic lesion whose fibrous wall is lined by well-differentiated, presumably benign, columnar mucinous epithelium
2. Usually occurs in smokers in their 50s to 60s; equal distribution among the sexes
3. Usually located at or near the periphery of the lung
4. Filled with clear gelatinous material
5. The cysts may have areas of borderline malignancy or adenocarcinoma.
6. Treatment is complete resection.

### B. NODULAR AMYLOID

1. These occur in three types—tracheobronchial, nodular pulmonary, and diffuse (interstitial) pulmonary.
2. Nodular pulmonary amyloidosis is a focal collection of amyloid in the lung usually with a giant cell reaction around it.
3. May be solitary or multiple nodules
4. Most patients are in their 70s.
5. Most patients are asymptomatic and are discovered incidentally.

41

BENIGN TUMORS OF THE LUNG

6. Long-term follow-up is needed because of the possibility of malignant lymphoma.
7. These lymphomas are identified by lymphatic tracking of the lymphocytic infiltrate, pleural infiltration, and sheetlike masses of plasma cells.

## RECOMMENDED READING

Chang AC, Martin J, Rusch VW: Lung neoplasms. In Mulholland MW, Lillemoe KD, Doherty GM, et al (eds): *Surgery, Scientific Principles & Practice,* 4th ed. Philadelphia, Lippincott Williams & Wilkins, 2006, pp 1367–1395.

Brinckerhoff LH, Mitchell JD: Carcinoma of the lung. In McIntyre RC, Stiegmann GV, Eiseman B (eds): *Surgical Decision Making,* 5th ed. Philadelphia, Elsevier, 2004, pp 84–85.

Schraufnagel DE: American Thoracic Society on line: http://www.thoracic.org/sections/clinical-information/best-of-the-web/pages/pathology/pulmonary-pathology-images.html

Shields TW, Robinson PG: Benign tumors of the lung. In Shields TW, Locicero J, Ponn RB, Rusch VW (eds): *General Thoracic Surgery,* 6th ed. Lippincott Williams & Wilkins, Philadelphia, 2005, pp 1778–1800.

# Carcinoma of the Lung

*Ryan A. LeVasseur, MD*

## I. EPIDEMIOLOGY

### A. GENERAL

1. 100,000 men (approximately 34/100,000/year) and 80,000 women (approximately 27/100,000/year) are affected in the United States each year.
2. Overall prevalence is about 125 per 100,000 people per year.
3. Estimated new cases per year in the United States: 172,570 (93,010 male and 79,560 female) cases

### B. MORTALITY

1. Primary lung malignancies are the leading cause of cancer deaths in men, accounting for 13% of all new cancers and 31% of all cancer deaths; in women, it accounts for 17% of all new cancers and 27% of all cancer deaths.
2. Estimated deaths per year in the United States: 163,510 (90,490 male and 73,020 female) deaths

## II. CAUSATIVE FACTORS

### A. CIGARETTE SMOKING

1. Overall risk for lung cancer in smokers versus nonsmokers is 20 to 25 times greater.
2. Only 10% of patients with lung cancer are nonsmokers, but 25% to 50% of these patients have significant second-hand smoke exposure.

### B. OCCUPATIONAL EXPOSURE

1. Asbestos
2. Ionizing radiation
3. Arsenic
4. Nickel
5. Chromium
6. Mustard gas
7. Chloromethyl ethers

## III. SOLITARY PULMONARY NODULE

### A. GENERAL

1. A solitary pulmonary nodule (SPN) is defined as <3 cm on radiograph with no adenopathy, atelectasis, or pleural effusion.
2. A lesion >3 cm is a lung mass.
3. One in 500 chest radiographs will demonstrate an SPN.

42

## B. DIFFERENTIAL DIAGNOSIS
1. Lung malignancy
2. Inflammation
3. Infection—fungal ball
4. Congenital lesion—hamartoma
5. Vascular
6. Trauma

## C. RADIOGRAPHIC CHARACTERISTICS OF BENIGN NODULE
1. Small, smooth, with sharply circumscribed margins
2. Benign calcification—laminar, central, diffuse, and popcorn patterns
3. Stable in size over 2-year period—doubling time is 40 to 360 days for malignant tumors.

## D. MANAGEMENT OF SPN
1. Depends greatly on size of the lesion and if the lesion has increased in size, patient's age and smoking history, and characteristics on chest computed tomography (CT) scan (calcification, spiculations)
2. Positron emission tomography (PET) scan
   a. Sensitivity 96%, specificity 74%
   b. False negative—bronchoalveolar carcinoma, carcinoid tumors, tumors <1 cm
   c. False positive—inflammation or infection
3. High-risk patients will get a tissue diagnosis via bronchoscopy, fine-needle aspiration (FNA), or video-assisted thoracic surgery (VATS) with wedge biopsy.

## IV. PATHOLOGY

## A. HISTOLOGIC CLASSIFICATION
Malignant epithelial lung tumors according to World Health Organization (1981):
1. Small-cell carcinoma—15%
2. Non–small-cell carcinoma—85%
   a. Adenocarcinoma—40%
   b. Squamous cell carcinoma—30% to 50%
   c. Large cell carcinoma—10%
      (1) Giant-cell carcinoma
      (2) Clear-cell carcinoma

## B. LOCATION OF PRIMARY TUMORS
1. "Central" tumors—squamous and small-cell carcinomas, carcinoid
2. "Peripheral" tumors—adenocarcinoma and large-cell carcinomas

## V. CLINICAL FEATURES

### A. RESPIRATORY
1. Cough—usually dry, persistent (common)
2. Dyspnea with or without wheezing (common)
3. Hemoptysis—may be small and recurrent or sudden and massive.
4. Symptoms of acute pneumonia (that is slow to resolve)

### B. ASSOCIATED SYNDROMES
1. Eaton–Lambert syndrome—proximal muscle group wasting
2. Endocrine abnormalities
a. Syndrome of inappropriate secretion of antidiuretic hormone
b. Hypercalcemia
c. Ectopic adrenocorticotropic hormone
3. Neurologic—peripheral neuropathies, cerebellar degeneration, degeneration of the cerebral cortex, pseudodementia
4. Musculoskeletal—clubbing, hypertrophic pulmonary osteoarthropathy, polymyositis
5. Vascular—anemia, thrombocytosis, thrombocytopenia, migratory thrombophlebitis, marantic thrombosis
6. Cutaneous—dermatomyositis, acanthosis nigricans

### C. EVIDENCE OF METASTATIC OR LOCALLY ADVANCED DISEASE
1. Mediastinal invasion
a. Tracheal obstruction with stridor and dyspnea
b. Dysphagia
c. Hoarseness (ipsilateral involvement of recurrent laryngeal nerve)
d. Horner syndrome
   (1) Tumor involving cervical and first thoracic segment of sympathetic trunk
   (2) Ptosis, meiosis, anhidrosis of the affected side
e. Superior vena cava syndrome
   (1) Compression or direct invasion of great veins of thoracic outlet
   (2) Dyspnea, severe headaches, and periorbital, facial, and neck edema
2. Metastatic disease/locally advanced disease
a. Pleural effusions
b. Bone pain
c. Weight loss
d. Neurologic symptoms
e. Chest pain and chest wall involvement

### D. METHOD OF SPREAD
1. Invades lymphatics and blood vessels, resulting in early metastasis
2. Small-cell carcinoma is most aggressive.
3. Thirty to 50% of patients with lung cancer have lymphatic or hematogenous spread at initial presentation.

42

CARCINOMA OF THE LUNG

4. Metastases in order of preference—regional lymph nodes, liver, adrenals, brain, bone, and kidneys
5. Contralateral pulmonary metastases at postmortem examination— 10% to 14%

## VI. CARCINOID (1–2%)

### A. GENERAL
1. Neuroendocrine family
2. All ages
3. Sixty percent to 70% found in central airways

### B. PATHOLOGIC LESIONS
1. Typical occur in 80% to 85% of patients
a. Lymph node metastasis in <15% of patients
2. Atypical
a. Older patients
b. Lymph node metastasis in 30% to 50% of patients
c. Histology—mitotic activity >2 or <10/2 HPF, cellular heterogenicity, necrosis, nuclear pleomorphism

### C. DIAGNOSIS
1. Chest CT scan
a. Atelectasis
b. Postobstructive pneumonia
c. Endobronchial mass
d. SPN
2. Bronchoscopy
3. PET—frequently false negative
4. Octreotide scan

### D. TREATMENT
1. Complete resection
2. Typical—wedge or segmentectomy if peripheral
3. Atypical—lobectomy, lymph node dissection
4. Bronchoplastic resection

### E. SURVIVAL
1. Typical—5-year survival rate of 90% to 100%
2. Atypical—5-year survival rate of 40% to 70%

## VII. SMALL-CELL LUNG CANCER (20%)

### A. GENERAL
1. Comprise 20% of malignant epithelial lung tumors
2. "Central tumors"—originate in the bronchial mucosa and grow into the walls of bronchi, peribronchial spaces, and lung parenchyma.

3. Noted for its rapid growth and early metastasis, with clinical features commonly caused by metastases
4. Invasion of the superior vena cava is common.

## B. PATHOLOGIC LESIONS
1. Some describe small-cell lung cancers on a spectrum, including Kulchitsky I (starting with well-differentiated, benign carcinoid tumor ranging to less-differentiated atypical carcinoids), Kulchitsky II (neuroendocrine tumors), and Kulchitsky III (undifferentiated small cell carcinomas).

## C. DIAGNOSIS
1. Chest CT—most appear as hilar abnormalities with wide mediastinum.

## D. STAGING
Based on TNM (tumor, node, metastases)—includes imaging of brain and bone marrow biopsy
1. Limited—disease limited to one radiation field.
2. Extensive—disease spread beyond one radiation field.

## E. TREATMENT
1. Widely spread at time of diagnosis—often not amenable to surgery or thoracic radiation alone
2. Systemic chemotherapy is treatment of choice (usually combination of the following: cyclophosphamide, cisplatin, etoposide, doxorubicin, and vincristine) with or without radiation for local control of tumor.
3. Small role for surgery in solitary peripheral nodules with no evidence of metastatic disease.

## VIII. NON–SMALL-CELL LUNG CANCER (85%)
### A. SUBTYPES
1. Adenocarcinoma—occurs in 40% of cases.
a. Increasing in both men and women
b. Arises mostly in the periphery of lung parenchyma
c. May be related to focal scars or regions of fibrosis
d. Grows rapidly and metastasizes early to mediastinal, periaortic, supraclavicular, and cervical lymph nodes
e. Present with metastases to adrenals, liver, bone, and brain
2. Squamous cell carcinoma—most common primary malignant epithelial lung tumor.
a. Occurs in the segmental, lobar, or main-stem bronchi in 90% of cases
b. Relatively slow growing and late to metastasize
c. Spread pattern is as follows:
   (1) Endobronchial growth and invasion of peribronchial lung parenchyma, soft tissue, and lymph nodes
   (2) Peripheral tumors commonly invade chest wall.

42

CARCINOMA OF THE LUNG

d. Pathologic lesions
   (1) Well-differentiated tumors produce keratin, epithelial pearls, and squamous pattern.
   (2) Poorly differentiated tumors with less obvious keratinization
3. **Large-cell carcinoma—10% of cases**
   a. Most tumors occur in a peripheral and subpleural location.
   b. Rapid growth and early metastasis
   c. Poor prognosis
   d. Pathologic lesions:
      (1) Do not show definitive squamous or glandular differentiation
      (2) Grow in sheets without organization or pattern
      (3) Necrosis and hemorrhage are dominant features of these tumors.
   e. Ten percent have mediastinal widening on chest radiograph.
4. **Bronchoalveolar**

## B. DIAGNOSIS
1. **Radiology**
   a. Chest radiograph—abnormalities suspicious of malignancy include the following:
      (1) Atelectasis or lobar emphysema
      (2) Enlarged hilum or hilar mass
      (3) Atelectasis or lobar emphysema
      (4) Enlarged upper or middle mediastinum
      (5) Evidence of bony erosion caused by metastases
   b. CT scan
      (1) May show additional pulmonary nodules
      (2) Evaluate spread to pleural and mediastinal structures
      (3) Direct percutaneous transthoracic needle biopsy
      (4) Use of CT scanning for screening of SPN is being studied.
   c. PET scanning
      (1) May differentiate benign from malignant lung tumor and evaluate metastatic mediastinal lymph node and distant spread
      (2) Based on high rate of glycolysis by uptake of fluorodeoxyglucose in malignant tumors
2. **Sputum cytology**
   a. Seventy percent to 80% sensitive with multiple specimens and central tumors
   b. May perform bronchial brushings to improve yield in peripheral tumors
   c. Cytology most diagnostic for squamous-cell carcinoma, intermediate for adenocarcinoma, and least for small-cell carcinoma.
3. **Bronchoscopy**
   a. Best for central tumors
   b. Complications are rare.
   c. Allows transbronchial biopsies, brush cytology, and bronchial washings for cytology

4. **Mediastinoscopy**
a. Fifty percent of patients have involved mediastinal lymph nodes at initial presentation.
b. Mediastinoscopy is used in patients with mediastinal nodes >1 cm before thoracotomy to evaluate resectability and staging.
c. May access anterior superior mediastinal or subcarinal lymph nodes for biopsy
d. Lymph nodes are positive for metastatic disease in 50% to 65% of patients.

5. **Needle biopsy**
a. False-negative result in 10% of patients
b. May be performed transbronchoscopically or via percutaneous approach with CT guidance
   (1) Transbronchoscopic approach is indicated for extrabronchial tumors without bronchial wall abnormalities.
   (2) CT guidance is used for peripheral lesions >1 cm.
c. Contraindications
   (1) Bleeding disorders or anticoagulation
   (2) Bullous disease near the lesion
d. Complications
   (1) Pneumothorax—20% to 25% of cases; only 10% require chest tube placement.
   (2) Minor hemoptysis—6% of cases

6. **Video-assisted thoracoscopic surgery**
a. May excise peripheral nodule, biopsy lymph nodes, and evaluate effusion
b. Proceed directly to video-assisted thoracoscopic surgery for wedge biopsy of peripheral lesion for diagnosis.

## C. CLASSIFICATION AND STAGING
1. Determines treatment options and prognosis
2. TNM classification for lung carcinoma (1986 International Staging System)
a. Primary tumor (T):
   **T0:** No tumor
   **Tx:** Positive cytology
   **Tis:** Carcinoma in situ
   **T1:** <3 cm, no main bronchial invasion, no invasion of visceral pleura
   **T2:** >3 cm or any size that invades visceral pleura, or main bronchus >2 cm from carina, atelectasis extending to hilum
   **T3:** Invades main bronchus <2 cm from carina, parietal pleura, chest wall, diaphragm, or pericardium
   **T4:** Invades mediastinum, great vessels, trachea, esophagus, carina, vertebral body, malignant effusion, or satellite tumor nodule in the same lobe
b. Regional lymph nodes (N):
   **N0:** No nodes
   **N1:** Ipsilateral nodes (peribronchial or hilar)

**N2:** Ipsilateral nodes (mediastinal) or subcarinal nodes
**N3:** Contralateral nodes (mediastinal) or hilar; ipsilateral or contralateral scalene or supraclavicular nodes
c. Distant metastases (M):
  **M0:** No metastasis
  **M1:** Metastasis
3. Staging for lung cancer:
  **Occult carcinoma:** Tx N0 M0
  **Stage Ia:** T1 N0 M0
  **Stage Ib:** T2 N0 M0
  **Stage IIa:** T1 N1 M0
  **Stage IIb:** T2 N1 M0, T3 N0 M0
  **Stage IIIa:** T3 N1 M0, T1-3 N2 M0
  **Stage IIIb:** any T N3 M0, T4 any N M0
  **Stage IV:** any T, any N, M1
4. Regional lymph node stations (American Thoracic Society):
  **2R:** Right upper paratracheal (suprainnominate) nodes
  **2L:** Left upper paratracheal (supraaortic) nodes
  **4R:** Right lower paratracheal nodes
  **4L:** Left lower paratracheal nodes
  **5:** Aortopulmonary nodes
  **6:** Anterior mediastinal nodes
  **7:** Subcarinal nodes
  **8:** Paraesophageal nodes
  **9:** Pulmonary ligament nodes
  **10R:** Right main bronchial nodes
  **10L:** Left main bronchial nodes
  **11:** Intrapulmonary nodes

## D. TREATMENT
1. Preoperative evaluation
a. Assess resectability if primary tumor
b. Rule out distant metastasis
c. Assess mediastinal lymph node spread
  (1) Staging
    (a) Noninvasive
      (1) Chest CT (lymph node >1 cm suspicious): 57% sensitive, 82% specific
      (2) PET scan: 84% sensitive, 89% specific
    (b) Mediastinoscopy
      (1) Gold standard
      (2) False-negative results in 8% of tests
      (3) Less than 1% rate of major complications
    (c) Endoscopic ultrasound with fine-needle aspiration
    (d) VATS with wedge biopsy
  (2) MUST obtain tissue

(a) Positive N2/N3 lymph nodes on CT, PET, or both
(b) Negative N2/N3 lymph nodes on CT and PET, but:
  (1) T2-T4 lesion
  (2) Suspicious N1 lymph nodes
  (3) Synchronous primary cancers
  (4) Solitary brain and adrenal metastasis
d. Assess patient's ability to tolerate resection.
  (1) Pulmonary function tests: $FEV_1$ (forced expiratory volume in 1 second) >60% and $DL_{CO}$ (diffusing capacity of the lung for carbon monoxide) >40%, patient can tolerate surgery—lobectomy

## 2. Surgical resection

a. General
  (1) Stage I and II cancers
  (2) Five-year survival rate after resection is 50%.
  (3) Adjuvant chemotherapy in stage II; may have some role in stage IB
  (4) Role for surgery in stage IIIA disease:
    (a) N2 disease
    (b) Neoadjuvant chemoradiation followed by surgery
    (c) Good risk patients
    (d) Surgically resectable primary
    (e) Absence of bulky or multilevel N2 disease
    (f) Absence of persistent N2 disease after induction
b. Lobectomy and mediastinal lymph node sampling
  (1) Procedure of choice for disease confined to one lobe
    (a) In Lung Cancer Study Group (1995), lobectomy versus limited resection showed 75% increase in local recurrence and 50% increase in cancer-related death when limited resection performed.
  (2) Includes entire first-level lobar lymphatics
  (3) Mortality rate of 0% to 8%
  (4) Sleeve lobectomy for peribronchial tumor or lymph node involvement at resection site
  (5) VATS lobectomy
    (a) Same operation as open with no difference in cancer-free survival
    (b) Advantages
      (1) No rib spreading means less postoperative pain.
      (2) Shorter hospital stay
      (3) Improved pulmonary function
      (4) Decreased inflammatory response
    (c) Contraindications
      (1) Central tumors
      (2) Tumor >6 cm
      (3) Extensive hilar calcification
      (4) T3 lesions
      (5) N2 disease

42

CARCINOMA OF THE LUNG

   c. Pneumonectomy
     (1) Indications—hilar involvement or tumor extension across oblique fissure
     (2) Can result in poor pulmonary reserve with significant change in lifestyle
     (3) Mortality rate of 5% to 10%

**3. Nonsurgical therapy**
a. Stage III
     (1) Radiation and chemotherapy (cisplatin-based)
     (2) Five-year survival rate of 10%
     (3) Median survival of 12 to 14 months
b. Stage IV
     (1) Chemotherapy only
     (2) Five-year survival rate of <1%
     (3) Surgical resection in very select patient:
       (a) Isolated adrenal or brain metastasis
       (b) No involvement of N2 lymph nodes

**4. Surveillance after curative-intent therapy**
a. Most lung cancer recurrence will be during the first 2 years after curative treatment.
b. Patient will have 1% to 2% yearly risk for development of a new primary lung cancer.
c. Follow-up includes the following: radiograph study (chest CT or chest radiograph), history and physical examination every 6 months for 2 years, then annually.

## IX. THE FUTURE

- Defining the role of CT screening
- Biological markers and defining which patients may benefit from adjuvant chemotherapy after surgical resection
- Defining the role of surgery in stage III disease

# Thymus

*Benjamin C. McIntyre, MD*

The thymus gland is an important structure for cell-mediated immunity, and accordingly, disease states that affect this organ reflect abnormalities in this pathway and preclude patients to several autoimmune disorders. Malignancy can also develop in the gland, resulting in the primary thymic tumor known as thymoma. Its location in the anterior mediastinum can make the diagnosis difficult because several other tumors are known to arise in this location.

**43**

## I. ANATOMY AND EMBRYOLOGY

- The thymus gland originates from the third and fourth pharyngeal pouches (along with the lower parathyroid glands) and typically descends into the anterior mediastinum.
- It can be found extending to both pleural reflections, from the hyoid bone, down along the diaphragm and as deep as the carina.
- Weight at birth approximates 10 to 35 g and grows until puberty, at which time it reaches a maximal weight of 20 to 50 g. It then involutes at an unspecified time in adulthood to become replaced with fibrofatty cells.
- The thymus gland itself is a pyramid-shaped, bilobed gland. Each lobe is subdivided into lobules that are surrounded by a fibrous cortex and a central medulla.

## II. PATHOLOGY

From a surgical standpoint, there are two clinical entities that are relevant: (1) thymoma and (2) myasthenia gravis.

### A. THYMOMA

1. Epidemiology
   a. Most common mediastinal neoplasm (20%) in adults
   b. Most common anterior mediastinal neoplasm (50%)
   c. Overall, it is a rare tumor (incidence of 0.15/100,000 people based on SEER [surveillance, epidemiology, end results] data).
   d. Equal distribution among the sexes
   e. Age group—40 to 60 years
   f. Epithelial tumor that tends to be slow-growing but has a propensity to be locally invasive and to disseminate to the pleural cavities

2. Symptoms
   a. Cough or vague chest discomfort are the most common symptoms.
   b. Thirty percent of patients are symptomatic on discovery.
   c. Locally invasive tumors may present with phrenic nerve paralysis, superior vena cava syndrome, pleural effusions, and shortness of breath from lung involvement.

    d. Several autoimmune disorders are associated with thymoma.
- (1) Myasthenia gravis is the most common autoimmune disorder.
  - (a) Thirty percent to 65% of patients with thymoma have myasthenia.
  - (b) Ten percent to 15% of patients with myasthenia will have thymoma.
- (2) Red cell aplasia is the second most common autoimmune disorder.
- (3) Lupus erythematosus
- (4) Hypogammaglobulinemia

**3. Differential diagnosis**

a. Malignant germ cell tumors, thyroid neoplasms, and lymphoma

b. Computed tomography scan with intravenous contrast is the examination of choice.
- (1) Precisely identifies great vessel, pericardial, and tracheal invasion
- (2) Droplet metastasis to either lung base can also be seen, which is highly suggestive of thymoma.

c. Malignant germ cell tumors usually occur in young males and are either $\alpha$-fetoprotein or $\beta$ subunit of human chorionic gonadotropin positive.

d. Thyroid lesions are usually seen to be contiguous with the thyroid gland, but if question exists, I-131 thyroid scanning can be done.

e. Patients with lymphoma tend to be younger than patients with thymoma, and they have associated lymphadenopathy and constitutional symptoms including fevers, night sweats, weight loss, and malaise.
- (1) Inguinal or axillary adenopathy can be biopsied for diagnosis.

**4. Staging (Masaoka clinical staging of thymoma)**

a. Stage I—macroscopically and microscopically unencapsulated

b. Stage II
- (1) Microscopic transcapsular invasion
- (2) Macroscopic invasion into surrounding fatty tissue

c. Stage III—macroscopic invasion into neighboring organs (i.e., pericardium, great vessels, lung)
- (1) Without invasion of great vessels
- (2) With invasion of great vessels

d. Stage IV
- (1) Pleural or pericardial dissemination
- (2) Lymphogenous or hematogenous metastasis

**5. Surgical treatment**

a. Stages I and II
- (1) Transsternal or VATS assisted thymectomy with complete en bloc thymectomy
- (2) Important to avoid intrapleural spread and phrenic nerve injury
- (3) If no clear plane exists between tumor and pericardium, then pericardial resection is indicated.
- (4) Radiation typically done in stage II disease as adjuvant therapy.

b. Stages III and IVA
    (1) Usually large tumors (>10 cm) with close proximity to major organs
    (2) Neoadjuvant chemotherapy usually done with PAC (cisplatinum, doxorubicin, and cyclophosphamide +/- prednisone) or ADOC (cisplatinum, etoposide, and epirubicin)
    (3) After chemotherapy, patients are restaged with computed tomography.
    (4) If operable, then median sternotomy or "clamshell" thoracotomy is performed with resection of adjacent pleura, lung, and pericardium, arteries, and veins as needed.
    (5) Bilateral phrenic nerve involvement is considered inoperable.
    (6) Superior vena cava or innominate veins can be resected with reconstruction.
    (7) Close margins or positive margins should be clipped for postoperative radiation therapy.
    (8) Even with great vein resection, 5- and 10-year survival approaches 77% and 59%, respectively.
    (9) For patients found to have large tumor deposits in both pleura intraoperatively, maximal surgical debulking should be performed.
    (10) There is no role for surgical debulking outside of this circumstance.
c. Unresectable stage III or IV disease
    (1) Unresectable tumors have the following characteristics: invasion of trachea, heart, bilateral phrenic nerve, extensive pleural spread, and extrathoracic metastatic disease.
    (2) Patients typically given chemotherapy followed by radiation
    (3) Recurrent thymoma should be resected if it appears resectable by computed tomography.

## B. MYASTHENIA GRAVIS

### 1. Epidemiology
a. Incidence in United States is 20 in 100,000 people.
b. Tends to occur in younger women (<40) and older men (>60), but it can occur in all ages, all races, and both sexes.
c. Men have a slightly increased incidence when compared with women.

### 2. Pathophysiology
a. Occurs largely as a result of autoantibodies to the acetylcholine receptor at the neuromuscular junction
b. This is thought to be a result of cross-reaction of antigens with the acetylcholine receptor produced by helper T-/B-cell interactions in the thymus.
c. The thymus is clearly involved because nearly 70% of thymic gland specimens have germinal centers indicating an active immune response.
d. Thymoma occurs in 10% to 15% of patients with myasthenia.
e. Patients with thymoma usually have more severe disease and are less likely to respond to thymectomy.

43

THYMUS

**3. Symptoms**

a. Related to blockage of the neuromuscular junction

b. Diplopia, ptosis, dysarthria, aspiration, dysphagia, and neck and shoulder girdle weakness are the most common.

c. Onset may be insidious.

**4. Diagnosis**

a. Tensilon test—Tensilon (edrophonium), an acetylcholinesterase inhibitor, is given and the patient is observed for improvement in weakness.

b. Acetylcholine receptor antibodies—present in 74% of patients with myasthenia and 54% of those patients with ocular myasthenia gravis

c. Muscle-specific tyrosine kinase antibodies are present in 50% of patients with myasthenia.

d. Anti-striated muscle antibodies are found in 90% of patients with thymoma with myasthenia.

e. Approximately 10% of patients have no detectable antibodies and are called *seronegative-type myasthenia gravis.*

f. Computed tomography scanning of the chest should always be done to evaluate for thymoma.

**5. Treatment**

a. Medical

   (1) Mestinon (pyridostigmine) is an analogue of neostigmine with fewer side effects and appears to be longer acting.

   (2) Steroids

   (3) Intravenous immunoglobulins

   (4) Plasmapheresis

   (5) Immunosuppressants such as mycophenolate mofetil (CellCept)

   (6) Thymic irradiation

b. Surgical

   (1) With en bloc thymectomy, drug-free remission can be expected in 42% of cases, and improvement in symptoms can be expected in 94%.

   (2) Should be done in all patients with mild disease and in patients with respiratory or oropharyngeal symptoms. Not as effective in those patients with only ocular symptoms.

   (3) Preoperative and perioperative support is critical.

      (a) Mestinon should be continued up until 8 hours before surgery because early discontinuation can result in myasthenic crisis, whereas continuing medications can result in cholinergic crisis after surgery, especially in those patients with mild symptoms.

      (b) Steroid coverage should be given perioperatively if patients are taking steroids before surgery.

      (c) If patients have marginal respiratory status before surgery, then plasmapheresis or intravenous immunoglobulin may be considered.

(d) Nondepolarizing paralytics should be avoided if possible because their use can result in a prolonged period of postoperative respiratory weakness.

(e) Patients may be extubated intraoperatively but must be initially observed in an intensive care unit.

(4) The goal of surgery is complete en bloc thymectomy, including all adjacent fat and lymphatic tissue.

(a) Typically done through a median sternotomy, although VATS and robotic-assisted techniques are becoming more common.

(b) The mediastinal dissection begins at the diaphragm.

(c) Mediastinal fat is elevated bilaterally and superiorly.

(d) Both phrenic nerves should be identified and preserved.

(e) If possible, the inferior parathyroids and thyroid gland should be preserved and their blood supply left intact.

(5) Surgical removal of the thymus offers the patient with myasthenia gravis the only hope of cure and of being medication free.

(a) Results are gradual after surgery and the maximal benefit may not be seen for 2 to 5 years.

(b) Younger patients with recent-onset disease tend to see more rapid improvement in their symptoms after surgery.

### RECOMMENDED READING

Dillon FX: Anesthesia issues in the perioperative management of myasthenia gravis. *Semin Neurol* 24:83–94, 2004.

Jaretzki A, Steinglass KM, Sonett JR: Thymectomy in the management of myasthenia gravis. *Semin Neurol* 24:49–62, 2004.

Nussbaum MS: Transternal, transcervical, and thoracoscopic thymectomy for benign and malignant disease. In Fischer JE (ed): *Mastery of Surgery,* 5th ed. Philadelphia, Lippincott Williams & Wilkins, 2006, pp. 451–455.

Wright CD, Kessler KA: Surgical treatment of thymic tumors. *Thorac Cardiovasc Surg* 17:20–26, 2005.

# Malignant Esophagus

*Jaime D. Lewis, MD*

## I. EPIDEMIOLOGY

Cancers of the esophagus account for approximately 1.5% of newly diagnosed malignancies in the United States, affecting 13,900 individuals annually. It leads to 2% of cancer-related deaths with an overall survival rate of only 14%. Adenocarcinoma accounts for more than 50% of cases in the United States, whereas squamous cell carcinoma accounts for 70% of cases worldwide. The incidence in the Western hemisphere is approximately 5 per 100,000 people but may reach 100 to 500 per 100,000 people in endemic areas such as northern China, South Africa, Iran, Russia, and India.

**44**

## II. CAUSATIVE FACTORS

**A. SQUAMOUS CELL AND ADENOCARCINOMA ACCOUNT FOR MORE THAN 90% OF ALL ESOPHAGEAL CANCERS. RARELY, MELANOMA, LYMPHOMA, LEIOMYOSARCOMA, AND CARCINOID MAY OCCUR.**

**B. INCIDENCE**
1. Men are affected more frequently than women.
2. Incidence increases with age and peaks at 67 years in the United States.

**C. SEVERAL RISK FACTORS ARE ASSOCIATED WITH THE DEVELOPMENT OF SQUAMOUS CELL CARCINOMA OF THE ESOPHAGUS.**
1. Social
   a. Tobacco use—source of nitrosamines
   b. Alcohol consumption—may increase esophageal epithelial cell proliferation and vulnerability to carcinogens.
2. Endemic regions
   a. Diets deficient in vitamins A, $B_2$ (riboflavin), C, zinc, magnesium, and protein.
   b. Diets with excessive nitrates and nitrosamines (secondary to fungal infestation).
   c. Thermal effect of hot liquids and foods
3. Environmental factors
   a. Asbestos and silica
   b. Radiation exposure including fallout and therapeutic radiotherapy to the mediastinum
   c. Human papillomavirus, particularly subtypes 16 and 18
4. Other associations
   a. Caustic injury to the esophagus
   b. Achalasia and esophageal diverticula causing stasis and increased exposure to carcinogens

c. History of head and neck cancer

d. Nonepidermolytic palmoplantar keratoderma (tylosis)—90% to 95% risk by 65 years of age

e. Plummer–Vinson syndrome

**D. ADENOCARCINOMA**

1. Barrett's esophagus

a. Associated with 70% of resected adenocarcinomas of the gastric cardia

b. Diagnosis portends a 30- to 40-fold increase in the risk for development of esophageal cancer.

2. **Risk factors associated with squamous cell cancer are usually absent.**

## III. PATHOLOGY

**A. ADENOCARCINOMA—90% DEVELOP IN THE DISTAL ESOPHA-GUS AND MAY EXTEND INTO THE STOMACH.**

**B. SQUAMOUS CELL CANCER**

1. Twenty percent of cases involve the upper third of the esophagus.

2. Fifty percent of cases involve the middle third of the esophagus.

3. Thirty percent of cases involve the lower third of the esophagus but rarely involve the stomach.

## IV. PREVENTION, SURVEILLANCE, AND SCREENING

**A. PREVENTION**

1. Encourage smoking cessation and moderation of alcohol consumption

2. Substitute fresh fruits and vegetables for preserved foods

**B. SURVEILLANCE AND SCREENING**

1. Population-based screening not advocated except in endemic regions.

2. Barrett's esophagus

a. Screening endoscopy every 3 to 5 years in absence of epithelial dysplasia

b. Screening endoscopy more frequently if low-grade dysplasia

c. Treatment with proton-pump inhibitors may cause reversion to normal mucosa.

## V. DIAGNOSIS AND STAGING

**A. HISTORY AND PHYSICAL**

1. Seventy-four of patients report dysphagia.

2. Seventeen percent of patients report odynophagia.

3. Fifty-seven percent of patients report weight loss.

4. Twenty-one percent of patients report long-standing gastroesophageal reflux disease.

5. Dyspnea, cough, hoarseness, pain, and neurologic symptoms suggest metastatic disease.

## B. IMAGING STUDIES

1. Posteroanterior and lateral chest radiographs provide assessment of the pulmonary parenchyma.
2. Double-contrast barium esophagogram and upper endoscopy are the primary studies used for evaluating esophageal lesions.
a. Barium swallow
   (1) Delineates the degree of esophageal compromise
   (2) May demonstrate an associated tracheoesophageal fistula
   (3) Limited use for TNM staging
b. Upper gastrointestinal endoscopy
   (1) Obtain tissue diagnosis
   (2) Facilitate intervention (i.e., dilation, stent) if indicated
c. Endoscopic ultrasound performed during endoscopy
   (1) Most accurate method for assessing locoregional tumor size (T) and nodal involvement (N)
   (2) May be used to perform fine-needle aspiration of suspicious nodes and liver lesions
3. Computed tomography scan of the chest and abdomen
a. Efficient means of evaluating for local extension and metastases
b. Less accurate than endoscopic ultrasound for T and N staging
c. May be used for reevaluation after cytoreductive therapy before possible surgical resection
4. Magnetic resonance imaging—offers no advantage when endoscopic ultrasound and computed tomography scanning are available.
5. Positron emission tomography—increasing role in evaluating for metastatic disease

## C. SURGICAL STAGING

1. Minimally invasive approach combines video-assisted thoracoscopy and laparoscopy
a. Thoracoscopy usually performed via the right chest
b. May use laparoscopic ultrasound to evaluate liver parenchyma
c. Efficacy, accuracy, and cost are under evaluation.

## VI. TNM STAGING (Table 44-1)

Primary tumor (T)
   TX—Primary tumor cannot be assessed
   T0—no evidence of primary tumor
   Tis—carcinoma in situ
   T1a—invades lamina propria
   T1b—invades submucosa
   T2—invades muscularis propria
   T3—invades adventitia
   T4—invades adjacent structures
Regional lymph nodes (N)

44

MALIGNANT ESOPHAGUS

STAGES AND SURVIVAL OF ESOPHAGEAL CANCER

| Stage | T | N | M | 5-Year Survival Rate (%) |
|-------|-----|-------|-----|--------------------------|
| 0 | Tis | N0 | M0 | >95 |
| I | T1 | N0 | M0 | 50–80 |
| IIA | T2-3 | N0 | M0 | 30–40 |
| IIB | T1-2 | N1 | M0 | 10–30 |
| III | T3 | N1 | M0 | 10–15 |
| | T4 | Any N | M0 | |
| IVA | Any T | Any N | M1a | <5 |
| IVB | Any T | Any N | M1b | <1 |

    NX—regional lymph nodes cannot be assessed
    N0—no regional lymph nodes metastasis
    N1—regional lymph nodes metastasis
Distant metastasis (M)
    MX—distant metastasis cannot be assessed
    M0—no distant metastasis
    M1—distant metastasis
Tumors of the lower thoracic esophagus
    M1a—metastasis in celiac lymph nodes
    M1b—other distant metastasis
Tumors of the midthoracic esophagus
    M1a—not applicable
    M1b—nonregional lymph nodes or other distant metastasis
Tumors of the upper thoracic esophagus
    M1a—metastasis in cervical lymph nodes
    M1b—other distant metastasis

## VII. THERAPY

### A. SURGICAL PRINCIPLES

1. **Stomach is ideal conduit for anastomosis.**
a. Complete mobilization is necessary.
b. Blood supply based on right gastroepiploic artery.
2. **Alternative conduits—jejunum, colon**
3. **Truncal vagotomy inevitable**
a. Fifteen percent to 30% experience delayed gastric emptying.
b. Gastric drainage procedure, either pyloromyotomy or pyloroplasty, is recommended.
4. **Ten-centimeter proximal margin recommended when possible because of submucosal lymphatic spread of disease—reduces risk for anastomotic recurrence rate to 7%.**
5. **Extent of lymphadenectomy controversial—clinical outcome may not be affected by more extensive nodal dissection.**

## B. TRANSTHORACIC ESOPHAGECTOMY

1. Right thoracic and laparotomy incision (Ivor–Lewis operation)
a. Provides full exposure to chest and abdomen
b. Excellent for middle and lower-third esophageal resections
2. Cervical, right thoracic, and abdominal incision with anastomosis in neck (three-field or McKeown technique)
3. Left transthoracic incision
a. Useful for gastroesophageal junction tumors
b. Perform entire procedure through seventh interspace incision
c. Usually extended to thoracoabdominal incision—allows for anastomosis in midchest, exposure for pyloric drainage procedure, and jejunostomy feeding tube placement
4. Advantages
a. Entire dissection performed under direct visualization—superior in cases of possible aortic or tracheal invasion.
b. No apparent difference in physiologic and function outcomes of intra-thoracic versus cervical anastomoses.
5. Disadvantages of transthoracic techniques
a. Thoracotomy incision may lead to increased rates, prolonged postoperative ventilatory requirements, and pneumonia.
b. Intrathoracic esophagogastric anastomosis
   (1) Disruption leads to mediastinitis and sepsis.
   (2) Mortality rates of 15% to 20% if leak occurs

## C. TRANSHIATAL ESOPHAGECTOMY

1. Indications
a. Elective esophagectomy in patients with Barrett's disease with high-grade dysplasia
b. Some suggest this is the preferred mode of resection for middle and lower-third esophageal tumors but can be considered in all patients with esophageal cancer.
2. Performed via upper abdominal and left cervical incisions
3. Entire intrathoracic esophagus resected regardless of level of tumor.
4. Advantages
a. Thoracotomy is avoided.
b. Intrathoracic anastomosis avoided.
   (1) If leak occurs, salivary fistula easily managed by opening and packing wound.
   (2) Leak (5–10%) often not a fatal complication (3–5%)
5. Disadvantages
a. Controversy exists regarding completeness of resection.
b. Risk for hemorrhage or injury to membranous trachea
c. Risk for recurrent anastomotic stricture
d. Risk for recurrent laryngeal nerve injury
e. Increased risk for conduit gangrene

44

MALIGNANT ESOPHAGUS

## D. RADICAL RESECTION
1. En bloc dissection—removal of esophagus and surrounding lymphatics and soft tissue with a 10-cm margin on either side of tumor
2. May require cervical, thoracic, and abdominal incisions
3. Benefits are controversial.

## E. CHEMOTHERAPY AND RADIOTHERAPY
1. Chemotherapy
   a. Fifty percent of patients respond.
   b. Two percent to 5% of patients will experience complete remission.
2. Chemotherapeutic agents
   a. Taxanes
      (1) Paclitaxel, docetaxel
      (2) May be used alone or combined with platinum agents
   b. Platinum agents
      (1) Cisplatin is among the most active as single agent.
      (2) Addition of 5-fluorouracil greatly improves response rates in locally advanced disease when combined with radiotherapy.
3. Radiotherapy
   a. Useful alone for palliation of obstructive symptoms
   b. May be curative in a small percentage of patients
   c. Most useful when combined with chemotherapy for patients who are not operative candidates
4. Data suggest that neoadjuvant chemotherapy in addition to radiotherapy may improve survival in certain stages.
   a. Chemotherapy may act systemically to eradicate micrometastatic disease.
   b. Preoperative radiotherapy proposed benefits
      (1) Down-stage tumors and improve the resectability of marginally resectable tumors
      (2) Reduce the risk for microscopic tumor spread during surgery
      (3) Treat microscopic tumor that extends beyond margins of resection
   c. Agents such as 5-fluorouracil, paclitaxel, and cisplatin may act synergistically with radiation to improve response.
   d. Consider neoadjuvant therapy for patients undergoing resection if preoperative staging reveals T2, T3, or N1 lesion.
5. Postoperative radiotherapy
   a. No significant impact on overall survival
   b. May improve local control of disease

## VIII. PALLIATIVE CARE
## A. DYSPHAGIA AND OBSTRUCTION
1. Radiotherapy
2. Esophageal dilation and stenting
   a. Dilation may be performed using bougies, wire-guided dilators, or balloon dilators.

  b. Stents—usually placed after dilation
- (1) Self-expanding metal stents
- (2) Plastic stents
- (3) May be placed using "pull-through" technique (during a laparotomy) or "push-through" (without a laparotomy)

**3. Local tumor ablation**
- a. Cryotherapy
- b. Intralesional injection of necrotizing agents
- c. Nd:YAG photoablative therapy
- d. Photodynamic therapy

**4. Chemotherapy**

## B. ESOPHAGEAL-AIRWAY FISTULA
1. May be precipitated by radiotherapy
2. Esophageal bypass not well tolerated by most patients
3. Most patients are treated with esophageal stents with or without endobronchial stents.

**44**

**MALIGNANT ESOPHAGUS**

# PART IX

# Hepatobiliary Surgery

# Cirrhosis and Portal Hypertension

*Prakash K. Pandalai, MD*

Cirrhosis is defined by the formation of scar tissue within the liver parenchyma and is the end result of progressive injury to hepatocellular elements,
which leads to architectural destruction and ultimately failed hepatocyte
regeneration. With scar formation, there is a change in liver architecture
such that resistance to blood flow, especially portal blood flow, increases.
The result is portal hypertension and the formation of spontaneous compensatory portosystemic shunts and hepatocellular failure.

**45**

## I. PATHOPHYSIOLOGY

1. Either acute or chronic injury initiates inflammatory responses associated with cytokine release and elaboration of toxic substances. Progressive destruction of hepatocytes, bile ducts, and vascular endothelial cells results in cellular proliferation, regeneration, and fibrous scar
   formation.
2. The primary cell implicated in the stimulus for fibrosis is the
   stellate cell (Ito cell) located in the perisinusoidal space of
   Disse.
   a. Ito cells normally function in storage of vitamin A.
   b. In response to various stimuli, they secrete and express various pro-
      proliferative cytokines (transforming growth factor-β, platelet-derived
      growth factor, interleukin-1, interleukin-6, endothelium-derived growth
      factor [EDGF]), leading to obliteration of the perisinusoidal space by
      fibrotic scar and setting the stage for nutrient depletion from normal
      hepatocytes.
3. Morphology
   a. Micronodular—smaller than 3-mm nodules uniformly
      distributed throughout the liver and indicative of early
      disease
   b. Macronodular—larger than 3-mm nodules; may be posthepatitis
      versus postnecrotic depending on septation patterns
   c. Mixed—micronodular and macronodular present in equal
      proportions

## II. CAUSATIVE FACTORS

### A. ALCOHOL

Ethanol abuse is responsible for up to 70% of cases of cirrhosis in the United
States. Characteristically, micronodular cirrhosis is seen in alcoholics. Only
10% to 30% of alcoholics go on to experience development of cirrhosis.
Acetaldehyde is the substrate of ethanol responsible for the majority of cellular
and biochemical damage.

## B. VIRAL HEPATITIS (B AND C)

Viral hepatitis is the most common cause of cirrhosis worldwide. Whereas hepatitis types A, B, C, D, and E have all been shown to cause acute hepatitis, only B, C, and D have been shown to progress to chronic hepatitis.

1. Hepatis virus type B (HBV)—chronic infection with HBV develops in less than 5% of those with acute HBV infection. Cirrhosis develops in 10% to 20% of chronic infection, leading to an overall rate of cirrhosis of less than 1%.

2. Hepatis virus type C (HCV)—90% become chronically infected, 60% progress to chronic hepatitis, and 30% experience development of cirrhosis. Overall rate of cirrhosis is 10% in those with HCV infection. Interferon-$\alpha$–based therapy may eradicate infection in 15% to 30% of patients.

3. Hepatis virus type D (HDV)—an RNA virus, requires HBV to be pathologic. HBV and HDV superinfection leads to cirrhosis in 80% of patients.

## C. NONALCOHOLIC STEATOHEPATITIS

## D. HEREDITY

1. Hemolytic anemia, cystic fibrosis, glycogen storage diseases, and $\alpha$1-antitrypsin deficiency are some of many inherited disorders that may lead to cirrhosis.

## E. CHOLESTASIS

Defined as decreased bile flow into the duodenum caused by intrahepatic or extrahepatic biliary obstruction, or a decrease in hepatocyte excretion of bile, resulting in proliferation of bile ducts and eventually fibrosis and biliary cirrhosis from exposure of hepatocytes to toxic elements of biliary elements.

1. Intrahepatic cholestasis—primary biliary cirrhosis, primary sclerosing cholangitis, lymphoma, amyloidosis, Alagille syndrome, and cystic fibrosis.

2. Extrahepatic cholestasis—choledocholithiasis, pancreatic cancer, cholangiocarcinoma, pancreatic and choledochal cystic disease, acquired immune deficiency syndrome, bile duct strictures, biliary atresia.

3. Hepatocellular cholestasis—alcoholic hepatitis, viral hepatitis, inherited deficiencies

## F. PRIMARY BILIARY CIRRHOSIS

1. 95% of patients are women; antimitochondrial antibody (+)

## G. AUTOIMMUNE HEPATITIS

## H. OCCUPATIONAL EXPOSURE

1. Chemical exposure, for example, carbon tetrachloride, beryllium, and vinyl chloride; all may result in cirrhosis.

## I. SCHISTOSOMIASIS

1. Endemic in sub-saharan Africa

### J. NUTRITIONAL
1. Cirrhosis can result from long-term total parenteral nutrition

### K. VENO-OCCLUSIVE DISEASE
1. Obstruction of the hepatic veins from chronic right-sided heart failure, constrictive pericarditis, and Budd–Chiari syndrome

### L. HEMOCHROMATOSIS
### M. WILSON'S DISEASE

## III. DIAGNOSIS
### A. HISTORY
1. Cirrhosis is a chronic disease process.
2. Patients are often aware of their diagnosis and have a history consistent with the causative factor.

### B. PHYSICAL EXAMINATION
1. Examine for the stigmata of hepatocellular failure and portal hypertension—jaundice, dark urine, muscle wasting, ascites, peripheral edema, purpura, encephalopathy, splenomegaly, spider angiomata, caput medusae, asterixis, gynecomastia, testicular atrophy, "venous hum" over the right upper quadrant, palmar erythema, loss of body hair, and Dupuytren's contractures.
2. Liver may be enlarged because of vascular congestion or shrunken because of chronic disease. Patients should also be evaluated for hemorrhoids (less specific finding).

### C. LIVER FUNCTION TESTS
1. Bilirubin
a. Direct hyperbilirubinemia—due to excess conjugated bilirubin caused by overproduction or underexcretion.
b. Indirect hyperbilirubinemia—an excess of unconjugated bilirubin primarily caused by enzymatic deficiency in conjugating bilirubin.
c. Clinical jaundice is apparent when total bilirubin level is greater than 2 mg/dl.
d. Conjugated bilirubin is water soluble and excreted by the kidney.
2. Serum enzymes
a. Alkaline phosphatase
   (1) Produced in bone, placenta, and liver
   (2) Excreted in bile
   (3) Increased alkaline phosphatase can signal obstruction of bile ducts (in the absence of bone disease and pregnancy).
b. Transaminases
   (1) Aspartate aminotransferase (serum glutamic-oxaloacetic transaminase)
   (2) Alanine aminotransferase (serum glutamic-pyruvic transaminase)
   (3) Alanine aminotransferase greater than aspartate aminotransferase in viral hepatitis

    (4) Aspartate aminotransferase greater than alanine aminotransferase in alcoholic hepatitis

    (5) Transaminase may be normal in long-standing disease, despite acute exacerbation.

**3.** Serum proteins (measure synthetic function)

a. Albumin—low level when hepatic function is impaired.

b. Coagulation factors

    (1) Prothrombin time reflects adequate fibrinogen, prothrombin, and coagulation factor (V, VII, IX, X) production.

    (2) Prothrombin time is prolonged when fat absorption, and subsequent vitamin K absorption, is impaired (i.e., biliary obstruction, malnutrition, and hepatocellular insufficiency).

    (3) Thrombocytopenia, a common finding, is reflective of hypersplenism and portal hypertension.

## D. RADIOLOGIC PROCEDURES

**1.** Ultrasound—may be 90% sensitive in diagnosing cirrhosis when the findings of multiple nodular irregularities along the ventral surface of the liver are demonstrated. Hepatic ductal anatomy may also be visualized.

**2.** Computed tomography/magnetic resonance imaging—assess size, ascites, and presence of varices.

**3.** Angiography—can directly measure hepatic artery pressures and define portal vein flow during the venous phase (see section IV). Computed tomographic angiography can be useful in determining portal and systemic vessel patency, as well as hepatobiliary pathology.

## E. PERCUTANEOUS LIVER BIOPSY

**1.** Permits histologic diagnosis

**2.** Contraindications—coagulopathy, thrombocytopenia, cholangitis, tense ascites

**3.** Complications—bile leak or peritonitis, pneumothorax, bleeding, pain

## F. PARACENTESIS

**1.** Relieves dyspnea and anorexia caused by increased intraabdominal pressure.

**2.** Cytologic examination of ascitic fluid—can distinguish cause (cancer vs. cirrhosis) and diagnose spontaneous bacterial peritonitis.

**3.** Complications—infection, bleeding, perforation of viscus

## IV. CIRRHOSIS AND LIVER FUNCTION

It is important to understand that the liver is the "metabolic clearinghouse" and regulates almost every aspect of metabolism to appreciate the impact of cirrhosis. Although cirrhosis implies nothing about the state of hepatic function, a cirrhotic liver is metabolically dysfunctional.

## V. PATHOPHYSIOLOGY

Alterations in liver function and the development of portosystemic venous shunting result in the pathophysiologic disease processes that characterize a patient with cirrhosis.

### A. PORTAL HYPERTENSION

1. Defined as portal venous pressure greater than 12 to 15 mm Hg by direct measurement, or a wedged hepatic vein pressure more than 5 mm Hg greater than inferior vena caval pressure; usually becomes clinically significant when wedged hepatic vein pressure more than 12 mm Hg greater than inferior vena caval pressure.

2. Portal hypertension is commonly classified by the level of venous obstruction.

a. Prehepatic (presinusoidal)—portal vein, superior mesenteric vein, splenic vein thrombosis, primary biliary cirrhosis, schistosomiasis, congenital hepatic fibrosis, and external compression

b. Intrahepatic (sinusoidal)—alcoholic, steatohepatitis, Wilson's disease, posthepatitis cirrhosis, hemochromatosis, and so forth

c. Posthepatic (postsinusoidal)—Budd–Chiari syndrome, vena caval web, right heart failure, and constrictive pericarditis

d. In the absence of obstruction, portal hypertension can occur with high flow states, that is, arteriovenous fistula or massive splenomegaly.

3. Portal vein pressure is decompressed through collateral veins in the systemic circulation forming portosystemic shunts.

a. Esophagogastric varices (esophageal venous plexus, coronary vein, splenophrenic, short gastric veins)

b. Abdominal wall (umbilical vein)

c. Hemorrhoidal (inferior mesenteric vein, veins of Retzius)

d. Diaphragm (diaphragmatic veins of Sappey and splenophrenic veins)

4. Diagnosis

a. Portal venography—obtained by venous phase imaging during mesenteric arteriography.
   (1) Defines size and location of dilated veins, and provides qualitative estimate of hepatic portal perfusion
   (2) Hepatopetal flow (away from liver) versus hepatofugal flow (toward liver)

b. Hepatic vein wedge injection
   (1) Visualize portal vein if hepatopetal flow present.
   (2) Used to determine adequacy of portal perfusion

c. Measurement of portal pressure
   (1) Direct—measured during operation or venography.
   (2) Indirect—wedged hepatic vein pressure; compare with inferior vena caval pressure (see V.A.1).

45

CIRRHOSIS AND PORTAL HYPERTENSION

## B. ASCITES

1. Portal hypertension—increased hydrostatic pressure
2. Lymphatic outflow obstruction—ascitic fluid can be seen weeping from surface of liver at surgery.
3. Hypoalbuminemia—results in low intravascular oncotic pressure, with water loss into the extravascular space.
4. Secondary hyperaldosteronism
   a. Caused by increased secretion and/or decreased inactivation of aldosterone by the impaired liver
   b. Results in increased total body water and sodium caused by augmented sodium resorption in the distal tubule
5. Increased antidiuretic hormone secretion
   a. Caused by relative hypovolemia, as detected by the carotid body and the central nervous system
   b. Results in decreased free water clearance

## C. CARDIOVASCULAR CHANGES

1. High cardiac output and low systemic vascular resistance may cause cardiac failure.
2. Low systemic vascular resistance is not completely understood, but several contributing factors are hypothesized:
   a. Peripheral shunting (splanchnic, muscle, skin)
   b. Putative vasodilatory agents include prostaglandins, γ-aminobutyric acid, vasoactive intestinal polypeptide, substance P, insulin, glucagon, and bile acids.
   c. Decreased estrogen metabolism
   d. Accumulation of "false" or "weak" neurochemical transmitters (phenylethylamine, tyramine, octopamine), displacing sympathetic adrenergic transmitters (norepinephrine)

## D. RENAL DYSFUNCTION

Hepatorenal syndrome may result (Table 45-1), including oliguria with increased blood urea nitrogen and creatinine levels.

1. Type 1—resolved by relief of ascites and improved volume status/ renal perfusion.
2. Type 2—resolved by improved hepatic function and increased systemic vascular resistance.
3. Urine sodium concentration less than 10 mEq/L

## E. ENCEPHALOPATHY

1. Characterized by altered consciousness, asterixis ("liver flap"), rigidity, hyperreflexia, and electroencephalographic changes
2. May be seen in acute or chronic hepatic dysfunction
3. Causative factors—shunting of portal blood containing toxins and nutrients metabolized by healthy hepatocytes around the liver. Factors implicated include ammonia, mercaptans, aromatic amino acids, and others.

**TABLE 45-1**

CLASSIFICATION OF HEPATORENAL SYNDROME

| Characteristic | Type 1 | Type 2 |
|---|---|---|
| Blood pressure | Normal or low | Increased |
| Cardiac index | Normal or decreased | Increased |
| Peripheral resistance | Normal or increased | Decreased |
| Intravascular volume | Low | Normal |
| Urinary sodium | <10 mEq/L | <10 mEq/L |
| Pathophysiology | Effective hypovolemia Portorenal reflex | Maldistribution of blood flow |
| Associated findings | Intractable ascites Pressure gradient between inferior vena cava and right atrium High hepatic vein wedge pressure | Hepatic encephalopathy Acute hepatic insult |
| Therapy | Volume infusion Ascites reinfusion (rare) Peritoneal-atrial shunt Side-to-side portal decompression | α-Adrenergic agents and levodopa—neither of these results in survival unless hepatic function improves |

**4. Precipitating factors**

a. Gastrointestinal hemorrhage

b. Portosystemic shunting procedure

c. Infection, especially spontaneous bacterial peritonitis

d. Excessive dietary protein

e. Constipation

f. Narcotics and sedatives

## VI. CHILD'S CLASSIFICATION

Patients with cirrhosis are at increased risk during any kind of surgery. When elective surgery is being considered, prophylactic treatment for the complications of cirrhosis should be considered. Child's classification (Table 45-2) originally was designed as a prognostic guide for patients receiving portal decompressive surgery. It has been modified to extrapolate surgical risk in patients with cirrhosis receiving other surgical procedures. With proper preoperative intervention (i.e., nutritional support, bowel preparation with antibiotics), liver function can be improved (as indicated by improved Child's class) and the risk for surgery reduced.

### A. THE CUMULATIVE SCORE DETERMINES THE CHILD'S CLASSIFICATION:

Child's A = 5 to 7 points (2% mortality rate)

Child's B = 8 to 10 points (10% mortality rate)

Child's C ≥11 points (>50% mortality rate)

**45**

**CIRRHOSIS AND PORTAL HYPERTENSION**

---

**TABLE 45-2**

CHILD–TURCOTTE–PUGH MODIFIED CLASSIFICATION OF CIRRHOSIS

| Characteristics | 1 Point | 2 Points | 3 Points |
|---|---|---|---|
| Ascites | None | Controlled | Uncontrolled |
| Bilirubin (mg/dl) | <2.0 | 2.0–2.5 | >3.0 |
| Encephalopathy | None | Minimal | Refractory |
| Prothrombin time (seconds) | 1–4 | 4–6 | >6 |
| Albumin (g/dl) | >3.5 | 3.0–3.5 | <3.0 |

## VII. TREATMENT OF COMPLICATIONS OF CIRRHOSIS

Primary complications of cirrhosis are ascites, variceal bleeding, encephalopathy, and hepatorenal failure.

### A. PROPHYLAXIS

1. **Meticulous fluid and electrolyte management**
a. Sodium and water restriction
b. Cautious diuresis—overdiuresing can result in intravascular dehydration and prerenal acute renal failure.
2. **Maintain nutritional status.**
a. Patients are hypermetabolic and require as much as 1.1 g protein/kg/day to maintain nitrogen balance.
b. HepatAmine is a specifically defined total parenteral nutrition solution that is high in branched-chain amino acids and low in aromatic amino acids that can be used in patients with liver dysfunction. Low-sodium enteral diet is still the preferred primary source of nutrition.
3. **Prevent gastrointestinal bleeding, which increases intraluminal protein load.**
a. H2 blockers
b. Neutralize gastric pH.
4. **Reduce intestinal flora to decrease bacterial production of ammonia.**
a. Neomycin 500 mg orally every 6 hours to decrease intraluminal bacterial counts
b. Lactulose 15 to 30 ml orally twice daily is metabolized to organic acids in the colon; $NH_3$ (easily absorbed and delivered to the liver via the portal circulation) is readily converted to $NH_4^+$, which is poorly absorbed, because of the change in colonic pH.

### B. GASTROINTESTINAL BLEEDING

1. Ten percent of all cases presenting with upper gastrointestinal bleeding are a result of variceal hemorrhage; 20% to 70% of patients with cirrhosis have varices depending on the severity of their cirrhosis, and up to 30% of them will experience variceal bleeding. A 20% to 50% mortality rate is associated with the first episode of bleeding. Of those

who survive, 30% experience rebleeding within 6 weeks, and up to 70% rebleed within 1 year.
2. Bleeding is rare unless wedged hepatic vein pressure is greater than 12 mm Hg.
3. Diagnosis
a. Nasogastric lavage to establish upper gastrointestinal bleed and endoscopy (esophagogastroduodenoscopy) to identify source
b. In patients with cirrhosis, 50% to 90% of upper gastrointestinal bleeds are due to variceal hemorrhage.
c. Remaining percentage is caused by Mallory–Weiss tears, portal hypertensive gastropathy, peptic ulceration, or gastric or esophageal neoplasm.
4. Treatment
a. Airway—adequate airway protection is the number one priority.
b. Bleeding—nasogastric tube with saline lavage in the emergency department will allow rapid diagnostic information.
c. Circulation—large-bore peripheral intravenous access, initial crystalloid volume resuscitation followed by early packed red blood cells, fresh frozen plasma, cryoprecipitate, and platelets as appropriate
d. Pharmacologic therapy for variceal bleeding
   (1) Octreotide 250 μg intravenous bolus, followed by continuous infusion of 25 to 50 μg/hr for 2 to 4 days
   (2) Vasopressin 20 units intravenous bolus over 20 minutes, followed by infusion of 0.2 to 0.4 units/min. Mechanism of action thought to be splanchnic vasoconstriction and controls bleeding in 50% to 75% of patients. After bleeding stops, wean off by 0.1-unit increments over 48 hours; watch closely, because rebleeding is common. May need to be combined with nitroglycerin 50 mg/min intravenously to protect against cardiac ischemia if symptomatic.
e. Endoscopic treatment
   (1) Sclerosant injection or band ligation is the standard therapy for variceal hemorrhage and achieves initial success in 75% to 95% of patients. Up to 50% rebleeding rates have been reported.
   (2) Sclerosant injection
      (a) 5% sodium morrhuate (prevalent in United States)
      (b) 5% ethanolamine (Canada and Europe)
      (c) Complications of sclerotherapy include esophageal stricturing, chest pain, esophageal perforation, hemorrhagic esophageal ulceration, and bacteremia.
   (3) Variceal banding has shown better long-term results with less rebleeding and fewer long-term complications (esophageal stricture) and has been the preferred method of endoscopic management.
f. Esophageal balloon tamponade (Sengstaken–Blakemore, Minnesota tubes)
   (1) Initial success rate is high, but rebleeding occurs in 40% to 70% of patients. Basic principle is direct upward pressure on varices at gastroesophageal junction.

**45**

CIRRHOSIS AND PORTAL HYPERTENSION

(2) Prophylactic endotracheal intubation to prevent aspiration is an absolute.

(3) Insert tube into stomach and inflate gastric balloon with 40 to 50 ml of air. Using fluoroscopy, verify position of gastric tube in stomach and then position balloon at gastroesophageal junction. Then instill another 200 to 300 ml of air into the gastric balloon and apply upward traction. If hemorrhage is not controlled, esophageal balloon may be inflated to 35 to 40 mm Hg. Apply suction to both gastric and esophageal ports to minimize aspiration risk and to monitor hemorrhage.

(4) Gastric erosion, gastric and esophageal perforation, and aspiration pneumonia are complications. Treatment-related mortality rate is 20%.

g. Transjugular intrahepatic portosystemic shunting—a minimally invasive technique of creating an intrahepatic portosystemic fistula for decompression of the portal system; first performed in 1982.

(1) Ultrasound confirmation of patency of portal vein

(2) Cannulation of hepatic vein via right internal jugular (usually right hepatic vein)

(3) Passage of needle from hepatic vein into portal vein branch through the liver parenchyma

(4) Seldinger technique used to pass guidewire from hepatic vein into portal vein branch, and subsequent dilation of needle tract and stent placement creating hepatic vein-portal vein fistula.

(5) Ninety percent success rate at controlling acute variceal hemorrhage; 10% rebleeding incidence rate is reported

(6) Complications include hepatic encephalopathy (25%) and accelerated liver failure (5%).

h. Surgical decompression of portal hypertension. Surgical therapy is the most effective method of controlling portal hypertension and preventing recurrent variceal hemorrhage. Surgical options fall into three categories: 1) portosystemic shunt procedures; 2) esophagogastric devascularization; and 3) orthotopic liver transplantation.

(1) Portosystemic shunt procedures involve decompression of the hypertensive portal circulation into the low-pressure systemic venous system.

(a) Deprives the liver of important hepatotrophic growth factors and routes cerebral toxins directly into the systemic circulation.

(b) Principal complication is the development of accelerated hepatic failure and hepatic encephalopathy.

(2) Nonselective shunt (Fig. 45-1)—eliminates portal venous flow; most effective at controlling bleeding but followed by a high rate of encephalopathy and hepatic failure.

(a) Portacaval end-to-side shunt (Eck fistula) and side-to-side portacaval shunts are the gold standard by which other shunts are evaluated.

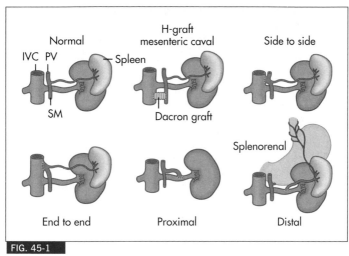

**FIG. 45-1**

Normal portacaval circulation *(top, left)* and types of portosystemic shunts. IVC = inferior vena cava; SM = superior mesenteric; PV = portal vein.

(1) Prospective, randomized trials have shown a significant decrease in rebleeding in surgical patients versus medical management (9–25% vs. 68–98%). In addition, there are trends to increased survival, but currently there are no statistically significant data to support decreased mortality with surgical treatment.

(2) Highly effective in preventing recurrent variceal hemorrhage (>90%). Hepatic encephalopathy occurs in about 15% to 30% of cases, whereas hepatic failure is a major cause of postshunt mortality (13–18%).

(3) The failure to show significant survival benefit has significantly decreased use of total portosystemic shunts. Currently, the most common indications include the use of an end-to-side shunt in acute variceal hemorrhage and a side-to-side shunt in the treatment of refractory ascites.

(4) Relative contraindication is Budd–Chiari syndrome, anticipation of orthotopic liver transplant, and refractory ascites.

(b) Interposition H-graft shunts—mesocaval, portacaval, and mesorenal

(1) Grafts larger than 10 mm in diameter are generally considered total shunts.

(2) Increased frequency of late thrombosis compared with conventional portacaval shunts

(3) Useful in patients who are transplant candidates

     (c) Central splenorenal shunt (Linton shunt)
       (1) Includes splenectomy with anastomosis of portal side of splenic vein to the left renal vein
       (2) Physiologically and hemodynamically similar to a side-to-side portacaval shunt
       (3) Results similar to those with portacaval shunts but probably has a greater thrombosis rate

(3) Selective portosystemic shunts—preserve portal venous flow to the liver via the mesenteric veins while decompressing esophagogastric flow.

(4) Distal splenorenal (Warren–Zeppa) shunt
     (a) Prototypical selective shunt used in United States. Splenic vein ligated near hilum and end-to-side anastomosis to left renal vein. Spleen remains in situ, and the coronary vein is ligated.
     (b) Varices are decompressed via the short gastric veins. It decompresses the varices while maintaining portal perfusion in 90% of patients.
     (c) Operative mortality (7–10%) and long-term survival are similar to nonselective shunts in patients with alcoholic cirrhosis. Survival seems to be improved in patients with nonalcoholic cirrhosis.
     (d) Possibly lower incidence of late hepatic failure and encephalopathy compared with nonselective shunts.
     (e) Long-term survival (60% 5-year survival rate) after distal splenorenal shunt is similar to that of endoscopic sclerotherapy. Rate of rebleeding is greater in sclerotherapy, whereas shunting may lead to progression of liver dysfunction.
     (f) Splenic vein must be greater than 7 mm in diameter, and ascites must be absent or medically controlled.

(5) Esophageal transection (including stripping of coronary veins [Sugiura procedure]) has met with limited success in the United States when compared with Japan.

(6) Orthotopic liver transplantation
     (a) Definitive treatment for portal hypertension and its complications
     (b) Donor limitations prevent routine employment.
     (c) Seventy percent 5-year survival rate in major centers for predominantly nonalcoholic patients with cirrhosis
     (d) Avoid portacaval shunt in patients awaiting transplant—use banding, sclerotherapy, transjugular intrahepatic portosystemic shunting, or selective shunting when possible to preserve portal anatomy for transplant purposes.

(7) Splenopneumopexy—anastomosis of spleen to lung through the diaphragm to decompress varices through pulmonary circulation

## C. SURGICAL TREATMENT OF ASCITES

1. Peritoneovenous shunt is the surgical treatment of choice for ascites.
2. Allows drainage of intraperitoneal fluid directly into the superior vena cava.
3. LeVeen shunt has a one-way valve that opens when intraabdominal pressure exceeds 3 cm $H_2O$.
4. Denver shunt incorporates a subcutaneous pump that prevents clogging by active pumping.
5. Complications—sepsis, congestive heart failure, disseminated intravascular coagulation, hypokalemia, shunt malfunction, air embolism, and superior vena cava thrombosis
6. Monitor for disseminated intravascular coagulation after surgery with serial fibrinogen levels, fibrin degradation products, and platelet counts. Shunt must be ligated if disseminated intravascular coagulation cannot be controlled with coagulation factors.

# Jaundice

Janice A. Taylor, MD

*We still consider phosphate of soda our best hepatic stimulant,
and I believe we are justified by the best authorities.*
—Dr. E. H. Pomeroy, regarding the treatment of jaundice, 1898

## I. BACKGROUND

### A. BILIRUBIN METABOLISM

46

1. Hemoglobin (Hgb), myoglobin → biliverdin → bilirubin
2. Seventy percent to 90% from Hgb, red blood cell breakdown; 10% to 30% from myoglobin breakdown, liver enzymes, non-Hgb heme, and non-Hgb porphyrin
3. Indirect (unconjugated)—bilirubin complexed with albumin; water insoluble
4. Direct (conjugated)—bilirubin conjugated with glucuronide; water soluble
5. Conjugation occurs in the liver.

### B. ENTEROHEPATIC CIRCULATION

1. Approximately 300 mg total bilirubin produced per day in healthy adults.
2. Conjugated bilirubin excreted by liver → biliary system → duodenum.
3. Bilirubin is reduced to urobilinogen by small-bowel bacteria.
4. Ten percent to 20% absorbed by terminal ileum and re-excreted by liver and kidneys.

### C. CLINICAL JAUNDICE

1. Observed when total bilirubin level >2 mg/dl
2. Total bilirubin level >3 mg/dl: Typically, both direct and indirect bilirubin levels are increased. Start to note changes in stool (light) and urine (dark) color.
3. Total bilirubin level >5 mg/dl points to liver disease or biliary obstruction.
a. Abdominal pain is experienced before systemic symptoms.
4. Courvoisier's sign—painless jaundice with palpable gallbladder indicates cancer distal to the cystic duct.
5. Charcot's triad—jaundice, fever, right upper quadrant pain; indicates extrahepatic obstruction with ascending cholangitis.
a. At minimum, need intravenous antibiotics and fluids; possibly vasopressor support
b. If no improvement and/or with continual deterioration, treat with endoscopic or surgical biliary decompression.

6. Reynolds' pentad—Charcot's triad + shock and mental status changes
a. Treatment as with Charcot's triad presentation

## II. CAUSATIVE FACTORS

### A. PREHEPATIC CAUSES

1. **Hemolysis**
a. Increased unconjugated bilirubin, which is bound to albumin, cannot be excreted in the urine.
b. Production of bile pigments will increase total bilirubin by 3 mg/dl; further increase indicates additional liver or biliary pathology, as stated earlier.

2. **Gilbert's disease**
a. Autosomal recessive disorder
b. Defect in hepatocyte uptake of unconjugated bilirubin
c. Intermittent jaundice but no hemolysis or liver parenchymal disease
d. Mild hyperbilirubinemia ($<6$ mg/dl)

3. **Crigler–Najjar syndrome**
a. Autosomal recessive disorder
b. Decreased bilirubin conjugation caused by impaired enzyme production or function
c. Type 1—neonatal unconjugated hyperbilirubinemia with kernicterus
d. Type 2—hyperbilirubinemia not as high as in type 1

### B. HEPATIC CAUSES

1. **Viral hepatitis**
a. Loss of appetite; fever, fatigue, headache, nausea, cough, and photophobia develop slowly, before patient reports abdominal pain.
b. Large liver, tender to palpation
c. Draw serologic markers to determine disease state (see section IV).

2. **Alcoholic hepatitis**
a. History of long-term alcohol abuse
b. Hepatocyte necrosis, fatty infiltration, hyaline inclusions, and cirrhosis develop in liver.

3. **Drug-related hepatitis**
a. Acute overdose or toxic levels built up over time
b. Cause 2% to 5% of hospital admissions for jaundice
c. Acetaminophen, halothane, erythromycin, isoniazid, chlorpromazine, $17\alpha$-alkyl substituted anabolic steroids, chlorpropamide, methimazole, valproic acid, and amoxicillin-clavulanic acid are causative agents.

4. **Cirrhosis (see Chapter 45 for a detailed discussion).**
a. Diffuse nodular fibrosis of liver
b. Common end-point state for hepatitis subtypes

5. **Dubin–Johnson syndrome**
a. Autosomal recessive disorder
b. Impaired hepatic excretion of conjugated bilirubin

c. Jaundice and hepatosplenomegaly are major findings on physical examination.

## C. POSTHEPATIC (OBSTRUCTIVE) CAUSES

**1. Choledocholithiasis (see Chapter 47 for a detailed discussion)**

a. Common bile duct stones caused by formation in duct or lodged gallstones passing through cystic duct

b. Risk factors to formation of duct stones are bile stasis and/or sludging, electrolyte imbalances, and increased bilirubin level.

**2. Cholangitis (see Chapter 47 for a detailed discussion)**

a. Infection of static bile and, as a result, the biliary tree.

b. Major risk factors are choledocholithiasis and duct manipulation for procedures.

c. As high as 85% mortality rate if untreated

**3. Sclerosing cholangitis**

a. Cause is unknown. Noninfectious, inflammatory changes to bile duct cause strictures. Condition is an extraintestinal manifestation of ulcerative colitis.

b. Typically presents in men aged 20 to 50

c. Symptoms include fatigue, weight loss, loss of appetite, slow onset of jaundice and pruritus, and intermittent right upper quadrant pain.

d. Diagnosis made with endoscopic retrograde cholangiopancreatography (ERCP) and biopsy.

e. Natural progression of disease, even with treatment, is often secondary biliary cirrhosis, ascites, varices with eventual liver failure, and need for transplantation.

f. Medical treatment—steroids, immunosuppression, long-term antibiotics for cholangitis prophylaxis, bile-acid–binding agents

g. Surgical treatment—decompression via transhepatic stent or T-tube placement in bile duct

**4. Benign biliary strictures**

a. Causative factors—95% surgical trauma; 5% abdominal trauma, chronic pancreatitis, impacted stone

b. History—intermittent cholangitis, jaundice

c. Diagnosis—percutaneous transhepatic cholangiography or ERCP

d. Treatment—antibiotics for cholangitis; choledochoduodenostomy versus choledochojejunostomy versus end-to-end bile duct anastomosis

e. Complications if strictures not treated—cholangitis, abscesses, sepsis, cirrhosis, portal hypertension

**5. Klatskin's tumor (bile duct carcinoma)**

a. Seen in patients older than 70 years; male sex predisposition

b. Associated with ulcerative colitis, *Clonorchis sinensis* (oriental liver fluke) infection, chronic typhoid carriers, choledochal cysts, and sclerosing cholangitis

c. Diagnosis—computed tomography and percutaneous transhepatic cholangiography or ERCP

d. Treatment—usually metastatic at presentation
   (1) Resect for cure—wide resection with biliary tract reconstruction; rarely an option secondary to metastasis.
   (2) Resect for palliation—to decompress; cholecystojejunostomy versus choledochojejunostomy versus stent.
   (3) Radiation—may help improve survival; performed after surgery or as sole mode of palliation.
e. Five-year survival rate is 10% to 15%.

6. **Pancreatic head carcinoma (see Chapter 56 for a detailed discussion)**
a. Painless jaundice is a hallmark sign of the disease.
b. May present with hepatomegaly, palpable gallbladder, and complaints of pruritus.

7. **Ampullary carcinoma (ampulla of Vater)**
a. Local spread, slow metastasis
b. Presentation—early jaundice, hemoccult-positive stools
c. Diagnosis—abdominal computed tomography scanning, ERCP with biopsy
d. Treatment—Whipple procedure (pancreaticoduodenectomy); 5% to 10% operative mortality rate
e. Five-year survival rate is 40% with favorable histology.

8. **Choledochal cysts**
a. Congenital cysts in intrahepatic or extrahepatic biliary tree. One third of cases diagnosed before age 10. If untreated, progress to biliary obstruction, cholangitis, secondary biliary cirrhosis, rupture, and carcinoma.
b. Presentation—female/male ratio is 4:1; right upper quadrant mass, jaundice, pain
c. Five types
   (1) Type I—>50% of cases. Cystic dilation of entire common hepatic and common bile duct. Excise cyst and perform Roux-en-Y hepaticojejunostomy.
   (2) Type II—<5% of cases. Diverticulum of common bile duct. Excise diverticulum.
   (3) Type III—5% of cases. Cystic dilation of distal common bile duct (choledochocele). Marsupialize the diverticulum with a long sphincteroplasty or divide the common bile duct with Roux-en-Y choledochojejunostomy.
   (4) Type IV—5% to 10% of cases. Type IVA refers to multiple extrahepatic and intrahepatic biliary cystic dilations. Type IVB refers to multiple dilations of extrahepatic biliary ducts. Excise cysts and perform Roux-en-Y hepaticojejunostomy with transhepatic stent.
   (5) Type V—1% of cases. Multiple intrahepatic biliary duct dilations (Caroli's disease). Excise cysts and perform Roux-en-Y hepaticojejunostomy with transhepatic stent.

## III. PRESENTATION
### A. HISTORY
1. Abdominal pain, nausea, vomiting, diarrhea
2. Fever
3. Pruritus
4. Acholic (light-colored) stools, dark ("Coca-Cola") urine
5. Alcohol abuse, intravenous drug abuse

### B. PHYSICAL EXAMINATION
1. Clinical jaundice—evaluate color of skin, sclera, oral mucosa.
2. Tender abdomen
3. Organomegaly—liver, spleen
4. Palpable gallbladder
5. Stigmata of liver disease
a. Varices—spider veins, palmar erythema, caput medusa
b. Ascites, muscle wasting
c. Asterixis, encephalopathy

## IV. LABORATORY TESTS
### A. COMPLETE BLOOD CELL COUNT
1. Leukocytosis, but is nonspecific
2. Microcytic anemia and increased reticulocyte count, indicating hemolysis

### B. BILIRUBIN LEVEL (TABLE 46-1)
1. When jaundice is secondary to hemolysis or hepatic disease, indirect bilirubin is 90% to 95% of total serum levels.
2. When jaundice is secondary to obstruction, direct bilirubin is at least 50% of total bilirubin.

### C. TRANSAMINASES
1. Alanine serum transaminase = serum glutamic-pyruvic transaminase
2. Aspartate serum transaminase = serum glutamic-oxaloacetic transaminase

**46**

**JAUNDICE**

**TABLE 46-1**

CAUSES OF JAUNDICE AND THEIR DIFFERENCES

| | Reference Values (mg/dL) | Hemolysis | Hepatocellular Disease | Bile Duct Obstruction |
|---|---|---|---|---|
| **Serum bilirubin** | | | | |
| Indirect | 0.2–1.3 | Increased | Increased | Normal |
| Direct | 0–0.3 | Normal | Increased | Increased |
| **Urine** | | | | |
| Urobilinogen | 2–4 | Increased | Increased | Absent |
| Bilirubin | Negative | Negative | Positive | Positive |
| **Fecal** | | | | |
| Urobilinogen | 40–280 | Increased | Decreased | Absent |

3. Increased in cases of hepatocellular injury, regardless of hepatitis causative factor
4. Alanine serum transaminase is more specific for liver.
5. Aspartate serum transaminase is found in liver, heart, skeletal muscle, kidney, and pancreas.

### D. ALKALINE PHOSPHATASE
1. Increased in intrahepatic and extrahepatic obstruction secondary to increased production by proliferating terminal biliary ductules
2. Also increased in hepatic spread of tuberculosis, sarcoid, or lymphoma; liver abscess or neoplasm; bone disease; and pregnancy
3. Found also in bone, placenta, kidney, intestine, and white blood cells

### E. GAMMA-GLUTAMYL TRANSFERASE
1. More sensitive and specific than alkaline phosphatase
2. Found throughout body except in muscle; greatest levels in liver, kidney, and prostate

### F. AMYLASE/LIPASE
1. Increased when the source of jaundice is pancreatic (pancreatic head lesion) or when the ampulla of Vater is obstructed (periampullary cancer)
2. Use in conjunction with liver function tests to assist in determining origin of jaundice

### G. UROBILINOGEN
1. Increased in stool and urine with hemolysis
2. Absent in stool and urine in complete biliary obstruction

### H. HEPATITIS PANEL
1. Hepatitis A
a. Usually contracted from eating contaminated food; positive travel history; fecal-oral transmission
b. IgM anti–hepatitis A virus—seen in acute disease; transiently positive.
c. IgG anti–hepatitis A virus—persists after recovery; positive result implies immunity.
2. Hepatitis B (Fig. 46-1)
a. Major risk factor for hepatocellular carcinoma
b. Transmission via blood, needles, sexual intercourse
c. HBsAg—surface antigen; appears first; negative 3 months after infection.
d. HBcAg—core antigen
e. HBeAg—marker of active viral replication; when positive, patient is highly infectious
f. HBsAb—surface antibody; persists chronically; positive after vaccination
g. HBcAb—core antibody; positive during "window" phase when HBsAg and HBsAb levels are too low to be detectable
   (1) IgM—acute disease

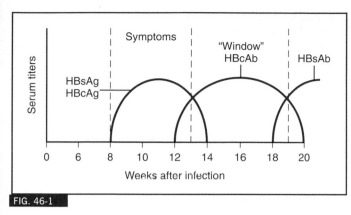

Symptoms
"Window"
HBcAb
HBsAb

HBsAg
HBcAg

Serum titers

0   6   8   10   12   14   16   18   20
Weeks after infection

FIG. 46-1

    (2) IgG—positive result indicates past infection and immunity; negative result after vaccination.

### 3. Hepatitis C
a. Major risk factor for hepatocellular carcinoma
b. History of intravenous drug abuse or blood transfusions
c. Leading cause of chronic hepatitis and cirrhosis in the United States
d. Half of patients will experience development of chronic hepatitis, and virus will not be detectable in 10% to 20% of these patients.
e. Anti-hepatitic C virus antibody—positive in acute, chronic, and resolved disease.

### 4. Hepatitis D
a. History of intravenous drug abuse or hemophilia
b. Can develop in patients positive for HBsAg

### 5. Hepatitis E
a. Infection caused by oral transmission via contaminated water.
b. Does not lead to chronic infection

### V. IMAGING
#### A. ABDOMINAL RADIOGRAPH
1. Fifteen percent of gallstones are radiopaque.
2. Gas in biliary tree is seen in gallstone ileus, cholangitis caused by gas-producing bacteria, and after surgical anastomosis with gastrointestinal tract.
3. Emphysematous cholecystitis (gas in gallbladder wall)—rare

#### B. ULTRASOUND
1. Gallstones, common duct stones. Procedure of choice for gallstone detection.

2. Dilated intrahepatic and extrahepatic ducts
3. Liver and pancreatic masses
4. Quality of results dependent on technician skill and patient body habitus.

## C.  COMPUTED TOMOGRAPHY
1. To evaluate liver/pancreatic masses, anatomy of obstructed bile ducts
2. Ninety-five to 100% gallstones visualized on computed tomography scanning.

## D.  PERCUTANEOUS TRANSHEPATIC CHOLANGIOGRAPHY
1. To determine cause, site, and extent of biliary duct obstruction
2. Contraindications
a. Coagulopathy—increased prothrombin time/partial thromboplastin time, platelet count <40,000 per liter
b. Ascites—inhibits ability to tamponade liver puncture site.
c. Hepatic sepsis
d. Disease of right lower lung or pleura
3. Complications
a. Bile peritonitis, hemobilia, bleeding
b. Pneumothorax, bilothorax
c. Sepsis

## E.  ERCP
1. To evaluate upper gastrointestinal tract, ampulla of Vater, and biliary and pancreatic ducts
2. Can both treat (place stent across ampulla to decompress) and diagnose (biopsy, cytology)
3. Complications
a. Iatrogenic pancreatitis
b. Pancreatic or biliary sepsis

## F.  NUCLEAR BILIARY SCAN (HYDROXY IMINODIACETIC ACID [HIDA] SCAN)
1. To visualize biliary system
2. Ability to see duodenum rules out complete bile duct obstruction.
3. Highly sensitive (95%) for acute cholecystitis
4. Less reliable when bilirubin level >20 mg/dl because of decreased hepatic secretion of tagging agent

## G.  LIVER SCAN
1. Identifies hepatic parenchymal disease better than HIDA scan
2. Can evaluate liver and spleen size, particularly masses >2 cm

## H.  LIVER BIOPSY
1. Open versus percutaneous
2. Histologic evaluation of liver parenchyma

## RECOMMENDED READING

Baron TH: Palliation of malignant obstructive jaundice. *Gastroenterol Clin North Am* 35:101–112, 2006.

Beck PD: Approach to the patient with jaundice or abnormal liver tests. In Goldman L (ed): *Cecil Textbook of Medicine.* Philadelphia, Saunders, 2004.

Lidofksy SD: Jaundice. In Feldman M (ed): *Sleisenger & Fordtran's Gastrointestinal and Liver Disease.* Philadelphia, Saunders, 2002.

Navarro VJ, Senior JR: Drug-related hepatotoxicity. *N Engl J Med* 354:731–739, 2006.

46

JAUNDICE

# Gallbladder and Biliary Tree

*Jocelyn M. Logan-Collins, MD*

## I. ANATOMY

### A. GALLBLADDER

1. Divided into four anatomic portions
a. Fundus—blind end, extends beyond liver margin.
b. Body—major storage area.
c. Infundibulum (Hartmann's pouch)—dilatation of the gallbladder as it empties into the neck.
d. Neck—funnel shaped, usually curved, connects with the cystic duct.
2. Supplied by the cystic artery
a. Originates from the right hepatic artery
b. Two millimeters in diameter
c. Courses superiorly and posteriorly to the cystic duct until it reaches the peritoneal surface of the gallbladder and divides
3. Venous drainage
a. Cystic vein drains to right portal vein.
b. Small veins drain directly into liver.
4. Cystic duct
a. Connects the gallbladder to the common duct system
b. Sits just anterior to the right hepatic artery
c. Valves of Heister—mucosal folds at the gallbladder/cystic duct junction.
d. Highly variable in length and anatomic course
5. Calot's triangle
a. Common hepatic duct, liver, cystic duct define the boundaries.
b. Cystic artery, right hepatic artery, and the cystic duct lymph node (Calot's node) lie within this triangle.

### B. BILE DUCTS

1. Left and right hepatic ducts join to form a common hepatic duct.
a. Left is longer than right and is at increased risk for dilatation from distal obstruction.
b. Joined by the cystic duct to form the common bile duct (CBD)
2. CBD is about 8 to 11.5 cm in length and 2 to 10 mm in diameter.
3. There are three portions to the CBD: suprapancreatic, intrapancreatic, and intraduodenal.
4. CBD empties into the duodenum in one of two patterns:
a. Unites with the pancreatic duct outside the duodenum and enters the duodenum as a single duct (75%)
b. Exits into the duodenum via a separate orifice (25%)

### C. ANOMALIES

Awareness of the highly variable nature of the gallbladder and associated structures is critical in the approach to the patient undergoing gallbladder or biliary surgery.

1. Gallbladder—duplication, intrahepatic, left-sided, or bilobed
2. Cystic duct—short or absent, long with alternative course, double cystic duct, accessory cystic duct, ducts of Luschka (drain directly from liver into gallbladder and may require clipping to prevent postoperative biloma)
3. Cystic artery and hepatic arteries—double cystic artery, accessory left hepatic artery, replaced right hepatic artery

## II. CHOLELITHIASIS

### A. INCIDENCE
1. Found in 12% of general population
2. Majority (80%) are asymptomatic.
3. Predisposing conditions
a. Sex distribution—twice as common in women
b. Age—found in 20% of adults older than 40 years and 30% of adults older than 50
c. Medical—obesity, pregnancy, rapid weight loss, total parenteral nutrition, diabetes, pancreatitis, chronic hemolytic states, malabsorption, Crohn's disease, spinal cord injuries, increased triglycerides, decreased high-density lipoprotein
d. Drugs—exogenous estrogens, clofibrate, octreotide, ceftriaxone
e. Ethnic factors—Pima Indians, other Native Americans, Scandinavians, persons living in Chile

### B. CAUSATIVE FACTORS
Three principal defects contribute to gallstone formation.
1. Cholesterol supersaturation—most critical to stone formation.
a. Three major constituents in bile:
   (1) Bile salts—primary: cholic and chenodeoxycholic acids; secondary: deoxycholic and lithocholic
   (2) Phospholipids—90% lecithin
   (3) Cholesterol—bile containing excess cholesterol relative to bile salts and lecithin is predisposed to gallstone formation.
2. Accelerated nucleation
a. Mucin and bilirubin are pronucleators associated with increased stone formation.
3. Gallbladder hypomotility

### C. TYPES OF GALLSTONES
1. Mixed (75%)
a. Most common, relatively small in size, usually multiple
b. Cholesterol predominates (at least 50% of content).
2. Pure cholesterol (10%)
a. Often solitary with large, round configuration
b. Usually not calcified
3. Pigment (15%)

a. Result from bilirubin precipitation
b. More common in women and Asian individuals
c. Black pigment—associated with cirrhosis and chronic hemolytic states.
d. Brown pigment—usually associated with biliary infection.

## D. TREATMENT OF ASYMPTOMATIC CHOLELITHIASIS
1. Prophylactic cholecystectomy is not indicated in most patients (only 20% become symptomatic).
2. Certain subgroups may benefit from prophylactic cholecystectomy.
a. American Indians with gallstones who have a greater rate of gallbladder cancer.
b. Heart and lung transplant patients because the complications of acute cholecystitis are severe in this subgroup (kidney transplant candidates do not appear to benefit).
c. Diabetes is *no longer* considered an indication for prophylactic cholecystectomy.
d. Gastric bypass with prophylactic cholecystectomy—controversial, does not appear to improve outcome.

## III. SYMPTOMATIC CHOLELITHIASIS
### A. BILIARY COLIC
Pain arising from the gallbladder without inflammation
1. Pathology—results from intermittent obstruction of the cystic duct by stone.
2. Natural history
a. Rate of recurrence is between 50% and 70% after first episode.
b. Risk for development of biliary complications is 1% to 2% per year.
3. Clinical manifestations
a. Severe pain, often visceral in nature, involving right upper quadrant
b. May radiate to back or below right scapula
c. Often follows a fatty meal
d. Pain lasts between 1 and 6 hours (if >6 hours, think cholecystitis).
e. Pain is steady, not undulating like that of renal colic.
f. Associated with nausea and vomiting
4. Physical examination—usually normal, only mild-to-moderate tenderness during an attack or mild residual tenderness lasting for a few days after an attack.
5. Diagnosis
a. Reference laboratory values
b. Ultrasound is 95% sensitive, 90% specific for diagnosis of cholelithiasis—diagnostic procedure of choice.
c. Plain radiography detects only 10% to 15% of cholesterol stones (50% of pigment stones).
d. Oral cholecystogram (Graham–Cole test)—rarely used today.
   (1) Oral contrast is given the evening before the test, is absorbed by the intestine, taken up by the liver, and secreted into bile.

**47**

GALLBLADDER AND BILIARY TREE

(2) Previously used to determine presence or absence of stones
(3) Currently used to confirm cystic duct patency in patients in whom medical dissolution therapy or lithotripsy is planned

6. Complications
a. Prolonged obstruction can lead to acute cholecystitis.
b. Stones may pass into the CBD, resulting in choledocholithiasis, cholangitis, or pancreatitis.
7. **Treatment: Patients with biliary colic and documented gallstones are generally treated with an elective laparoscopic cholecystectomy (lap chole).**

## B. ACUTE CALCULOUS CHOLECYSTITIS
Pain arising from inflammation of the gallbladder wall
1. Pathology
a. Impacted stone in the cystic duct results in prolonged obstruction.
b. Stasis of bile damages gallbladder mucosa, resulting in the release of enzymes and inflammatory mediators.
c. Histology ranges from mild acute inflammation to edema to necrosis and perforation of the gallbladder wall.
d. Forty percent of bile cultures are positive for bacteria in this setting.
   (1) Usually single-organism growth
   (2) Most likely organisms include *Escherichia coli, Klebsiella, Enterococcus, Enterobacter*
2. Natural history
a. Seventy-five percent of cases report previous attack of biliary pain.
b. If untreated, 80% resolve within 7 to 10 days.
c. Complications develop in approximately 17%.
3. Clinical manifestations
a. As inflammation progresses, visceral pain gives way to parietal pain localized to right upper quadrant.
b. Duration of pain beyond 6 hours
c. Nausea and vomiting are more common than in biliary colic.
4. Physical examination
a. Fevers are common.
b. Murphy's sign—during palpation of the right upper quadrant and deep inspiration, the inflamed gallbladder comes in contact with the examiner's hand, resulting in pain and inspiratory arrest.
c. The gallbladder is palpable in one third of the patients.
d. Mild jaundice in 20% of cases
5. Diagnosis
a. Laboratory tests—leukocytosis is common; increases in alkaline phosphatase and serum aminotransferase, serum bilirubin level between 2 and 4 mg/dl can also occur.
b. Ultrasound is useful in diagnosing acute cholecystitis.
   (1) Sonographic Murphy's sign in the presence of stones predicts acute cholecystitis 90% of the time.

(2) Thickened gallbladder wall and pericholecystic fluid in up to 50% of patients with acute cholecystitis.

(3) These findings also lose specificity in patients with ascites or hypoalbuminemia.

c. CT scan—useful in diagnosing complications of acute cholecystitis (empyema, perforation, or emphysematous cholecystitis).

d. Cholescintigraphy (i.e., HIDA scan)

(1) Intravenous administration of gamma-emitting $^{99m}$Tc-labeled hydroxyl iminodiacetic acid, which is rapidly taken up by the liver and secreted into bile

(2) Nonfilling of the gallbladder with preserved excretion into the CBD and small bowel indicates an obstructed cystic duct.

(3) Accuracy in diagnosing acute cholecystitis is 95%, superior to ultrasound.

**6. Complications**

a. If left untreated and the cystic duct remains obstructed, the gallbladder can fill with a clear mucoid fluid—*hydrops of the gallbladder.*

(1) This can lead to ischemia/necrosis/perforation of gallbladder wall.

b. Results in gangrenous cholecystitis 7% of the time, gallbladder empyema 6%, perforation 3%, and emphysematous cholecystitis less than 1%

**7. Treatment**

a. Intravenous hydration, correction of electrolyte imbalance may be necessary.

b. Antibiotics

(1) Not necessary in mild acute cholecystitis

(2) Coverage for gram-negative organisms can be initiated if severe or complicated cholecystitis is suspected (first- or second-generation cephalosporin is first choice).

(3) Patients who have more severe complications or are toxic in appearance should be given broad-spectrum antibiotics, including anaerobic coverage.

c. Cholecystectomy is the definitive treatment for acute cholecystitis and its complications.

(1) Usually can be performed laparoscopically

(2) Cholecystectomy within 72 hours of symptom onset is optimal.

(3) Patients who are immunosuppressed (steroid use, diabetes) should have immediate cholecystectomy.

(4) Delayed cholecystectomy (initial conservative management with intravenous fluids and antibiotics followed by cholecystectomy on an elective basis) is justified in some patients who are at high surgical risk.

(5) In patients who are not stable enough to undergo anesthesia, ultrasound or CT-guided percutaneous cholecystostomy with external drainage can be performed to decompress the gallbladder; followed by cholecystectomy when the patient is more stable.

d. Intraoperative cholangiogram can be helpful to define ductal anatomy when dissection is difficult due to inflammation or biliary tract variation.

## IV. CHOLEDOCHOLITHIASIS

Choledocholithiasis is the occurrence of stones in the bile ducts.

### A. CAUSATIVE FACTORS/NATURAL HISTORY

1. **Fifteen percent of patients with gallstones have CBD stones.**
2. **Primary CBD stones**
   a. Brown pigment stones often form as a result of bacterial action on phospholipids and bile, and form de novo in the duct.
   b. Those with a history of biliary sphincterotomy are at greater risk.
3. **Secondary CBD stones**
   a. Cholesterol stones and black pigment stones form in the gallbladder and pass into the CBD.
4. **Retained stones after cholecystectomy, CBD exploration, or endoscopic sphincterotomy**
   a. Can be followed conservatively to see if they pass over time (4–6 weeks) but need cholangiography to confirm passage
   b. Require removal if stones persist
5. **CBD stones may remain asymptomatic for years and pass silently into the duodenum.**
6. **Laboratory values can be normal; however, increases in serum bilirubin, alkaline phosphatase, or amylase are often seen.**

### B. TREATMENT

Complications of CBD stones such as acute pancreatitis or cholangitis can be life-threatening; therefore, all stones, even if asymptomatic, require removal.

1. **If choledocholithiasis is identified before cholecystectomy, there are two alternatives:**
   a. Lap chole with intraoperative cholangiogram and either transcystic duct or direct CBD exploration results in fewer procedures and a shorter overall stay. The majority of CBD can be removed at the same setting as the lap chole.
   b. Endoscopic retrograde cholangiography (ERC) with endoscopic papillotomy to clear the CBD before cholecystectomy is also acceptable. However, reliance on preoperative ERC is unnecessary in most settings.
      (1) Exceptions—suspicion of neoplasm, worsening pancreatitis, severe cholangitis, unfit for surgery
2. **When choledocholithiasis is identified on cholangiogram during cholecystectomy, there are three alternatives:**
   a. Laparoscopic transcystic duct or direct CBD exploration
      (1) Stone clearance rate is 95% in experienced hands.
      (2) Operative mortality rate is 0.5%.
   b. Convert to open procedure and perform CBD exploration.

      (1) Initial attempt—transcystic approach

      (2) If this fails, choledochotomy is required (T-tube or antegrade stent is necessary).

c. Complete cholecystectomy and ERC with endoscopic sphincterotomy to clear stones

      (1) Sphincterotomy is technically successful in 90% of patients.

      (2) Complete clearance of CBD stones possible in only 70% to 80% of patients

      (3) In such cases, a second attempt at stone clearance may be necessary.

**3. Retained CBD stones**

a. If T-tube in place, cholangiogram can be performed 4 to 6 weeks after surgery, or earlier if obstructive symptoms occur, to evaluate for retained stones.

b. If retained stones persist, they can be removed percutaneously using basket through a mature T-tube tract (4 weeks) under fluoroscopic control (>90% success rate).

c. ERC with sphincterotomy or transduodenal "basket" removal of stones for unstable patients, malfunctioning T-tubes, or unsuccessful percutaneous extraction

d. Percutaneous transhepatic approach

e. Reoperation

f. Extracorporeal shockwave lithotripsy

## V. CHOLANGITIS

### A. CAUSATIVE FACTORS/PATHOPHYSIOLOGY

1. Eighty-five percent of cases are caused by impacted stone in the bile ducts, resulting in stasis of bile in the presence of bacteria.

2. Pus under pressure in the bile ducts leads to rapid bacteremia and sepsis.

3. Other causes include neoplasm, strictures, parasitic infections, and congenital abnormalities.

4. Most common organisms include *E. coli, Klebsiella, Pseudomonas,* enterococci, *Proteus.*

a. Anaerobic organisms *(Bacteroides and Clostridium)* in 15% of cases

### B. CLINICAL FEATURES/DIAGNOSIS

1. *Charcot's triad*—fever (95%), right upper quadrant pain (90%), jaundice (80%)

a. Full triad present in only 70% of cases.

2. *Reynolds' pentad*—Charcot's triad plus altered mental status and hypotension

a. Occurs in severe suppurative cholangitis

b. Elderly patients may present solely with delirium or an altered mental status.

3. Intrahepatic abscess can present as a late complication.

47

GALLBLADDER AND BILIARY TREE

4. Laboratory/radiographic evaluation
a. Leukocytosis is common—a normal white blood cell count can be accompanied by a severe left shift.
b. Bilirubin level is increased to more than 2 mg/dl in 80% of cases, although it can initially be normal.
c. Serum alkaline phosphatase concentration is usually increased.
d. CBD dilatation on ultrasonography in 75% of cases
e. Abdominal CT—useful in diagnosing complications such as abscess and pancreatitis.
f. ERC is the standard for diagnosis and is also useful in treatment of cholangitis.

## C. TREATMENT

1. If suspected, blood cultures should be taken and antibiotics started as indicated for the severity of infection.
2. Aggressive resuscitation with intensive care unit admission is often necessary.
3. The patient's condition should improve within 6 to 12 hours of starting antibiotics, with defervescence, white blood cell count decline, and relief of discomfort occurring within 2 to 3 days.
4. If the patient's condition declines within 6 to 12 hours, immediate CBD decompression must be undertaken.
a. ERC with endoscopic decompression, sphincterotomy, and stent placement is the treatment of choice (mortality rate of 5–6%).
b. Percutaneous transhepatic biliary drainage can also be used with reasonable success if ERC unsuccessful or unavailable (mortality rate of 9–16%).
c. Emergency laparotomy with open CBD exploration associated with high mortality rates (up to 50% mortality rate).

## VI. ACALCULOUS CHOLECYSTITIS

### A. EPIDEMIOLOGY/PATHOGENESIS

1. Most cases occur in the setting of prolonged fasting, immobility, and hemodynamic instability.
a. With prolonged fasting, the gallbladder is not stimulated by cholecystokinin to empty and bile stagnates in the lumen.
b. Dehydration can lead to formation of extremely viscous bile, which may obstruct or irritate the gallbladder.
c. Bacteremia may result in the seeding of the stagnant bile.
d. Septic shock with resultant mucosal hypoperfusion can result in ischemia of the gallbladder wall.
2. Less commonly, it may occur in children, patients with vascular disease or systemic vasculitis, bone marrow transplant recipients, immunocompromised patients, and patients receiving cytoxic drugs via the hepatic artery.

## B.  NATURAL HISTORY

1. Patients are often in the intensive care unit with multiple medical problems, resulting in a difficult and often delayed diagnosis.
2. By the time diagnosis is made, gangrene, perforation, empyema, bacterial superinfection, or cholangitis has occurred in 50% of patients.
3. Mortality rate is reported to be as high as 50%.

## C.  CLINICAL MANIFESTATION/DIAGNOSIS

1. A high degree of suspicion is required.
2. Right upper quadrant tenderness is helpful but is absent in three fourths of patients initially.
3. Fevers and hyperamylasemia are often the only signs.
4. Ultrasound
a. Bedside availability is a major advantage in this setting.
b. Thickened gallbladder wall (>4 mm) and pericholecystic fluid in the absence of hypoalbuminemia and ascites.
c. Sonographic Murphy's sign is reliable when the patient is cooperative.
d. Sensitivity ranges between 62% and 90%; specificity greater than 90%.
5. CT scan
a. Gallbladder wall thickening, pericholecystic fluid, subserosal edema, intramural gas, and sloughed gallbladder mucosa can be detected.
b. Often detects gallbladder disease in patients with a normal ultrasound.
c. Patient must be stable enough to travel to the CT scanner.

## D.  TREATMENT

1. Cholecystectomy, laparoscopic or open, is the definitive treatment; however, patients are often too unstable.
2. Percutaneous cholecystostomy under radiographic guidance can be performed, followed by definitive cholecystectomy when the patient is stable.

## VII. OTHER DISORDERS OF THE GALLBLADDER

## A.  GALLSTONE DISEASE IN PREGNANCY

1. Lap chole can be undertaken with minimal fetal and maternal morbidity.
2. Indications include severe biliary colic, acute cholecystitis, gallstone pancreatitis, and when the underlying disease poses a threat to the pregnancy.
3. Surgery traditionally is considered to be safest during the second trimester; however, several series demonstrate that lap chole is safe at all stages of pregnancy.

## B.  BILIARY DYSKINESIA

1. Delayed gallbladder emptying in the absence of stones or sludge is predictive of pain relief after cholecystectomy.

47

GALLBLADDER AND BILIARY TREE

2. Low gallbladder ejection fraction also predicts outcome.
a. Ejection fraction less than 35% is considered abnormal.
b. Cholecystectomy improves symptoms 67% to 90% of the time.
3. Both delayed emptying and gallbladder ejection fraction can be detected with HIDA scan.

### C. BILIARY SLUDGE
1. Generally a complication of biliary stasis
2. Pathogenesis, natural history, and treatment are similar to gallstones.
3. Commonly found in patients in the intensive care unit
4. Less chance of recurrence after single episode of colic

### D. MIRIZZI SYNDROME
1. Stone impacted in the gallbladder neck or cystic duct compresses the common hepatic duct, resulting in bile duct obstruction and jaundice.
2. Found in 1% of patients undergoing cholecystectomy
3. Presents as recurrent bouts of abdominal pain, fever, and jaundice
4. Ultrasound shows stones in a contracted gallbladder with moderate dilatation of the hepatic bile ducts.
5. Type I—compression of hepatic duct by large stone
a. Subsequent inflammation can result in a stricture of the hepatic duct.
6. Type II—cholecystocholedochal fistula from stone erosion into the hepatic duct
7. Treatment
a. Mirizzi syndrome type I—cholecystectomy with or without CBD exploration. If severe inflammation is present, partial cholecystectomy with postoperative endoscopic sphincterotomy to ensure clearance of CBD stones.
b. Mirizzi syndrome type II—partial cholecystectomy and cholecystocholedochoduodenostomy

### E. GALLSTONE ILEUS
Bowel obstruction resulting from impaction of gallstone in the intestinal lumen.
1. Cause of obstruction in less than 1% of patients younger than 70 years; 5% in patients older than 70
2. Results from erosion of a large gallstone (>2.5 cm) into the intestinal lumen via a *cholecystenteric fistula*
a. Most commonly into the duodenum, but also can erode into the colon or stomach
3. Classic symptoms and signs of bowel obstruction (cramping abdominal pain, vomiting, abdominal distention, small bowel dilatation on radiograph)
4. Described as a *tumbling ileus*—as the stone passes through the length of the gut, symptoms wax and wane, intermittently obstructing the bowel lumen

5. Complete obstruction generally occurs in the terminal ileum where the bowel lumen is the narrowest.
6. Pneumobilia is present on radiograph in 50% of patients.
7. *Bouveret syndrome*—gallstone impaction in pylorus or duodenum resulting in symptoms of gastric outlet obstruction.
8. Ultrasound can confirm presence of gallstones and, on occasion, can identify the fistula.
9. Treatment involves laparotomy with removal of the stone via a small enterotomy proximal to the point of obstruction.
a. Resection is only necessary if perforation or ischemia.
b. The cholecystenteric fistula is left alone because many close spontaneously and recurrence rate is only 5%.

## F. EMPHYSEMATOUS CHOLECYSTITIS
1. Infection of the gallbladder wall with gas-forming bacteria, usually anaerobes
2. More common in individuals with diabetes and can rapidly progress to gangrene and perforation
3. Prompt cholecystectomy is imperative.

## G. CALCIFIED "PORCELAIN" GALLBLADDER
1. Intramural calcification of the gallbladder wall
2. Seen on CT or abdominal radiograph
3. Gallbladder carcinoma in 20%
4. Treat prophylactically with open or lap chole.

## VIII. MEDICAL TREATMENTS
### A. ORAL DISSOLUTION THERAPY
1. Chenodeoxycholic acid is effective in reducing the cholesterol-to-bile salt ratio.
2. For small (<10 mm), noncalcified cholesterol stones in patients with a functioning gallbladder
3. Therapy takes 6 to 12 months.
4. Five-year recurrence rate is about 50%.

### B. EXTRACORPOREAL SHOCK WAVE LITHOTRIPSY
1. Uses high-energy sound waves to physically fragment gallstones into pieces small enough to be passed into the duodenum.
2. Outcomes and overall effectiveness are no better than dissolution therapy alone.

## IX. LAPAROSCOPIC CHOLECYSTECTOMY
Laparoscopic cholecystectomy is a safe and well-tolerated procedure with reduced perioperative morbidity and improved cost-effectiveness when compared with the open approach.

47

GALLBLADDER AND BILIARY TREE

## A. SETUP
1. Antibiotics—first-generation cephalosporin or clindamycin. May be unnecessary in uncomplicated biliary colic or cholecystitis.
2. Place patient on fluoroscopy-compatible table for possible intraoperative cholangiogram.

## B. TECHNIQUE (FIGS. 47-1 AND 47-2)
1. Four trocars traditionally placed (see Fig. 47-1).
a. Veress or Hassan technique via infraumbilical or supraumbilical 11-mm port. Use an angled (30-degree) laparoscope for best visualization.
2. Assistant, standing on the right, elevates the gallbladder toward the ipsilateral diaphragm and retracts the infundibulum of the gallbladder toward the right hip.
3. Surgeon, standing on the left, dissects the cystic artery and duct from the gallbladder wall.
4. Dissection of the peritoneum over Calot's triangle reveals the "critical view" (see Fig. 47-2D) where the cystic duct and artery can be seen at their junction with the gallbladder.
a. This view is crucial to avoid inadvertently mistaking the CBD for the cystic duct or the right hepatic artery for the cystic artery.
5. Metallic clips are placed across the cystic duct at the gallbladder origin, and a small incision is made in the cystic duct for cholangiogram catheter placement.
a. Cholangiography is performed to confirm ductal anatomy (difficult dissection, abnormal appearance of structures) or to exclude choledocholithiasis (increased liver function tests, history of pancreatitis or jaundice).
b. If available, laparoscopic biliary ultrasound is also an effective modality for visualizing the biliary tree.
6. The cystic duct and artery are secured with metal clips and divided.
7. Gallbladder is dissected off the liver bed with cautery and removed in an EndoCatch bag via the periumbilical port.

## C. POSTOPERATIVE CARE
1. Patients can generally go home the day of surgery on a regular diet and mild oral analgesics.
2. Full physical activity can be resumed within 1 week.

## D. COMPLICATIONS
1. Overall morbidity rate is 7%.
2. Operative mortality rate of 0.12%
3. Bile duct injury in 0.35% of cases

## X. GALLBLADDER CANCER
### A. GENERAL CONSIDERATIONS
1. 1.2 cases per 100,000 people annually in the United States
2. Found in 1% of all cholecystectomy specimens

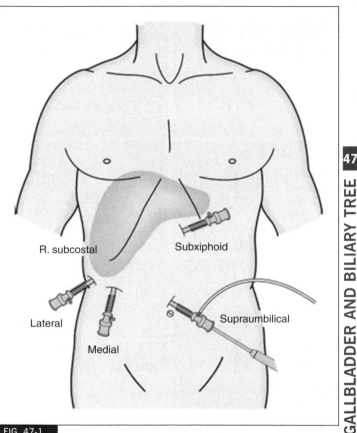

**FIG. 47-1**

Trocar placement for laparoscopic cholecystectomy. The laparoscope is placed through a 10-mm port just above the umbilicus. Additional ports are placed in the epigastrium and subcostally in the midclavicular and near the anterior axillary lines. *(Reproduced with permission from Cameron J: Atlas of Surgery, vol. 2. Philadelphia, BC Decker, 1994.)*

3. Associated with gallstones in more than 90% of cases (large > small)
4. Increased incidence in certain ethnic groups—Alaskan, Native Americans
5. Other factors—porcelain gallbladder, cholecystenteric fistulas, anomalous pancreaticobiliary junction, inflammatory bowel disease, Mirizzi syndrome

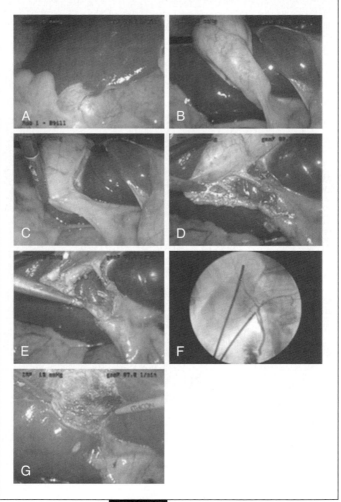

**FIG. 47-2**
For legend see opposite page.

Laparoscopic cholecystectomy. *A,* Gallbladder in situ. *B,* Cephalad retraction of the fundus toward the right shoulder exposes the infundibulum of the gallbladder. *C,* Retraction of the infundibulum toward the right lower quadrant opens up the hepatocystic triangle. The hepatocystic triangle is the area bordered by the cystic duct, gallbladder edge, and liver edge. *D,* Division of the peritoneum overlying the anterior and posterior aspects of the hepatocystic triangle exposes "the critical view." *E,* Cholangiogram catheter in the cystic duct. *F,* Normal cholangiogram. *G,* Gallbladder removed from the gallbladder fossa with electrocautery. *(Reproduced with permission from Feldman M: Sleisenger & Fordtran's Gastrointestinal and Liver Disease, 8th ed. Philadelphia, Saunders, 2006, by permission. Copyright © 2006 Saunders, an Imprint of Elsevier.)*

**47**

6. Male/female ratio of 1:2
7. Adenocarcinoma is the most common cell type—82% of cases.
8. Prognosis is grave, with 5-year survival rates of less than 5% in untreated patients.

## B.  PRESENTATION
1. Usually found incidentally at the time of elective cholecystectomy
a. Loss of clear dissection planes in the gallbladder bed or near the hilum is common.
2. Symptoms include right upper quadrant pain, jaundice, and symptoms secondary to metastasis.
3. CEA or CA 19-9 may be increased.

## C.  TREATMENT
1. If carcinoma is suspected before surgery, do open cholecystectomy with hepaticoduodenal lymphadenectomy.
2. Carcinoma in situ and T1 tumors (invades lamina propria or muscle layer).
a. Cholecystectomy alone is adequate therapy—survival rate approaches 100%.
3. T2 lesions (invades perimuscular connective tissue but not beyond serosa or into liver)
a. Incidence rate of lymph nodes metastasis is 56%.
b. Extended cholecystectomy with resection of gallbladder and portal lymph nodes
c. Wedge resection of gallbladder bed (segments IVb and V) is also done at some centers but remains controversial.

GALLBLADDER AND BILIARY TREE

4. Locally advanced tumors, T3 (perforates serosa/invades liver and/or invades one other adjacent organ) or T4 (invades hepatic artery, portal vein, or multiple extrahepatic organs)
   a. Associated with long-term 5-year survival rates less than 5%
   b. Often present with lymph node or peritoneal metastasis and are therefore unresectable
   c. Some studies report improved 5-year survival rates as high as 21% to 44% in patients who underwent radical resection with tumor-free margins.
5. Adjuvant chemotherapy has been largely ineffective.
6. Radiation therapy has been used with some success to reduce tumor size and relieve jaundice.

# Benign and Malignant Liver Lesions

*Andreas Karachristos, MD, PhD*

The presence of solid asymptomatic liver lesions is increasingly recognized because of the availability of sophisticated imaging. Management depends on knowledge of the pathology, radiologic appearance, and clinical behavior of each lesion. Generally, liver lesions can be morphologically differentiated into solid and cystic. The most common diagnosis of each category is described in this chapter, and a common clinical problem for each is discussed briefly.

**48**

## I. SOLID LIVER LESIONS

Most importantly, one must differentiate between malignant and benign disease, and if benign (which is far more common), whether the patient needs any further follow-up or treatment.

### A. BENIGN

1. Hemangioma
   a. This is the most common benign tumor; prevalence rate is 7% to 20% in ultrasound and autopsy series. Female/male ratio is 3:1.
   b. Vascular malformation that enlarges by ectasia
   c. Generally remains stable over time but occasionally may demonstrate growth. Rapid expansion may cause symptoms by stretching of Glisson's capsule or pressure on neighboring organs.
   d. In contrast-enhancing computed tomography (CT), during the arterial phase, the tumor appears as a sharply defined mass with sequential globular opacification from "outside in." In magnetic resonance imaging (MRI), the tumor appears higher in signal density on T2-weighted images.
   e. *Technetium-99m pertechnate-labeled red blood cell* scan can usually provide definitive diagnosis.
   f. The majority of patients can be managed by *observation alone*.
   g. Resection or enucleation is indicated in symptomatic patients or inability to exclude malignancy. Usually hemangiomas smaller than 10 cm do not produce symptoms.
   h. Kasabach-Merritt syndrome is a rare entity of giant hemangioma associated with diffuse intravascular coagulopathy. Patients need urgent therapy including embolization or resection with concomitant treatment of coagulopathy.

2. Focal nodular hyperplasia (FNH)
   a. FNH is the second most common benign liver tumor. Autopsy series show a prevalence rate of 0.31%. Occurs in male and female individuals but more common in female sex.

b. Developmental vascular malformation that induces a vascular hyperplastic process. Unclear relation with oral contraceptives.

c. Majority of patients are and remain asymptomatic; however, symptoms occur in up to 10% of patients.

d. In contrast-enhanced CT, it appears as homogenous hyperattenuating in arterial phase with *central scar and radiating bands*. In MRI, T1-weighted images appear isointense or slightly hypointense, and T2-weighted images appear isointense or slightly hyperintense.

e. *Technetium-99m–labeled sulfur colloid* scan may be useful in confirming diagnosis.

f. The lesion that resembles FNH is fibrolamellar carcinoma.

g. The majority of patients can be managed by observation alone. In asymptomatic patients, *if definite diagnosis is provided by imaging, no further follow-up is necessary*.

### 3. Hepatocellular adenoma (HA)

a. Rare, benign proliferation of hepatocytes

b. The annual incidence is approximately 1 in 1,000,000 people in non-contraceptive users, and the risk is increased 500-fold in women who are long-term users.

c. Female/male ratio is up to 11:1.

d. *Documented link with long-term oral contraceptive use*

e. More patients with HA are symptomatic than with FNH. Up to one third can present with acute rupture.

f. *HAs can undergo malignant transformation,* although the exact risk is not well defined.

g. Usually are solitary but can be multiple in up to 30% of cases

h. In contrast-enhanced CT, adenomas often demonstrate moderate enhancement during the arterial phase that tends to be less than that seen in FNH. In MRI, the majority of adenomas are hyperintense in T1-weighted images and isointense or hyperintense on T2-weighted images. There is overlap with FNH, and it sometimes is difficult to differentiate the tumor.

i. *Most HAs should be resected*. Discontinuation of oral contraceptives should be advised.

j. Behavior of HAs during pregnancy is unpredictable; therefore, it may be advisable to resect them before pregnancy.

k. Ruptured adenomas are often surgical emergencies. Embolization may be helpful to stabilize the patient.

## B. MALIGNANT

### 1. Metastatic lesions to the liver

a. Metastatic lesions are the most common malignant lesions to the liver, mainly from colorectal, lung, pancreas, breast, carcinoid, neuroendocrine, and urogenital cancer. Metastasis from colorectal cancer is the most common form, and resection in selected patients provides a survival advantage.

b. The liver is the second most common site of colorectal metastases after the lymph nodes: 25% of all patients with colorectal cancer will have hepatic metastases at presentation, and 50% will experience development of them in the future.

c. Nearly 10% of these patients will be amenable to aggressive surgical treatment.

d. *Keep in mind that in a patient with known malignancy, the likelihood of a solitary liver mass ≤1 cm being a metastasis is less than 20%.*

e. Most metastases, including colorectal, are hypovascular and appear to be hypoattenuating on portal venous CT images. During the arterial phase, they most commonly appear with a ringlike peripheral enhancement.

f. Hypervascular metastases are renal cell carcinoma, carcinoid tumors, adrenal tumors, thyroid carcinoma, pancreatic islet cell tumors, and neuroendocrine tumors.

g. Colorectal liver metastases are associated with elevated carcinoembryonic antigen.

h. Previously, colorectal liver metastases were considered resectable under the following circumstances: four or fewer lesions occupying one lobe, with a margin of at least 1 cm.

i. Recently, improved combination chemotherapy has significantly improved survival.

j. Criteria for resection include:
  (1) Patient is fit for surgery.
  (2) All detectable liver tumors can be removed, leaving adequate liver parenchyma, as long as a clear margin can be achieved.
  (3) At the University of Cincinnati, the following algorithm is applied:
    (a) For patients with resectable metachronous metastases, immediate surgical resection is an attractive option.
    (b) For patients with questionably resectable lesions or in whom negative margins may be difficult to achieve, as well as in those patients with synchronous metastases or recurrent disease, neoadjuvant chemotherapy followed by restaging and resection, if possible, is a better option.
    (c) For patients who are surgically resectable but do not have adequate hepatic reserve, portal vein embolization (which is thought to increase the size of the remaining liver) is an attractive adjunct before resection.
    (d) Finally, in those patients who remain unresectable despite all these measures, radiofrequency ablation should be strongly considered.

2. **Primary hepatocellular carcinoma (HCC)**

a. This is one of the most common cancers worldwide. Its incidence in the United States is relatively low: approximately 6 cases (of liver and intrahepatic biliary cancers) per 100,000 people. Male/female ratio is 3:1. Consensus exists among experts that the incidence is increasing.

48

BENIGN AND MALIGNANT LIVER LESIONS

b. The most common *causative factor is the presence of cirrhosis*.
Hepatocellular injuries related to alcohol, hepatitis C infection, hepatitis B infection, and fatty liver disease (nonalcoholic steatohepatitis) are the leading causes in the United States. Other causes are hemochromatosis, Wilson's disease, tyrosinemia, α-1-antitrypsin deficiency, and Budd-Chiari syndrome.

c. Symptoms of malignancy are common at the time of presentation and may include anorexia, weight loss, lethargy, nausea, right upper quadrant pain, and symptoms related to cirrhosis, such as ascites, jaundice, and encephalopathy.

d. The radiologic appearance of HCC is quite variable. In contrast-enhanced CT, it most commonly appears as a transiently heterogeneously hyperattenuating mass in the arterial phase. Vascular invasion or vein thrombosis may be present.

e. *α-Fetoprotein level is increased in approximately 75% of HCCs*, but it is nonspecific and related to size. Percutaneous biopsy of a suspicious lesion should be performed with caution because of the risk for needle seeding (approximately 2%). α-Fetoprotein level >200 ng/ml together with an imaging study showing a hypervascular mass is considered diagnostic of HCC.

f. Options that improve survival include liver resection or liver transplantation. Management depends on the extent of the disease. Important preoperative determinants are presence of vascular invasion, multiple tumors, and presence of hepatic fibrosis, as well as the general condition of the patient. In general, Child A and early B (Child–Pugh–Turcotte score ≤8) patients are offered resection, and late B and C patients are best treated by transplantation. The best outcomes in liver transplantation are achieved when there is one tumor less than 5 cm or no more than three tumors, none of them more than 3 cm, without vascular invasion (Milan criteria).

g. Recently, radiofrequency ablation has been shown to have comparable results with resection for small HCCs. Other treatment options for inoperable patients used at the University of Cincinnati are transarterial chemoembolization and transarterial yttrium-90 theraspheres.

h. Fibrolamellar carcinoma is a variant of HCC that is more common in young women. α-Fetoprotein is usually normal, is not associated with liver disease, and has better prognosis than HCC. Therapy is complete surgical resection. *Must be differentiated from FNH*.

**3. Intrahepatic cholangiocarcinoma**

a. This is the second most common liver cancer after HCC. Originates from intrahepatic bile ducts.

b. In most patients, the tumor is discovered incidentally.

c. Most patients *do not* have underlying liver disease.

d. On CT, usually appears as a large hypovascular tumor with central necrosis. It is important to identify before surgery the extent of the portal or hepatic artery involvement.

e. Resection with negative margins remains the only viable therapy. Chemotherapy or radiotherapy has *not* been shown to improve survival.

**Clinical scenario:** *A 39-year-old woman after injury during exercise had persistent right upper quadrant pain. Her primary care physician ordered an ultrasound that showed a 4-cm solid mass in the right lobe of the liver. The patient was referred for further management.*

*In differentiating between the above entities, one must consider the age of the patient, history or clinical signs of liver disease, or any history of malignancy. A breast examination, liver palpation for presence of hepatomegaly, and rectal examination are of paramount importance. Laboratory tests are in order: a complete blood cell count, liver function tests, and serology for hepatitis B and C viruses, as well as tumor markers α-fetoprotein, carcinoembryonic antigen, and CA 19-9. In one study, all patients with asymptomatic liver lesion and age older than 55, with increased alkaline phosphatase level and hepatomegaly, had cancer. An imaging study should be ordered next. At the University of Cincinnati, a triple-phase liver CT is the modality of choice and provides helpful insight. If malignancy cannot be excluded by imaging, then one should proceed with laparoscopic or open biopsy and/or resection. Percutaneous biopsy of benign lesions often gives indeterminate results. In addition, when HCC is suspected, percutaneous biopsy should be avoided because of the risk for seeding. This particular patient had no history of liver disease, normal laboratory tests, and a CT suggestive of FNH. An MRI scan confirmed the result. The patient will be managed with another MRI in 6 months, and if the lesion is unchanged, no further follow-up is necessary. She was advised to avoid oral contraceptives, and the pain resolved with symptomatic therapy.*

## II. CYSTIC LESIONS

Cystic lesions of the liver are also quite common. Most are benign. Cystic neoplasms are complex lesions and rare. Following is an outline of the most common cystic lesions.

### A. BENIGN
1. Pyogenic hepatic abscess
a. Results from bacterial infection of the liver parenchyma
b. Most common cause is *ascending cholangitis* (caused by lithiasis, cancer, or manipulation), followed by *pyelophlebitis* (complicated appendicitis, diverticulitis, pancreatitis, inflammatory bowel disease) or any other cause of intraabdominal sepsis, septicemia, direct extension, or trauma.
c. *No clear causative factor can be identified in 20% to 45% of cases.*
d. Most common organisms are aerobic gram-negative (*Escherichia coli, Klebsiella* spp, *Enterococcus* spp), *Streptococcus* spp, *Staphylococcus aureus,* and anaerobes (*Bacteroides* sp, Clostridia). Fungal abscesses are common in immunocompromised patients.
e. Blood cultures are positive in only 50% of patients at presentation.

f. Clinical presentation is often subacute, and mild symptoms may precede admission. Fever, right upper quadrant pain, and hepatomegaly are common symptoms and signs.

g. Characteristic contrast CT appearance is that of a round or irregularly shaped hypoattenuating mass with a peripheral capsule that shows enhancement.

h. Once the diagnosis has been made, broad-spectrum antibiotics (piperacillin/tazobactam) should be started and modified according to available cultures.

i. *Antibiotic therapy is not enough.* Percutaneous catheter drainage is the usual treatment modality. If lithiasis or biliary strictures are present, they should be treated with ERCP or surgery. The underlying source, if present, should be treated.

j. Surgical drainage is indicated when percutaneous drainage has failed (48 hours after percutaneous drainage without improvement), location inaccessible to percutaneous drainage, multiloculated abscesses, or concomitant pathology that requires surgery.

k. Mortality rate has significantly declined since the late 1980s, reaching 2% to 6% in many recent series. Ruptured hepatic abscess carries a high mortality rate of 30% to 43%.

## 2. Amebic hepatic abscess

a. Caused by entamoeba histolytica. Travels to the liver from the intestines via the portal blood.

b. A concomitant hepatic abscess is found in only one third of patients with amebic colitis. Male/female ratio is 10:1. Usually patients have a history of *traveling to a tropical area*.

c. Typically, the onset of the illness is abrupt with right upper quadrant pain, fever, anorexia, and acute colitis.

d. Diagnosis is made by serum indirect hemagglutination assay.

e. Findings in CT are nonspecific and usually appear as solitary, round, hypoattenuating mass with an enhancing ring; 70% to 80% of the abscesses occur exclusively in the right lobe.

f. Usually therapy with metronidazole (750 mg three times daily for 5–10 days) is effective, with a 95% success rate.

## 3. Echinococcal cysts

a. Hydatid disease is caused by the dog tapeworm *Echinococcus granulosus,* with sheep being the usual intermediate host.

b. Humans ingest ova shed in the feces of the host. The ova penetrate the intestinal wall, pass the portal circulation, enter the liver, and from there the lungs, brain, and bones.

c. *E. granulosus* has an active cyst wall consisting of a germinal layer and a laminar layer. A reactive fibrous layer surrounds the active cyst, called the *pericyst,* which becomes calcified in 50% of liver cases. The germinal layer produces the *daughter cysts.*

d. Liver cells undergo liquefaction necrosis and produce a cavity filled with pus appearing as *"anchovy paste."*

e. Diagnosis is made by enzyme-linked immunosorbent assay or indirect hemagglutination tests. Eosinophilia is present in 40% of cases.

f. Classic ultrasonographic or CT findings are a thick wall, often with calcifications and with daughter cysts.

g. Most cysts are asymptomatic at presentation. Patients with complicated conditions present with cholangitis from rupture into a bile duct or with acute abdomen and anaphylaxis from rupture into the peritoneal cavity.

h. Medical therapy with albendazole (the best regimen) has a less than 30% success rate.

i. Definitive therapy includes complete *excision of living parasites.*

j. Extreme caution should be used to avoid spillage, and all surrounding tissues should be packed with 20% normal saline–soaked gauze. Open cyst evacuation with aspiration of the contents and removal of the active cyst lining, complete pericystectomy, or liver resection are acceptable options.

k. If the patient presents with jaundice or cholangitis, then ERCP with sphincterotomy should precede surgery.

4. **Simple hepatic cyst**

a. Prevalence rate of asymptomatic liver cysts in ultrasound or CT series is approximately 3% in adults. Equal distribution among sexes, although symptomatic cysts are more common in female individuals.

b. Adult polycystic kidney disease is associated with liver cysts in approximately 60% of patients.

c. In general, these cysts grow slowly, lack septa, and do not have malignant potential. In most cases, they are asymptomatic and only large cysts produce symptoms. Therefore, any patient with abdominal pain and simple liver cysts *should be evaluated for other pertinent pathology.*

d. Most patients do *not* require any treatment. In *symptomatic* patients, laparoscopic or open fenestration and rarely partial liver resection are acceptable treatments.

5. **Hepatic cystadenoma**

a. Uncommon single, usually large tumor

b. Abdominal pain or discomfort is common presenting symptom because of size.

c. Ultrasonography is probably the best modality and shows a single large fluid-filled cyst with irregular margins, septations, and mural nodules.

d. Must be differentiated from hydatid cyst and simple cyst

e. Treatment is complete surgical resection.

## B. MALIGNANT

### 1. Cystic subtypes of primary liver neoplasms

These lesions are rare and usually are the result of central necrosis or systemic or local treatment. The two most common neoplasms that can present as cystic lesions are *HCC* and *giant hemangioma.* Characteristic CT features of the mass and liver parenchyma will help identify the nature of these lesions.

## 2. Cystic metastases

Cystic metastases may be seen in mucinous adenocarcinomas from colorectal or ovarian origin. Also, hypervascular metastases, such as carcinoid, neuroendocrine, sarcoma, and melanoma, may have cystic appearance because of central necrosis.

**Clinical scenario:** *A 42-year-old man presents to the emergency department with a 1-week history of malaise and currently fever up to 102°F, upper abdominal discomfort, diaphoresis, and tachycardia. An upper abdominal ultrasound showed at least two separate large (7 and 3 cm) cystic lesions in the right lobe of the liver.*

*Again, history and physical examination are of paramount importance. History of recent travel to tropical areas, pathology related to the liver, and recent therapeutic interventions to the liver and bile ducts, as well as recent history of intraabdominal infections, should be defined in detail. A triple-phase CT should be ordered to better delineate the lesion. At the same time, serology for hydatid and amebic disease should be ordered. Our patient was resuscitated, and intravenous broad-spectrum antibiotics were started immediately. CT showed lesions compatible with pyogenic abscesses that were subsequently percutaneously drained. His condition did not improve and a new CT scan 30 hours later showed that the abscesses were enlarged. He underwent a formal right lobectomy. Gallbladder was significantly inflamed. He had an uneventful postoperative course.*

## RECOMMENDED READING

Blumgart LH (ed): *Surgery of the Liver and Biliary Tract,* 4th ed. Saunders, 2007, Philadelphia.
Cameron JL (ed): *Current Surgical Therapy,* 9th ed. Mosby, 2004, St. Louis.
Lee JKT, Sagel SS, Stanley RJ, Heiken JP (eds): *Computed Body Tomography with MRI Correlation,* 4th ed. Lippincott Williams & Wilkins, 2006.

# PART X

# Transplant Surgery

# Renal Transplantation

*Dong-Sik Kim, MD*

## I. EVALUATION OF CANDIDATES FOR TRANSPLANTATION

### A. QUALIFICATIONS

**1. Criteria**
a. End-stage renal disease from a variety of causes
b. Patient life expectancy longer than graft half-life

**2. Absolute contraindications**
a. Malignancy
b. Current infection
c. Hepatitis
d. Human immunodeficiency syndrome

**3. Relative contraindications**
a. History of noncompliance
b. Malnutrition
c. Severe cardiovascular disease
d. Substance abuse
e. High likelihood of recurrent renal disease (e.g., primary oxalosis)

### B. PATIENT EVALUATION

**1. Detailed history and physical examination with special emphasis on:**
a. Underlying renal disease
b. Estimated urine output
c. Cardiovascular history
d. History of infectious disease

**2. Routine pretransplant studies**
a. Routine screening laboratory studies; renal panel, liver function tests, complete blood cell count, coagulation screen, urinalysis, calcium, phosphorus, magnesium
b. Hepatitis screen, human immunodeficiency syndrome, Venereal Disease Research Laboratory, viral titers (cytomegalovirus, Epstein–Barr virus, varicella), throat and urine cultures, tuberculin skin test
c. Chest radiograph, electrocardiogram
d. Blood typing, human leukocyte antigen (HLA), panel-reactive antibodies

**3. Indication for pretransplantation native nephrectomy**
a. Chronic renal parenchymal infection
b. Infected stones
c. Heavy proteinuria
d. Intractable hypertension
e. Polycystic kidney disease that is massive, recurrently infected, or bleeding
f. Acquired renal cystic disease with suspicion of adenocarcinoma
g. Infected reflux

49

## II. IMMUNOLOGY OF RENAL TRANSPLANTATION

### A. ABO ANTIGENS

1. The ABO blood group antigens behave as strong transplantation antigens, and transplantation across ABO barriers usually leads to irreversible hyperacute rejection.
2. Disproportionate percentage of waiting patients who are type O or B generally mandates that ABO identity (same blood type) rather than ABO compatibility (B → B or O) determines the distribution of deceased donor kidneys.
3. For living-related donor transplantation, ABO compatibility is adequate.
4. A2 kidneys can be safely transplanted into O or B recipients with low preoperative titers of isoagglutinin.
5. ABO-incompatible transplants may be performed if isoagglutinins are removed by splenectomy and plasmapheresis.

### B. HLA MATCHING IN TRANSPLANTATION

1. Class I antigens consist of A, B, or C loci antigens located on the surface membranes of all nucleated cells.
2. Class II antigens consist of DP, DQ, and DR loci found primarily on immune, dendritic, and endothelial cells.
3. In clinical transplantation, the most important major histocompatibility genes are HLA-A, -B, and -DR.
4. HLA-DR matching provides a greater benefit than class I antigen matching.

### C. PANEL-REACTIVE ANTIBODY

1. The patient's serum is incubated separately with B and T cells from a panel of donors selected to represent the HLA antigens commonly found in the local population.
2. The results are usually expressed as the percentage of panel cells that are killed by the serum.
3. The anti-HLA antibodies that are detected are called *panel-reactive antibodies.*
4. The finding of 60% of panel-reactive antibodies suggests that 60% of donors will be unacceptable for the patient because there are circulating antibodies that react with one or more of the donor's HLA antigens.

### D. CROSS-MATCH

1. The cross-match test is the final pretransplant immunologic screening step.
2. The presence of cytotoxic IgG antidonor HLA antibodies is a strong contraindication to transplantation.
3. Preliminary cross-match is performed by testing donor lymphocytes with stored sera of patients at the time of donor HLA typing.

Sensitized patients with a positive cross-match are excluded, but those with a negative preliminary cross-match and 80% or more panel-reactive antibody receive special consideration in the ranking of candidates.
4. When the preliminary cross-match is negative, a final cross-match is performed with recent or fresh sera.

## III. IMMUNOSUPPRESSION

### A. IMMUNOSUPPRESSIVE AGENTS IN CURRENT CLINICAL USE
1. Calcineurin inhibitors: cyclosporine (Sandimmune or Neoral) and tacrolimus (Prograf)
2. Antimetabolites: mycophenolate mofetil (CellCept) and azathioprine
3. Target of rapamycin inhibitors: sirolimus (Rapamune) and everolimus
4. Corticosteroids
5. Monoclonal and polyclonal antibodies: muromonab-CD3 (OKT3), antithymocyte globulin (Thymoglobulin), basiliximab (Simulect), daclizumab (Zenapax)

### B. IMMUNOSUPPRESSIVE PROTOCOLS
1. Conventional immunosuppressive protocols consist of a calcineurin inhibitor, an adjunctive agent, corticosteroids, and the possible addition of antibody induction.
2. Conventional immunosuppressive protocols that can provide 90% to 95% 1-year graft survival rate and 10% to 20% incidence rate of acute rejection include:
a. Cyclosporin/mycophenolate mofetil/steroids
b. Tacrolimus/mycophenolate mofetil/steroids
c. Cyclosporin/sirolimus/steroids
d. Tacrolimus/sirolimus/steroids

## IV. KIDNEY DONATION

### A. LIVING DONOR KIDNEY TRANSPLANTATION
1. Risks of donation
a. The risk rate for mortality as a result of donor nephrectomy is estimated to be 0.03%.
b. The reoperation rate and the readmission rate are both less than 1%.
c. The incidence rate of other postoperative complications approximates 3%.
d. A follow-up of more than 356 donors for at least 20 years reported one case of chronic renal failure in an aged patient.
2. Exclusion criteria for living kidney donation include:
a. Inadequately treated psychiatric disease
b. Active drug or alcohol abuse
c. Evidence of renal disease

49

RENAL TRANSPLANTATION

d. Abnormal renal anatomy
e. Recurrent nephrolithiasis or bilateral kidney stones
f. Collagen vascular disease
g. Diabetes
h. Hypertension
i. Prior myocardial infarction or treated coronary artery disease
j. Moderate-to-severe pulmonary disease
k. History of cancer
l. Active infection
m. Chronic active viral infection (hepatitis B or C, human immunodeficiency syndrome, human T-cell lymphocytic virus)
n. Significant chronic liver disease
o. Significant neurologic disease
p. Disorders requiring anticoagulation
q. Current pregnancy
r. History of thrombotic disease with risk factors for future events (such as anticardiolipin antibody, factor V Leiden mutation)

## B. DECEASED DONOR KIDNEY TRANSPLANTATION
**1.** Donor age is an important determinant of long-term graft function.
**2.** Expanded criteria for donor kidney
a. Kidneys from donors older than age 60 years
b. Age 50 to 59 years with two additional risk factors, including a history of hypertension, death as a result of cerebrovascular accident, or an increased terminal serum creatinine concentration >1.5 mg/dl
c. Approximately 15% of transplantations are deceased donor kidneys.
d. At least a 70% increased risk for failure within 2 years when compared with standard criteria kidneys. (On the positive side, this means that if a standard kidney has a 2-year graft survival rate of 88%, an expanded criteria donor [ECD] kidney has an estimated survival at 2 years of approximately 80%.)

## V. SPECIFIC OPERATIVE CONSIDERATIONS
### A. LIVING DONOR NEPHRECTOMY
**1.** Left kidney is preferred because of longer renal vein and better access to arteries.
**2.** Laparoscopy-assisted nephrectomy technique is used preferentially in many centers.
**3.** Procedure
a. The donor is placed in lateral decubitus position and pneumoperitoneum obtained.
b. Colon is reflected medially, away from the kidney.
c. The spleen or the liver is mobilized and retracted away from the upper pole of the kidney.
d. The perinephric tissues are freed, and the ureter and periureteral tissues are then mobilized.

e. The renal artery and vein are carefully identified and isolated.
f. The renal artery and vein are divided with a vascular stapler.
g. The ureter is ligated distally and kidney is brought out through hand port.
h. The kidney is flushed with preservation solution, placed on ice, and transported to the recipient room.

## B. TRANSPLANT PROCEDURE

1. Kidney graft is placed in pelvic cavity (heterotopic) because of less surgical burden and easier access for evaluation after transplant.
2. Generally, the right iliac fossa is favored for transplant site because the vessels are more superficial.
3. Oblique incision cranial to inguinal ligament—muscles are divided; then the peritoneum is exposed and retracted medially to expose the iliac vessels.
4. Vascular anastomoses are performed as follows:
a. Renal artery to external iliac artery (end to side)
b. Renal artery to hypogastric artery (end to end)
c. Renal vein to external iliac vein (end to side)
d. Accessory renal arteries can be anastomosed end to side to the largest renal artery and then anastomosed to the recipient vessels. This is usually done ex vivo on ice.
5. Ureteroneocystostomy
a. Tension-free suture
b. Water-tight suture
c. One-centimeter submucosal tunnel to prevent reflux

## VI. POSTOPERATIVE CONSIDERATIONS

### A. POSTOPERATIVE CARE

1. Observation and documentation of hourly urine output is critical to determine the early degree of initial function of the graft.
2. Beware of volume depletion caused by posttransplant diuresis. This can be avoided by replacing urine output milliliter per milliliter every hour with intravenous fluid of similar electrolyte composition.
3. Central venous pressure monitoring is a useful guide to intravascular volume status.
4. It is not uncommon for electrolyte abnormalities to develop, including hyperkalemia or hypokalemia, hypocalcemia, and hypomagnesemia.
5. Sutures or wound clips are generally left in place for 21 days because of delayed wound healing in patients with renal failure and immuno-suppressed patients.
6. Foley catheters are left in place for 2 to 5 days after surgery.

### B. ASSESSMENT OF GRAFT FUNCTION

1. Urine output—nonspecific; decreased urine output may indicate hypovo-lemia, urinary obstruction, ureteral compromise, vascular compromise, acute tubular necrosis, rejection.

49

RENAL TRANSPLANTATION

2. Creatinine and blood urea nitrogen—nonspecific.
3. Ultrasound—demonstrates patency of artery and vein, detects fluid collection and hydronephrosis; first-step study after laboratory abnormality.
4. Radionucleotide imaging—can image flow and function.
5. Renal biopsy—may yield definitive pathologic diagnosis in cases of dysfunction; it is difficult to assess cyclosporine nephrotoxicity.

## VII. COMPLICATIONS

### A. SURGICAL COMPLICATIONS

1. Wound infection rate <1%
2. Lymphocele—many are asymptomatic, some present with mass effects, lymph fistula; diagnosed by sonography; percutaneous drainage or intraperitoneal window.
3. Bleeding
4. Graft thrombosis—most often within the first 2 to 3 days after transplantation; sudden cessation of urine output and rapid increase of creatinine; diagnosed by Doppler ultrasound or isotope flow scan; most of the time, kidney will be lost.
5. Renal artery stenosis—usually occurs 3 months to 2 years after transplantation; presents with refractory hypertension, unexplained increase in creatinine concentration; diagnosed by Doppler sonography or angiography; percutaneous transluminal angioplasty offers the safest mode of treatment.
6. Urine leaks
   a. Incidence rate of 3% to 10%
   b. Related to ureteral ischemia, anastomotic tension
   c. Usually in first month after transplant
   d. Symptoms—pain with graft swelling, fever, sepsis, and urine fistula
   e. Diagnosis—CT scan, ultrasonogram may demonstrate fluid collection
   f. Management
      (1) Percutaneous nephrostomy and stenting
      (2) Ureteroneocystostomy revision
      (3) Boari flap, donor-recipient pyeloureterostomy
7. Ureteral stenosis
   a. This is the most common urinary complication.
   b. Causative agents include hematoma, kinking, or edema.
   c. Late-onset obstruction is related to fibrosis from ischemia.
   d. Presentation depends on degree of obstruction.
   e. Oliguria, increased creatinine concentration, sepsis, anuria
   f. Diagnosis by sonography, antegrade pyelography (most sensitive), renal venography (less sensitive)

g. Management
    (1) Percutaneous nephrostomy and surgical correction
    (2) Percutaneous transluminal dilation and stenting

## B. MEDICAL COMPLICATIONS
### 1. Infections
a. First month
    (1) Cause related to surgical procedure.
    (2) Wound infections, urinary tract infection, infections related to
        indwelling catheters
    (3) Pneumonia
    (4) Also infections transmitted with graft (human immunodeficiency
        syndrome, cytomegalovirus, hepatitis)
b. Months 1 to 6—high mortality because of degree of immunosuppression.
   Viral infections are common.
c. After 6 months—risk is reduced because of reduced
   immunosuppression.

### 2. Malignancy
a. Immunosuppression predisposes to the development of malignancy.
b. The incidence of nonskin malignancies in renal transplant recipients is
   up to 3.5-fold greater than that of age-matched control subjects.
c. Posttransplant lymphoproliferative disorders and Kaposi's sarcoma tend
   to occur early after transplant; other tumors tend to occur later.
d. The cumulative incidence of skin cancer is much greater, but few patients
   die of skin cancer after renal transplantation.
e. Decision regarding cancer screening should be made on an individual
   basis.

## VIII. STATISTICS OF RENAL TRANSPLANTATION
### A. SURVIVAL BENEFIT OF RENAL TRANSPLANTATION
1. Survival benefit of transplantation versus remaining on the waiting list
   (Fig. 49-1). Note that in the early period after a transplant, the risk for
   death is greater for transplant recipients than for wait-listed patients.
   Within a short period, somewhat longer for recipients of marginal
   kidneys, the risk of death and chances of survival equalize. Thereafter,
   transplantation has a persistent survival benefit.
2. The longer patient receives dialysis, the greater the risk for posttransplant morbidity, mortality, and graft loss.

### B. SURVIVAL
1. Graft versus patient survival is shown in Figure 49-2.

49

RENAL TRANSPLANTATION

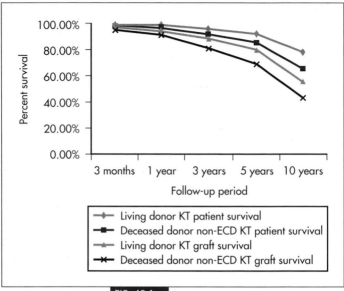

**FIG. 49-1**

Survival after kidney transplant.

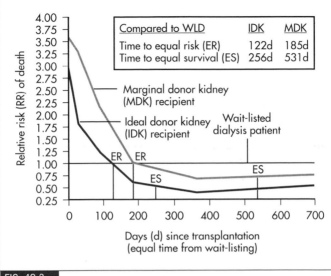

FIG. 49-2

Relative risk of death after kidney transplant compared with remaining on waiting list.

## RECOMMENDED READING

Danovitch GM: *Handbook of Kidney Transplantation,* 4th ed. Philadelphia, Lippincott Williams & Wilkins, 2005.

Stuart FP, Abecassis MM, Kaufman DB: *Organ Transplantation,* 2nd ed. Georgetown, TX, Landes Bioscience, 2003.

Organ Procurement and Transplantation Network: 2005 OPTN/SRTR Annual Report. Available at http://www.optn.org/AR2006/default.htm

Ojo AO, Hanson JA, Meier-Kriesche HU, et al: Survival in recipients of marginal cadaveric donor kidneys compared wih other recipients and wait-listed transplant candidates. *J Am Soc Nephrol* 12:589, 2001.

# Liver Transplantation

*Mubeen A. Jafri, MD*

## I. GENERAL CONSIDERATIONS

### A. HISTORY

1. 1967—Starzl performed the first successful liver transplant.
2. 1983—venovenous bypass was introduced for use during anhepatic phase; cyclosporin approved for transplant immunosuppression.
3. 1984—Broelsch and associates introduced the reduced-size liver transplantation.
4. 1989—first successful living-related transplant
5. Today, almost 6500 liver transplants are performed yearly in the United States.

## 50

### B. INDICATIONS AND LISTING PROCESS FOR TRANSPLANTATION

For a patient to be placed on the waiting list, he/she must have a Child–Turcotte–Pugh score of 7 or greater. Generally, patients are transplanted for complications of portal hypertension, encephalopathy, hepatic synthetic dysfunction, or growth failure (children). Organs in each geographic area are distributed by United Network for Organ Sharing based on the patient's MELD (Model for End-stage Liver Disease) score. MELD score is based on the following factors: creatinine, bilirubin, and international normalized ratio.

### C. SPECIFIC INDICATIONS AND CONTRAINDICATIONS

1. Alcoholic cirrhosis—most common causative factor of liver failure in the United States.
2. Hepatitis—virtually all patients with chronic hepatitis B or C ultimately become reinfected, with variable outcomes.
3. Acute fulminant hepatic failure—secondary to drug toxicity, hepatitis, Wilson's disease, pregnancy, Budd-Chiari syndrome, mushroom intoxication, and others. Acetaminophen toxicity is the most common cause.
4. Inborn errors of metabolism—glycogen storage disease, Wilson's disease, $\alpha$1-antitrypsin deficiency, protein S deficiency, among others
5. Biliary disease—primary biliary cirrhosis, primary sclerosing cholangitis, extrahepatic biliary atresia (most common causative factor in children)
6. Primary hepatic malignancy—controversial indication, associated with high likelihood of recurrent disease. Milan criteria for transplant for hepatocellular carcinoma: 1 nodule $\leq$5 cm or $\leq$3 nodules of 3 cm or less.
7. Contraindications—extrahepatic malignancy, active infection, severe organ impairment (excluding renal), acute substance abuse, poor social support, inability to comply with medical regimen, fixed pulmonary hypertension (does not respond to prostaglandin $E_1$)

### D. ORGAN SELECTION

In general, standard criteria apply, including a hemodynamically stable donor with no evidence of sepsis or non–central nervous system primary malignancy, and ABO compatibility.

1. Cadaveric whole organ
2. Cadaveric reduced-sized grafts—full right, full left, or left lateral lobe graft. With a left lateral lobe, a size discrepancy of 10:1 can be overcome.
3. Living related liver donation—increases the limited pool of pediatric-sized livers; graft and patient survival rates as high as 95%.

## II. SPECIFIC OPERATIVE CONSIDERATIONS

### A. TRADITIONAL OPERATIVE TECHNIQUE

1. Bilateral subcostal incision with midline extension to xiphoid process
2. Mobilization of the native liver. Isolation of the suprahepatic and infrahepatic venae cavae. Skeletonization of the hilar structures—portal vein, bile duct, and hepatic artery.
3. Establishment of venous-venous bypass to decompress the splanchnic venous system; selectively used with intestinal edema, hypotension after test clamping of the vena cava, extensive portal hypertension bleeding, and difficult hepatectomy. Cannulas (percutaneous or cut-down) from the portal and femoral veins drain blood into the axillary vein.
4. Recipient hepatectomy
5. Vascular anastomoses—suprahepatic vena cava, infrahepatic vena cava, hepatic artery, and portal vein
6. Biliary anastomosis—end-to-end bile duct anastomosis or choledochojejunostomy
7. Abdominal fascial closure with nonabsorbable sutures

### B. PIGGYBACK TECHNIQUE

1. Recipient hepatectomy altered to leave the recipient retrohepatic vena cava intact.
2. Hilar dissection performed as in traditional technique.
3. Recipient liver remains attached to vena cava only by hepatic veins.
4. Recipient hepatectomy
5. Vascular anastomosis—donor suprahepatic vena cava to recipient inferior vena cava in end-to-side fashion, donor infrahepatic vena cava ligated, hepatic artery and portal vein.
6. Remainder of procedure done as in traditional technique.

## III. POSTOPERATIVE CONSIDERATIONS

### A. POSTOPERATIVE CARE

1. Hemodynamic monitoring and resuscitation with the aid of pulmonary artery catheter
2. Correction of coagulopathy with blood products

3. Ventilatory support often for 24 to 48 hours after transplantation
4. Electrolyte management—correction of glucose, calcium, potassium, magnesium, and phosphate are particularly important.
5. Infection surveillance and prophylaxis—trimethoprim/sulfamethoxazole, fluconazole, and ganciclovir
6. Immunosuppression—protocols vary among institutions.
a. Antilymphocyte induction therapy available but has not been widely used.
b. Calcineurin inhibitors remain the baseline postoperative immunosuppression. Tacrolimus (Prograf; FK506) is the most widely used agent. Renal toxicity is an important adverse effect.
c. Steroids are generally given as intravenous methylprednisolone sodium succinate (Solu-Medrol) after surgery, and patients are transitioned to oral prednisone as advancement of diet permits.
d. Mycophenolate mofetil (CellCept) is a commonly used third baseline immunosuppressive agent.
7. Disease-specific consideration
a. Hepatitis B recurrence occurs in 80% to 90% of patients and should be treated at time of operation with hepatitis B immunoglobulin.
b. Transplant for hepatocellular carcinoma should include neoadjuvant chemotherapy to improve survival.

## B. ASSESSMENT OF GRAFT FUNCTION
1. Routine laboratory tests: Transaminase levels, alkaline phosphatase, factor V function (best predictor of early graft function), serum bilirubin, and coagulation parameters are nonspecific but are usually used to follow trends in graft function.
2. Radionuclide imaging can be used to assess hepatocellular function and continuity of biliary drainage.
3. Liver biopsy: This is most specific for differentiating rejection from recurrent hepatitis, steatosis, ischemia, or other causes of graft dysfunction.

## C. COMPLICATIONS
1. Primary nonfunction—has become a relatively rare cause of graft dysfunction since the introduction of UW (University of Wisconsin) solution. Manifested by failure to regain hepatic function in the early postoperative period. Urgent retransplantation is usually indicated.
2. Rejection—occurs at some time in 60% of liver transplant patients. Diagnosis is made by biopsy of graft.
3. Hepatic artery thrombosis—diagnosis is made by angiogram, after screening with ultrasound/Doppler examination; increased risk with pediatric transplant.
4. Portal vein thrombosis—usually requires retransplantation but may respond to thrombolytic therapy. It is less common than arterial complications.

5. Biliary complications—manifested by fever and increasing bilirubin and alkaline phosphatase levels; diagnosed by cholangiogram; biliary stricture (resulting from technical error with anastomosis or hepatic artery thrombosis/stenosis) managed by conversion to choledochojejunostomy or stent placement.
6. Vena caval obstruction
7. Renal dysfunction
8. Infection and immunosuppressive drug complications
9. Recurrence of native disease
10. Hyperlipidemia and obesity in up to 60% of patients after transplant

D. **RESULTS (UNITED NETWORK FOR ORGAN SHARING DATA 1997–2004, PRIMARY LIVER TRANSPLANT)**
1. Patient survival rates at 1 and 5 years are 88% and 74%, respectively.
2. Graft survival rates at 1 and 5 years are 83% and 68%, respectively.

## RECOMMENDED READING

Abecassis M, Blei A, Koffron A, et al: Liver transplantation. In Stuart FP, Abecassis MM, Kaufman DB (eds): *Organ Transplantation,* 12th ed. Georgetown, TX, Landes Bioscience, 2003, pp 205–243.

USTransplants.org. Scientific Registry of Transplant Recipients. Available at: http://www.ustransplant.org. Accessed September 30, 2006.

# Pancreas Transplantation

*Mubeen A. Jafri, MD*

## I. GENERAL CONSIDERATIONS
### A. HISTORY
1. 1921—Banting and Best report the discovery of insulin.
2. 1966—Kelly and Lillehei perform the first pancreas transplant.
3. 1986—Corry and associates develop technique of urinary bladder diversion of exocrine secretions.
4. 1999—Edmonton protocol increases success of pancreatic islet transplant.
5. Currently, approximately 1500 pancreas transplants are performed yearly in the United States. The majority (85%) occur simultaneously with kidney transplant (simultaneous pancreas-kidney transplant [SPK]), followed by those (10%) that occur after kidney transplant (pancreas alone after kidney transplant), and a minority (5%) occur alone (pancreas transplant alone [PTA]).

### B. INDICATIONS FOR PANCREAS TRANSPLANTATION
Insulin-dependent diabetes mellitus is associated with increased risk for blindness (25 times), kidney disease (17 times), gangrene (20 times), and heart disease or stroke (2 times each) compared with patients without diabetes. Pancreas transplant is performed in three categories of patients:
1. SPK—patient with insulin-dependent diabetes with end-stage renal disease who is also in need of kidney transplant.
2. Pancreas alone after kidney transplant—patient with functioning renal transplant, to prevent the development of nephropathy in the transplanted kidney; may improve kidney graft survival.
3. PTA—nonuremic, labile diabetic with hypoglycemic unawareness. The risks of surgery and immunosuppression must be balanced against the likelihood of development of secondary complications of diabetes.

### C. SPECIFIC INDICATIONS AND CONTRAINDICATIONS
1. Insulin-dependent diabetes mellitus documented by absence of circulating C peptide.
2. Microalbuminuria with a creatinine clearance of <60 ml/min
3. Proteinuria with a projected dialysis requirement
4. Autonomic neuropathy
5. Retinopathy
6. Labile diabetes and failure of medical management (brittle diabetes)
7. Absence of coronary artery disease
8. Absence of gangrene or ongoing sepsis
9. Age 18 to 50 years

51

## D. ORGAN SELECTION

Most are performed from cadaveric donors. In addition to standard criteria for donor selection, specific contraindications to pancreas transplantation include the following:

1. Presence of diabetes mellitus
2. Chronic pancreatitis
3. Pancreatic damage secondary to trauma
4. History of alcohol abuse or relapsing pancreatitis (center specific)

## II. SPECIFIC OPERATIVE CONSIDERATIONS

1. The recipient bed is prepared in the right iliac fossa.
2. Venous drainage is first established by portal vein-external iliac vein anastomosis.
3. Arterial inflow is determined by manner of donor harvest. With the whole graft, the celiac axis and superior mesenteric artery are preferentially removed together on an aortic patch that is anastomosed end to side to the recipient external iliac artery.

## A. MANAGEMENT OF EXOCRINE SECRETIONS

1. Diversion into the bowel with anastomosis to the second portion of the donor duodenum, which is harvested en bloc with the pancreas, is the preferred technique at the University of Cincinnati.
2. Diversion to the urinary bladder has the advantage of using urinary amylase to monitor graft function but is associated with cystitis and acid-base abnormalities.
3. Pancreatic duct occlusion with injectable synthetic polymer completely blocks exocrine secretion but can lead to severe inflammation and fibrosis, and is rarely practiced.

## III. POSTOPERATIVE CONSIDERATIONS

### A. POSTOPERATIVE CARE

1. Vascular thrombosis is the most common cause of early graft loss, necessitating some form of perioperative anticoagulation. Suggested protocols include aspirin, systemic heparinization, and low-molecular-weight dextran.
2. Graft function can be monitored by amylase levels and glucose homeostasis. Because 90% of the pancreas may be lost before glucose homeostasis is impaired, this is not sensitive. Use of insulin is generally avoided.
3. No reliable technique exists for the diagnosis of rejection. In the patient undergoing SPK, rejection is usually monitored by following serum creatinine levels. Increases in serum creatinine levels precede a decrease in pancreatic exocrine function 90% of the time. Rejection demonstrated on biopsy of the renal allograft is also an indication of pancreatic rejection.

4. Immunosuppressive regimens vary, but most centers use induction with antilymphocyte globulin or muromonab CD3 (OKT3) and maintenance with cyclosporine or tacrolimus (FK506), prednisone, and azathioprine or mycophenolate mofetil. Rejection accounts for up to 32% of graft loss in the first year.
5. Radionuclide perfusion scans can be used to evaluate blood flow to the allograft.

## B. ASSESSMENT OF GRAFT FUNCTION
1. Urinary or systemic amylase
2. Concomitant renal function (creatinine) to assess rejection
3. Transplant biopsy

## C. COMPLICATIONS
1. Graft pancreatitis
a. Occurs in 3% to 5% of transplants
b. Secondary to preservation injury and ischemia
c. Suggested by hyperamylasemia and local graft pain
d. May require drainage of peripancreatic collections or operative debridement of necrotic pancreas
2. Graft thrombosis
a. Most common cause of sudden early graft loss—10% to 20% of cases
b. Attributed to the fact that the pancreas is a low-flow organ
c. If confirmed by radionuclide scan, the graft must be removed urgently to prevent septic or vascular complications.
3. Anastomotic failure (3.5–6%)
a. Presents with fever, leukocytosis, and drainage of clear fluid from the operative wound
b. Rare with bladder drainage of the exocrine pancreas, but it can be fatal if not addressed early.
4. Sepsis—almost always related to the development of graft pancreatitis or anastomotic failure.
5. Bleeding (5%)
a. Site is usually gastrointestinal tract.
b. Usually related to the use of anticoagulation in perioperative period
6. Peripheral hyperinsulinemia—result of systemic venous delivery of insulin. Limited trials are under way to assess the viability of portal venous drainage.
7. Rejection

## D. RESULTS (UNITED NETWORK FOR ORGAN SHARING DATA 1997–2004)
1. SPK patient survival rate at 1 and 5 years is 95% and 86%, respectively.
2. SPK graft survival rate at 1 and 5 years is 92% and 76%, respectively.

3. Pancreas alone patient survival rate at 1 and 5 years is 94% and 83%, respectively.
4. Pancreas alone graft survival at 1 and 5 years is 79% and 53%, respectively.
5. Insulin independence at 1 year—SPK, 81%; pancreas alone after kidney transplant, 71%; PTA, 62%
6. Insulin independence improves quality of life. Data support potential reversal of diabetic neuropathy, decreased recurrence of nephropathy in SPK for end-stage renal disease. Advanced, secondary diabetic complications such as retinopathy and vascular disease are unlikely to be improved. Increased rate of thrombosis and rejection after solitary pancreas transplant.

## IV. ISLET CELL TRANSPLANTATION
### A. BACKGROUND
1. Currently, PTA is performed rarely for patients with diabetes with labile disease who do not experience symptoms of life-threatening hypoglycemia.
2. PTA occurs less commonly than SPK and pancreas alone after kidney transplant because of the need for immunosuppression and the high perioperative morbidity.
3. By isolating insulin-producing beta cells within the islets of Langerhans, organ transplantation may be obviated.

### B. INDICATIONS
1. Autotransplantation after pancreatectomy for carcinoma or refractory pancreatitis
2. Allotransplantation in patients with type I diabetes with hypoglycemic unawareness or inability to tolerate major transplant operation

### C. TECHNIQUE
1. Pancreatic tissue obtained from pancreatectomy or cadaveric source is enzymatically digested. Usually requires two cadaveric pancreas grafts to harvest about 1 million islets or 300,000+ islet cell equivalents in autotransplant.
2. Islet cells are extracted and purified via gradient separation.
3. Microencapsulation to decrease immunogenicity in allotransplant
4. Islet tissue infused into hepatic parenchyma via injection into portal vein or directly into liver.

### D. RESULTS
Multiple challenges must be overcome before islet cell transplantation can become routinely successful. Paramount is the creation of an ideal microencapsulation vehicle that may ultimately facilitate further xenotransplantation efforts.

1. Insulin independence at 1 year up to 80% (with repeat infusions), but less than 40% at 3 years with allotransplant.
2. Insulin independence at 1 year with autotransplant with >300,000 islets up to 75%, with <300,000 islets only 20%.

## RECOMMENDED READING

Nadey H, Stratta R, Gray D: *Pancreas and Islet Transplantation.* New York, Oxford University Press, 2002.

51

PANCREAS TRANSPLANTATION

# PART XI

# Surgical Oncology

# Malignant Skin Lesions

*Amy T. Makley, MD*

The skin is the largest organ of the human body and one of the most important structures of the immune system. It is the barrier for all chemical and physical trauma, and it provides the body with the most efficient form of thermoregulation. More recently, it has become the subject of dedicated research involving wound healing and synthetic skin substitutes. As the most common malignancies of the human body, skin carcinomas are discovered on a regular basis in everyday surgical practice. The three most common skin carcinomas are basal cell carcinoma, squamous cell carcinoma, and malignant melanoma.

**52**

## I. BASAL CELL CARCINOMA

### A. GENERAL
1. Most common skin malignancy
2. Associated with ultraviolet exposure
3. Clinical presentation
   a. Waxy or cream-colored
   b. Classically described with pearly, rolled borders
   c. Central ulceration common
   d. Slow growing
   e. Local destruction; rarely metastatic disease
4. Types
   a. Nodular—classic type
   b. Superficial—slow growing, scaly, pink plaque
   c. Sclerosing/Morpheaform—rarest form, resembles scar

### B. DIAGNOSIS
1. Punch biopsy
2. Excisional biopsy for smaller lesions

### C. TREATMENT
1. Surgical excision with 2- to 4-mm margins ideal.
2. Curettage/laser ablation for smaller lesions/premalignant lesions
3. Mohs micrographic surgery
   a. For cosmetically sensitive areas
   b. Serial excision of tumor with immediate evaluation of frozen sections until normal tissue margins obtained.
4. Radiation therapy
5. Topical treatment with 5-fluorouracil/imiquimod cream for multiple lesions.

## II. SQUAMOUS CELL CARCINOMA

### A. GENERAL

1. Second-most common skin malignancy.
2. Squamous cell carcinoma >2 cm has increased likelihood of metastasis compared with basal cell carcinoma of similar size.
3. Associated with ultraviolet exposure, chronic scars, and irradiated skin
4. Clinical presentation
   a. Arise in sun-exposed areas (i.e., face, extremities)
   b. Erythematous, scaly plaque, ulcerated mass or nodule
5. Bowen's disease
   a. Squamous cell carcinoma in situ
   b. Five percent develop into invasive squamous cell carcinoma.
6. Marjolin's ulcer—squamous cell carcinoma arising in burn scar.
7. Erythroplasia of Queyrat—in situ squamous cell carcinoma of penis.

### B. DIAGNOSIS—PUNCH BIOPSY VERSUS EXCISIONAL BIOPSY

### C. TREATMENT

1. Surgical excision with 2- to 4-mm margins
2. Regional lymph node dissection if palpable lymphadenopathy
3. Sentinel lymph node biopsy if large tumor or carcinoma arising in chronic wounds

## III. MALIGNANT MELANOMA

### A. GENERAL

1. Increasingly more common diagnosis
2. No increase in mortality—reflects increases in detection and treatment.
3. Risk factors
   a. Previous melanoma
   b. Large number of dysplastic nevi
   c. Ultraviolet exposure
   d. Fair complexion, light-colored eyes
   e. Family history (6–14% of melanomas with some family history)

### B. CLINICAL PRESENTATION

1. A—asymmetry
2. B—border irregularity
3. C—color variation
4. D—diameter >6 mm
5. E—evolution

### C. TYPES OF MELANOMA

1. Superficial spreading (70%)
   a. Long radial growth phase before vertical growth
2. Nodular (15–30%)

a. Predominately vertical growth phase
b. More aggressive lesion
c. Equal mortality with superficial spreading type of equivalent depth
3. **Lentigo maligna (4–15%)**
a. Increased incidence in elderly adults
b. Targets face/neck/dorsum of hands
c. Best prognosis given thin depth
4. **Acral lentiginous (2–8%)**
a. Palms/soles/subungual region
b. Predominant subtype in dark-skinned individuals
c. "Hutchinson's sign"—pigmented proximal/lateral nail folds
d. Most aggressive but least common type

**D. PROGNOSTIC FACTORS**
1. Depth of invasion is most important prognostic factor.
2. Presence of ulceration increases aggressiveness.
a. Ulceration shown to correlate with increased angiogenesis.
3. Vertical growth phase and mitotic rate are inversely related to prognosis.
4. Findings of regression on pathology signifies worse prognosis.
5. Anatomic location—extremities more favorable than trunk/face.
6. Sex—female patients have increased survival with respect to male counterparts.

**E. STAGING**
1. Clark level of staging—based on anatomic depth.
a. Level I—superficial to basement membrane (in situ)
b. Level II—papillary dermis
c. Level III—papillary and reticular junction
d. Level IV—reticular junction
e. Level V—subcutaneous fat
2. Breslow level of staging—based on vertical thickness.
a. More important than Clark level for prognosis
b. <1 mm—thin
c. 1–4 mm—intermediate
d. >4 mm—thick
3. TNM staging system—most current staging system, developed by American Joint Committee on Cancer.
a. Primary tumor thickness (T)
Each T stage is subgrouped into "a" and "b" denoting the absence or presence of ulceration, respectively:
T1: <1.0 mm
T2: 1.01 to 2.0 mm
T3: 2.01 to 4.0 mm
T4: >4.01 mm
b. Nodal status (N).

N1: 1 node positive

    N1a—micrometastasis

    N1b—macrometastasis

N2: two to three nodes positive

    N2a—micrometastasis

    N2b—macrometastasis

    N2c—negative nodes with in-transit metastases

N3: 4+ nodes positive or in-transit metastases with positive nodes

c. Metastases (M)

  M0: no evidence of metastatic disease

  M1: distant skin, subcutaneous, or nodal disease with normal LDH

  M2: lung metastases with normal LDH

  M3: all other visceral metastases

d. Stages

  Stage 1a: T1a, N0, M0

  Stage 1b: T1b, N0, M0

     T2a, N0, M0

  Stage IIa: T2b, N0, M0

     T3a, N0, M0

  Stage IIb: T3b, N0, M0

     T4a, N0, M0

  Stage IIc: T4b, N0, M0

  Stage III: any T, N1-3, M0

  Stage IV: any T, any N, M1-3

## F. DIAGNOSIS

1. Excisional biopsy
2. Punch biopsy
3. Shave biopsy not recommended—may not measure thickness of lesion accurately.

## G. TREATMENT

1. **Wide local excision of remaining lesion and biopsy scar**
a. Lesions with 1-mm depth or less require 1-cm margins.
b. Lesions 1 to 2 mm in thickness require 1- to 2-cm margins.
c. Lesions with >2-mm depth require 2-cm margins.
d. Must excise to the level of underlying fascia.
2. **Lymph-node evaluation**
a. Regional lymph nodes most common site of metastatic disease.
b. All palpable lymphadenopathy requires therapeutic nodal dissection.
c. Sentinel lymph node dissection.
   (1) Appropriate for clinically node-negative disease in most lesions >1 mm, and in select patients with thin lesions
   (2) Techniques: Radiolabeled isotope is injected before surgery around the lesion, using a gamma probe intraoperatively to detect sentinel lymph nodes; 1% isosulfan blue dye is also injected around the

targeted lesion, highlighting the appropriate sentinel lymph node for excision.

3. Any positive node mandates therapeutic nodal dissection.
4. Additional treatment options
a. Interferon-$\alpha$2b
   (1) Only Federal Drug Administration–approved adjuvant for stage IIB/III disease
   (2) Proven increase in disease-free survival
b. Radiation therapy is adjunct treatment of choice for nodal basins with multiple involved lymph nodes.
c. Hyperthermic regional chemoperfusion/infusion
   (1) Melphalan
   (2) Used only if the extremity lesion is not amenable to surgical excision or if many in-transit metastases are present.
   (3) Risks for vascular damage, compartment syndrome, and thromboembolic events
   (4) Isolated brain, lung, or gastrointestinal metastases may be surgically excised for cure.
   (5) High dose interleukin-2 may lead to cure in less than 10% of patients with stage IV disease.
   (6) Many immunotherapy trials are currently under way with potentially promising results.

52

MALIGNANT SKIN LESIONS

# Diseases of the Breast

*Kelly M. McLean, MD*

## I. ANATOMY AND PHYSIOLOGY

### A. ANATOMY BASICS

1. Modified sweat gland of ectodermal origin that lies cushioned in fat and enveloped by superficial and deep layers of superficial fascia of the anterior chest wall
2. Each mammary gland consists of 15 to 20 lobules drained by lactiferous ducts that may coalesce. The nipple has 5 to 20 orifices.
3. Fibrous septa (Cooper's ligaments) interdigitate the mammary parenchyma and extend from the deep pectoral fascia to the superficial layer of fascia within the dermis. These provide structural support to the breast.
4. The base of the breast extends from the second to the sixth rib. Medial border = lateral margin of sternum; lateral border = midaxillary line. Axillary tail of Spence pierces deep fascia and enters axilla.

### B. LYMPHATIC DRAINAGE

1. Lymph node involvement is the most important prognostic factor for survival.
2. Any part of the breast can drain to any set of nodes.
3. Axillary nodes—75% of drainage from ipsilateral breast; contains up to 40 to 50 nodes. Axillary nodes secondarily drain to supraclavicular and jugular nodes.
4. Levels of axillary nodes—all nodes are below the axillary vein.
   **Level I**—lateral to pectoralis minor; includes external mammary, subscapular, axillary vein, and central nodal groups.
   **Level II**—deep to pectoralis minor muscle; includes central nodal groups.
   **Level III**—medial to pectoralis minor and extending up to apex of axilla; includes central nodal groups.
5. Internal mammary nodes—account for up to 20% of drainage; contain about four nodes per side, with one node in each of the first three interspaces and another in the fifth or sixth interspace.
6. Interpectoral (Rotter's) nodes—lie between pectoralis major and pectoralis minor muscles.
7. Abdominal and paravertebral nodes—account for 5% of drainage.

### C. NERVES

1. Intercostobrachial nerve—traverses the axilla from chest wall to supply cutaneous sensation to upper medial arm. Sacrificing this nerve results in anesthesia of upper medial arm. Runs below the axillary vein.

2. Long thoracic nerve (of Bell)—arises from roots of C5, C6, and C7. Courses close to chest wall along medial border of axilla to innervate serratus anterior muscle. Injury results in a "winged" scapular deformity. Runs with lateral thoracic artery, also to serratus anterior.

3. Thoracodorsal nerve—arises from posterior cord of brachial plexus (C5, C6, C7). Courses along lateral border of axilla to innervate latissimus dorsi muscle. Loss weakens arm adduction and pull-ups. Thoracodorsal artery supplies the latissimus dorsi.

4. Lateral pectoral nerve—arises from lateral cord of brachial plexus. Innervates pectoralis major muscle only. Exits medial to the medial pectoral nerve.

5. Medial pectoral nerve—arises from the medial cord of the brachial plexus. Innervates both the pectoralis minor and major muscles. Emerges lateral to the lateral pectoral nerve.

## D. BLOOD SUPPLY

1. The internal thoracic artery, intercostal arteries, thoracoacromial artery, and lateral thoracic artery supply blood to the breast.

2. Batson's plexus—valveless venous drainage that allows metastasis to the spine.

## E. PHYSIOLOGY

1. Phases of breast development are dependent on pituitary and ovarian hormones.

a. Estrogen—promotes ductal development and fat deposition in preparation for lactation, growth of glandular tissue.

b. Progesterone—promotes lobular-alveolar development and prepares breast for lactation, maturation of glandular tissue.

c. Prolactin (from the anterior pituitary)—involved in milk production.

d. Oxytocin (from the posterior pituitary)—involved in milk ejection.

2. Menopause: Menstrual cycle allows for cyclic growth. Declines in both estrogen and progesterone levels lead to cellular apoptosis, resulting in involution of breast tissue with atrophy of lobules, loss of stroma, and replacement with fatty tissue.

## II. HISTORY

### A. AGE

1. Fibrocystic changes increase with age after puberty and until menopause.

2. Fibroadenoma is most common breast lesion in women younger than 30 years.

3. Risk for breast cancer increases with increasing age—rare (<1%) in patients younger than 30 years of age; more than 70% of all cases occur in patients older than 50 years.

## B. MASS
1. Determine when first noted, how first noted, tender or nontender, and any change in size with time and in relation to the menstrual cycle, fixed or mobile.

## C. NIPPLE DISCHARGE (TABLE 53-1)
1. Bloody—benign intraductal papilloma most common. Rule out invasive papillary cancer. Discharge cytology notoriously poor for determining cancer because dying cells usually look atypical. Need to excise papilloma.
2. Milky (galactorrhea)—pregnancy, lactation, pituitary adenoma, acromegaly, hypothyroidism, stress, drugs (oral contraceptives, antihypertensives, certain psychotropic drugs). Evaluation should include urine or serum pregnancy tests and prolactin levels.
3. Serous—normal menses, oral contraceptives, fibrocystic change, early pregnancy
4. Yellow/green—fibrocystic change, galactocele
5. Purulent—superficial or central breast abscess

## D. BREAST PAIN (MASTODYNIA)
1. Rarely a symptom of breast cancer. Pain can be cyclic or continuous. Associated with menstrual irregularity, premenstruation, exogenous ovarian hormones during or after menopause, or fibrocystic change.
2. Query regarding its type, relation to menses, duration, and location.
3. Discontinue caffeine and nicotine.
4. Treat with evening primrose oil or nonsteroidal antiinflammatory drugs. If symptoms are debilitating, danazol (Danocrine) may be used for a maximum of 4 to 6 months.

## E. GYNECOLOGIC HISTORY (SEE SECTION VII)
1. Woman's age at the birth of her first child, age of menarche, age at menopause, use of oral contraceptives, and use of estrogen replacement

53

DISEASES OF THE BREAST

TABLE 53-1

CHARACTERISTICS OF NIPPLE DISCHARGE

| Physiologic | Pathologic |
| --- | --- |
| Bilateral | Unilateral |
| Clear/milky | Bloody |
| Multiple ducts/quadrants | Single duct/quadrant |
| Not spontaneous | Spontaneous |
| Negative for occult blood | Positive for occult blood |
| No mass | Palpable mass |

## F. MEDICAL HISTORY

1. History of benign breast disease (i.e., fibrocystic change), breast cancer, and radiation therapy to the breast or axilla

## G. SURGICAL HISTORY

1. History of breast biopsy, lumpectomy, mastectomy, axillary node dissection, hysterectomy, oophorectomy, or adrenalectomy

## H. FAMILY HISTORY

1. Note any family history of breast disease, especially in mother, sisters, or daughters. Also include history of breast, ovarian, or prostate cancer on either maternal or paternal side.

## I. CONSTITUTIONAL SYMPTOMS

1. Include anorexia, weight loss, dyspnea, cough, chest pain, hemoptysis, headache, and bone pain.

# III. PHYSICAL EXAMINATION

## A. INSPECTION

1. Examine the patient seated with her arms at her side, seated with her arms raised over her head, seated with her hands on her hips, and supine.
2. Note breast size, shape, contour, and symmetry; skin coloration, skin dimpling, edema, erythema, peau d'orange, and excoriation, as well as nipple inversion, retraction, symmetry, or discharge.

## B. PALPATION

1. With the patient in the sitting position, support the patient's arm and palpate each axilla to detect axillary adenopathy. Also palpate the supraclavicular fossae and cervical region. Note node size, character, and mobility.
2. Palpation of the breast is performed with the patient in the supine position with the arms stretched above the head and with the arms at her sides. Identify any masses, noting location, size, shape, consistency, tenderness, skin dimpling, and mobility. *Use the 4 D's to distinguish a true lump from a lumpy area: dominant, discrete, dense, and different.* Carcinoma is typically firm, nontender, poorly circumscribed, and relatively immobile. Use the flat portion of your fingers for the examination.
3. Nipples, including pressing on the areola, should be palpated to identify any discharge.

## C. SCREENING (CURRENT AMERICAN CANCER SOCIETY RECOMMENDATIONS)

1. Mammography and clinical breast examination: Emphasize breast self-examination. Most breast masses are found by patients themselves.

2. Breast self-examination on monthly basis beginning at 20 to 25 years of age. Breast self-examination should be performed about 5 days after completion of menses in the premenopausal woman and at the same time each month in the postmenopausal woman.
3. Physician examination every 1 to 3 years depending on risk factors. In general, every 3 years beginning at age 18 and annually beginning at age 40.
4. Baseline mammogram for women by age 40 years or 10 years before the youngest age of diagnosis in first-degree relative. The density of breast tissue in young women limits the interpretation of early mammograms.
5. Perform mammogram yearly thereafter.

## IV. RADIOGRAPHIC STUDIES

### A. MAMMOGRAPHY
1. Sensitivity and specificity varies with breast density, around 90% for both.

### B. MAMMOGRAPHIC FINDINGS SUGGESTIVE OF MALIGNANCY
1. Irregularly marginated stellate or spiculated mass
2. Architectural distortion with retraction and speculation
3. Asymmetrical localized fibrosis
4. Fine pleomorphic microcalcifications with a linear, branched, or rodlike pattern, especially when focal or clustered. Increased likelihood of cancer with increased number of microcalcifications.
5. Increased vascularity
6. Altered subareolar duct pattern
7. Unclear border with the rest of breast tissue
8. BIRADS (breast imaging reporting and data system) classification—recommendations are changing rapidly (Table 53-2).

### C. ULTRASONOGRAPHY
1. Useful for distinguishing between cystic and solid masses
2. Effective for lesions larger than 0.5 cm in diameter
3. Helpful in evaluating young women whose breast tissue is too dense for mammogram

## V. EVALUATION OF BREAST MASS

### A. NIPPLE DISCHARGE
1. Evaluation
a. Physical examination
b. Ultrasound
c. Mammogram
d. Occult blood
e. Galactogram

**TABLE 53-2**

BIRAD (BREAST IMAGING REPORTING AND DATA SYSTEM) CLASSIFICATION

| Class | Interpretation | Recommendations |
| --- | --- | --- |
| 0 | Unable to determine | Additional studies needed |
| 1 | Negative—no abnormalities seen | Routine follow-up |
| 2 | Benign | Routine follow-up |
| 3 | Probably benign | Repeat mammogram in 3–6 months May biopsy |
| 4 | Suspicious | Strongly consider biopsy |
| 5 | Probably malignant | Biopsy |

2. Treatment—excise intraductal lesion on ultrasound or galactogram or persistent discharge.

## B. PALPABLE LESIONS

1. Cystic—well-demarcated, mobile, firm, and fluctuates with menstrual cycle. Most common in women in their 40s. Perform fine-needle aspiration (FNA).
   a. Premenopausal
      (1) Nonbloody fluid and mass disappears—requires no further workup
      (2) Bloody fluid, mass remains, or cyst recurs more than twice—excisional biopsy. Send fluid for cytology.
   b. Postmenopausal
      (1) Reexamine in 4 to 6 weeks for recurrence.
      (2) A simple cyst on ultrasound does not require further workup.
2. Solid
   a. Proceed immediately to excisional biopsy (only 20% reveal malignancy).
   b. Triple-diagnosis strategy—serial clinical breast examinations, mammography, and FNA; monitor the mass for at least 1 year in 3- to 6-month intervals. If all modalities indicate mass is benign, then have 95% confidence of being benign. DOES NOT RULE OUT CANCER.

## C. FNA BIOPSY

1. Accuracy rates approach 90% to 94%.
2. Nondiagnostic cytology (no epithelial cells present in aspirate)—excisional biopsy.
3. Diagnostic cytology—discuss cancer treatment options.
4. Inconsistent with mammogram—perform excisional biopsy.

## D. CORE NEEDLE BIOPSY (PERCUTANEOUS)

1. Used for palpable masses, nonpalpable masses, or calcifications
2. Can be used in conjunction with image guidance such as mammogram or ultrasound for nonpalpable masses

3. Papilloma has 10% sampling error rate.
4. Atypia has 25% chance of missing adjacent cancer.

## E. EXCISIONAL BIOPSY

1. Definitive method for tissue diagnosis
2. Nonpalpable lesion—image-guided core biopsy or excision with wire localization. If core shows papilloma or atypical cells, then must excise. Obtain postbiopsy radiograph of the specimen to confirm the adequacy of the biopsy. Postbiopsy mammogram in 3 to 6 months to confirm removal of the lesion.
3. Biopsy incisions—plan incision with regard to natural skin tension lines: curvilinear incisions in the upper hemisphere of the breast, radial incisions in the lower hemisphere of the breast, and circumareolar incisions for masses just beneath the areola. Incision should be made so that subsequent mastectomy can incorporate biopsy site. All breast biopsies should be performed with the assumption that the lesion is malignant.
4. The entire mass with a surrounding 1-cm rim of normal tissue should be excised. The specimen should be processed for hormone receptor analysis, human epidermal growth factor receptor 2 (HER-2)/neu, and flow cytometry.

## VI. BENIGN BREAST DISEASE

### A. GALACTORRHEA

1. Differential includes increased prolactin, oral contraceptives, tricyclic antidepressants, phenothiazines, metoclopramide, $\alpha$-methyldopa, reserpine.
2. Can be induced by frequent nipple stimulation
3. Often associated with amenorrhea

### B. FIBROCYSTIC CHANGES

1. Encompass a wide spectrum of clinical and histologic findings, including cyst formation, breast nodularity, stromal proliferation, and epithelial hyperplasia. May represent an exaggerated response of normal breast stroma and epithelium to circulating and locally produced hormones and growth factors.
2. Three categories—nonproliferative lesions, proliferative lesions, and atypia
3. Incidence greatest around age 30 to 40 years but may persist into 8th decade of life.
4. Usually presents as breast pain, swelling, and tenderness associated with focal areas of nodularity, induration, or gross cysts. Frequently bilateral. Varies with menstrual cycle.
5. Not associated with an increased risk for breast cancer unless gross cysts are combined with family history of breast cancer.
6. Treatment

53

DISEASES OF THE BREAST

a. Rule out carcinoma by aspiration or excisional biopsy of any discrete mass. Any sampling biopsy should be interpreted in light of examination and imaging. Any discordance requires excisional biopsy.
b. Frequent breast examinations (physician and self-examination)
c. Baseline mammogram for ages 35 to 39 years and annual mammogram for age older than 40 years to identify any new or changing lesions
d. Patient should avoid xanthine-containing products (coffee, tea, chocolate, cola drinks) and nicotine.
e. Danazol, a weak androgen, may be prescribed for severe mastalgia. Must be continued for 2 to 3 months to see a potential effect. Administer for maximum of 4 to 6 months. Recurrence rate of 50% within 1 year of discontinuing drug.
f. Tamoxifen, which binds to estrogen receptors, has been used for severe symptoms, although it is not FDA approved for this indication. Adverse effects include hot flashes, thrombosis, cataracts, and increased risk for uterine cancer.

## C. FIBROADENOMA

1. Most common breast lesion in women younger than 30 years. Present in 9% to 10% of women. Comprises 50% of breast biopsies and 75% of those in women younger than 20 years.
2. Round, well-circumscribed, firm, rubbery, mobile, nontender mass 1 to 5 cm in diameter that is usually solitary. Lesions larger than 5 cm, referred to as giant fibroadenomas, must be differentiated from cystosarcoma phyllodes. Usually solitary but may be multiple and bilateral. Hormonally dependent; may increase in size with normal menses, pregnancy, lactation, and use of oral contraceptives.
3. It increases risk for breast cancer, especially if a family history of breast cancer is present or if postmenopausal.
4. Treatment—excisional biopsy to remove the tumor and establish the diagnosis, or combination of physical examinations, ultrasonography, and FNA.

## D. PHYLLODES TUMOR/CYSTOSARCOMA PHYLLODES

1. Differentiated from fibroadenoma by the number of mitoses per high-power field
2. May occur at any age, but mean patient age is 30 to 40 years
3. Presents as a smooth, rounded, multinodular, painless mass. Overlying skin is red, warm, and shiny, with venous engorgement. The tumor itself is smooth, well circumscribed, and freely mobile, with a median size of 4 to 5 cm. Characterized by rapid growth.
4. Spreads hematogenously
5. Contains both mesenchymal and stromal components. Approximately 90% are benign. Malignancy is based on occurrence of metastases.

6. High rate (30%) of local recurrence after simple excision or enucleation
7. Treatment—wide local excision (WLE) with at least 1-cm margins for smaller tumors; simple mastectomy for larger tumors

## E. INTRADUCTAL PAPILLOMA
1. It is a benign, solitary polypoid lesion involving epithelium-lined major subareolar ducts.
2. May present as bloody nipple discharge in premenopausal women. Although most do not cause discharge, it is the most common lesion to cause serous or serosanguineous discharge.
3. Major differential diagnosis is between intraductal papilloma and invasive papillary carcinoma.
4. Treatment—excision of involved duct after localization by physical examination.
5. Diffuse papillomatosis—involves multiple ducts of both breasts. Increased risk for breast cancer.

## F. FAT NECROSIS
1. Presents as an occasionally ecchymotic, tender, firm, ill-defined mass, often accompanied by skin or nipple retraction. Almost impossible to differentiate from carcinoma by physical examination or mammography. Usually located in superficial breast tissue, averaging only 2 cm in diameter. More common in overweight women or those with pendulous breasts.
2. History of antecedent trauma may be elicited in about 65% of patients. Can also be caused by surgery, infection, duct ectasia, and aseptic saponification.
3. Treatment: If a clear history of trauma, observe; otherwise, excise to rule out malignancy.

## G. PLASMA CELL MASTITIS/PERIDUCTAL MASTITIS
1. It is a subacute inflammation of ductal system characterized by dilated mammary ducts (mammary duct ectasia) with inspissated secretions, marked periductal inflammation, and infiltration of plasma cells causing yellowish white viscous nipple discharge.
2. Occurs at or after menopause. History of difficult nursing may be elicited.
3. Presenting symptoms include noncyclical, focal breast pain (mastodynia) associated with nipple retraction or discharge, and subareolar masses.
4. A benign lesion that is difficult to differentiate from carcinoma clinically or radiographically. Excisional biopsy is indicated to rule out carcinoma. Multiple biopsies may be required because of the diffuse nature of the lesion. Curative treatment usually requires subareolar duct excision.

## H. GALACTOCELE

1. Occurs after cessation of lactation secondary to an obstructed lactiferous duct filled with inspissated milk and desquamated epithelial cells
2. Presents as round, well-circumscribed, mobile, tender subareolar mass associated with milky yellow or greenish yellow nipple discharge
3. Treatment—needle aspiration; excision indicated if cyst cannot be aspirated or cyst becomes infected

## I. MASTITIS AND BREAST ABSCESS

1. Common in lactating women after the third week, possibly because of inspissation of milk, obstruction, and secondary infection. May develop generalized cellulitis of breast tissue or abscess.
2. Patients present febrile and with a hard, painful, erythematous breast.
3. Progression from mastitis to abscess formation occurs in 5% to 10% of cases.
4. Most common causative organisms in lactating women are *Staphylococcus aureus* and *Staphylococcus epidermidis;* less common are *Streptococcus* and diphtheroid organisms.
5. Most common causative organisms in nonlactating women are *S. aureus* and anaerobes such as *Bacteroides* and *Peptostreptococcus.*
6. Treatment
a. Culture breast milk; begin broad-spectrum antibiotics (dicloxacillin or amoxicillin and clavulanate potassium [Augmentin] for 2 weeks; add metronidazole [Flagyl] if abscess). Traditionally, cessation of breast-feeding was encouraged to prevent reinfection. More recent evidence, however, shows that breast-feeding may accelerate recovery.
b. Incision and drainage if fluctuant and not improved with appropriate antibiotic therapy
c. Recurrent infection best treated by excision of diseased subareolar ducts
7. Differential diagnosis includes inflammatory carcinoma. When incision and drainage is performed, send biopsies of abscess cavity in all patients.

## J. MONDOR'S DISEASE

1. Superficial thrombophlebitis of the thoracoepigastric vein. Usually secondary to trauma or surgery.
2. It presents as local pain associated with a tender, palpable, subcutaneous area or linear skin dimpling.
3. Finding of palpable cord along the inframammary fold is diagnostic. Vein is deep to breast.
4. Treatment—nonsteroidal antiinflammatory drugs for pain. Resolves spontaneously. Mammogram if patient is older than 35 years.

## K. GYNECOMASTIA
1. Physiologic
a. Benign proliferation of male breast glandular tissue; prevalence rate of 34% to 65%. In an adult, defined as larger than 2 cm in diameter.
b. Newborns—caused by exposure to maternal estrogens.
c. Pubertal (ages 13–17 years)—may be bilateral or unilateral; greatest prevalence in adolescence beginning at 10 to 12 years of age with complete involution by age 16 or 17. Treat with reassurance.
d. Senescent (age >50 years)- –caused by male "menopause" with relative estrogen increase; frequently unilateral; breast tissue is enlarged, firm, and tender; usually regresses spontaneously within 6 to 12 months.
2. Drug induced (10–20%)—associated with use of estrogens, digoxin, thiazides, phenothiazines, phenytoin, theophylline, cimetidine, antihypertensives (reserpine, spironolactone, methyldopa), diazepam, tricyclics, antineoplastic drugs, marijuana, anti–human immunodeficiency virus medication. Treatment is discontinuation of offending drug or surgery.
3. Pathologic—associated with cirrhosis, renal failure, malnutrition, hyperthyroidism, adrenal dysfunction, testicular tumors, hermaphrodism, hypogonadism (e.g., Klinefelter syndrome).
4. Any dominant or suspicious mass should undergo biopsy to rule out carcinoma, especially in the senescent male individual.
5. Resect if causing social problems or if disfiguring.

## L. POLAND SYNDROME
1. Hypoplasia of chest wall and shoulder, absence of breast, secondary to absence of pectoralis major muscle, which is necessary for the developmental induction of breast tissue.

## VII. BREAST CANCER
## A. EPIDEMIOLOGY
1. Most common nonskin cancer in U.S. women—12% of women in the United States (1/8 or 180,000 U.S. women each year) will experience development of breast cancer during their lifetime, and 3.5% (44,000 U.S. women each year) will die of the disease; constitutes 30% of cancers diagnosed in women.
2. It is a disease of developed nations.
3. Incidence increases with increasing age.
4. Leading cause of death in U.S. women 40 to 55 years of age.
5. Age-adjusted incidence appears to be increasing whereas age-adjusted death rate appears to be decreasing.
6. Screening decreases mortality rate by 25% because of diagnosis at an earlier age.

## B. RISK FACTORS
1. Sex—female-to-male ratio for breast cancer is 100:1 to 150:1.
2. Age—risk increases with increasing age.

**53**

**DISEASES OF THE BREAST**

3. Family history of breast cancer—overall risk depends on number of first-degree relatives with breast cancer, their ages at diagnosis, and whether the disease was unilateral or bilateral.
4. Genetic mutations—account for 10% of all breast cancers. Breast cancer invariably develops in patients with Li–Fraumeni syndrome, a rare disorder involving a germline mutation in the tumor suppressor gene *p53*.
   a. *BRCA1* gene—chromosome 17q, associated with ovarian, prostate, and colon cancer; breast cancer at earlier age (40–50 years)
   b. *BRCA2* gene—chromosome 13, associated with male breast cancer, bladder cancer, and pancreatic cancer; breast cancer at older age (>50 years)
5. History of breast cancer
6. History of breast biopsy regardless of underlying pathology
7. Atypical ductal or lobular hyperplasia identified on breast biopsy
8. Noninvasive carcinoma (ductal carcinoma in situ [DCIS])
9. Cumulative duration of menstruation, early menarche (<12 years of age) or late menopause (>55 years of age). Risk is increased for women who menstruate for more than 30 years.
10. Nulliparity or age older than 30 years at first delivery
11. Exogenous hormone use. Current use of oral contraceptives. Risk declines to baseline within months after discontinuation.
12. Exposure to low-dose ionizing radiation between 13 and 30 years of age
13. Alcohol consumption, especially before 30 years of age

## C. CLINICAL PRESENTATION

1. Nonpalpable, suspicious lesion on mammogram requires needle localization biopsy or stereotactic FNA biopsy for diagnosis.
2. Palpable mass—most are detected by patient on routine self-examination. Typically nontender, firm, irregular, relatively immobile, most commonly located in upper outer quadrant of breast (50%). May be multifocal, multicentric, or bilateral.
3. Skin changes—skin dimpling (tethering of Cooper's ligaments), nipple retraction or inversion, erythema, warmth, edema, peau d'orange (dermal lymphatic invasion), ulceration, eczema or excoriation of superficial epidermis of nipple (as in Paget's disease), en cuirasse (leather-like changes).
4. Nipple discharge—bloody; most commonly caused by intraductal papilloma, but invasive papillary carcinoma must be ruled out.
5. Metastatic spread—spreads via lymph nodes to bone, lungs, brain, liver; may present with anorexia, weight loss, cachexia, dyspnea, cough, hemoptysis, bony pain (especially vertebral), pathologic fractures.

## D. TNM CLASSIFICATION

1. Primary tumor (T)
   **TX:** Primary tumor cannot be assessed

**T0:** No evidence of primary tumor

**Tis:** Tis (ductal) or Tis (lobular)—ductal or lobular carcinoma in situ, does not cross the basement membrane. Tis (Paget's)—Paget's disease of nipple without tumor.

**T1:** Tumor ≤2 cm

**T2:** Tumor >2 cm but ≤5 cm

**T3:** Tumor >5 cm

**T4:** Tumor of any size with involvement of chest wall or skin, including inflammatory carcinoma

2. Lymph nodes (N):

**NX:** Lymph nodes cannot be assessed

**N0:** No regional lymph node metastases

**N1:** Metastases to movable ipsilateral axillary lymph nodes or microscopic metastases to ipsilateral internal mammary nodes

**N2a:** Metastases to fixed or matted ipsilateral axillary lymph nodes

**N2b:** Clinically apparent metastases to ipsilateral internal mammary nodes without clinically apparent axillary node involvement

**N3a:** Metastases to ipsilateral infraclavicular lymph nodes

**N3b:** Clinically apparent metastases to ipsilateral internal mammary nodes with clinically apparent axillary node involvement

**N3c:** Metastases to ipsilateral supraclavicular lymph nodes

3. Distant metastases (M):

**MX:** Metastases cannot be assessed

**M0:** No distant metastasis

**M1:** Distant metastasis—includes cervical or contralateral internal mammary lymph nodes

**E. STAGING**

**Stage 0**—Tis N0 M0

**Stage I**—T1 N0 M0

**Stage IIa**—T0 N1 M0, T1 N1 M0, T2 N0 M0

**Stage IIb (sum of 3)**—T2 N1 M0, T3 N0 M0

**Stage IIIa**—T1-3 N2 M0 + T3 N1 M0

**Stage IIIb**—T4 N0-2 M0

**Stage IIIc**—any N3 M0

**Stage IV**—any M1

**F. PATHOLOGIC LESIONS**

1. Growth patterns

a. May be broadly divided into epithelial tumors arising from cells lining ducts or lobules versus nonepithelial tumors arising from supporting stroma (i.e., angiosarcoma, malignant cystosarcoma phyllodes, primary stromal sarcomas). Nonepithelial tumors are much less common.

b. May be noninvasive (DCIS or lobular carcinoma in situ [LCIS]) or invasive (infiltrating ductal or lobular carcinoma). Noninvasive refers to the absence of invasion through the basement membrane.

c. May be multifocal (disease within same quadrant as dominant lesion), multicentric (disease in distant quadrant within the same breast), or bilateral (disease in both breasts).

**2. Common histologic types of breast cancer (Table 53-3)**

a. Noninvasive

   (1) DCIS—proliferation of malignant epithelial cells completely contained within breast ducts. Does not invade the basement membrane.

   (a) A premalignant lesion, more common than LCIS. Risk for subsequent invasive ductal carcinoma is 25% to 30% and usually occurs within 10 years of diagnosis.

   (b) Solid, cribriform, papillary, micropapillary, and comedo subtypes; comedo subtype poorest prognosis—most likely to recur.

   (c) Average age at diagnosis is mid-50s.

   (d) Although occasionally may present with palpable mass, 80% of DCIS lesions are nonpalpable and appear as clustered microcalcifications on screening mammography. Prevalence has increased as screening mammography has improved.

   (e) It tends to be multicentric (35%).

   (f) Occult invasive carcinoma may coexist with in situ lesion in 11% to 21% of cases.

   (g) Van Nuys classification: (1) non–high-grade DCIS without comedo necrosis, (2) non–high-grade DCIS with comedo-type necrosis, and (3) high-grade DCIS with or without comedo-type necrosis.

   (2) LCIS—traditionally considered a marker for malignancy and not a premalignant condition, although this is currently the subject of debate.

   (a) Risk for subsequent invasive carcinoma (usually ductal) is increased 7 to 10 times in both the ipsilateral and the contralateral breast. The risk rate for development of breast cancer is 1% per year. Invasive carcinoma usually occurs more than 15 years after diagnosis.

**TABLE 53-3**

**COMMON HISTOLOGIC TYPES OF BREAST CANCER**

| Characteristics | DCIS | LCIS |
|---|---|---|
| Age | Postmenopausal | Premenopausal |
| Mass | Rare | None |
| Mammogram | Microcalcifications | None |
| Risk | Invasive ductal cancer Same breast | Invasive ductal or lobular cancer Either breast |
| Nodes | Rare | None |
| Treatment | Lump ± radiation or simple mastectomy No ALND | Observation vs. prophylactic bilateral simple mastectomy No ALND |

ALND = axillary lymph node dissection; DCIS = ductal carcinoma in situ; LCIS = lobular carcinoma in situ.

      (b) Mean age of diagnosis is 44 to 46 years with 80% to 90% of cases in premenopausal women. Estrogens are hypothesized to play an important role in the pathogenesis of LCIS.

      (c) Does not form a palpable mass and is not visible on mammogram. Usually discovered incidentally on biopsy for another abnormality; identified in 4% of biopsy specimens obtained for benign disease.

      (d) Tends to be bilateral and multicentric (60–80% of cases). LCIS is identified in the contralateral breast in 25% of cases.

b. Invasive

  (1) Infiltrating ductal carcinoma

      (a) Most common breast malignancy (80%)

      (b) Originates from ductal epithelium and infiltrates supporting stroma. Less common forms include medullary carcinoma, colloid carcinoma, tubular carcinoma, and papillary carcinoma.

      (c) Most commonly presents as a palpable mass or mammographic abnormality.

  (2) Invasive lobular carcinoma

      (a) Accounts for 5% to 10% of all invasive breast malignancies

      (b) Originates from lobular epithelium and infiltrates supporting stroma

      (c) Similar prognosis to invasive ductal carcinoma

      (d) Presents as a palpable mass or mammographic abnormality. Does not form microcalcifications. Thirty to 40% of lesions are bilateral.

  (3) Paget's disease of the nipple

      (a) Accounts for 1% to 3% of all breast malignancies

      (b) Usually associated with intraductal carcinoma (DCIS) or invasive carcinoma just beneath the nipple. Caused by invasion of malignant cells across epithelial-epidermal junction into the epidermis of the nipple.

      (c) Presents initially as erythema and mild eczematous changes that become erosions and ulcerations

      (d) Rapid and lethal malignancy

      (e) Diagnosis by scrape cytology, shave biopsy, punch biopsy, or nipple excision

      (f) Treat with mastectomy or, if limited to retroareolar area, excision of nipple-areolar complex.

  (4) Inflammatory breast carcinoma

      (a) Accounts for 1% to 4% of all breast malignancies

      (b) Characterized by peau d'orange of the skin as a consequence of dermal lymphatic invasion. Presents as diffuse induration, erythema, warmth, edema.

      (c) Axillary lymphadenopathy is almost always present.

      (d) Distant metastases common at time of diagnosis (17–36%).

      (e) Most rapid and lethal malignancy; usually poorly differentiated

**53**

**DISEASES OF THE BREAST**

(f) Start with chemotherapy. Combined-modality therapy has 30% to 40% 10-year survival rate.

c. Staging is more important than histology in determining prognosis.

d. Other prognostic indicators include nuclear and histologic grade, presence or absence of estrogen and progesterone receptors, HER-2/neu DNA content, and proliferative fraction (S-phase).

## G. SURGICAL TREATMENT OPTIONS

1. WLE, lumpectomy, and partial mastectomy—breast-conserving therapy

a. Two major objectives are as follows:

(1) Complete excision of tumor with tumor-free margins

(2) Good cosmetic result

b. Usually accompanied by sentinel lymph node biopsy and/or axillary node dissection and radiation therapy to the whole breast

c. Eligibility criteria for stage I or II include the following:

(1) Tumor size smaller than 4 cm

(2) Appropriate tumor size-to-breast size ratio

(3) No fixation of tumor to underlying muscle or chest wall

(4) No involvement of overlying skin

(5) No multicentric cancer; may be multifocal

(6) No fixed or matted axillary nodes

d. Contraindications to breast-conserving therapy

(1) Absolute

(a) Two or more primary tumors in separate quadrants (multicentricity)

(b) Diffuse malignancy with microcalcifications

(c) History of breast irradiation

(d) Scleroderma

(e) Persistent positive surgical margins

(2) Relative

(a) Collagen vascular disease other than scleroderma

(b) Pregnancy

(c) Tumors larger than 4 cm in diameter

(d) Multiple tumors in the same quadrant

(e) Large breast size

2. Subcutaneous mastectomy—removes breast tissue only, sparing nipple-areolar complex, skin, and nodes. Not a cancer operation.

3. Simple mastectomy (total mastectomy)—often performed for DCIS or LCIS. Removes breast tissue, nipple-areolar complex, and skin without axillary node dissection.

4. Modified radical mastectomy (MRM)—removes breast tissue, pectoralis fascia, nipple-areolar complex, skin, and axillary lymph nodes in continuity. Spares pectoralis major muscle.

5. Radical mastectomy (Halsted)—removes breast tissue, nipple-areolar complex, skin, pectoralis major and minor, and axillary lymph nodes in continuity. Leaves bare chest wall with significant cosmetic and

functional deformity. Clinical trials comparing MRM with radical mastectomy report no significant difference in disease-free survival, distant disease-free survival, or overall survival. Used only when tumor significantly invades muscle.

6. Sentinel lymph node biopsy

a. Combined technetium sulfur colloid injected 2 to 16 hours before surgery and Lymphazurin blue injected into tumor area at time of surgery.

b. Collect the hottest nodes and all nodes that have emitted counts greater than 10% of the hottest node.

c. Lymphazurin blue dye may cause type I hypersensitivity reaction or skin necrosis (1–3%).

d. If the sentinel node(s) is negative, then a formal axillary lymph node dissection (ALND) is not required.

e. If no radioactive nodes are found, then a formal ALND is required.

f. If clinically positive nodes are present, a formal ALND must be performed.

g. It is contraindicated during pregnancy, multicentric disease, previous axillary surgery, and neoadjuvant therapy.

7. **ALND**

a. Collect all level I and II nodes.

b. Adequate if more than 10 nodes collected

c. Boundaries of axilla—lateral border latissimus dorsi muscle (posterior), axillary vein (superior), lateral border pectoralis major (anterior), infra-mammary fold (inferior), pectoralis minor muscle (superficial), chest wall (deep)

d. Complications

    (1) Axillary vein thrombosis—sudden, early postoperative swelling; rare

    (2) Lymphedema—slow swelling of upper extremity or breast/chest over 18 months

    (3) Lymphangiosarcoma (Stewart–Treves syndrome)—dark purple bruiselike discoloration on arm about 10 to 20 years after surgery

    (4) Intercostal brachiocutaneous nerve—most commonly injured nerve, paresthesia of lateral chest wall and inner arm

## H. SURGICAL TREATMENT BY STAGE

1. Stage 0

a. DCIS—total ipsilateral mastectomy versus WLE with 2- to 3-mm margin plus radiation therapy. Mastectomy if multicentric, multifocal, comedo type, larger than 2.5 cm, or unable to obtain clear margins. No ALND.

b. LCIS—prophylactic treatment: bilateral total mastectomy versus tamoxifen coupled with close observation. No ALND.

c. Clinically occult invasive carcinoma—MRM versus WLE with axillary node dissection plus radiation therapy.

d. Paget's disease—total mastectomy versus MRM. About 95% will be coupled with invasive disease within the breast.

2. Stages I and II—represent 85% of breast cancers.

a. Current treatment recommendations—MRM versus WLE with axillary assessment (sentinel lymph node biopsies and/or axillary node dissection) plus radiation therapy.

b. Clinical trials have shown WLE with axillary assessment plus radiation therapy to be equivalent to MRM in terms of disease-free survival, distant disease-free survival, and overall survival.

c. Adjuvant chemotherapy is indicated for node-positive patients and high-risk, node-negative patients. Preoperative chemotherapy may have a role in converting tumors to make breast conservation surgery possible.

d. Factors associated with high risk for recurrence include the following:

    (1) Age younger than 35 years

    (2) Tumor size larger than 2 cm

    (3) Poor histologic (scirrhous) and nuclear grade (II, III)

    (4) Absence of estrogen and progesterone receptors

    (5) Aneuploid DNA content

    (6) High-proliferative fraction (S-phase)

    (7) Overexpression of epidermal growth factor receptor II

    (8) Presence of cathepsin D

    (9) Amplification of Her-2/neu *(c-erb-b2)* oncogene

    (10) Lymphatic or vascular invasion

    (11) p53 or Ki67

    (12) Extensive DCIS component (>25% of tumor)

e. Five-year survival rates for stage I and II breast cancers are 95% and 85%, respectively.

**3. Stages III and IV**

a. Multimodality therapy including surgery, radiation therapy, and systemic therapy is usually used.

b. Surgical therapy must be individualized based on extent of tumor and technical ease of resection.

c. Preoperative chemotherapy followed by MRM and chest wall local radiation therapy is the mainstay of treatment for inflammatory breast carcinoma.

d. Five-year survival rates for stage III and IV breast cancers are 45% and 15%, respectively.

## I. RADIOTHERAPY TO CHEST/BREAST

1. Lumpectomy
2. Greater than four nodes
3. Skin or chest wall involvement
4. Positive margins
5. Tumor larger than 5 cm
6. Inflammatory cancer
7. Fixed axillary or internal mammary nodes

## J. CHEMOTHERAPY AND HORMONAL THERAPY

1. Surgery and radiation therapy are used to achieve locoregional control, whereas chemotherapy and hormonal therapy are used to achieve systemic control.
2. Adjuvant therapy
   a. The decision to offer systemic therapy for metastatic disease should be based on the extent and rate of progression of metastatic disease, prognostic factors, degree and progression of symptoms, and the patient's ability to tolerate therapy without significant toxicity.
   b. Chemotherapy should be considered for patients with hormone receptor–negative tumors, aggressive metastatic disease, and the ability to tolerate adverse effects of cytotoxic drugs.
   c. Hormonal therapy should be considered for patients with hormone receptor–positive tumors and relatively indolent metastatic disease. Tamoxifen is the treatment of choice for premenopausal patients. Aromatase inhibitors are the drugs of choice for postmenopausal women unless osteoporotic.
3. Cytotoxic chemotherapy
   a. Combination chemotherapy is more effective than single-agent chemotherapy.
   b. Associated with greater toxicity than hormonal therapy; may be poorly tolerated by elderly or debilitated patients.
   c. Premenopausal patients tend to have better response to cytotoxic chemotherapy, whereas postmenopausal patients tend to have better response to hormonal therapy.
   d. Options
      (1) CMF—cyclophosphamide, methotrexate, 5-fluorouracil
      (2) CA—cyclophosphamide, adriamycin
      (3) Often given serially with taxane (Taxol, Taxotere)
4. Hormonal therapy
   a. Indications
      (1) Adjuvant therapy for hormone receptor–positive, premenopausal, or postmenopausal, node-positive or high-risk, node-negative patients
      (2) Palliative therapy for relatively indolent metastatic disease in premenopausal or postmenopausal patients with hormone receptor–positive tumors
   b. Response to hormonal therapy is dependent on the status of hormone receptors.
   c. Tamoxifen versus aromatase inhibitors (anastrozole, letrozole)
      (1) Tamoxifen is a competitive antagonist of estrogen that binds to estrogen receptors and prevents binding of estrogen. It is effective in premenopausal women. It is as effective as oophorectomy.
      (2) Aromatase inhibitors block estradiol formation. It is effective in postmenopausal women.

       (3) Prophylactic tamoxifen reduces breast cancer incidence rate by approximately 50% to 60%.
   d. Alternatives to tamoxifen
      (1) Aromatase inhibitors
      (2) Estrogen receptor down-regulators (fulvestrant)
      (3) Oophorectomy—only indication is in the treatment of metastatic breast cancer in premenopausal, hormone receptor–positive patients. Tamoxifen, however, has been shown to be equally effective.
   e. Herceptin (trastuzumab)—synthetic monoclonal antibody to HER-2. Used only with HER-2 overexpression in tumor.
   f. Treatment scheme is presented in Table 53-4.

## K.  BREAST CANCER AND PREGNANCY
1. Diagnosis is more difficult and frequently delayed because of breast engorgement, tenderness, and increased nodularity.
2. Suspicious masses detected during pregnancy should undergo FNA or core biopsy.

---

**TABLE 53-4**

INDICATIONS FOR HORMONAL THERAPY

| Nodes | Menopausal Status | Estrogen Receptor Status | Therapy |
|---|---|---|---|
| Positive | Premenopausal | Positive | Chemotherapy + tamoxifen |
| | | Negative | Chemotherapy |
| | Postmenopausal | Positive | Chemotherapy + aromatase inhibitor |
| | | Negative | Chemotherapy |
| Negative | Premenopausal | Positive: | |
| | | Low risk (tumor <1 cm) | Tamoxifen |
| | | High risk | Chemotherapy + tamoxifen |
| | | Negative: | |
| | | Low risk (tumor <0.5 cm) | None |
| | | High risk | Chemotherapy |
| | Postmenopausal | Positive: | |
| | | Low risk (tumor <2 cm) | Aromatase inhibitor vs. tamoxifen |
| | | High risk (tumor ≥2 cm) | Aromatase inhibitor vs. tamoxifen + chemotherapy |
| | | Negative: | |
| | | Low risk | None |
| | | High risk | Chemotherapy |

3. If malignancy is identified, subsequent treatment decisions are influenced by specific trimester of pregnancy. The goal of treatment is the cure of breast cancer without injury to the fetus.

a. Radiation is contraindicated during pregnancy.

b. Studies have demonstrated that termination of pregnancy, in hopes of decreasing hormonal tumor stimulation, has no added benefit.

c. For cancer detected during first and second trimesters, MRM is the treatment of choice. However, immediate breast reconstruction should not be performed because a symmetrical result is impossible until the postpartum appearance of the contralateral breast is known.

d. In the second and third trimesters, preoperative adjuvant chemotherapy can be given followed by breast conservation with radiation therapy deferred until after delivery. Studies have shown no increased risk of fetal malformation for chemotherapy administered during the second and third trimesters. An increased incidence of spontaneous abortion and congenital malformation is associated with chemotherapy given during the first trimester.

e. For cancer detected during the third trimester, WLE and axillary node dissection may be safely performed, with radiation therapy delayed until after delivery.

## L. MALE BREAST CANCER

1. Incidence rate is 1% of all breast cancers.

2. Increased risk may be associated with hyperestrogenic states—Klinefelter syndrome, liver disease, and exogenous estrogen use (metastatic prostate cancer, transvestites). Low-dose radiation is also implicated. Twenty-six percent of men with breast cancer have the *BRCA2* mutation.

3. Usually diagnosed at a later age than in women—mean age at diagnosis is 60 to 65 years.

4. Because of scant breast tissue in men, the skin and pectoralis major muscle is more often involved than in women. Delay in diagnosis may result in more advanced stage at presentation and worse prognosis.

5. Infiltrating ductal carcinoma is most common histologic type of breast cancer in men.

6. Node-negative disease—prognosis similar to that in women. Node-positive disease has a significantly worse prognosis than in women.

7. Treatment—depends on stage and local extent of tumor.

a. DCIS—simple mastectomy

b. Invasive carcinoma—total mastectomy with axillary assessment. If underlying pectoralis major muscle is involved, then radical mastectomy is recommended.

c. Postoperative radiation therapy improves local control but does not affect survival.

d. Node-positive or high-risk, node-negative patients—adjuvant chemotherapy or hormonal therapy. Greater than 80% of male breast cancers are hormone receptor positive; therefore, tamoxifen may play an important role.

## M. BREAST RECONSTRUCTION AFTER MASTECTOMY

1. No evidence to suggest that breast reconstruction after mastectomy compromises efficacy of adjuvant chemotherapy, increases incidence of local recurrence, or delays diagnosis of recurrence on chest wall
2. Significantly improves patient's concept of body image
3. With early cancers, may be performed immediately. If advanced, delay until after radiation therapy is completed.
4. Types of reconstructive procedures
   a. Prosthetic breast implant—filled with silicone or saline, inserted subpectorally after expansion
   b. Myocutaneous flap reconstruction—more complicated procedure but better long-term cosmetic results
      (1) Transverse rectus abdominis flap—based on superior mesenteric artery and vein; entire contralateral rectus abdominis muscle is transposed with transverse ellipse of skin and subcutaneous tissue from lower abdomen.
      (2) Latissimus dorsi flap—based on thoracodorsal artery and vein.
      (3) Free rectus abdominis flap—thoracodorsal or anterior serratus vessels are anastomosed to internal mammary or axillary vessels to maintain blood supply to the flap.
      (4) Greater omentum pedicle flap covered with a skin graft
      (5) Gluteus maximus free flap
   c. Nipple-areolar reconstruction may be performed after prosthetic breast implant or myocutaneous flap reconstruction once the reconstructed breast attains its final shape and position, typically in 6 to 12 weeks.
5. Complications of breast reconstruction
   a. Infection
   b. Tissue loss, especially because of vascular compromise. More common in smokers.
   c. Poor cosmetic result
   d. Slippage of prosthetic implant or capsular contraction
   e. Fat necrosis

# Breast Reconstruction

*T. Kevin Cook, MD*

## I. HISTORY

One in nine women is affected by breast cancer during her lifetime. Breast cancer is second only to lung cancer as the principal source of cancer deaths in women. Thus, it is a disease that warrants aggressive medical and surgical therapy. Although the techniques of mastectomy have changed since Halsted's time, significant disfigurement occurs without reconstruction. Breast reconstruction can profoundly help a woman's healing and self-image as she is treated for breast cancer. Currently, approximately 15% of mastectomy patients choose to undergo reconstruction.

**54**

### A. INITIAL ATTEMPTS AT RECONSTRUCTION

1. The first recorded attempt at breast reconstruction involved transplantation of a lipoma by Czerny in 1895.
2. In 1905, Ombredanne of France used the pectoral muscle to mimic the breast mound.
3. Tanzini, an Italian surgeon, performed the first recorded myocutaneous flap transposition for breast reconstruction with a pedicled latissimus dorsi flap in 1906.
4. Despite the development of these and other techniques, breast reconstruction lay stagnant for 60 years because it was discouraged by Halsted's principle of local control of the disease.

### B. FURTHER ADVANCEMENTS

1. The modern age of breast reconstruction began in 1963 with the use of silicone gel implants by Cronin and Gerow. The initial approach was a delayed reconstruction after mastectomy.
2. Snyderman and Guthrie modified this technique with the introduction of immediate silicone implantation in 1971. Subsequently, breast reconstruction has continued to advance, with the advent of expander technology and autologous tissue transfers.
3. In 1979, Holstrom described free tissue transfer of abdominal myocutaneous flap for breast reconstruction.

## II. RELEVANT ANATOMY FOR RECONSTRUCTION

### A. VASCULAR SUPPLY (FIG. 54-1)

1. Internal mammary artery/vein (most preferred)
2. Thoracoacromial trunk vessels
3. Lateral thoracic artery and vein
4. Thoracodorsal artery and vein
5. Intercostal perforators

### B. INNERVATION

1. Supraclavicular nerve

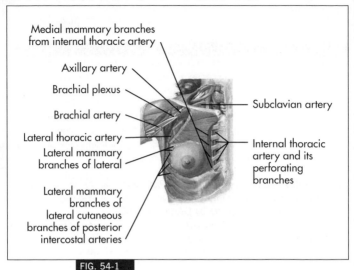

Medial mammary branches
from internal thoracic artery

Axillary artery

Brachial plexus

Brachial artery

Lateral thoracic artery

Lateral mammary
branches of lateral

Lateral mammary
branches of
lateral cutaneous
branches of posterior
intercostal arteries

Subclavian artery

Internal thoracic
artery and its
perforating
branches

**FIG. 54-1**

Arterial blood supply of the breast.

2. Intercostobrachial nerve
3. Anteromedial intercostal nerves

### III. PREOPERATIVE EVALUATION

#### A. GOALS OF RECONSTRUCTION

1. Desire for natural-appearing breast mound
a. Ample breast volume
b. Appropriate projection
2. **Optimize skin envelope reconstruction.**
a. Skin-sparing mastectomy—conserving skin if it does not compromise the oncologic treatment will improve the ultimate aesthetic outcome.
b. Non–skin-sparing mastectomy—leads to techniques of expansion versus autologous tissue transfer.
3. **Symmetry**
a. May need augmentation or reduction of contralateral breast
b. Some patients choose prophylactic mastectomy of disease-free contralateral breast to prevent new primary disease, which can improve symmetric outcome during reconstruction.
4. **Nipple areolar complex reconstruction**
a. Matching pigmentation to contralateral breast
b. Nipple projection corresponding to contralateral breast

## B. TIMING
1. Immediate—occurring during initial breast resection procedure
a. Allows inframammary fold to be preserved
b. Provides psychological benefits to patients
2. **Delayed reconstruction indications**
a. Postoperative radiation
   (1) Impaired wound healing
   (2) Stimulates fat necrosis of transposed tissue
   (3) Increases incidence and severity of prosthetic capsular contracture
b. Chemotherapeutic agents
   (1) Impaired wound healing

## C. CURRENT TECHNIQUES
1. Temporary expander to be replaced later with permanent implant
2. Permanent expander with removable injection port
3. Autologous tissue transfer with implant or expander
4. Pedicled latissimus dorsi flap
5. Pedicled transverse rectus abdominis musculocutaneous flap (TRAM)
6. Free tissue transfer such as TRAM or gluteal flaps

## D. TECHNIQUE SELECTION CRITERIA
1. Laxity and thickness of chest skin
2. Condition of serratus and pectoralis muscle
3. Size of opposite breast
4. Availability of donor sites for free tissue transfer

## IV. TECHNIQUES
## A. RECONSTRUCTION USING IMPLANTS AND EXPANDERS
1. Implants
a. Placement
   (1) Subpectoral
b. Indications
   (1) Sufficient skin envelope
   (2) Planned contralateral procedure for symmetry
   (3) Patient's personal preference contraindicates creation of donor-site wound for purposes of autologous tissue reconstruction.
c. Contraindications
   (1) Postoperative radiation planned leading to common complications
      (a) Greater rate of capsular contracture
      (b) Chance of implant extrusion
      (c) Subsequent poor aesthetic outcome and poor patient satisfaction
   (2) Artificial implant unacceptable to patient
d. Advantages
   (1) Decreased operative time
   (2) Second procedure not necessary
   (3) No donor site morbidity

54

BREAST RECONSTRUCTION

e. Disadvantages
  (1) Capsular contracture
  (2) Implant rupture
  (3) Decreasing patient satisfaction with time
**2. Expanders**
a. Type
  (1) Removable expander with indwelling injection port
  (2) Implant/expander with removable injection port
b. Stages of expansion
  (1) Placement of expander either during initial surgery or at a later date
  (2) Tissue is expanded with serial injections over a few months' time.
  (3) If expander is intended to be removed, an exchange for an implant after sufficient expansion has been achieved is performed.
  (4) If expander is permanent, then injection port is removed.
c. Positioning
  (1) Subpectoral
d. Indications
  (1) Skin envelope sufficient
  (2) Planned contralateral procedure for symmetry
  (3) Patient's personal preference contraindicates creation of donor-site wound for purposes of autologous tissue reconstruction.
e. Contraindications
  (1) Unstable skin envelope secondary to surgical procedure or postsurgical radiation therapy
  (2) Patient wishes reconstructed breast to match contralateral large or ptotic breast.
  (3) Permanent foreign body such as implants unacceptable to patient.

## B. AUTOLOGOUS TISSUE TRANSFER
**1. Pedicle-based flaps (Fig. 54-2)**
a. Latissimus dorsi myocutaneous flap
  (1) Vascular supply—thoracodorsal artery and venae comitantes
  (2) May be combined with an implant to provide adequate volume
  (3) In event of significant skin envelope loss secondary to mastectomy or radiation, it provides significant tissue for reconstruction.
b. TRAM
  (1) Vascular supply—perforators from deep superior epigastric artery
  (2) Rectus abdominis muscle is raised with its pedicle and tunneled through subcutaneous tissue to transverse breast pocket.
  (3) May be performed in a delayed fashion to increase vascular perfusion
  (4) Delayed technique involves ligation of inferior epigastric vessels with a resulting increase in perfusion pressure three times reference levels.

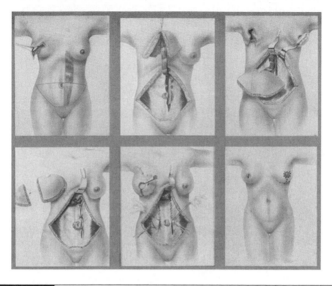

**FIG. 54-2**

Pedicle transverse rectus abdominis musculocutaneous flap procedure. Flap is raised, then tunneled to the mastectomy. *(From Thorne CH: Grabb and Smith's Plastic Surgery, 6th ed. Philadelphia, Lippincott Williams & Wilkins, p 642, 2007.)*

   c. Pedicle flap common complications
      (1) Fat/skin necrosis at distal ends of pedicle—5% to 16% of cases
      (2) Abdominal hernias (TRAM flap)—8% of cases
      (3) Wound dehiscence—6% of cases
      (4) Vessel thrombosis varies with surgical experience/technique
**2. Autologous free tissue flaps and vessels**
   a. TRAM (Fig. 54-3)
      (1) Deep inferior epigastric perforator
      (2) Superficial epigastric perforator
   b. Gluteus maximus
      (1) Superior gluteal artery perforator
      (2) Inferior gluteal artery perforator
   c. Internal mammary artery is vessel of choice for blood supply to the free tissue flap.

## C.  NIPPLE AREOLAR COMPLEX RECONSTRUCTION (FIG. 54-4)
**1. Anatomic considerations**

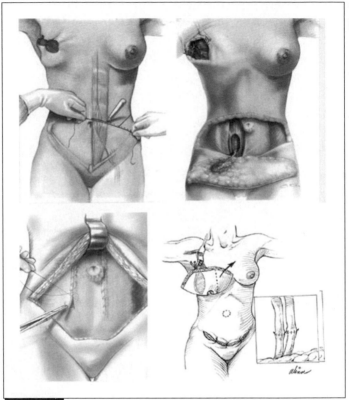

**FIG. 54-3**

Free transverse rectus abdominis musculocutaneous flap. Flap is raised and then transposed to the mastectomy defect where microvascular anastomoses are performed. *(From Thorne CH: Grabb and Smith's Plastic Surgery, 6th ed. Philadelphia, Lippincott Williams & Wilkins, p 642, 2007.)*

a. Ideal location is at the most prominent point of breast mound, or at or above inframammary crease.

b. Areola has an average diameter of ~35 to 45 mm.

c. Nipple projects an average of 5 mm.

d. Tattooing of skin to match color of contralateral nipple

**2. Goals**

a. Appropriate position to provide symmetric result in comparison with contralateral breast

b. Color

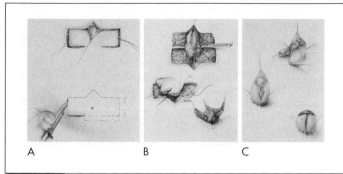

**FIG. 54-4**

Penny flap for nipple reconstruction: *(A)* flap design; *(B)* flap elevation; *(C)* flap formation. *(From Thorne CH: Grabb and Smith's Plastic Surgery, 6th ed. Philadelphia, Lippincott Williams & Wilkins, p 659, 2007.)*

c. Projection
d. Sensitivity
3. **Techniques**
a. Skin grafts
b. Tattoo
c. Prosthesis
   (1) Polyurethane
   (2) Silicone ectoprosthesis—mold of native breast created and silicone impression is then glued to the reconstructed breast.
d. Local flaps
   (1) Skate flap
   (2) Star flap
   (3) Bell flap
4. **Complications**—rate of complication will vary with technique used.
a. Loss of projection
b. Dehiscence
c. Necrosis

## V. ONCOPLASTIC SURGERY
### A.  DEFINITION
1. Defined as the surgical approach of malignant breast tissue excision providing maximum margins while allowing for glandular tissue to be reapproximated with an aesthetically pleasing outcome.

### B.  CONSIDERATIONS (FIG. 54-5)
1. Location of tumor

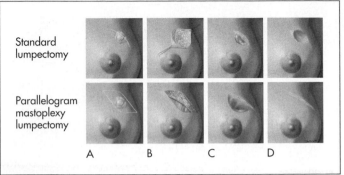

Standard lumpectomy

Parallelogram mastoplexy lumpectomy

A        B        C        D

**FIG. 54-5**

Comparison of standard lumpectomy (top row) versus parallelogram oncoplastic approach (bottom row). *(From Anderson B, Masetti R, Silverstein M: Oncoplastic approaches to partial mastectomy: An overview of volume-displacement techniques. Lancet Oncol 6:145–157, 2005.)*

2. Distribution of tumor
a. Localized—involves only one major duct
b. Segmental extension—involves more than one major duct

### C. TECHNIQUES
1. Batwing mastopexy (Fig. 54-6)
a. Centrally located tumor
b. Localized
2. Donut mastopexy
a. Upper or lateral breast
b. Segmental extension
3. Radial segmentectomy
a. Lateral breast
b. Segmental extension

## VI. POSTRECONSTRUCTION FOLLOW-UP
1. Serial evaluations of postoperative reconstruction to monitor wound healing and aesthetic outcome
2. Coordinated surveillance of reconstructed breasts for any signs of breast cancer recurrence, for example, mammography
3. Revision of reconstruction if necessary
a. Poor implant position
b. Implant capsular contracture
c. Autologous tissue flaps requiring contouring with liposuction for better aesthetic appearance and symmetry with contralateral breast

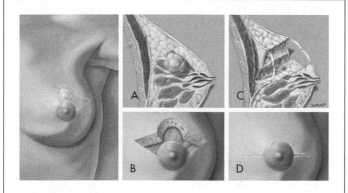

**FIG. 54-6**

Batwing mastopexy: *(A)* preoperative view; *(B)* excision of mass; *(C)* flap advancement; *(D)* final result. *(From Anderson B, Masetti R, Silverstein M: Oncoplastic approaches to partial mastectomy: An overview of volume-displacement techniques.* Lancet Oncol *6:145–157, 2005.)*

## RECOMMENDED READING

Beckenstein MS, Grotting JC: Breast reconstruction with free tissue transfer. *Plast Reconstr Surg* 108:1345–1353, 2001.

Hidalgo DA: Aesthetic refinement in breast reconstruction: Complete skin sparing mastectomy with autogenous tissue transfer. *Plast Reconstr Surg* 102:63–70, 1998.

Mathes SJ: *Plastic Surgery,* vol 6. Philadelphia, Saunders, pp 631–789, 2006.

Spear SL, Spittler CJ: Breast reconstruction with implants and expanders. *Plast Reconstr Surg* 107:177–187, 2001.

Thorne CH: *Grabb and Smith's Plastic Surgery,* 6th ed. Philadelphia, Lippincott Williams & Wilkins, pp 621–657, 2007.

# Gastric Tumors

*Jocelyn M. Logan-Collins, MD*

## I. ADENOCARCINOMA OF THE STOMACH

### A. EPIDEMIOLOGY

1. Comprises 95% of all gastric tumors
2. Third most common gastrointestinal (GI) malignancy in North America (after colorectal and pancreatic cancer)
3. Declining incidence (10/100,000 people in the United States)
4. Seventy percent of patients are older than 50 (peak in seventh decade of life).
5. Male/female ratio is 2:1.
6. Incidence is greatest in Japan (80 times greater than in the United States).
7. Sixty-five percent of gastric cancers in the United States present at an advanced stage (T3/T4).
a. Recurrence rate is 40% to 65%.

### B. RISK FACTORS

1. Environmental factors
a. Diet (rich in salt, smoked or poorly preserved foods, nitrates, nitrites, and secondary amines)
b. Smoking
c. Low socioeconomic status
d. Occupational hazards (metal, rubber, wood, asbestos)
2. Genetic factors
a. p53 mutations (deletion or down-regulation) are present in more than 55% of tumors.
b. Eight percent to 10% of gastric cancers have an inherited component.
c. Hereditary diffuse gastric cancer—germline mutation of *CDH-1* encoding *E-cadherin*
   (1) Autosomal dominant, 70% penetrance
d. BRCA1 and BRCA2, hereditary nonpolyposis colon cancer syndrome, familial adenomatous polyposis, and Peutz–Jeghers syndrome
e. Blood type A (relative risk, 1.2)
f. Ethnicity—Asians, Native Americans, Latinos, and blacks have increased incidence versus whites.
3. Infectious factors
a. *Helicobacter pylori*
   (1) Fivefold increased risk
   (2) Common in patients with distal cancer, not proximal cancer
b. Epstein-Barr virus
4. Other risk factors
a. Chronic atrophic gastritis (conditions associated with decreased acid production)

      (1) Hypertrophic gastropathy (Metenier's disease)—hypertrophic disease of the gastric epithelium

      (2) Pernicious anemia (10% lifetime risk for development of gastric cancer)

  b. Gastric polyps—rarely precursors of cancer

      (1) Villous adenomas (2% of all polyps) are associated with an increased risk for malignancy.

      (2) Smaller than 2 cm (2–4% risk); ≥2 cm (20–40% risk)

      (3) Hyperplastic polyps are not precursors to malignancy.

  c. History of gastric surgery for benign disease

      (1) Relative risk is 1.5 to 3.

      (2) Average latency of 15 years

## C.  PATHOLOGIC CLASSIFICATIONS

**1. Macroscopic classification**

a. Ulcerative (75%)

b. Polypoid (10%)

c. Scirrhous (10%)

d. Superficial (5%)

**2. The Lauren classification is based on microscopic configuration and growth.**

a. Intestinal

    (1) Arise from gastric mucosa, glandular formation

    (2) Most common type worldwide

    (3) Associated with Erb-2 and Erb-3 overexpression

    (4) Usually well to moderately differentiated

    (5) Tends to spread hematogenously

    (6) Distal stomach

    (7) Older patients

    (8) Associated with *H. pylori* (90%), chronic atrophic gastritis, and intestinal metaplasia

b. Diffuse

    (1) Arises from lamina propria, lacks organized gland formation

    (2) More common in the United States

    (3) Usually poorly differentiated with many signet ring cells

    (4) Invasive growth pattern; spreads transmurally in the submucosa

    (5) Lymphatic invasion and peritoneal metastasis more common

    (6) Proximal stomach

    (7) Younger patients

    (8) Associated with obesity

    (9) Associated with *H. pylori* in only 30% of cases

**3. *Linitis plastica (10%)***

a. Entire stomach involved.

b. Malignant cells infiltrate beyond mass.

c. Dismal prognosis

**4. Early gastric cancer**

a. Tumor confined to mucosa or submucosa.
b. Diagnosed on endoscopy
c. Almost 50% of gastric cancer cases are in Japan (where there is aggressive early screening).
d. Ten percent to 15% of cases associated with positive lymph nodes.

## D. CLINICAL MANIFESTATIONS

1. Often produces no specific symptoms when it is superficial and potentially curable
2. Up to 50% of patients may have nonspecific GI complaints such as dyspepsia.
3. Other symptoms include abdominal pain, nausea, vomiting, early satiety with bulky tumors, dysphagia, hematemesis, and melena.
a. Patients with these symptoms are often in the late or advanced stage of disease and are incurable.
4. Physical examination
a. Unhelpful in early gastric cancer
b. Palpable abdominal mass, cachexia, bowel obstruction, ascites, hepatomegaly, or lower extremity edema are signs of advanced disease.
c. Peritoneal seeding may result in a mass palpated on rectal examination (Blumer's shelf) or periumbilical mass (Sister Mary-Joseph's node).
d. Distant lymph node involvement can result in supraclavicular lymph node (Virchow's node) or left axillary lymph node (Irish's node).

## E. SCREENING

1. Cost-effective only in high incidence areas such as China and Japan
2. In the United States, endoscopic surveillance is recommended in high-risk individuals (history of gastric polyp, familial adenomatous polyposis, hereditary nonpolyposis colon cancer syndrome, Peutz–Jeghers syndrome, Metenier's disease) every 1 to 2 years.

## F. DIAGNOSIS/STAGING

1. Endoscopy is the modality of choice for diagnosis.
a. All gastric ulcers seen on endoscopy should undergo biopsy and be followed to ensure they resolve.
b. Four to six biopsies are sufficient. Biopsies should be taken from the mucosa at the edge of the ulcer.
c. Repeat biopsy may be necessary if ulcer remains despite medical therapy.
d. Less than 3% of gastric ulcers are malignant.
2. Endoscopic ultrasound is the most useful tool for preoperative staging.
a. Eighty percent to 90% accurate in assessing depth of tumor invasion
b. Sixty-five percent accurate in determining lymph-node status
   (1) Endoscopic ultrasound–guided node biopsy can improve accuracy of preoperative staging.
3. CT scan used for staging—can demonstrate primary tumor extent (invasion into surrounding structures) and presence of metastatic

55

GASTRIC TUMORS

disease. Accuracy of determining tumor stage is 50% to 70% and node stage is 25% to 86%.

4. Laparoscopy—valuable in further staging given the low sensitivity of CT scan.

a. Peritoneal surfaces examined

b. Liver, omentum visualized

c. The lesser sac can be visualized to evaluate extent of locoregional disease.

d. Cytologic analysis of peritoneal washings can aid in staging.

e. Suspicious lymph nodes should undergo biopsy.

f. Can prevent patients with micrometastatic disease not found on CT scan from undergoing nontherapeutic laparotomy

## G. AMERICAN JOINT COMMITTEE ON CANCER TNM (TUMOR, LYMPH NODE, METASTASIS) CLASSIFICATION

1. T = Primary tumor

   **Tis**—Carcinoma in situ—no invasion of lamina propria

   **T1**—Tumor invades lamina propria or submucosa

   **T2**—Tumor invades muscularis propria or subserosa

   **T3**—Penetrates serosa

   **T4**—Tumor invades adjacent structures

2. N = Regional lymph nodes involved

   **N0**—No regional lymph nodes involved

   **N1**—Metastasis in 1 to 6 regional lymph nodes

   **N2**—Metastasis in 7 to 15 regional lymph nodes

   **N3**—More than 15 regional nodes involved

3. M = Distant metastasis

   **Mx**—Distant metastasis cannot be assessed

   **M0**—No distant metastasis

   **M1**—Distant metastasis

## H. CLASSIFICATION OF SURGICAL RESECTIONS WITH RESPECT TO FINAL PATHOLOGY

1. R0—no residual tumor

2. R1—microscopic residual disease only

3. R2—gross residual disease

4. Long-term survival is expected only if there is an R0 resection.

## I. SURGICAL TREATMENT

1. Curative resection—macroscopic margin of 5 to 6 cm is recommended together with a D1 lymphadenectomy (see later).

a. Cardia, fundus (50% of all gastric carcinomas, usually advanced with poorer prognosis)

   (1) Total gastrectomy with reconstruction by Roux-en-Y esophagojejunostomy

   (2) Proximal subtotal gastrectomy is an alternative for lesions confined to the cardia.

(3) Esophagogastrectomy for tumors of the gastroesophageal junction
b. Body (15–30%): Total gastrectomy is almost always required to obtain adequate margins.
c. Antrum and pylorus (35%)
    (1) Distal subtotal gastrectomy is associated with improved quality of life over total gastrectomy and identical survival outcomes.
    (2) At least 1-cm margin in the first part of the duodenum and a 5-cm margin in the proximal stomach are needed.
    (3) Obtain frozen section of margin before anastomosis.
    (4) Optimal reconstruction is by antecolic gastrojejunostomy.

## 2. Lymphadenectomy
a. Fifteen lymph nodes required for adequate staging.
b. "D" nomenclature for extent of resection/lymphadenectomy
    (1) D1—all lymph nodes within 3 cm of the primary tumor
    (2) D2—D1 plus hepatic, splenic, celiac, and left gastric lymph nodes
    (3) D3—D2 plus omentectomy, splenectomy, distal pancreatectomy, clearance of porta hepatis lymph nodes and paraaortic lymph nodes
c. Extent of lymphadenectomy is controversial.
    (1) Japanese advocate D2 dissections with improved survival and low mortality rate (<2%).
    (2) United States/Europe: D2 dissections are not associated with improved survival and may be associated with increased morbidity. The current standard is a D1 dissection (perigastric nodes); however, some specialized centers are performing D2 dissections with success rates similar to those in Japan.

## 3. Palliative surgery—for obstruction or bleeding in patients deemed unresectable for cure
a. Endoscopic dilatation and/or stenting
    (1) Least invasive method of palliation
    (2) Benefits patients who are poor surgical candidates and who have a short life expectancy
b. Resection
    (1) Subtotal gastrectomy can improve quality of life in patients with excellent preoperative performance status.
    (2) Total gastrectomy or esophagogastrectomy is less likely to improve quality of life given the high associated morbidity and poor prognosis in these patients.
c. Gastrointestinal bypass—for patients who can tolerate a laparotomy and are not candidates for gastric resection

## 4. Endoscopic mucosal resection for early gastric cancer
a. Incidence of lymph node metastasis in early gastric cancer is less than 10% if the following criteria are met:
    (1) Well or moderately differentiated histology
    (2) Confined to gastric mucosa

    (3) Polypoid or protruding tumor less than 2 cm in diameter
    (4) Nonulcerated, no evidence of ulcer scar
    (5) Flat or depressed lesions less than 1 cm in diameter
b. Cure rate is greater than 90%.
c. Close endoscopic follow-up is necessary.
d. If submucosal invasion is seen on permanent sectioning, gastrectomy with D1 lymphadenectomy is required.

## J. ADJUVANT THERAPY

1. Postoperative chemotherapy only: Results are inconsistent. Few trials or studies demonstrate any significant survival benefit.
2. Radiation therapy alone: Some studies report improved local recurrence rates but no evidence of improvement in overall survival.
3. Combined chemoradiation: Intergroup 0116 trial demonstrated that postoperative 5-fluorouracil/leucovorin–based chemoradiation significantly improves overall and disease-free survival.
a. Trial demonstrated a decrease in local recurrence; however, many of the surgeries were suboptimal (54% had less than a D1 lymphadenectomy).
b. This should be considered in all patients with stage II or greater disease.

## K. NEOADJUVANT THERAPY

1. Rationale
a. Attempt to down-stage tumors before surgery to improve chance for curative resection
b. Greater rates of tolerance and compliance versus postoperative adjuvant therapy
2. Potential adverse effects—delay in definitive local control with surgery, allowing tumor progression if patient is a nonresponder.
3. Candidates—patients at high risk for recurrence, T2-T4, N (any), M0
4. Results
a. Unresectable disease: Phase II trials demonstrate down-staging or complete responses to neoadjuvant chemotherapy to allow for curative resections with improvements in overall survival.
b. Resectable disease: MAGIC trial (prospective, randomized) demonstrated that preoperative and postoperative chemotherapy with epirubicin, cisplatin, and fluorouracil (ECF) improves overall and disease-free survival compared with surgery alone.
    (1) Five-year survival rate of 36% versus 23% (surgery alone)

## L. PROGNOSIS (5-YEAR SURVIVAL, WESTERN SERIES)

1. Overall 5-year survival rate: 10% to 21%
2. Patients after R0 resection: 35% to 60%
3. Patients with T1 cancer: 90%
4. Patients with cancer of the cardia: <10%
5. Patients with *linitis plastica*: <5%

## II. GASTRIC LYMPHOMA

### A. GENERAL CONSIDERATIONS
1. Second most common malignancy of the stomach after adenocarcinoma
2. Two percent of all non–Hodgkin's lymphoma, most common extranodal lymphoma
3. Strongly associated with *H. pylori*
4. Average age at presentation is 60 years.
5. Five-year survival rate of 80% for stage I and II tumors

### B. CLINICAL PRESENTATION
1. Indistinguishable from gastric adenocarcinoma at presentation
2. Forty-two percent present as emergencies (bleeding, perforation, obstruction).

### C. PATHOLOGY
1. B-cell non–Hodgkin's lymphoma is most common, with histiocytic subtype.

### D. DIAGNOSIS
1. Endoscopy with biopsy and brush cytology—80% accuracy
2. Staging—chest radiograph, chest and abdominal CT, bone marrow biopsy, biopsy of enlarged lymph nodes, routine laboratory tests, lactate dehydrogenase

### E. TREATMENT
1. Chemotherapy regimen (doxorubicin and cyclophosphamide) produce complete response in 80% of all gastric lymphomas.
2. Radiation therapy and surgery if incomplete response to chemotherapy or recurrence
3. Bone marrow transplant if aggressive disease
4. Mucosal-associated lymphoid tissue (MALT) lymphoma can often be eradicated by *H. pylori* treatment alone.
a. If this treatment fails, radiation or chemotherapy is usually sufficient to eradicate the tumor.

## III. GASTROINTESTINAL STROMAL TUMORS

### A. GENERAL CONSIDERATIONS
1. Comprise less than 1% of all GI malignancies
2. Previously described as leiomyoma, leiomyoblastoma, and epithelioid leiomyosarcoma
3. Stomach is most common site of gastrointestinal stromal tumors—52% of cases.
4. One percent to 3% are primary gastric malignancies.

### B. OTHER CHARACTERISTICS
1. Ninety-five percent of gastrointestinal stromal tumors express CD117 (c-kit).

2. Appears to arise from the interstitial cell of Cajal that variably expresses CD117 (94%) and histologic features of smooth muscle and neural tissue
3. Mutation of c-kit proto-oncogene results in ligand-independent activation of the Kit receptor tyrosine kinase and unopposed cell cycle.
4. Tumor develops submucosally.
5. Presents as bulky mass with central necrosis

### C.  DIAGNOSIS
1. Upper GI—smooth-lined filling defect with sharp borders
2. Endoscopy—endophytic lesion on gastric wall. Overlying mucosa usually intact; ulceration/bleeding can occur.
3. Endoscopic ultrasound—hypoechoic mass contiguous with muscularis propria

### D.  PATHOLOGIC LESIONS
1. Heterogenous ranging from well-differentiated tumors (myoid, neural, or ganglionic) to incomplete or mixed differentiation
2. Hematogenous spread is common; liver is frequently involved.

### E.  TREATMENT
1. R0 resection is treatment of choice—5-year survival rate is 55%.
2. Patients with unresectable or metastatic disease are given imatinib mesylate (Gleevec), an oral tyrosine kinase inhibitor that targets c-kit, and then reevaluated for potential resection if they respond to this treatment.
3. Patients who do not respond to Gleevec can be given sunitinib (Sutent).

## IV. GASTRIC CARCINOID
### A.  GENERAL CONSIDERATIONS
1. Comprise 8.7% of all gastrointestinal carcinoids
2. Arise from proliferating enterochromaffin-like cells of the fundus
3. Neoplastic change is induced by increased gastrin levels.

### B.  CLASSIFICATION
1. Type I—most common type (70–80%)
a. Associated with type A chronic atrophic gastritis
b. More common in women
c. Usually small (<1.5 cm), multifocal, and confined to the fundus
d. Usually well differentiated and benign in nature, rarely metastasize
e. Gastrin level is high, gastric acid level low, secretin test negative.
2. Type II (8%)
a. Associated with multiple endocrine neoplasia type I syndrome with Zollinger-Ellison syndrome
b. Usually small (<1 cm), multifocal, and confined to the fundus

c. Usually well differentiated, benign, metastasis rare
d. Gastrin level is high, gastric acid level high, *secretin test positive.*

### 3. Type III (23%)

a. Sporadic
b. Eighty percent of cases occur in men.
c. Tumors are larger (2–5 cm), solitary, and found in the antrum or fundus.
d. More aggressive in nature; hepatic metastasis in 50%, lymph node involvement in 57%
e. *Gastrin level is normal,* gastric acid level normal, secretin test negative.

## C. CLINICAL PRESENTATION

### 1. Types I and II

a. Dyspepsia, abdominal pain, bleeding
b. Often seen incidentally as a yellow nodule on endoscopy workup for other symptoms
c. Rarely present with carcinoid syndrome

### 2. Type III

a. Atypical carcinoid syndrome is common—flushing, bronchospasm, itching, lacrimation.
   (1) Results from unregulated histamine release from enterochromaffin-like cells

## D. DIAGNOSIS

### 1. Endoscopy with endoscopic ultrasound—to evaluate size, location, and number of tumors

a. Biopsy is necessary to obtain histologic diagnosis.
   (1) Histologic chromogranin, features of dysplasia, mucosal atrophy, degree of invasion
b. If gastric carcinoid found, the duodenum should be inspected for carcinoid presence.

## E. TREATMENT

### 1. Type I or II

a. If less than three to five tumors, less than 1 cm in diameter → polypectomy and endoscopic surveillance every 6 months
b. If larger tumors, more than five tumors, or recurrence → antrectomy *or* local tumor excision
   (1) This will decrease gastrin levels and frequently lead to regression of other tumors.
c. For diffuse or recurrent disease → complete gastrectomy

### 2. Type III

a. En bloc resection with lymphadenectomy
b. Can reduce symptoms and improve survival even if hepatic metastasis present

c. Chemotherapeutic agents (cyclophosphamide, doxorubicin, etoposide, 5-fluorouracil) have reduced tumor size by 20% to 40%; however, side effects may outweigh its benefit.

## F. PROGNOSIS (5-YEAR SURVIVAL RATE)
1. Types I and II—60% to 75%
2. Type III—<50%

# Malignant Pancreas Disease

*Joshua M. V. Mammen, MD*

## I. PANCREATIC ADENOCARCINOMA

### A. EPIDEMIOLOGY

1. Eighth most common malignancy, fifth most common cause of adult cancer mortality
2. Approximately 32,000 new cases nationally with similar mortality
3. Incidence in white male individuals has decreased in past several decades.
4. Slight male sex predominance; 1.3:1 male/female ratio
5. Slightly greater incidence in blacks than whites
6. Dramatically increases after age 50; peaks in seventh and eighth decades of life

### B. CAUSATIVE FACTORS (UNCLEAR)

1. Cigarette smoking (twofold to threefold increase)—increases with duration and amount; risk remains for approximately one decade after cessation.
2. Familial (5% of all cases)—*BRCA2* is most commonly implicated gene; p16 mutation also reported.
3. Chronic pancreatitis—extent of risk is controversial but may be up to 15-fold increase.
4. Others factors are less clear.
   a. Diabetes mellitus
   b. Caffeine
   c. Alcohol
   d. Organic solvents
   e. Petroleum products
   f. Obesity

### C. PATHOLOGIC LESIONS

1. Ductal adenocarcinoma—90% of cases
2. Giant-cell carcinoma—4% of cases
3. Adenosquamous carcinoma—3% of cases
4. Mucinous carcinoma—2% of cases
5. Mucinous cystadenocarcinoma—1% of cases
6. Acinar-cell carcinoma—1% of cases

### D. PRESENTATION

1. Weight loss—90% of cases at presentation; because of a combination of malnutrition from malabsorption and anorexia
2. Pain—usually poorly localized and of low intensity; increases in intensity and is in lower back in advanced disease, invading celiac and superior mesenteric neural plexuses.

3. New-onset diabetes—a concern in patients younger than 40 years
4. Painless jaundice—occurs in tumors of the pancreatic head or uncinate process.
5. Gastric outlet obstruction
6. Courvoisier's sign

## E. EVALUATION FOR THERAPY

1. Dynamic, thin-section, computed tomographic (CT) scan (pancreas protocol) of abdomen
a. Provides information regarding the tumor, extension, lymph-node involvement, and vascular invasion
b. Assists in delineating variations in arterial anatomy for surgical planning
c. Greater than 80% accuracy in predicting resectability
2. Chest radiograph—evaluate for metastatic disease.
3. Endoscopic retrograde cholangiopancreatography (ERCP)
a. Useful when CT is equivocal because rarely have a normal pancreatogram with pancreatic cancer
b. Stent can be used to palliate when surgery is not an option immediately or if needed to resolve symptoms or sepsis.

**Pearl:** *A greater wound infection rate exists for patients with a stent placed before surgery.*

c. Consider magnetic resonance cholangiopancreatography if ERCP not technically possible.
d. Brushings can be obtained if strictures are present.
4. Endoscopic ultrasound
a. Provides information regarding vascular and lymph-node involvement with accuracy similar to CT scan
b. Can be combined with fine-needle aspiration (tissue is needed only to direct neoadjuvant therapy)
5. Magnetic resonance imaging—useful in patients allergic to CT contrast dye.
6. Positron emission tomography scan—questions regarding sensitivity and specificity of modality
7. Tumor markers—serum CA 19-9
8. Laparoscopy
a. Current indications—tumor larger than 4 cm, located in the body or tail, and suspicion of extrahepatic disease
b. Usefulness of peritoneal washings has not been demonstrated in era of high-resolution CT.

## F. SURGICAL THERAPY

1. Guidelines for resection
a. No extrapancreatic disease

b. Superior mesenteric artery and celiac axis lack direct tumor extension (at least a fat plane being present between vessels and tumor).

c. Patent superior mesenteric vein/portal vein confluence

2. Palliative surgery has largely been replaced by endoscopic and percutaneous means, thereby avoiding the morbidity of a laparotomy.

3. If the patient is deemed unresectable at the time of laparotomy, biliary diversion is only performed if obstruction is deemed inevitable; gastric diversion is performed routinely because of the 10% to 15% incidence rate of eventual gastric outlet obstruction; alcohol splanchnicectomy can be done concomitantly with other procedures to alleviate pain, but the endoscopic alternative has replaced it as a separate procedure.

4. Initial step of any definitive procedure is a thorough intraabdominal metastatic evaluation, which includes examining the liver, peritoneum, paraaortic lymph nodes, and mesentery.

5. Eighty percent of patients present with disease that is not resectable; 5-year survival rate in patients who undergo resection is 20%, with median survival of 15 to 19 months.

6. Operative procedures.

a. Pancreaticoduodenectomy (i.e., Whipple procedure)—consider for pancreatic head disease.

b. Distal pancreatectomy—consider for pancreatic body and tail disease.

c. Regional pancreatectomy—involves an extensive lymphadenectomy dissection with possibly high morbidity and mortality rates; has not demonstrated a survival advantage.

d. Total pancreatectomy—consider if anastomosis not possible or unable to get negative margins.

7. Unclear if need for superior mesenteric vein reconstruction results in poor prognosis

8. Marked difference in survival between low- and high-volume centers

## G. ADJUVANT THERAPY

1. Traditionally has been 5-fluorouracil–based chemoradiation

2. Gemcitabine adjuvant regimen appears to provide superior results to 5-fluorouracil (may double disease-free survival).

3. Controversy about the role of chemoradiation

## H. SURVEILLANCE

Follow-up three to four times annually after resection for clinical examination, chest radiograph, CA 19-9 level, and abdominal CT scan

## I. PRECURSOR LESIONS

1. Pancreatic intraepithelial neoplasia (PanIn) is a pancreatic ductal lesion that does not penetrate the basement membrane.

2. Graded from 1 to 3 based on number of mitoses, necrosis, nuclear atypia, and papillary component

3. PanIn grade 3 lesions are found in half of individuals with invasive pancreatic cancer.

## J.  ADVANCED DISEASE
1. Most common regimen is 50 to 60 Gray radiation with 5-fluorouracil infusion.
2. Gemcitabine is considered if the patient can tolerate further treatment; can consider gemcitabine also in lieu of chemoradiation.
3. Role of neoadjuvant chemoradiation has not been defined but is currently performed with several theoretical advantages to adjuvant therapy
a. Allows for early treatment of metastases
b. Patients that progress to unresectable disease during treatment are spared unnecessary surgery.
c. Blood supply to tumor is unchanged.
d. Opportunity to down-stage before resection; includes converting unresectable lesions to resectable

## K.  CYSTIC NEOPLASMS
1. Usually located in the tail of the pancreas
2. Three times more common in women than men
3. Serous lesions (seen as multiple small cysts on CT scan) have a much lower malignant potential than mucin-containing lesions (small number of large cysts on CT scan).
4. Fluid should be aspirated and tested for mucin, cytology, amylase, carcinoembryonic antigen (CEA), and CA 15-3 to differentiate among an inflammatory pseudocyst, serous cystadenoma, and mucinous neoplasm.
5. All mucinous lesions should be resected, but serous cystadenoma can be closely followed in select cases.
6. Intraductal papillary mucinous neoplasms
a. Mucin-producing tumors from the epithelium of the pancreatic duct; often detected by endoscopic aspiration of mucin
b. Can progress to invasive carcinoma and should be resected

## L.  CLINICAL STAGING
1. TNM classification
a. Primary tumor (T):
   **Tx**—Primary tumor cannot be assessed
   **T0**—No evidence of primary tumor
   **T1**—Tumor limited to pancreas and $\leq 2$ cm in diameter
   **T2**—Tumor limited to pancreas and $>2$ cm in diameter
   **T3**—Tumor extends beyond pancreas; celiac axis and superior mesenteric artery not involved
   **T4**—Tumor involves celiac axis or superior mesenteric artery
b. Regional lymph nodes (N):
   **Nx**—Regional lymph nodes cannot be assessed
   **N0**—Regional lymph nodes not involved
   **N1**—Regional lymph nodes involved

c. Distant metastasis:

**Mx**—Distant metastasis cannot be assessed

**M0**—No evidence of distant metastasis

**M1**—Distant metastasis present

2. TNM (tumor, lymph node, metastasis) staging system:

**Stage 1A**—T1, N0, M0

**Stage 1B**—T2, N0, M0

**Stage IIA**—T3, N0, M0

**Stage IIB**—T1-3, N1, M0

**Stage III**—T4, any N, M0

**Stage IV**—any T, any N, M1

3. R classification (residual tumor after resection):

**R0**—No residual tumor

**R1**—Microscopic residual tumor

**R2**—Macroscopic residual tumor

**56**

### RECOMMENDED READING

Neoptolemos JP, Stocken DD, Friess H, et al: A randomized trial of chemoradiotherapy and chemotherapy after resection of pancreatic cancer. *N Engl J Med* 350:1200–1210, 2004.

Oettle H, Post S, Neuhaus P, et al: Adjuvant chemotherapy with gemcitabine vs observation in patients undergoing curative-intent resection of pancreatic cancer. *JAMA* 297:267–277, 2007.

Royal RE: The multimodality treatment of patients with pancreatic cancer. *Cancer* 16:1–16, 2004.

Tempero MA, Behrman S, Ben-Josef, E, et al: Pancreatic adenocarcinoma. *J Natl Compr Canc Netw* 3:598–625, 2005.

MALIGNANT PANCREAS DISEASE

# Colorectal Cancer

*Konstantin Umanskiy, MD*

## I. POLYPS

### A. CHARACTERIZED BY:
1. Histology, presence of dysplasia or cancer, and anatomy (polypoid or sessile)

### B. BROADLY CLASSIFIED AS FOLLOWS:
1. Nonadenomatous: Hyperplastic and hamartomatous polyps have no malignant potential.
2. Adenomatous: Adenomas, tubular adenomas, and tubulovillous and villous adenomas are mostly premalignant, although 1% to 2% of all polyps will harbor an invasive cancer.

### C. PREDICTORS OF INVASIVE CARCINOMA WITHIN A POLYP
1. Size
   a. One to 2 cm—2% to 9%
   b. Larger than 2 cm—20% to 50%
2. Villous or tubulovillous histology
3. Left-sided location
4. Age >60 years

### D. HAGGITT CLASSIFICATION OF MALIGNANT NONSESSILE POLYPS:
1. Level 0—carcinoma in situ
2. Level 1—invasion into submucosa but limited to the head of the polyp
3. Level 2—invasion into the neck of the polyp
4. Level 3—carcinoma invading stalk
5. Level 4—invasion into submucosa below the stalk

### E. MANAGEMENT OF POLYPS
1. Polypectomy using endoscopic forceps or a snare is appropriate for all polyps found during colonoscopy.
2. For adenomatous polyps not amenable to endoscopic treatment (usually because of size or sessile anatomy), biopsies should be obtained and a formal colectomy should be performed.

### F. MANAGEMENT OF MALIGNANT POLYPS REMOVED ENDOSCOPICALLY.
1. Haggitt levels 1, 2, and 3 have less than 1% chance of nodal metastases and no further therapy is required, except in cases of lymphovascular invasion, poor differentiation, or cancer being present less than 2 mm to resection margin.
2. Haggitt level 4 has 12% to 25% risk for nodal metastases and requires colectomy.

3. Most sessile polyps harboring a malignancy are managed with colectomy.

## II. PREOPERATIVE EVALUATION

### A. COMPLETE HISTORY
With emphasis on personal and family history of malignancies or polyps

### B. COLONOSCOPY
With complete visualization of entire colon to cecum
1. Synchronous cancers are present in 2% to 9% of patients.
2. If unable to perform complete colonoscopy before surgery because of obstruction, a computed tomography colonography or double-contrast enema should be obtained when possible, or a complete colonoscopy should be performed 3 to 6 months after surgery.

### C. IN CASES OF RECTAL CANCER
1. Endorectal ultrasound is used to determine tumor invasion and to detect enlarged lymph nodes.

### D. CARCINOEMBRYONIC ANTIGEN (CEA)
1. Increased level is an independent prognostic factor of decreased disease-free survival and increased risk for metastases.

### E. CHEST, ABDOMINAL, AND PELVIC CT SCAN
1. Evaluates for metastatic disease
2. Determines local tumor extension
3. Can detect regional lymphadenopathy
4. Useful in operative planning if synchronous resection of metastases is considered

### F. RISK FACTORS
1. Personal history of colorectal cancer or polyps
2. Age—increase in incidence after age 50.
3. Heredity—up to 20% of patients have family history of colorectal cancers; genetic syndromes account for less than 5% of colorectal cancers.
4. Environmental and dietary factors
   a. Low-fiber, high-fat diet increases risk for colorectal cancer.
   b. High-fiber, calcium, selenium, vitamins A, C, and E, carotenoids, and plant phenols appear to be protective.
   c. Cigarette smoking is associated with increased risk, especially more than 35 years of smoking.
5. Inflammatory bowel disease—after 10 years, the risk for cancer in left-sided colitis or pancolitis is 1% to 2% per year. The risk appears to be similar between ulcerative colitis and Crohn's proctocolitis.

## III. PATHOGENESIS

### A. LOSS OF HETEROZYGOSITY PATHWAY—80% OF CASES

1. *APC* (adenomatous polyposis coli) gene first studied in familial adenomatous polyposis. Present in 80% of sporadic colorectal cancers.
2. *K-ras*—protooncogene; mutation leads to uncontrolled cell division.
3. *DCC* (deleted in colorectal carcinoma)—tumor suppressor gene. Mutation present in more than 70% of colorectal cancers.
4. *p53*—gene crucial for initiation of apoptosis. Mutations present in 75% of colorectal cancers.

### B. REPLICATION ERROR REPAIR PATHWAY—20% OF CASES.

1. Mismatched repair genes—*hMSH2, hMLH1, hPMS1, hPMS2, hMSH6/GTPB.*
2. Mutations result in microsatellite instability—variable lengths of short-base-pair segments repeated several times.
3. Tumors of replication error repair pathway tend to be right-sided and have overall better prognosis.

### C. ADENOMATOUS POLYPOSIS SYNDROMES

1. Familial polyposis—adenomatous polyposis of the colon with a 100% risk for malignancy; may also occur in the proximal gastrointestinal tract; autosomal dominant inheritance. Associated with *APC* mutation.
2. Gardner syndrome—polyposis associated with exostoses, soft-tissue tumors, and osteomas; also has a 100% incidence rate of malignant degeneration.
3. Turcot syndrome—polyposis of the colon associated with central nervous system tumors; autosomal recessive inheritance.
4. Cronkhite–Canada syndrome—gastrointestinal polyposis with alopecia, nail dystrophy, hyperpigmentation; minimal malignant potential; no inheritance pattern.

### D. NONADENOMATOUS POLYPOSIS SYNDROMES

1. Peutz–Jeghers syndrome—hamartomatous polyps of the entire gastrointestinal tract with mucocutaneous deposition of melanin in lips, oral cavity, and digits; hamartomas do not have malignant potential, but increased rate of gastrointestinal tract cancers are a common comorbidity; autosomal dominant inheritance.
2. Juvenile polyposis syndrome—hamartomatous polyps found in the colon and rectum, but can be diffuse; hamartomas do not have malignant potential but increase risk for colorectal cancer; autosomal dominant inheritance.

### E. NONPOLYPOSIS SYNDROMES

1. Hereditary nonpolyposis syndrome (Lynch syndromes)—replication error repair pathway and the most common inheritable colorectal cancer syndrome account for 2% to 7% of all colorectal cancers.

**57**

**COLORECTAL CANCER**

a. Lynch syndrome I—colorectal cancer only
b. Lynch syndrome II—colorectal cancer, endometrial and ovarian cancer, transitional cell cancer of the ureter and renal pelvis, gastric cancer, pancreatic cancer

## F.　SUMMARY OF MAJOR RISK FACTORS
1. Hereditary polyposis syndromes
2. Hereditary nonpolyposis syndromes
3. Previous colorectal cancer
4. Adenomatous polyps
5. Inflammatory bowel disease
6. Family history of colorectal cancer
7. Age older than 50 years

## IV. SCREENING GUIDELINES FOR COLORECTAL CANCER

### A.　AVERAGE-RISK PATIENT, STARTING AT AGE 50—ANY OF THE FOLLOWING SCREENING MODALITIES ARE ACCEPTED:
1. Colonoscopy every 10 years (preferred method)
2. Annual fecal occult blood test and flexible sigmoidoscopy every 5 years
3. Air contrast barium enema every 5 years
4. Yearly fecal occult blood test

### B.　ADENOMATOUS POLYPS
1. Colonoscopy every 3 years
2. If no further polyps, may increase interval to 5 years; otherwise, continue at 3-year intervals.

### C.　COLORECTAL CANCER AFTER RESECTION
1. Colonoscopy 1 year after resection
2. Repeat at 3 years
3. Continue with 5-year interval if no new lesions found

### D.　INFLAMMATORY BOWEL DISEASE—INITIAL COLONOSCOPY AT DIAGNOSIS
1. Colonoscopy with biopsies every 1 to 2 years after 8 years for pancolitis
2. Colonoscopy after 15 years for left-sided colitis

### E.　FAMILIAL ADENOMATOUS POLYPOSIS
1. Annual colonoscopy starting at 10 to 12 years of age

### F.　HEREDITARY NONPOLYPOSIS COLORECTAL CANCER
1. Colonoscopy every 1 to 2 years starting at 20 to 25 years of age

### G.　FAMILY HISTORY
1. Screening every 5 years at 40 years or 10 years before the age of youngest affected relative

## V. DIAGNOSIS

### A. SIGNS AND SYMPTOMS

1. Right-sided lesions are typically bulky, fungating, ulcerative lesions that project into the lumen.
   a. Anemia—microcytic; chronic, intermittent occult blood loss in the stool
   b. Systemic complaints—anorexia, fatigue, weight loss, or dull, persistent abdominal pain; abdominal mass with more advanced tumors
   c. Obstruction is rare secondary to the liquefied consistency of the stool and the large diameter of the bowel.
   d. Triad—anemia, weakness, right lower quadrant mass
2. Left-sided lesions—annular, "napkin ring" lesions that often obstruct the bowel
   a. Change in bowel habits—obstipation, alternating constipation and diarrhea, small-caliber "pencil" stools
   b. Obstructive symptoms are more prominent because of growth pattern of tumor, small caliber of bowel, and solid stool.
3. Rectal cancer
   a. Blood streaking in stools, tenesmus
   b. This finding must not be attributed to hemorrhoids without further investigation.
   c. Obstruction is uncommon but is a poor prognostic sign when present.

### B. SIGNS OF LOCAL EXTENSION OR METASTASIS

1. Abnormal liver function tests, jaundice, or hepatomegaly
2. Fistula formation
3. Mass fixed to sacrum on rectal examination

### C. STAGING—AMERICAN JOINT COMMITTEE ON CANCER (AJCC) STAGING SYSTEM

1. Primary tumor (T):
   **Tx**—primary tumor cannot be assessed
   **T0**—no evidence of primary tumor
   **Tis**—intraepithelial, carcinoma in situ
   **T2**—tumor invades the muscularis propria
   **T3**—tumor invades into the subserosa or nonperitonealized pericolic structures
   **T4**—tumor directly invades other organs or perforates
2. Regional lymph nodes (N):
   **Nx**—regional lymph nodes cannot be assessed
   **N0**—no regional lymph node metastasis
   **N1**—metastasis in one to three pericolic lymph nodes
   **N2**—metastasis in four or more pericolic lymph nodes
   **N3**—other distant lymph node metastasis

57

COLORECTAL CANCER

3. Distant metastasis (M):

**Mx**—presence of metastases cannot be assessed
**M0**—no distant metastases
**M1**—distant metastases

4. Five-year survival rates by American Joint Committee for the Cancer/TNM stage:

**Stage I:** T1-2, N0, M0—93%
**Stage IIA:** T3, N0, M0—85%
**Stage IIB:** T4, N0, M0—72%
**Stage IIIA:** T1-2, N1, M0—83%
**Stage IIIB:** T3-4, N1, M0—64%
**Stage IIIC:** any T, N2, M0—44%
**Stage IV:** any T, any N, M1—8%

## VI. TREATMENT OF COLON CANCER

### A. GENERAL PRINCIPLES

1. An adequate cancer operation requires resection of tumor-containing bowel with 2- to 5-cm margins and resection of the mesentery at the origin of the arterial supply, including the primary lymphatic drainage of the tumor.
2. At least 12 to 15 lymph nodes are required for adequate staging.
3. Ten percent of primary lesions are unresectable.
4. Only 70% of colorectal cancer patients can undergo resection for cure at presentation.
5. Forty-five percent of patients are cured by primary resection.
6. Synchronous colon cancers can be addressed by segmental resections.

### B. PREOPERATIVE PREPARATION

1. Mechanical bowel preparation and oral antibiotics are unnecessary but continue to be used in an effort to prevent infectious complications after surgery; recent randomized trials support no such benefit.
2. Perioperative systemic antibiotics (e.g., cefazolin and metronidazole) decrease the incidence of infectious complications.

### C. SURGICAL THERAPY (FIG. 57-1)

1. Lesions of the cecum and ascending colon are treated by resection of the distal ileum to the midtransverse colon, including the ileocolic, right colic, and right branch of the middle colic vessels with accompanying mesentery.
2. Tumors in the left transverse colon and splenic flexure require resection of the transverse and proximal descending colon. The middle and left colic arteries are removed.
3. Tumors in the descending and sigmoid colon require removal from the splenic flexure to the rectosigmoid. The inferior mesenteric artery is removed.

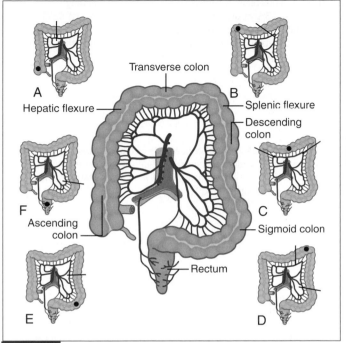

**FIG. 57-1**

Anatomic resection commonly used for cancer at different sites within the large bowel. *A,* Right hemicolectomy. *B,* Extended right hemicolectomy. *C,* Transverse colectomy. *D,* Left hemicolectomy. *E,* Sigmoid colectomy. *F,* Abdominal perineal resection. *Black circles* signify the location of the cancer.

## D. LAPAROSCOPIC COLORECTAL SURGERY

1. Laparoscopic surgery for colon and rectal cancer is appropriate for most patients and is equivalent oncologically when performed by an expert surgeon.
2. Less postoperative pain, more rapid return of bowel function, and a shorter length of stay are the main benefits of this technique.

## E. STAGE-SPECIFIC THERAPY

1. Stage I resection alone is sufficient if all resection margins are negative.
2. Stage II—"low risk," same as stage I
3. Stage II—"high risk" (clinical obstruction or perforation at presentation, fewer than 12 nodes in surgical specimen, poorly differentiated or lymphovascular invasion), should be considered for adjuvant chemotherapy.

4. Stage III—resection, followed by systemic chemotherapy
5. Stage IV—15% of distant metastases limited to liver, of which 20% potentially resectable for cure. Treatment is tailored to the individual patient and could include surgery before or after multidrug chemotherapy.

### F. DISTANT METASTASES

1. Involve the liver, lung, bone, and brain (in order of frequency)
2. Thirty-five percent to 50% of all colorectal carcinoma patients experience development of hepatic metastases during the course of their disease.
3. Ten percent to 20% of patients with hepatic metastases may benefit from resection or radiofrequency ablation. After resection for cure, 5-year survival can be improved to 20% to 40%. Relative contraindications to resection are the following:
a. Positive hepatic nodes
b. Extrahepatic metastases
c. More than four hepatic metastases
4. Hepatic metastases found during operation for primary colorectal malignancy may be removed simultaneously or at second operation 2 to 3 months later.
5. No difference in survival has been demonstrated for lobectomy versus wedge resection.
6. Pulmonary metastases most often present as disseminated disease. For metastatic nodules, up to 38% 5-year survival has been demonstrated with surgical resection. Patients with solitary nodules and nodules smaller than 3 cm may have better survival rates.
7. For unresectable systemic disease, chemotherapy (5-fluorouracil/Leucovorin/Oxaliplatin [FOLFOX] or irinotecan/5-fluorouracil/Leucovorin [FOLFIRI with addition of bevacizumab]) is recommended.

### VII. RECTAL CANCER

### A. STAGE-SPECIFIC THERAPY

1. Carcinoma in situ and selected T1 lesions (well or moderately differentiated histology, Haggitt levels 1, 2, and 3) can be resected transanally either by standard approach or by transanal endoscopic microsurgical technique that allows excision of lesions up to 15 cm from anal verge. This method does not allow examination of lymph nodes, potentially resulting in understaging.
2. T1 and T2 lesions treated by radical resection. Transanal resection followed by chemoradiation can be used in selected patients who are at high risk for an abdominal operation.
3. T3 and T4 lesions treated by neoadjuvant chemoradiation given as 4500 cGy external beam radiation with concurrent administration of 5-fluorouracil. Neoadjuvant therapy may significantly down-stage tumors:

a. Improves resectability
b. Potential for sphincter preservation
4. Presence of nodal metastases requires treatment with neoadjuvant chemoradiation regardless of T stage, followed by adjuvant chemotherapy.
5. Distant metastatic disease treated with palliative procedure and approached similar to colon cancer.

## B. OPERATIVE APPROACH

1. Total mesorectal excision in the plane between the mesorectum and sacral fascia. This technique decreases local recurrence and blood loss, and minimizes injury to pelvic nerves.
2. Tumors in the upper third of the rectum are treated by a low anterior resection.
3. Lesions between 5 and 10 cm from the anal verge are treated by a low anterior resection or an abdominal-sacral resection (Kraske, York–Mason).
4. Lesions in the lower third of the rectum (2–5 cm) may be amenable to a low anterior resection with coloanal anastomosis using an end-to-end anastomosis (EEA) stapler if patient has good continence and no evidence of sphincter involvement by tumor. Abdominoperineal resection (Miles procedure) with a permanent end-sigmoid colostomy is offered to those patients who are not candidates for low anterior resection.
5. Bilateral oophorectomy is advised when one or both ovaries are grossly abnormal or involved with contiguous extension of colon cancer.
6. Direct adherence of the tumor to adjacent structures may result from inflammation rather than from tumor extension. A cure in the presence of local invasion may still be possible with en bloc resection of the involved structures, or if local invasion is more extensive, by total pelvic exenteration.

## VIII. POSTOPERATIVE FOLLOW-UP

Approximately 80% of recurrences occur within 2 years of resection, most often in the form of hepatic metastases or local recurrence.

## A. DIAGNOSIS AND TREATMENT

1. Careful history, physical examination, CEA screening, and stool guaiacs detect more than 90% of recurrent disease.
2. Follow-up protocol
a. Routine physical examination, complete blood cell count, liver function tests—every 3 months for 2 years, then every 6 months for 2 years, then annually
b. CEA—every 3 months for 2 years, then every 6 months for 2 years, then annually
c. Colonoscopy—1 year, then 3 years, then 5 years

d. Barium enema should be performed if complete visualization is not achieved by colonoscopy.
3. CEA helpful only if initially increased and returns to normal after resection.
4. An increase in CEA (>5 ng/ml) requires repeat level to confirm the result, followed by prompt investigation.
a. Computed tomography scan of the chest, abdomen, and pelvis
b. Colonoscopy
c. Positron emission tomography (PET) scan
   (1) When conventional imaging fails to identify the site of presumed recurrence, PET scan can be used as an adjunct.
   (2) In cases when resectable disease is found on standard imaging, PET scan can be used to rule out additional sites of disease.
   (3) If all imaging including PET scan is negative, follow up with repeat PET scan in 3 to 6 months.
   (4) If PET scan detects disease, determination of resectability can be made based on imaging alone.
d. Laparotomy is reserved for patients found to have resectable disease.

## B. TREATMENT OF LOCAL RECURRENT DISEASE
1. Should attempt a cure by resection in selected patients or to palliate symptoms whenever possible.
2. Debulking procedures (tumor resections with gross disease left behind) are rarely indicated.
3. Recurrence after low anterior resection usually requires an abdomino-perineal resection.
4. Pelvic recurrences after abdominoperineal resection are usually unresectable, but occasionally pelvic exenteration is possible.

# Tumor Biology

*Jaime D. Lewis, MD*

*The pathogenesis of human cancers is governed by a set of genetic and biochemical rules that apply to most and perhaps all types of human tumors.*

—W. C. Hahn and R. A. Weinberg

## I. SELF-SUFFICIENCY IN GROWTH SIGNALS

Cancer cells, in contrast with healthy cells, have a reduced dependence on external growth factors.

**58**

### A. GROWTH FACTORS
1. Platelet-derived growth factor and transforming growth factor-$\alpha$
2. Production by cancer cells obviates their dependence on other cells for the production of mitogens

### B. GROWTH-FACTOR RECEPTORS
1. Overexpressed or structurally altered in a diverse array of human tumors
2. Amplification of epidermal growth factor receptors such as human epidermal growth factor receptor 2/neu found in aggressive breast cancer.
3. High plasma levels of insulin-like growth factor receptor 1 and low levels of its inhibitor, insulin growth factor binding protein 3, are associated with increased risk for prostate, breast, and colorectal cancer.

### C. SOS/RAS/RAF/MITOGEN-ACTIVATED PROTEIN KINASE PATHWAY
1. Altered in about 25% of human cancers
2. *K-ras* mutations are found in lung, pancreatic, and colon cancers.
3. The *Ras* oncogene encodes mutant protein that continuously releases mitogenic signals.

### D. INTEGRINS
1. Cells may alter the type of extracellular matrix receptors (integrins) that they produce to favor those that transmit progrowth signals.

## II. INSENSITIVITY TO GROWTH-INHIBITORY SIGNALS
### A. THE RETINOBLASTOMA PROTEIN (pRB)
1. Central role in progression of cell through the G1-phase of the cell cycle
2. Action may be lost through deletion or inactivation.
3. Evidence suggests that alterations leading to the loss of growth suppression by pRB exist in the majority of human cancers.

## III. EVASION OF PROGRAMMED CELL DEATH

### A. THE p53 TUMOR-SUPPRESSOR PROTEIN

1. Responsible for temporary arrest of cell growth in response to damage to allow for repair or elimination by apoptosis.
2. Action may be lost via a diverse array of mechanisms.
3. Evidence suggests that alterations in the p53 pathway exist in the majority of human cancers.

### B. *BCL-2* AND *BAX*

1. Cancer cells resistant to chemotherapy and radiotherapy often have increased levels of antiapoptotic *Bcl-2.*
2. New therapies are aimed at up-regulating proapoptotic proteins such as *Bax* and down-regulating antiapoptotic proteins such as *Bcl-2.*

## IV. LIMITLESS REPLICATIVE POTENTIAL

### A. NORMAL CELLS CARRY AN INTRINSIC PROGRAM THAT LIMITS THEIR ABILITY TO REPLICATE.

1. Independent of cell-to-cell signaling pathways
2. Senescence reached once cells have divided a specified number of times.

### B. LOSS OF TUMOR SUPPRESSOR PROTEINS (p53 AND pRB) LEADS TO A CRISIS STATE.

1. Massive cell death
2. Karyotypic disarray
3. One in $10^7$ achieves the ability to divide ad infinitum, termed *immortalization.*

### C. MOST TUMOR CELLS PROPAGATED IN CULTURE APPEAR TO BE IMMORTALIZED.

### D. TELOMERE MAINTENANCE IS VITAL TO CONTINUED REPLICATION OF TUMOR CELLS.

1. Ongoing maintenance of protective telomere sequences on the ends of chromosomes allows for immortality of cells.
2. Reactivation of telomerase (suppressed in normal human cell types) and a telomerase-independent mechanism ("alternative lengthening of telomeres") allow for indefinite proliferation of cells.

## V. SUSTAINED ANGIOGENESIS

### A. TUMORS CANNOT EXCEED DIAMETERS OF 2 MM WITHOUT ACQUIRING A BLOOD SUPPLY.

### B. SOLID TUMORS SECRETE PROANGIOGENIC FACTORS.

1. Vascular endothelial growth factor and basic fibroblast growth factor
2. Factors bind to transmembrane tyrosine kinase receptors on endothelial cells

### C. TUMORS MAY ALSO DOWN-REGULATE ANTIANGIOGENIC PROTEINS.
1. Thrombospondin-1, which binds to CD36, and interferon-$\beta$

### D. INTEGRINS
1. Variably expressed on quiescent and sprouting capillaries, and growth may be disrupted by signal interference

## VI. TISSUE INVASION AND METASTASIS
### A. TETHERING MOLECULES ARE ALTERED.
1. Cell-cell adhesion molecules
a. E-cadherin, ubiquitously expressed on epithelial cells
   (1) Coupling of these proteins between cells leads to antigrowth signals.
   (2) Function is lost in the majority of epithelial cell tumors.
b. N-CAM
   (1) Expression changed from a highly adhesive form to a poorly adhesive form in Wilms' tumor, small-cell lung cancer, and neuroblastoma.
   (2) Reduced expression seen in invasive pancreatic and colorectal cancers.
2. Integrins link cells to extracellular matrix proteins.
a. Successful colonization of new sites is achieved through changes in integrin $\alpha$ and $\beta$ subunits on migrating cells.
b. Tumor cells facilitate invasion by expressing integrins that preferentially bind degraded stromal components produced by extracellular proteases.

### B. EXTRACELLULAR PROTEASES
1. Protease genes are up-regulated.
2. Protease inhibitors are down-regulated.
3. Inactive forms of protease zymogens are converted to active forms.
4. Expression may be induced by stromal and inflammatory cells rather than the cancer cells themselves.

## VII. GENETIC INSTABILITY
### A. THE PREVIOUS SIX (I–VI) CHARACTERISTICS MUST BE ACQUIRED THROUGH GENETIC ALTERATION
1. An occurrence unlikely to occur in any one cell over a human lifetime because of fastidious maintenance of genome integrity via a complex system of monitoring and repair

### B. MALFUNCTION OF THE "CARETAKER" SYSTEM
1. May allow for the mutability necessary for tumor progression
2. Loss of the p53 tumor suppressor protein occurs in nearly all human cancers.
3. No signal for cell to repair DNA damage or undergo apoptosis in case of excessive damage.

**58**

**TUMOR BIOLOGY**

4. Loss of other tumor suppressor proteins appears to allow for the rapid accumulation of genetic alteration leading to tumor growth and is the subject of ongoing research.

## VIII. PHARMACOTHERAPY

### A. TUMOR GROWTH AND KINETICS

1. Gompertzian growth
   a. Cell population decreasing because of cell death, increasing because of proliferation, and constant subpopulations that are not dead and not proliferating
   b. Sigmoid-shaped growth curve (Fig. 58-1)
   c. Maximum growth at 30% of maximum tumor volume
      (1) Nutrient and oxygen supply optimized
      (2) Point where drug efficacy may be best estimated
2. Cell cycle (Fig. 58-2)
   a. G0-phase—resting or nonproliferating
   b. S-phases—DNA synthesis

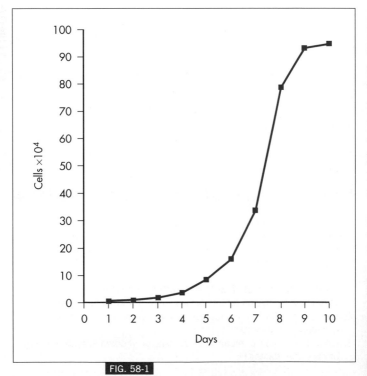

FIG. 58-1

Sigmoid-shaped curve of tumor growth.

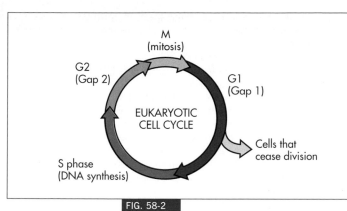

FIG. 58-2

Cell cycle of eukaryotic cell.

   c. G2-phase—postsynthetic
   d. M phase—mitosis
   e. G1 phase—postmitotic

## B. DRUG MECHANISMS AND THERAPEUTICS
### 1. Chemotherapy mechanisms
a. DNA damage
   (1) Alkylation
   (2) Cross-linking
   (3) Double-strand cleavage by topoisomerase I
   (4) Intercalation
   (5) Blockage of RNA synthesis
b. Spindle poisons may arrest mitosis.
c. Antimetabolites interrupt DNA synthesis.
d. Signal transduction inhibitors
e. Oncoviral therapy involves injection of tumor-specific replicating virus to cause cancer cell destruction.
f. Gene therapy involves the transfer of wild-type genes into tumor cells to restore or add expression of tumor suppressor or immunostimulatory genes or inhibit oncogene expression.
g. Antiangiogenesis therapy
h. Immune therapy to induce protective immunity.
   (1) Vaccines
   (2) Monoclonal antibodies
   (3) Cytokines
### 2. Drug resistance
a. Multiple mechanisms of drug resistance may develop during cancer progression.

       (1) *mdr* gene—codes for membrane-bound P-glycoprotein that serves as a channel for excretion of cellular toxins (i.e., chemotherapeutic agents)

       (2) Decreased drug transport into cells

       (3) Reduction of drug activation

       (4) Enhanced drug metabolism

       (5) Development of alternative metabolic pathways

       (6) Gene amplification to overcome drug inhibition of enzyme targets

       (7) Impairment of drug binding to target

  b. Normal human cells do not develop drug resistance.

  c. Drugs active as single agents may be used alone.

  d. When given in combination, use drugs with different dose-limiting toxicities and different patterns of resistance.

## IX. CHEMOTHERAPEUTIC AGENTS: MECHANISMS, USES, AND IMPORTANT TOXICITIES

### A. ALKYLATING AGENTS

1. Cyclophosphamide—may cause hemorrhagic cystitis.
2. Melphalan—melanoma limb perfusion/infusion

### B. ANTIMETABOLITES

1. 5-Fluorouracil—stomatitis, myelosuppression, nausea, vomiting, diarrhea
2. Methotrexate—mucositis, myelosuppression, pulmonary fibrosis, hepatotoxicities and nephrotoxicities, diarrhea

### C. ANTITUMOR ANTIBIOTICS

1. Bleomycin—pulmonary fibrosis
2. Doxorubicin—cardiotoxicity
3. Mitomycin C

### D. MITOTIC INHIBITORS

1. Etoposide (VP-16)
2. Paclitaxel (Taxol)—peripheral neuropathy
3. Vinblastine—myelosuppression
4. Vincristine—peripheral neuropathy

### E. HORMONAL AGENTS

1. Tamoxifen (antiestrogen)—hot flashes, blood clots, increased risk for uterine cancer
2. Aromatase inhibitors (i.e., anastrozole, letrozole)—osteoporosis

### F. MISCELLANEOUS

1. Mitotane—adrenal insufficiency
2. Streptozocin—hypoglycemia
3. Cisplatin—nephrotoxicity, neurotoxicity

4. Carboplatin
5. Oxaliplatin
6. Leucovorin

## G. TARGETED THERAPEUTICS
1. Monoclonal antibodies
a. Bevacizumab (Avastin)—colorectal cancer; small incidence of gastrointestinal perforation
b. Cetuximab (Erbitux)—colorectal cancer
c. Trastuzumab (Herceptin)—breast cancer
2. Growth factor receptor inhibitors
a. Erlotinib (Tarceva)—non–small-cell lung cancer
b. Gefitinib (Iressa)—non–small-cell lung cancer
c. Imatinib (Gleevec)—gastrointestinal stromal tumors
3. Cytokines
a. Interferon-α—melanoma, chronic hepatitis B and C
b. Interleukin-2—renal cell carcinoma, metastatic melanoma

# PART XII

# Endocrine Surgery

# Thyroid

*Thomas W. Shin, MD*

## I. EMBRYOLOGY

### A. THYROID

1. First of the endocrine organs to develop, at about 24 days of gestation
2. Originates as an outgrowth of the pharyngeal endoderm at the base of the tongue
3. Epithelialized endoderm migrates down the middle of the neck.
4. A tubular tract is left behind the migratory path of the thyroid. This tract, called the *thyroglossal duct,* solidifies and becomes obliterated by the 10th week of gestation.
5. Thyroglossal duct cyst can form if the migratory tract fails to obliterate.
6. Aberrant and ectopic thyroid tissue can form anywhere along the migratory tract.
7. Pyramidal lobe, found in about 50% of people, results from the failure of the inferior end of the thyroglossal duct to obliterate.

## II. ANATOMY

### A. HIGHLY VASCULAR

1. Weighs about 15 to 30 g in adults

### B. PRETRACHEAL LAYER OF THE DEEP CERVICAL FASCIA

1. Forms the capsule of the gland

### C. ARTERIAL SUPPLY (IN PAIRS)

1. Superior thyroid artery—first branch of the external carotid
2. Inferior thyroid artery—branch of the thyrocervical trunk

### D. "THYROID IMA"

1. Small, unpaired artery found in 10% of people. Arises from the brachiocephalic trunk/aorta/carotid artery. Runs anterior to the trachea.

### E. VENOUS DRAINAGE (IN PAIRS)

1. Superior and middle thyroid veins—drain to the internal jugular vein.
2. Inferior thyroid veins—drain to the brachiocephalic vein.

### F. NERVES

1. Recurrent laryngeal nerves innervate the intrinsic muscles of the larynx; 70% run in the tracheoesophageal groove. (Always identify them in surgery.)
2. Superior laryngeal nerves innervate the cricothyroid muscle and run along the superior thyroid artery.
3. Unilateral recurrent laryngeal nerve injury leads to hoarseness.
4. Injury to both recurrent laryngeal nerves leads to the closure of the vocal cords.

## III. PHYSIOLOGY

### A. IODINE METABOLISM
1. Starts with the absorption of iodide in the gut.

### B. IN THE THYROID CELL, IODIDE IS OXIDIZED TO IODINE
1. Added on to the tyrosine residue of the glycoprotein thyroglobulin (Tg) in a process called *organification*

### C. TYROSINE RESIDUE
1. With one iodine, the residue is called *monoiodotyrosine,* and the residue with two iodines is called *diiodotyrosine.*

### D. *COUPLING* OF TWO DIIODOTYROSINES
1. Results in tyroxine (T4)
2. Coupling of a monoiodotyrosine and a diiodotyrosine results in triiodothyronine (T3).

### E. THYROID PEROXIDASE
1. Catalyzes both the *organification* and *coupling* reactions

### F. THYROID-STIMULATING HORMONE (TSH)
1. Stimulates many aspects of thyroid hormone synthesis and release
2. Increases uptake of iodide by the thyroid cells
3. Increases formation of thyroid peroxidase and thyroglobulin
4. Increases release of thyroid hormone
5. Increases conversion of T4 to T3
6. Also stimulates thyroid cell proliferation and division

## IV. HYPERTHYROIDISM

### A. THYROTOXICOSIS
1. Caused by excessive thyroid hormone

### B. SIGNS/SYMPTOMS
1. Weight loss, heat intolerance, sweating, tremor, hyperreflexia, warm moist skin, palpitations, tachycardia

### C. *GRAVES' DISEASE (DIFFUSE TOXIC GOITER)*
1. Most common cause of hyperthyroidism; characterized by diffuse goiter, thyrotoxicosis, orbitopathy/ophthalmopathy, and occasional dermopathy
2. Pathophysiology/pathology
a. Autoimmune disorder—forms antibodies that bind and activate TSH receptor (TSHR).
b. Histology—diffuse lymphocytic infiltration of the gland is seen.
3. Clinical features
a. Presents between the ages of 30 and 40 years with female/male ratio of 6:1

b. Thyroid is diffusely enlarged, often two to three times the normal size.
c. Increased vascularity of the gland leads to thrill or audible bruits.
d. Various manifestations of thyrotoxicosis are seen.
e. Almost all patients with Graves' disease have some degree of infiltrative orbitopathy. Clinically apparent "eye" disorder is seen in about 50% of patients.
f. Five percent of patients have dermopathy. Often associated with severe eye disease.

4. **Diagnostic tests—not always needed when diagnosis can be established clinically.**
a. TSH level is low. Both free and total T3, T4 levels are increased.
b. Antibodies against the TSHR are present.
c. Increased I-121 uptake. (TSHR activating autoantibodies stimulate iodine uptake.)

5. **Treatment consists of three options: medication, radioiodine, and surgery.**
a. Medical therapy
   (1) Thionamides
      (a) Propylthiouracil and methimazole—most commonly used
      (b) Inhibit thyroid peroxidase
      (c) Have no effect on the release of the hormones—drug effect not seen until preformed hormones are depleted. This may take several weeks.
      (d) Medical therapy should be continued for at least 6 months.
      (e) Long-term remission seen in one third of patients.
   (2) Iodine
      (a) High dose rapidly decreases the hormone level by inhibiting release of T4/T3.
      (b) Suppressive effect of iodine is rapidly lost when the medication is discontinued.
      (c) Worsening of thyrotoxicosis may occur once iodine is discontinued.
      (d) Useful for acute treatment of severe thyrotoxicosis (thyroid storm) and in prevention of thyrotoxic crisis
      (e) Should be used with propylthiouracil or methimazole, both of which inhibit new T4/T3 synthesis
b. Radioiodine ablative therapy
   (1) Ablative therapy with I-131 is effective in treating Graves' disease.
   (2) Main drawbacks include:
      (a) High occurrence of hypothyroidism after treatment
      (b) Risk for exacerbating infiltrative orbitopathy after treatment
   (3) About 10% of patients may experience worsening of orbitopathy after treatment.
c. Surgery
   (1) In the United States, surgery is usually reserved for patients who are poor candidates for medical or radioiodine ablative therapy. These include:

(a) Patients with significant infiltrative orbitopathy
(b) Pregnant patients
(c) Young patients (want to avoid radiation treatment)
(d) Patients with large goiters—generally respond poorly to other modalities
(e) Patients with suspicious mass in the thyroid gland
(f) Patients who want surgery for treatment of their disorder

(2) Bilateral subtotal thyroidectomy is usually done (leaves 4–6 g of the gland).

(3) Advantages of surgery
(a) Rapid return to euthyroid state
(b) Lower risk for posttreatment hypothyroidism versus I-131 treatment

(4) Main surgical risks
(a) Injury to the recurrent laryngeal nerves (1%)
(b) Permanent hypoparathyroidism (1%)

(5) Similar to radioiodine treatment; surgery requires careful preoperative planning

(6) Important preoperative preparations include:
(a) Euthyroid state should be established with antithyroid medication.
(b) Once the euthyroid state is achieved, pharmacologic dose of iodine is started and maintained for 7 to 10 days. High doses of iodine (3 drops three times daily of saturated solution of potassium iodide or Lugol's solution) causes involution of the thyroid gland and decreases its vascularity.

(7) Thyroidectomy should not be scheduled until the patient is euthyroid.

## D. TOXIC ADENOMA (PLUMMER'S DISEASE)

1. Autonomously functioning follicular adenoma
2. Most are caused by somatic point mutations in the TSHR gene
3. Over period of years, adenoma will become larger and have increasing function leading to suppression of the normal thyroid tissue.
4. Clinical presentation
   a. Presents in the 30 to 40 years age group, often with a history of slow-growing neck mass
   b. Smooth, well-defined, firm mass that moves with swallowing
   c. Usually there is only a single adenoma.
   d. Patients have no evidence of infiltrative orbitopathy.
5. Diagnostic tests
   a. Thyroid hormone levels depend on the size and functioning capacity of the adenoma.
   b. Radioiodine uptake study will show uptake of iodine by the functioning adenoma with suppression of uptake in the normal surrounding thyroid tissue.

**6.** Treatment

a. Ablative therapy and surgery

b. Radioiodine therapy is associated with a high risk for posttreatment hypothyroidism.

c. Surgery, either nodulectomy or a lobectomy, avoids the risk for hypothyroidism and is the treatment of choice.

d. Pretreatment with iodine is not needed because the adenoma is not hypervascular.

e. Patient with thyrotoxicosis should be started on antithyroid medication to establish euthyroid state before operation.

### E. TOXIC MULTINODULAR GOITER

**1.** Arises from an existing nontoxic multinodular goiter that becomes autonomous

**2.** Clinical presentation

a. Patients are usually older than 50 years with a long history of nontoxic multinodular goiter.

b. The degree of thyrotoxicosis is milder than that of Graves' disease.

c. Cardiovascular symptoms such as atrial fibrillation and tachycardia are often seen.

d. Infiltrative orbitopathy does not occur with toxic multinodular goiter.

e. Large goiters may cause obstructive symptoms.

**3.** Diagnostic tests

a. TSH is suppressed and T4, T3 are increased in patients with thyrotoxicosis. In mild cases, only the suppression of TSH may be present.

b. Radioiodine uptake is usually not helpful (often normal or shows mild uptake).

c. Ultrasound of the gland will show multiple nodules.

**4.** Treatment

a. Radioiodine ablative therapy and surgery

b. Surgery—lobectomy on one side and subtotal lobectomy on the other side

### V. HYPOTHYROIDISM

### A. SIGNS/SYMPTOMS

**1.** Weight gain, lethargy, cold intolerance, hyporeflexia reflexes, constipation, coarse dry skin, brittle hair, slow mentation, irregular menses, bradycardia

### B. HASHIMOTO'S THYROIDITIS

**1.** Autoimmune disease marked by hypothyroidism and goiter (Table 59-1)

**2.** Pathophysiology/pathology

a. Formation of antithyroglobulin (Tg) and antithyroid peroxidase (TPO) antibodies

b. Apoptosis of thyroid cells leads to hypothyroidism.

c. Gland is marked by extensive infiltration by lymphocytes.

| TABLE 59-1 |
|---|

**CLASSIFICATION OF THYROID CANCER**

Well-differentiated thyroid cancers:
    Papillary thyroid cancer (80%)
    Follicular thyroid cancer (10%)
    Hürthle cell thyroid cancer (variant of the follicular thyroid cancer) (3%)
Undifferentiated thyroid cancer:
    Anaplastic thyroid cancer (1%)
Medullary thyroid cancer (5%)
Lymphoma of the thyroid (1%)

**3. Clinical presentation**
a. Most commonly seen in women between the ages of 40 and 60 who present with a progressively enlarging neck mass over a period of many years.
b. Gland is symmetrically enlarged, firm, and moves with swallowing.
c. Compressive symptoms may occur with large goiters.
d. Distinctive, palpable nodule is unusual and its presence should prompt further evaluation for possible neoplasm.

**4. Diagnostic tests.**
a. Once the hypothyroidism sets in, the patient will have decreased T4, T3 levels with increased TSH level.
b. Diagnosis confirmed by the presence of thyroid autoantibodies (antithyroid peroxidase [TPO] and antithyroglobulin [Tg] antibodies).

**5. Treatment**
a. Hormone replacement with levothyroxine
b. TSH level is the most sensitive method of monitoring the effectiveness of therapy.
c. Surgery reserved for the following conditions:
    (1) Goiters that continue to cause compressive symptoms
    (2) Appearance remains cosmetically unacceptable after medical therapy.

## VI. NONTOXIC GOITER (NONTOXIC MULTINODULAR GOITER, DIFFUSE NONTOXIC GOITER)

**A. DEFINITION:**
1. Enlarged thyroid gland without any evidence of hypothyroidism or hyperthyroidism

**B. TREATMENT**
1. Levothyroxine to suppress the TSH level to low-to-normal range
2. Levothyroxine treatment has been shown to cause regression of the goiter.

### C.  SURGERY/RADIOIODINE ABLATIVE THERAPY
1. For goiters that continue to cause compressive symptoms or remain cosmetically unacceptable after hormone therapy

## VII. THYROID NODULES

### A.  ABOUT 5% OF NODULES REPRESENT CARCINOMAS.
### B.  THYROID NODULES THAT REQUIRE EVALUATION INCLUDE:
1. A palpable solitary nodule
2. A dominant nodule within a multinodular gland
3. A palpable nodule in a diffuse goiter (e.g., Hashimoto's disease)
4. A nonpalpable nodule that is larger than 8 mm (see VII.N)

### C.  PHYSICAL FINDINGS THAT SUGGEST MALIGNANCY:
1. Firm, nontender nodule
2. Nodule that is fixed (does not move with swallowing)
3. Cervical lymphadenopathy

### D.  HISTORY THAT SUGGESTS MALIGNANCY:
1. History of external head/neck irradiation
2. Age younger than 20 years or older than 70 years
3. Recent onset of hoarseness
4. Family history of thyroid cancer or multiple endocrine neoplasia (MEN) type II

### E.  OBTAIN A TSH LEVEL (SEE DIAGRAM).
### F.  LOW TSH INDICATES TOXIC NODULE.
1. Confirm with I-121 scan. If "hot," treat with surgery or I-131 ablation therapy. Fine-needle aspiration (FNA) is *not* needed because almost all "hot" nodules are benign.

### G.  IF THE TSH LEVEL IS NORMAL/LOW:
1. Get an FNA of the nodule. (Do not get an I-121 scan in this setting because it will not be helpful.)
2. Insert a 20- to 22-gauge needle into the nodule.
3. Apply suction and fan needle to obtain sample.
4. Remove needle and place contents onto a slide for examination.

### H.  FNA IS EXCELLENT AT DIAGNOSING
1. Papillary and medullary cancers

### I.  FNA IS UNABLE TO DISTINGUISH
1. Follicular/Hürthle cell adenoma (benign) from carcinoma (malignant)

### J.  DIAGNOSIS OF FOLLICULAR (AND HÜRTHLE) CELL CARCINOMA
1. Requires the demonstration of vascular or capsular invasion by the tumor (not seen on FNA)

**59**

**THYROID**

## K. THE RESULTS OF THE FNA ARE SEPARATED INTO FOUR GROUPS:

1. Benign (70%)—include colloid nodules, thyroiditis
2. Malignant (5%)
3. Nondiagnostic (15%)
4. Suspicious/indeterminate (10%)—includes follicular neoplasms (follicular adenoma and carcinoma and Hürthle cell adenoma and carcinoma).

## L. MANAGEMENT BASED ON THE RESULTS OF THE FNA (SEE DIAGRAM).

1. Benign: Follow clinically. Enlargement of the nodule requires repeat FNA.
2. Malignant: Patients will need surgery (see section VIII).
3. Nondiagnostic: Repeat FNA. Consider ultrasound-guided FNA. If FNA is persistently nondiagnostic, consider either close follow-up or surgery. The latter should be pursued in patients at high risk for development of thyroid cancer.
4. Suspicious/indeterminate: Patients will need surgery because FNA is unable to differentiate follicular (and Hürthle cell) adenoma from carcinoma.
   a. About 20% of the FNA diagnosis of "follicular neoplasm" and "Hürthle cell neoplasm" represents carcinomas.
   b. Lobectomy and isthmectomy is performed initially. If the final histopathology shows carcinoma, a second operation will be needed to remove the remaining thyroid.
5. Factors that favor total thyroidectomy at the *initial* surgery include:
   a. History of head and neck irradiation
   b. A strong family history of thyroid cancer
   c. Evidence of local invasion
   d. Findings on ultrasound that strongly suggest malignancy
6. Nodule greater than 4 cm

## M. CYSTIC NODULES

1. All cystic fluid should be aspirated and sent for cytology. If palpable nodule remains, this solid component of the nodule must also be sent for examination.
2. The character of the fluid (bloody, clear, thick, etc.) has no bearing on the diagnosis.
3. Nondiagnostic FNA needs no further workup *if* the nodule does not recur.
4. Cystic nodule that recurs after a nondiagnostic FNA will need a repeat FNA.
5. Cystic nodules that require surgical resection include:
   a. Cystic nodule with FNA-containing malignant or suspicious cells
   b. Cystic nodule that recurs after two aspirations
   c. Cystic nodule with solid component that is nondiagnostic with FNA

## N. INCIDENTALOMA

1. Thyroid incidentalomas are subclinical/nonpalpable thyroid nodules that are discovered "incidentally" during evaluations related to the head and neck; often found on imaging studies such as computed tomography, magnetic resonance, and carotid duplex scans.
2. Currently, no clear guidelines exist for the management of incidentalomas.
3. Based on currently available studies, the following approaches to treatment of thyroid incidentaloma appear reasonable:
a. Incidentalomas larger than 15 mm should undergo ultrasound-guided FNA.
b. Hypoechogenic nodules between 8 and 15 mm with at least one feature commonly found in carcinoma should undergo ultrasound-guided FNA.
c. Lesions smaller than 8 mm with worrisome features should be considered for biopsy or undergo close clinical follow-up.
d. All incidentalomas found in patients with risk factors for thyroid cancer should undergo ultrasound-guided FNA regardless of the size or ultrasound features.

## VIII. THYROID NEOPLASM

### A. THYROID CANCER

1. Accounts for about 1.5 % of all cancers in the United States, with about 15,000 new cases diagnosed each year

### B. CLASSIFICATION OF THYROID CANCER IS PRESENTED IN TABLE 59-1.
### C. THYROID CANCER STAGING IS PRESENTED IN TABLE 59-2.
### D. PROGNOSTIC FEATURES

1. Used to form risk group analysis that predict patient outcome (Tables 59-3 and 59-4). AGES and MACIS are the most frequently used.
2. Based on the prognostic factors, patients can be grouped into high- or low-risk categories (Table 59-5).

**TABLE 59-2**

THYROID CANCER STAGING

Papillary or Follicular

| Stage | Age <45 Years | Age ≥45 Years | Medullary | Anaplastic |
|---|---|---|---|---|
| I | M0 (any T, N) | T1 | T1 | — |
| II | M1 | T2, T3 | T2, T3, T4 | — |
| III | — | T4 or N1 | N1 | — |
| IV | — | M1 | M1 | Any |

T1: tumor ≤1 cm. N0: no nodal involvement. M0: no metastasis.
T2: tumor >1 cm but ≤4 cm. N1: nodal involvement. M1: metastasis present.
T3: tumor >4 cm.
T4: Extrathyroidal invasion.

THYROID

59

| TABLE 59-3 | | | |
|---|---|---|---|
| **RISK GROUP ANALYSIS** | | | |
| Mayo Clinic (1987) | Mayo Clinic (1993) | Lahey Clinic | Sloan-Kettering |
| **AGES** | **MACIS** | **AMES** | **GAMES** |
| **A**ge | **M**etastasis | **A**ge | **G**rade |
| **G**rade | **A**ge | **M**etastasis | **A**ge |
| **E**xtracapsular tumor | **C**ompleteness of resection | **E**xtracapsular tumor | **M**etastasis |
| **S**ize | **I**nvasion (extracapsular tumor) | **S**ize | **E**xtracapsular tumor |
| | **S**ize | | **S**ize |

| TABLE 59-4 |
|---|
| **MACIS** |

Score = 3.1 (if <40 years) or 0.08 × age (if ≥40 years) (**A**ge)
  +0.3 × tumor size in centimeters in maximum diameter (**S**ize)
  +1 (if incompletely resected) (**C**ompleteness of resection)
  +1 (if locally invasive) (**I**nvasion/extracapsular tumor)
  +3 (if distant metastasis) (**M**etastasis)
Survival rate by MACIS score (20 years)
  <6 = 99%
  6–6.99 = 89%
  7–7.99 = 56%
  ≥8 = 24%

| TABLE 59-5 |
|---|
| **RISK GROUPS FOR WELL-DIFFERENTIATED THYROID CANCER** |
| **High Risk** |

Age ≥45 years
Extrathyroidal invasion
Major invasion of the tumor capsule (follicular)
Distant metastasis
Tumor size >4 cm
High grade (tall-cell variants, poorly differentiated)

**Low Risk**

Age <45 years
Tumor confined to the thyroid
No distant metastasis
Tumor size <4 cm
Well or moderately differentiated tumor

## E. FOUR IMPORTANT PROGNOSTIC FACTORS ARE:

1. *A*ge, *s*ize, *e*xtrathyroidal invasion, *m*etastasis
2. Lymph-node status is *not* an important prognostic factor in thyroid cancer.

## F. PAPILLARY THYROID CARCINOMA (PTC; 80% OF THYROID CANCER)

1. Usually presents between the ages of 20 and 40 years with female/male ratio of 2:1
2. Most common thyroid cancer associated with head and neck irradiation
3. Thyroid cancer most often seen in children
4. Diagnosis by FNA
5. Pathologic lesions
   a. PTC may be solitary but is often multifocal.
   b. Has areas of fibrosis and calcification (Psammoma bodies) and are often cystic
   c. Diagnosis is based on distinct nuclear features (Orphan Annie eye nuclei)
6. Clinical presentation
   a. Usually present with an asymptomatic neck mass, which moves with swallowing
   b. Thirty percent have clinical evidence of cervical lymphadenopathy at presentation.
7. Treatment
   a. Minimal papillary cancer (size <1 cm) without evidence of local invasion or metastasis is treated with lobectomy and isthmectomy.
   b. Patients in high-risk group need total thyroidectomy.
   c. Both lobectomy and total thyroidectomy are treatment options for low-risk patients.
   d. In comparison with lobectomy, total thyroidectomy has the following results:
      (1) Lower recurrence rate
      (2) More effective postoperative monitoring for recurrence
      (3) Increased risk for surgical complication
      (4) No clear difference in mortality or morbidity
   e. PTC has a tendency to spread to lymph nodes. In patients younger than 45 years, even the clinically apparent cervical node does not decrease survival; in high-risk patients, a modest increase occurs in local recurrence when nodal involvement is present.
   f. Routine/prophylactic neck dissection is not performed.
   g. Modified radical neck dissection should be done on the side with the palpable nodes to decrease the risk for local recurrence.

## G. FOLLICULAR THYROID CARCINOMA (FTC; 10% OF THYROID CANCER CASES) AND HÜRTHLE CELL CARCINOMA (3% OF THYROID CANCER)

1. Peak incidence at 40 to 50 years of age. Female/male ratio is 2:1.
2. In areas of iodine deficiency, the incidence of FTC is greater.
3. Hürthle cell carcinoma, a variant of FTC, has a greater propensity for multifocality, lymph-node involvement, and distant metastasis versus FTC (about 30% of them are bilateral and multifocal).
4. Only about 10% of Hürthle cell carcinoma cases take up iodine.

THYROID

59

5. FTC rarely invades the lymph nodes; usually spreads via blood vessels.
6. FNA establishes the diagnosis of follicular/Hürthle cell *neoplasm*.
7. Diagnosis of *carcinoma* requires the demonstration of either vascular/capsular/lymphatic invasion on sectioned specimen.
8. Pathologic lesions
   a. FTC is often a solitary lesion surrounded by a tumor capsule.
   b. Unlike PTC, follicular carcinoma has no distinct cellular features.
   c. There are two types of FTC: minimally invasive and widely invasive.
   d. Minimally invasive type has grossly intact tumor capsule.
   e. Widely invasive type has extensive capsular and vascular invasion.
9. Clinical presentation
   a. Patients usually present with a slow-growing, painless, solitary thyroid nodule.
   b. Some patients may have a long history of goiter.
   c. Cervical lymphadenopathy is uncommon.
10. Treatment
    a. Lobectomy is performed after diagnosis by FNA. Most patients (about 80%) will have a benign adenoma on final histopathology and require no further surgery.
    b. If the final histopathology shows carcinoma, second operation (usually performed within days to months after the first operation) is performed.
       (1) FTC
           (a) Wide invasive FTC—total thyroidectomy (completion thyroidectomy)
           (b) Minimally invasive FTC—either no further surgery or total thyroidectomy
           (c) Prophylactic neck dissection is not performed.
           (d) Modified radical neck dissection should be done on the side with palpable nodes.
       (2) Hürthle cell carcinoma
           (a) All Hürthle cell carcinomas require total thyroidectomy.
           (b) Central neck node dissection is always performed.
           (c) Central neck dissection involves the removal of pretracheal and paratracheal lymph nodes, which drain the thyroid.
           (d) Ipsilateral modified radical neck dissection is performed for clinically palpable cervical nodes.

## H. MEDULLARY CARCINOMA (MTC; 5% OF THYROID CANCER CASES)

1. MTC arises from the parafollicular cells (C cells). It is a neuroendocrine tumor.
2. MTC secretes calcitonin and carcinoembryonic antigen.
3. Eighty percent of MTC cases are sporadic and 20% are hereditary.
4. Hereditary type consists of familial MTC and those associated with MEN types IIa and IIb.
5. Diagnosis by FNA

**6.** Clinical presentation
a. Patients present with a firm neck mass that may be associated with neck swelling.
b. Unlike the differentiated thyroid cancer, MTC often causes neck pain.
c. MTC may secrete substances that can cause symptoms (cushingoid features from adrenocorticotropic hormone secretion and watery diarrhea from vasoactive intestinal polypeptide secretion).

**7.** Pathologic lesions
a. Solitary lesions often appear in sporadic cases, and multiple/bilateral lesions in familial cases.
b. Amyloid deposits, composed of modified calcitonin molecules, are seen.

**8.** Treatment
a. Total thyroidectomy and, at the least, central neck node dissection is performed.
b. Total thyroidectomy is done because MTC is often bilateral and multifocal.
c. Central neck node dissection is done because locoregional lymph-node involvement is common.
d. Ipsilateral modified radical neck dissection should be performed as well if the following is true:
  (1) Tumor is greater than 1 cm (larger tumors have greater risk for nodal spread).
  (2) Gross central lymph node involvement exists.
  (3) Gross cervical lymph node involvement exists.
e. Bilateral modified radical neck dissection should be done as well if the following is true:
  (1) Gross tumor exists on both lobes of the thyroid.
  (2) Extensive lymph-node involvement occurs.

## I. MEN TYPES IIA AND IIB/HEREDITARY MTC

**1.** Autosomal dominant with almost 100% penetrance
**2.** Caused by germline point mutations in the RET tyrosine kinase protooncogene
**3.** MEN types IIa and IIb are associated with other neoplasms/hyperplasia (Table 59-6).
**4.** Genetic testing is effective for detecting carriers of the RET mutation.
**5.** Carriers of RET mutation need prophylactic thyroidectomy.
**6.** For patients with RET gene mutation, diagnosed by genetic testing, the following protocol should be followed:
a. Need prophylactic total thyroidectomy because MTC will develop in all patients if left untreated.
b. Perform thyroidectomy at age 5 and 6 years for MEN type IIa, familial MTC.
c. MTC caused by MEN type IIb is aggressive—total thyroidectomy as soon as the diagnosis is confirmed regardless of age.

59

THYROID

**TABLE 59-6**

**MULTIPLE ENDOCRINE NEOPLASIA**

**MEN type I**

Pituitary, parathyroid, pancreatic neoplasms

**MEN type IIa**

Medullary thyroid carcinoma (100% of cases)
Pheochromocytoma (50% of cases)
Parathyroid neoplasm/hyperplasia (10–35% of cases)

**MEN type IIb***

Medullary thyroid carcinoma (100% of cases)
Pheochromocytoma (50% of cases)
Mucosal neuroma, gastrointestinal neuroma (>95% of cases)

*Patients with multiple endocrine neoplasia (MEN) type IIb often have a marfanoid habitus. Mucosal neuromas are often seen at the distal portion of the tongue, on the lips ("bumpy lip syndrome"), and subconjunctival areas.

   d. Patients with MEN type IIa or IIb should be checked for pheochromocytoma before the thyroid resection. If present, pheochromocytoma should be treated first.
   e. Routine central neck node dissection is not performed at the time of *prophylactic* thyroidectomy.
   f. Prophylactic central neck node dissection should be done if the following occurs:
      (1) Basal or stimulated calcitonin level is increased before surgery.
      (2) Preoperative ultrasound shows a thyroid mass, or a nodule is noted intraoperatively.
      (3) Evidence exists of lymph node involvement.

## J. ADJUVANT THERAPY
1. **Follow up for differentiated thyroid cancer (PTC, follicular, and Hürthle cell)**
   a. Thyroglobulin (Tg) level and whole-body radioiodine scan are used to detect recurrence.
   b. Tg is produced by normal and tumor follicular cells.
   c. Increase of Tg level after total thyroidectomy is a sensitive marker of recurrence.
   d. Whole-body radioiodine scan uses low-dose radioiodine to look for uptake. Positive uptake, after a total thyroidectomy, indicates recurrence.
   e. The usefulness of Tg level and iodine scan to detect recurrence is greatly diminished after limited thyroid resection.
   f. Two main adjuvant modalities after surgical resection are iodine-131 therapy and thyroid hormone suppressive therapy.
2. **Iodine-131 ablative therapy**
   a. Postoperative iodine ablative therapy has two goals:

    (1) Destroy any normal remaining thyroid tissue, thereby increasing the sensitivity of the whole-body iodine scan and the Tg level to detect recurrence

    (2) Destroy any occult microscopic cancer cells

b. Ablative therapy is needed after total thyroidectomy in high-risk patients.

c. Ablative therapy is not needed after lobectomy for minimal disease.

**3. Levothyroxine suppressive therapy**

a. TSH stimulates the growth of both normal and tumor thyroid cells.

b. Levothyroxine should be adjusted to keep the TSH concentration to less than 0.1 mU/L (reference range, 0.5–5 mU/L).

## K. ANAPLASTIC THYROID CANCER (1% OF THYROID CANCER CASES)

**1.** Rare, highly aggressive cancer that usually presents between 50 and 70 years of age

**2.** About 10% of patients have a history of long-standing goiter.

**3.** Twenty percent of patients have a history of being treated for a well-differentiated thyroid cancer.

**4.** Patients usually present with a rapidly enlarging neck mass together with symptoms of dysphonia, dyspnea, and dysphagia caused by tumor invasion and compression.

**5.** Diagnosis by FNA

**6.** Multimodality treatment with surgery, radiation, and chemotherapy is used.

**7.** Poor prognosis, with a median survival of only a few months

## L. THYROID LYMPHOMA (1% OF THYROID CANCER CASES)

**1.** Majority of cases are of the B-cell type that arises in patients with Hashimoto's thyroiditis.

**2.** Presents with a rapidly growing, painless neck mass and obstructive/compressive symptoms

**3.** Diagnosis may be established by FNA; surgical biopsy in equivocal cases.

**4.** Treatment of choice is chemotherapy combined with external beam radiation.

**5.** Surgery is reserved for relief of symptoms not responsive to medical therapy.

### RECOMMENDED READING

Brunicardi FC, Andersen DK, Billiar TR, et al (eds): *Schwartz's Principles of Surgery.* New York, McGraw-Hill, 2005, pp 1395–1429.

Caron NR, Clark OH: Papillary thyroid cancer. *Curr Treat Options Oncol* 7:309–319, 2006.

Dackiw APB, Zeiger M: Extent of surgery for differentiated thyroid cancer. *Surg Clin North Am* 84:817–832, 2004.

59

THYROID

Kebebew E, Clark OH: Medullary thyroid cancer. *Curr Treat Options Oncol* 1:359–367, 2000.

Larsen PR, Kronenberg HM, Melmed S, Polonsky KS (eds): *Williams Textbook of Endocrinology.* Philadelphia, Saunders, 2003.

Shaha AR, Shah JP, Loree TR: Low-risk differentiated thyroid cancer: The need for selective treatment. *Ann Surg Oncol* 4:328–333, 1997.

Silver RJ, Parangi S: Management of thyroid incidentalomas. *Surg Clin North Am* 84:907–919, 2004.

# Parathyroid

*Joshua M. V. Mammen, MD*

## I. PARATHYROID EMBRYOLOGY AND ANATOMY

### A. EMBRYOLOGY

1. Inferior parathyroids originate from the third branchial pouch (same as the thymus). Ultimate location is quite variable, anywhere from the base of the skull to the anterior mediastinum.
2. Superior parathyroids originate from the fourth branchial pouch (same as the trachea). They have a more consistent location but may be found as inferior as the posterior mediastinum.

### B. ANATOMY

1. A normal parathyroid gland weighs 40 to 50 mg and measures $3 \times 3 \times 3$ mm.
2. Inferior parathyroids are usually anterior to recurrent laryngeal nerve; superior parathyroids are usually posterior to recurrent laryngeal nerve.
3. Most individuals have 4 glands, but 13% have more and 3% have less.
4. Difficult to distinguish from surrounding fat; classically described to look like the "tongue of a jaundiced hummingbird"

## II. PRIMARY HYPERPARATHYROIDISM

### A. GENERAL

1. One or more parathyroid glands produce inappropriately high levels of parathyroid hormone (PTH).
2. Incidence of 1 in 1000 people
3. Hypercalcemia secondary to increased PTH hormone leads to increased enteral absorption of calcium, increased hydroxylation of vitamin D, and reduced renal calcium clearance.

### B. CAUSATIVE FACTORS

1. Cause is unclear; ionizing radiation and genetic inheritance have been implicated in a few cases.
2. Well-established inheritance pattern with multiple endocrine neoplasia types I and IIa
3. Forms
a. Adenoma in 80% of cases (up to 10% have double adenomas)
b. Hyperplasia in 15% to 20% of cases
c. Carcinoma in less than 1% of cases

### C. PRESENTATION

**Pearl:** *"Stones, bones, groans and psychic overtones."*

1. Seventy percent of cases found incidentally by laboratory studies; otherwise asymptomatic
2. "Stones"
   a. Twenty percent to 25% incidence of nephrolithiasis
   b. Usual stone composition of calcium phosphate or oxalate
   c. Less than 5% incidence rate of nephrocalcinosis
   d. Eighty percent of patients have some renal dysfunction.
3. "Bones"—osteopenia, osteoporosis, osteitis fibrosa cystica
   a. Incidence rate of 15%
   b. Symptoms include bone pain, tenderness, and pathologic fractures.
   c. Cortex resorbed (radius) with the medullary bone spared (vertebrae)
   d. Osteitis fibrosa cystica (<5%)—brown cysts prone to fracture develop in the bone because of increased osteolytic activity.
4. "Groans"
   a. Affects 20% of symptomatic patients
   b. Causative factor is commonly peptic ulcer disease, pancreatitis, or cholelithiasis.
5. "Psychic overtones"—fatigue, depression, anxiety, irritability, lack of concentration, and insomnia
   a. Occurs in 50% of symptomatic patients
   b. Severity does not correlate with calcium or PTH levels.
   c. Correction of underlying causes resolves all symptoms except anxiety.
6. Symptomatic hypercalcemia is more common with parathyroid carcinoma than in benign conditions.

## D. DIAGNOSIS
1. Physical examination—of limited usefulness; a palpable mass should raise suspicion of parathyroid carcinoma or thyroid anomaly.
2. Biochemical analysis
   a. PTH assay should be compared with serum ionized calcium level; increased PTH and low-to-normal calcium levels imply primary hyperparathyroidism.
   b. Serum phosphate levels—low in primary hyperparathyroidism, high in secondary hyperparathyroidism
   c. Chloride/phosphate ratio greater than 33 suggests primary hyperparathyroidism.
   d. Evaluation should be performed for other causes of hypercalcemia— malignancy, adrenal insufficiency, pheochromocytoma, vitamin D toxicity, granulomatous disease, immobility, drug induced (thiazides, mild-alkali syndrome, lithium).

## E. MANAGEMENT
1. Medical treatment
   a. May be necessary during a hypercalcemic crisis
   b. Symptoms of hypercalcemic crisis—anorexia, nausea, emesis, polyuria, polydipsia, abdominal pain, lethargy, bone pain, muscle weakness

c. Treat with normal saline fluid resuscitation.

d. After restoring isovolemia, initiate diuresis with a furosemide drip (10–20 mg/hr).

e. Dialysis to reduce calcium levels quickly

**2. Surgical treatment**

a. Indications

(1) Parathyroid carcinoma

(2) Asymptomatic patients with one of the following parameters:

  (a) Persistent calcium level of 1 to 1.6 mg/dl above normal

  (b) Calciuria >400 mg/24 hours

  (c) Decreased bone density greater than two standard deviations

  (d) Creatinine clearance 30% below normal

  (e) Age <50 years

(3) Hypercalcemia-associated diseases

  (a) Urolithiasis or nephrocalcinosis

  (b) Peptic ulcer disease

  (c) Musculoskeletal symptoms

  (d) Pancreatitis

  (e) History of severe hypercalcemic crisis

b. Management

(1) Ninety percent to 95% of explorations are successful without preoperative localization; localization (with sestamibi scan and ultrasonography) is mandatory with reoperation and leads to less invasive surgery.

(2) Adenoma—resection is curative.

(3) Hyperplasia—3½- or 4-gland resection with reimplantation of ½ gland in forearm or sternocleidomastoid

(4) Parathyroid cancer—wide en bloc excision including ipsilateral thyroid lobe and bilateral neck exploration; modified radical neck dissection for lymphadenopathy

(5) Ectopic locations of the glands

  (a) Thymus—20%

  (b) Posterior neck—5% to 10% of cases

  (c) Intrathyroid—5% of cases

  (d) Carotid sheath—1% of cases

  (e) Anterior mediastinum—1% to 2% of cases

(6) Intraoperative PTH: If PTH decreases by 50% within 10 minutes of resection and is within reference limits, more than 90% likelihood of successful resection

(7) Median sternotomy should not be performed at initial operation to find missing gland; must first get localization studies before proceeding.

c. Postoperative care

(1) Recurrent laryngeal nerve palsy 1% to 3% (one one-tenth permanent)

(2) Treat hypocalcemia with calcium carbonate 1 g orally every 6 hours; intravenous calcium only for severe hypocalcemia.
(3) Vitamin D supplementation for refractory hypocalcemia

## III. SECONDARY HYPERPARATHYROIDISM

### A. CAUSE IS USUALLY CHRONIC RENAL FAILURE
1. Poor renal excretion of phosphate leads to decreased serum calcium; less renal hydroxylation of vitamin D leads to decreased enteral calcium absorption and less renal clearance of PTH breakdown products.

### B. OTHER CAUSES
1. Osteogenesis imperfecta, paget's disease, multiple myeloma, malabsorption, or inadequate calcium intake

### C. SYMPTOMS
1. Psychiatric disorders, pruritus, headache, muscle weakness, weight loss, fatigue, renal osteodystrophy, and soft-tissue calcifications

### D. TREATMENT
1. Medical—phosphate-binding antacids, oral calcium, vitamin D, dialysis for severe cases
2. Surgical
a. Indications—calcium greater than 11 mg/dl with increased PTH, calciphylaxis, renal osteodystrophy, soft-tissue calcifications, or markedly increased calcium and phosphate levels
b. Dialysis day before surgery
c. Three-and-a-half-gland resection or four-gland parathyroidectomy with reimplantation for refractory cases; always perform cervical thymectomy concurrently

## IV. TERTIARY HYPERPARATHYROIDISM

### A. CAUSATIVE FACTOR
1. Persistent hyperparathyroidism after renal transplantation or resolution of underlying disorder; caused by parathyroid gland hyperplasia with autonomous PTH production

### B. TREATMENT
1. $3\frac{1}{2}$-gland resection or 4-gland parathyroidectomy with reimplantation for symptomatic patients or refractory cases 1 year after renal transplant

# Adrenal Gland

*Stacey A. Milan, MD*

## I. EMBRYOLOGY
### A. CORTEX
1. Derived from mesodermal tissue on adrenogenital ridge

### B. MEDULLA
1. Derived from ectodermal tissue arising from the neural crest

## II. ANATOMY
### A. GENERAL

## 61

1. Retroperitoneal
2. Superior and medial to kidney
3. Normal weight 4 to 5 g
4. Appears yellow because of high lipid content of cortex

### B. ARTERIAL SUPPLY
1. Inferior phrenic artery
2. Middle adrenal artery (derived from aorta)
3. Inferior adrenal artery (derived from renal artery)

### C. VENOUS DRAINAGE
1. Single major adrenal vein
2. Right adrenal vein—short, drains directly into inferior vena cava
3. Left adrenal vein—longer, empties into left renal vein

### D. CORTEX
Outer portion of adrenal gland composed of three zones (from superficial to deep)
1. Zona glomerulosa—produces mineralocorticoid aldosterone (salt)
2. Zona fasciculata—produces glucocorticoid cortisol (sugar)
3. Zona reticularis—produces androgens (sex)

### E. MEDULLA
Inner portion of adrenal gland
1. Produces catecholamine hormones epinephrine and norepinephrine
2. Often referred to as chromaffin cells because they stain with chromium salts

## III. PHYSIOLOGY AND PATHOPHYSIOLOGY—ADRENAL CORTEX
### A. MINERALOCORTICOIDS—ALDOSTERONE
1. Renin-angiotensin system—primary regulation for aldosterone secretion
2. Stimuli for renin secretion from juxtaglomerular cells in kidney
a. Decreased renal blood flow
b. Decreased plasma sodium

c. Increased sympathetic tone
3. Renin causes conversion of angiotensinogen to angiotensin I
4. Angiotensin I cleaved by angiotensin converting enzyme (produced in lungs) to angiotensin II.

**Pearl:** *Side effect of angiotensin-converting enzyme inhibitors is cough.*

5. **Angiotensin II**
a. Potent vasoconstrictor
b. Also leads to increased aldosterone synthesis and release
6. **Aldosterone**
a. Works at level of distal convoluted tubule
b. Increases sodium reabsorption
c. Increases potassium and hydrogen excretion
7. **Pathophysiology**
a. Conn syndrome (primary hyperaldosteronism)
b. Differential diagnosis for causes of hyperaldosteronism
    (1) Renal artery stenosis
    (2) Low-flow states such as cirrhosis or congestive heart failure
    (3) Adrenal adenoma, bilateral adrenocortical hyperplasia, or rarely, adrenocortical carcinoma
c. Symptoms
    (1) Hypertension, often long-standing and difficult to control despite multidrug therapy
    (2) Hypokalemia and related muscle weakness, fatigue
    (3) Other nonspecific symptoms such as polydipsia, polyuria, and headaches
d. Diagnosis of primary hyperaldosteronism
    (1) Laboratory tests—hypokalemia and metabolic alkalosis
    (2) Measurement of plasma aldosterone and renin levels
    (3) Important to adequately replace sodium and potassium before testing
    (4) Increased plasma aldosterone concentration and low plasma renin activity
    (5) Failure to suppress aldosterone levels with sodium loading
e. Radiologic studies
    (1) Computed tomography (CT) scan
    (2) Magnetic resonance imaging (MRI) less sensitive but more specific than CT scan, and it is useful for pregnant patients or those unable to tolerate intravenous contrast.
    (3) Selective venous catheterization
        (a) Requires an interventional radiologist to cannulate and sample blood from both adrenal veins and vena cava after adrenocorticotropic hormone (ACTH) administration
        (b) Blood sampled for aldosterone and cortisol levels
        (c) Greater than fourfold difference in aldosterone/cortisol ratios between adrenal veins is diagnostic.

(d) Invasive, risk for adrenal vein rupture
(e) Usually reserved when tumor cannot be localized or with bilateral adrenal enlargement
(4) Scintigraphy (nuclear medicine study)
(a) NP-59 $^{131}$I-6B-iodomethyl noriodocholesterol
(b) Taken up by adrenal cortex, similar to cholesterol, but does not undergo further metabolism
(c) Adrenal adenomas appear as hot nodules with suppressed contralateral uptake.
(d) Hyperplastic glands show bilaterally increased uptake.
f. Treatment
(1) Preoperative medical control of hypertension
(a) Spironolactone (aldosterone antagonist)
(b) Amiloride (potassium-sparing diuretic)
(c) Nifedipine (calcium-channel blocker)
(d) Captopril (angiotensin-converting enzyme inhibitor)
(2) Potassium supplementation
(3) Surgery
g. Postoperative considerations
(1) Patients may have transient hypoaldosteronism requiring mineralo-corticoid replacement.
(2) Adrenal insufficiency may occur 2 to 3 days after adrenalectomy.

## B. GLUCOCORTICOIDS—CORTISOL

1. Hypothalamic-pituitary-adrenal axis
2. Hypothalamus—secretes corticotrophin-releasing hormone
3. Anterior pituitary—secretes ACTH (derived from POMC [pro-opiomelanocortin hormone])
a. ACTH stimulates secretion of glucocorticoids, mineralocorticoids, and androgens.
b. Trophic for adrenal gland
c. ACTH secretion stimulated by stress, pain, hypoxia, hypothermia, trauma, and hypoglycemia
d. Secretion peaks morning, nadir late afternoon.
4. Adrenal cortex—secretes cortisol.
a. Cortisol controls secretion of corticotrophin-releasing hormone and ACTH via negative feedback loop.
b. Glucocorticoid hormones enter cell free and bind to receptors in cytosol.
c. Activated receptor-ligand complex is then transported to nucleus where it stimulates transcription of certain genes.
5. Cushing syndrome
a. Chronic glucocorticoid excess
b. Symptoms include hirsutism, purple striae, characteristic fat deposition (moon facies, buffalo hump, central obesity), diabetes, hypertension, amenorrhea.

   c. Different from Cushing's disease, which refers to a pituitary tumor that causes bilateral adrenal hyperplasia and hypercortisolism

   d. Causative agents of Cushing syndrome

     (1) ACTH dependent—pituitary adenoma, ectopic ACTH production, ectopic corticotrophin-releasing hormone production

     (2) ACTH independent—adrenal adenoma, carcinoma, hyperplasia

     (3) Iatrogenic—exogenous steroid administration (most common)

**6. Diagnostic tests: Cushing syndrome is characterized by increased glucocorticoid levels not suppressible by exogenous hormone administration and loss of diurnal variation.**

   a. Twenty-four-hour urinary cortisol measurement

   b. Low-dose overnight dexamethasone suppression: 1 mg dexamethasone given at 11 PM and cortisol levels measured at 8 AM the following morning. Normal physiologic response is suppression of ACTH and stop cortisol production; low-dose suppression test will not suppress excessive cortisol production from an autonomous adrenal gland.

   c. High-dose dexamethasone suppression test: Used to distinguish between the causes of ACTH-dependent Cushing syndrome (pituitary vs. ectopic): 8 mg dexamethasone given overnight with 24-hour urine collection for cortisol and 17-hydroxysteroids. Failure to suppress urinary cortisol by 50% confirms diagnosis of an ectopic ACTH-producing tumor.

   d. Bilateral petrosal vein sampling: This is helpful to distinguish between Cushing's disease and ectopic Cushing syndrome. Presence of a central-peripheral ACTH gradient is evidence for Cushing's disease (pituitary tumor).

**7. Radiologic tests include CT, MRI, and scintigraphy to image adrenals. MRI of brain for suspected pituitary adenoma**

**8. Treatment**

   a. No long-term effective medical treatments

   b. Adrenalectomy

## C. SEX STEROIDS

**1. ACTH stimulates adrenal gland to produce androgens from 17-hydroxypregnenolone.**

**2. Include dihydroepiandrosterone (DHEA), androstenedione, testosterone, and estrogen**

**3. During fetal development, adrenal androgens promote formation of male genitalia; adrenal androgen excess leads to precocious puberty in male individuals and virilization, acne, and hirsutism in female individuals.**

**4. Diagnostic tests—plasma or urine 17-ketosteroids (DHEA)**

**5. Treatment**

   a. Adrenolytic drugs such as mitotane, aminoglutethimide, and ketoconazole for control of symptoms in metastatic disease

   b. Adrenalectomy

## D. ADRENOCORTICAL CANCER

1. Rare—worldwide incidence of two occurrences per 1 million people
2. Bimodal age distribution—children and adults during fourth to fifth decades of life
3. Fifty percent of cancers are nonfunctioning.
4. Patients with functioning tumors often present with rapid onset of Cushing syndrome and virilizing features.
5. Diagnosis
   a. Renal panel—rule out hypokalemia.
   b. Low-dose dexamethasone suppression test
   c. Twenty-four-hour urine collection for cortisone, 17-ketosteroids, and catecholamines
   d. CT scan, MRI—large mass with heterogeneity, irregular margins and presence of hemorrhage, and adjacent lymphadenopathy or liver metastasis
6. Size greater than 6 cm is the most important criterion for likelihood of malignancy.
7. Once malignancy is diagnosed, obtain CT scan of chest and pelvis for staging.
8. Treatment
   a. En bloc resection with any involved lymph nodes or organs
   b. Subcostal or thoracoabdominal incision to permit wide exposure, control of vascular structures, and minimize chance of tumor spillage
   c. Mitotane (derivative of pesticide DDT) used in adjuvant setting, unresectable and metastatic disease
   d. Systemic chemotherapeutic agents—etoposide, cisplatin, doxorubicin, paclitaxel, but consistent responses are rare.
   e. External beam radiation for bony metastases
9. Prognosis
   a. Most important survival predictor is adequacy of resection.
   b. Complete resection median 5-year survival rate is 30% to 50%.
   c. Incomplete resection median survival time is less than 1 year.
10. Adrenal metastasis: Cancers that metastasize to adrenal gland include lung cancer (especially small-cell carcinoma), renal-cell carcinoma, melanoma, gastric adenocarcinoma, hepatocellular adenocarcinoma, esophageal adenocarcinoma, and breast cancer.

## IV. PHYSIOLOGY AND PATHOPHYSIOLOGY—ADRENAL MEDULLA

### A. GENERAL

1. Catecholamine hormones—epinephrine, norepinephrine, dopamine
2. Produced in central nervous system and adrenal gland
3. Metabolism in liver and kidneys forms metabolites metanephrines, normetanephrines, and vanillylmandelic acid.

### B. PHEOCHROMOCYTOMA—CATECHOLAMINE-SECRETING TUMOR

1. Peak incidence in fourth to fifth decades of life
2. Extraadrenal tumors may be found at sites of sympathetic ganglia in organ of Zuckerkandl, neck, mediastinum, abdomen, and pelvis.
3. Rule of 10's—10% bilateral, malignant, pediatric, extraadrenal, familial
4. Occur in multiple endocrine neoplasia types IIA and IIB, von Hippel–Lindau disease
5. Hereditary pheochromocytomas tend to be multiple and bilateral.
6. Symptoms
   a. Headache, palpitations, diaphoresis, anxiety, tremulousness, flushing, chest pain, nausea, vomiting
   b. Symptoms are often paroxysmal.
7. Diagnosis
   a. Twenty-four-hour urine catecholamines, metanephrines, vanillylmandelic acid
   b. Plasma metanephrines
   c. Extraadrenal sites secrete norepinephrine because they lack phenylethanolamine-$N$-methyltransferase, which converts norepinephrine to epinephrine, whereas adrenal tumors secrete epinephrine because this enzyme is present.
   d. CT scan without contrast (to minimize risk for precipitating hypertensive crisis)
   e. MRI and radiolabeled MIBG (metaiodobenzylguanidine i123) also useful
8. Treatment
   a. Preoperative volume repletion
   b. Alpha blockade with phenoxybenzamine (usually 1–3 weeks before surgery), then beta blockade after adequate alpha blockade and hydration (to avoid hypertensive crisis and congestive heart failure)
   c. Adrenalectomy—goal is minimal manipulation of tumor.
   d. Arterial line and central venous line with or without Swan–Ganz catheter for intraoperative monitoring
   e. After surgery, patients are prone to hypotension because of loss of adrenergic stimulation.
9. Malignancy
   a. Diagnosed by invasion into surrounding structures
   b. Common sites of metastasis include bone, liver, regional lymph nodes, lung, and peritoneum.

## V. INCIDENTALOMA

### A. DEFINITION:

1. Adrenal lesion found during imaging for unrelated reasons. Excludes tumors discovered on imaging studies for evaluation of hormone hypersecretion or staging of known cancers.

### B. INCIDENCE RATE OF INCIDENTALOMAS 0.4% TO 4%

## C. DIFFERENTIAL DIAGNOSIS

1. Benign functioning lesion—aldosteronoma, cortisol- or sex steroid–producing adenoma, pheochromocytoma
2. Malignant functioning lesion—adrenocortical cancer, malignant pheochromocytoma
3. Benign nonfunctioning lesion—cortical adenoma, myelolipoma, cyst, ganglioneuroma, hemorrhage
4. Malignant nonfunctioning lesion—metastasis

## D. DIAGNOSTIC WORKUP

1. Aimed at identifying patients who would benefit from adrenalectomy— functioning tumors (especially subclinical Cushing's syndrome) and increased risk for malignancy
2. Asymptomatic patients with imaging consistent with cysts, hemorrhage, myelolipoma, or diffuse metastatic disease need no further testing.
3. All other patients should be managed as follows:
   a. Low-dose dexamethasone suppression test or 24-hour urine cortisol to rule out subclinical Cushing syndrome
   b. Twenty-four-hour urine collection for catecholamines, metanephrines, and vanillylmandelic acid to rule out pheochromocytoma
   c. Serum electrolytes, plasma aldosterone, and renin to rule out aldosteronoma
4. Lesions greater than 6 cm have approximate 35% risk for malignancy; however, malignancy can present in masses smaller than 6 cm.
5. CT scan characteristics of adrenal malignancy—hyperattenuation, inhomogeneous, irregular borders, local invasion, adjacent adenopathy
6. Fine-needle aspiration biopsy useful in setting of patient with history of cancer and a solitary adrenal mass. *Note: Must appropriately rule out pheochromocytoma before biopsy.*

## E. MANAGEMENT

1. Patients with functioning tumors by biochemical testing or signs of malignancy should undergo adrenalectomy.
2. Nonoperative therapy with yearly CT scan follow-up is advised for lesions less than 4 cm.
3. Nonfunctional lesions 4 to 6 cm are more controversial. May be treated nonoperatively or operatively; the risks and benefits must be weighed for each patient.

## VI. ADRENAL SURGERY

### A. MANY SURGICAL OPTIONS

1. Open versus laparoscopic, anterior transabdominal, posterior approaches, multiple variations for each approach

### B. LAPAROSCOPIC ADRENALECTOMY

1. Standard procedure for all indications except cancer

C. **OPEN ADRENALECTOMY IS THE SAFEST OPTION FOR SUSPECTED OR KNOWN CANCERS AND MALIGNANT PHEOCHROMOCYTOMAS.**

## VII. ADRENAL INSUFFICIENCY

A. **PRIMARY (ADRENAL) OR SECONDARY (ACTH DEFICIENCY)**
B. **CAUSATIVE FACTORS**
1. Autoimmune disease, infections, metastatic deposits, hemorrhage (waterhouse–friderichsen syndrome from fulminant meningococce-mia), trauma, severe stress, exogenous steroid discontinuation

C. **SIGNS AND SYMPTOMS**
1. Patients with recent steroid intake
2. Suspect in stressed patients
3. May mimic sepsis
4. Fever, nausea, vomiting, lethargy, abdominal pain, hypotension

D. **DIAGNOSIS**
1. Hyponatremia, hypokalemia, hypoglycemia, eosinophilia
2. Cortisol levels
3. ACTH stimulation test with cortisol measurement

E. **TREATMENT**
Rests on volume replacement, steroid replacement, and correction of under-lying cause
1. Intravenous hydrocortisone 100 mg every 8 hours
2. Fludrocortisone (mineralocorticoid) may also be required.

# Neuroendocrine Tumors

*Joshua M. V. Mammen, MD*

## I. CARCINOID TUMORS

### A. DEMOGRAPHICS

1. Most common gastrointestinal (GI) neuroendocrine malignancy
2. Peak incidence in sixth to seventh decade of life

### B. LOCATION

1. Eighty-five percent of tumors are located in the GI tract.
2. Non GI locations include lungs (10%), larynx, pancreas, biliary tract, thymus, ovary, kidney, and skin.
3. GI locations are appendix (41%), small bowel (20%), and rectum (16%).

### C. PRESENTATION

1. Varies depending on physical characteristics, origin, and hormones produced
2. Ninety percent of patients are hormonally asymptomatic; hormonal products must obtain direct access to the systemic circulation (hepatic metastases, significant retroperitoneal disease, primary tumor is not in portal venous circulation).
3. Causes of common symptoms
   a. Flushing—bradykinin, hydroxytryptophan, prostaglandins
   b. Diarrhea—serotonin
   c. Cramping—serotonin
   d. Endocardial fibrosis—serotonin
   e. Pellagra—depletion of niacin stores because of serotonin
   f. Bronchospasm—bradykinin, histamine, prostaglandins
   g. Telangiectasia—vasoactive intestinal peptides, serotonin, prostaglandins, bradykinin
   h. Glucose intolerance—serotonin
   i. Arthropathy—serotonin
   j. Hypotension—serotonin
4. Symptoms can be induced by consumption of ethanol, chocolate, blue cheese, and by exertion.
5. Foregut carcinoids
   a. Atypical symptoms caused by secretion of nonserotonin peptides.
   b. Pulmonary carcinoid—often present with cough, chest pain, and recurrent pneumonia.
   c. Gastric carcinoid—associated with chronic atrophic gastritis (75%), Zollinger–Ellison syndrome (5–10%), sporadic (15–25%).
6. Midgut carcinoids
   a. Symptoms with bulky or metastatic disease
   b. Seventy-five percent of cases are located on distal appendix (rarely cause symptoms).

7. Hindgut carcinoid
a. Usually asymptomatic until quite advanced

## D. DIAGNOSIS
1. **Urinary 5-hydroxyindoleacetic acid**
a. Positive if more than 10 mg in 24 hours
b. Seventy percent sensitivity and 100% specificity
c. Avoid when performing test (bananas, avocados, chocolate, walnuts, pineapples, phenothiazines).
2. **Additional biochemical tests when 5-hydroxyindoleacetic acid is nondiagnostic.**
a. Urinary 5-hydroxytryptamine
b. Urinary 5-hydroxytryptophan
c. Plasma 5-hydroxytryptophan
d. Platelet 5-hydroxytryptophan
e. Serum chromogranin A
f. Serum neuron-specific enolase
g. Serum substance P
h. Serum neuropeptide K
3. **Localization**
a. Chest computed tomography (CT) scan—bronchial carcinoids
b. Endoscopy/barium studies—gastric, duodenal, colonic, and rectal carcinoids
c. Abdominal CT scan—liver metastases, and retroperitoneal and small-bowel (spoke-wheel appearance) carcinoids
d. Nuclear medicine scans (combination of indium-111 and MIBG [metaiodobenzylguanidine $I^{123}$])—sensitivity of 95%
e. Angiography/selective venous sampling—may be useful in difficult cases.

## E. MANAGEMENT
1. **Determined by size of primary tumor and incidence of metastatic spread**
2. **Appendiceal**
a. Less than 1 cm—appendectomy
b. One to 2 cm—controversial but appendectomy accepted if smaller than 1.5 cm
c. More than 1.5 cm, location at base of cecum, invasion of mesoappendix or lymph nodes—right hemicolectomy
3. **Small bowel (more likely to metastasize)**
a. Twenty percent to 40% multicentric—must examine all of small bowel and colon
b. Wide resection of small bowel and mesentery
4. **Rectal**
a. Less than 1 cm—wide local excision
b. One to 2 cm—abdominoperineal resection or low anterior resection
c. More than 2 cm—controversial, wide local excision because likely no benefit from more extensive surgery
5. **Metastatic disease**

a. Mild symptoms
   (1) Diarrhea—loperamide, diphenoxylate, cyproheptadine
   (2) Flushing—clonidine, phenoxybenzamine, types 1 and 2 histamine receptor antagonists
   (3) Bronchospasm and wheezing—aminophylline
b. Moderate-to-severe symptoms
   (1) Octreotide
   (2) Surgical intervention
      (a) Obstruction
      (b) Perforation
      (c) Severe symptoms and dominant mass identified
   (3) Chemotherapy—poor results
   (4) Interferon—poor results
   (5) Hepatic artery embolization—high complication rate
   (6) Radiofrequency ablation—promising results but early in experience

## F. PROGNOSIS
1. Localized disease—near 100%
2. Resectable metastatic disease—5-year survival rate of 68%
3. Unresectable metastatic disease—5-year survival rate of 38%

# II. GASTRINOMA
## A. DEMOGRAPHICS
1. Found in 0.1% of individuals with duodenal ulcers and 2% of individuals with ulcers refractory to medical therapy
2. Twenty-five percent of gastrinomas are associated with multiple endocrine neoplasia syndrome type I (MEN I; see section VIII).
3. Sex distribution: 60% male, 40% female
4. Mean onset of symptoms in sixth decade of life

## B. LOCATION
1. Eighty-five percent of gastrinomas are located in the gastrinoma triangle (see Fig. 62-1).
2. Common ectopic locations include splenic hilum, gastric wall, duodenum, mesentery, and liver.

## C. PRESENTATION
1. Symptoms are secondary to hypergastrinemia; increased gastrin leads to hypersecretion of acid by parietal cells.
2. Abdominal pain
a. Most common symptom
b. May be caused by ulcers that 90% of individuals have endoscopically confirmed in the upper GI tract
c. Ulcers may also lead to bleeding (30–50%) and perforation (5–10%).
3. Secretory diarrhea
a. Only symptom in 20% of cases

**62**

**NEUROENDOCRINE TUMORS**

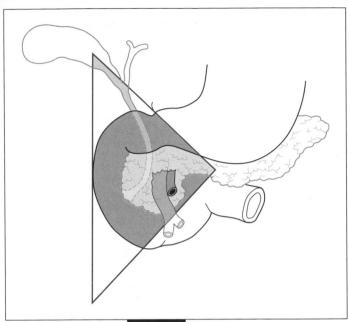

**FIG. 62-1**

The gastrinoma triangle.

b. Caused by acid hypersecretion, injury to small-bowel mucosa, malnutrition caused by inactivated enzymes, and increased motility
4. **Gastroesophageal reflux**

## D. DIAGNOSIS
1. Biochemical tests
a. Serum gastrin level
   (1) Increased in 90% of patients (reference range, 100–200 pg/ml)
   (2) Serum gastrin level greater than 1000 pg/ml suggests the diagnosis.
   (3) If serum gastrin level is 200 to 1000 pg/ml, will need to proceed to secretin stimulation testing.
b. Secretin stimulation test
   (1) Overnight fast
   (2) Administer secretin 2 units/kg intravenously.
   (3) Serum gastrin levels are to be checked 15 and 2 minutes before injection, and then 0, 2, 5, 10, and 20 minutes thereafter.
   (4) Positive if serum gastrin increases 200 pg/ml above baseline
c. Gastric acid hypersecretion
   (1) Acid hypersecretion must be documented to confirm gastrinoma.
   (2) Need to document gastric pH greater than 2.5.

2. Localization
a. Combination of somatostatin receptor scintigraphy and endoscopic ultrasound provides best localization.
b. Somatostatin receptor scintigraphy
   (1) Most gastrinomas have somatostatin receptors.
   (2) Sensitivity of 90%, specificity of 80%
   (3) High false-negative rate for duodenal wall gastrinomas
c. Endoscopic ultrasound—good for localization of duodenal and pancreatic gastrinomas

## E.  MANAGEMENT
1. Medical therapy
a. Initially should control acid hypersecretion with proton-pump inhibitor.
b. Octreotide may be added to decrease gastrin secretion.
2. Exploration
a. One third of patients will not have adequate localization before surgery.
b. For sporadic disease, exploration is indicated, but for MEN I, most experts believe that exploration is contraindicated because of general failure to resolve hypergastrinemia and less aggressive disease.
c. Exploration should be systematic.
   (1) Initial assessment for metastatic disease (found in 50% of cases)
   (2) Mobilization of pancreas with intraoperative ultrasound
   (3) Duodenotomy with bimanual palpation if fail to find tumor
   (4) Enucleation for small tumors less than 2 cm; resection for larger tumors
   (5) Resections without localization not indicated.
3. Metastatic disease
a. Debulking palliates disease by improving symptoms and extending life.
b. Hepatic artery embolization if surgery is contraindicated
c. Chemotherapy—best response with streptozocin, 5-fluoruracil, with or without doxorubicin

## III. INSULINOMA
### A.  DEMOGRAPHICS
1. Most common islet cell tumor
2. Slight female sex predominance
3. Age of presentation from fifth to sixth decade of life

### B.  PRESENTATION
1. Whipple's triad
a. Components
   (1) Symptoms of hypoglycemia at fast
   (2) Blood glucose level of less than 50 mg/dl at fast
   (3) Resolution of symptoms at glucose administration
b. Poor specificity
2. Common symptoms—visual disturbances, altered consciousness, weakness, seizures, diaphoresis, tremors, and tachycardia

62

NEUROENDOCRINE TUMORS

## C. DIAGNOSIS

1. Biochemical tests
a. Seventy-two-hour supervised fast (most reliable test)
   (1) Measure serum glucose and insulin levels every 4 hours.
   (2) When glucose level is less than 60 ml/dl, measure levels every hour.
   (3) Diagnosis confirmed with symptoms of hypoglycemia, serum insulin level greater than 6 μU/ml, and insulin/glucose ratio greater than 0.3.
b. C-peptide levels (not increased with surreptitious insulin)
c. Equivocal cases: Consider C-peptide suppression test and tolbutamide test.

2. Localization
a. Usually small (<2 cm) and single (90%)
b. Ten percent of patients have metastatic disease at diagnosis.
c. CT scan—detects majority of primary tumors and almost all metastatic disease.
d. Visceral angiography—used if disease is not seen on CT scan.
e. Selective portal sampling—used if not detected with visceral angiography.
f. Endoscopic ultrasound—useful in lesions in the head of the pancreas

## D. MANAGEMENT

1. Exploration
a. Pancreas should be completely mobilized.
b. Enucleation for small lesions away from the pancreatic duct
c. Distal pancreatectomy for body and tail near the duct, and pancreaticoduodenectomy for lesions in the head that are large
d. Resection without identification is not recommended.
e. Pancreatic biopsy if no tumor is found to evaluate for beta-cell hyperplasia and adult nesidioblastosis

2. Metastatic disease
a. Resection
   (1) Should be attempted because increased survival rate if complete section
   (2) Debulking may improve control of symptoms.
b. Medical therapy
   (1) Diazoxide—inhibits release of insulin.
   (2) Octreotide
   (3) Streptozocin

## IV. GLUCAGONOMA

### A. DEMOGRAPHICS

1. Rare, less than 100 cases have been reported

### B. PRESENTATION

1. Most commonly present with mild glucose intolerance (>90%)
2. Necrolytic migratory erythema
a. Occurs in 70% of patients
b. Located on lower abdomen, perineum, perioral, or feet

3. Other symptoms—weight loss, depression, deep venous thrombosis, cachexia, hypoaminoacidemia, anemia, and stomatitis

## C. DIAGNOSIS
1. Biochemical tests
a. Fasting serum glucagon level—positive if greater than 1000 pg/ml
2. Biopsy of skin rash has pathognomonic histology.
3. Localization
a. CT scan—usually identifies tumor because mostly large and located in body and tail of the pancreas.
b. Somatostatin receptor scintigraphy—reliable if CT scan fails.
c. Additional modalities—visceral angiography and portal venous sampling

## D. MANAGEMENT
1. Reverse catabolic state with octreotide and amino acid supplementation
2. Resection if possible
3. Metastatic disease
a. Found in more than two thirds of patients
b. Debulking assists symptomatic control
c. Medical therapy
   (1) Octreotide—control of diabetes and dermatitis
   (2) Dacarbazine
   (3) Streptozocin

## V. VASOACTIVE INTESTINAL POLYPEPTIDOMA
## A. DEMOGRAPHICS
1. Rare, approximately 200 cases described

## B. PRESENTATION
1. Usually presents with high-volume diarrhea exacerbated by enteral intake, but that does not resolve with fasting
2. Hypokalemia and acidosis from electrolyte imbalances

## C. DIAGNOSIS
1. Biochemical tests
a. Serum fasting vasoactive intestinal polypeptide level greater than 200 pg/ml with secretory diarrhea and pancreatic mass confirms diagnosis.
2. Localization
a. CT scan—usually identifies tumor because mostly large and located in tail of the pancreas.
b. Somatostatin receptor scintigraphy—reliable if CT scan fails
c. Additional modalities—visceral angiography and portal venous sampling

## D. MANAGEMENT
1. Initial resuscitation—rehydration and correct electrolytes
2. Control diarrhea

a. Octreotide is first agent.
b. Additional agents—steroids, nonsteroidal antiinflammatories, phenothiazines

3. **Exploration**
a. Complete resection via distal pancreatectomy if located in tail of pancreas
b. Fifty percent of disease is extrapancreatic; careful exploration of both adrenal glands is indicated.

4. **Metastatic disease**
a. Debulking assists with symptomatic control.
b. Medical therapy
   (1) Streptozocin
   (2) Interferon
   (3) Octreotide to control diarrhea

## VI. SOMATOSTATINOMA

### A. DEMOGRAPHICS
1. Rare

### B. PRESENTATION
1. Classic syndrome
a. Mild hypoglycemia, cholelithiasis, steatorrhea, and diarrhea
b. Seen with pancreatic tumors but not duodenal tumors
2. Duodenal tumors are associated with neurofibromatosis.

### C. DIAGNOSIS
1. Often incidental finding during invasive procedures including cholecystectomy
2. Biochemical tests—serum somatostatin level found that is 50-fold greater than reference value
3. Localization—CT scan usually identifies lesion.

### D. MANAGEMENT
1. Exploration
a. Resection is treatment of choice.
b. Always perform cholecystectomy because of high incidence of cholelithiasis.
2. Metastatic disease
a. Found in majority of patients
b. Debulking aids in symptomatic control
c. Poor results with chemotherapy

## VII. PANCREATIC POLYPEPTIDEOMAS

### A. DEMOGRAPHICS—RARE
### B. PRESENTATION—NONSPECIFIC SYMPTOMS SUCH AS DIARRHEA AND WEIGHT LOSS
### C. DIAGNOSIS

1. Increased serum pancreatic polypeptide (>300 pmol/L) and pancreatic mass
2. Localization with CT scan

### D. MANAGEMENT
1. Exploration—resection is treatment of choice.
2. Metastatic disease
a. Found in majority of patients
b. Streptozocin is preferred medical therapy.

## VIII. MULTIPLE ENDOCRINE NEOPLASIA (MEN) SYNDROMES
These syndromes have familial inheritance patterns of development of endocrine neoplasias; not all of the classic elements of each syndrome may be expressed in each individual.

### A. MEN I (WERMER SYNDROME)
1. General
a. (3 P's)—parathyroid hyperplasia, pancreatic islet cell neoplasms, and pituitary neoplasms
b. Additional manifestations—foregut carcinoid, adrenocortical tumors, thyroid tumors, lipomas, angiofibromas, and collagenomas
c. Autosomal dominant inheritance
d. Mutation of 11q13
2. Hyperparathyroidism
a. Usually first anomaly to occur and the most common
b. Presentation—usually asymptomatic
c. Diagnosis—serum calcium, phosphate, and parathyroid hormone levels
d. Management
   (1) Surgical excision (total excision with autotransplantation or $3\frac{1}{2}$-gland excision)
   (2) Always examine thyroid gland intraoperatively.
3. Pancreatic tumors
a. Sixty percent of individuals with MEN I
b. Most common are gastrinomas and insulinomas.
c. Tend to be multifocal and extrapancreatic
d. Resection is the treatment.
4. Pituitary tumors
a. Thirty percent to 50% of patients
b. Prolactinomas are most common tumor.
c. Presentation—caused by secreted hormones or mass effect.
d. Management
   (1) Bromocriptine is first line for prolactinoma.
   (2) Transsphenoidal hypophysectomy for nonprolactinoma or failure of bromocriptine

## B. MEN II (SIPPLE SYNDROME)

1. **Three subtypes (all mutation of RET protooncogene, 10q11.2):**
   a. MEN IIA—parathyroid hyperplasia, medullary thyroid carcinoma, and pheochromocytoma
   b. MEN IIB—multiple facial neuromas, diffuse ganglioneuromatosis, marfanoid habitus, medullary thyroid carcinoma, and pheochromocytoma
   c. Familial medullary thyroid carcinoma

2. **Medullary thyroid carcinoma**
   a. First endocrine anomaly to occur
   b. Origin: parafollicular cells (C cells)
   c. Secretes calcitonin, serotonin, adrenocorticotropic hormone, prostaglandins, melanin, and carcinoembryonic antigen
   d. Presentation
      (1) Secretory diarrhea (30%)
      (2) Often found on genetic/biochemical screening
   e. Diagnosis
      (1) Genetic test for anomaly in RET protooncogene
      (2) Provocative calcitonin testing to examine for recurrent disease
   f. Management
      (1) Exclude presence of pheochromocytoma and hyperparathyroidism because they take operative priority.
      (2) Treatment is total thyroidectomy with central neck dissection.
      (3) Provocative calcitonin testing as part of routine follow-up
      (4) Metastatic disease—controversy of whether repeat exploration is of benefit

3. **Pheochromocytoma**
   a. Diagnosed in second to fourth decade of life
   b. Usually benign, bilateral, and confined to adrenal medulla
   c. Presentation
      (1) Paroxysmal or sustained hypertension, often stimulated by activity or food containing tyramine
      (2) Other symptoms—diaphoresis, tremors, palpitations, anxiety, chest pain, glucose intolerance
   d. Diagnosis
      (1) Biochemical testing—urinary epinephrine, norepinephrine, and total metanephrines
      (2) CT or magnetic resonance imaging is first-line method of diagnosis; MIBG scan if equivocal results.
   e. Management
      (1) Adrenalectomy is treatment.
      (2) Controversy whether unilateral or bilateral resection should occur initially

4. **Hyperparathyroidism**
   a. Most individuals are asymptomatic.
   b. Management is similar to MEN I; diagnosis should be made before resection of medullary thyroid carcinoma.

# PART XIII

# Trauma

# Trauma Overview

*Colin A. Martin, MD*

*An expert is a man who has made all possible mistakes in a very narrow field.*
—Niels Bohr

## I. EPIDEMIOLOGY

### A. MORTALITY

Trauma is the fourth leading cause of death in the United States for all ages and the number one cause of deaths in persons younger than 44 years.

1. Fifty percent of deaths occur within minutes after injury.
2. Thirty percent of deaths occur within 2 days of injury.
3. The remainder of deaths occur days to weeks after injury.

### B. MECHANISMS OF INJURY

1. Motor vehicle crashes or collision (MVC)
a. Leading cause of death
b. Adolescents and young adults are at greatest risk for fatal MVCs.
c. Alcohol intoxication is a major factor in fatal MVCs in adolescents and young adults.
2. Firearms
a. Approximately 30,000 deaths occur secondary to firearms per year.
b. Fifty-seven percent of firearm deaths in male individuals aged 15 to 34 were homicides.
c. Suicide accounts for 39% of firearm deaths.
3. Falls
a. Leading cause of nonfatal injury in children younger than 5 years
b. Causes 23% of trauma deaths in adults older than 65 years
c. Twenty percent of adults older than 65 years will fall each year.
4. Industrial accidents and assaults are also significant.

## II. MANAGEMENT OF THE TRAUMA PATIENT

### A. PRIMARY SURVEY

Initial evaluation of the trauma patient

1. Brief history—mechanism of injury, time of injury, vital signs in the field, and medical history
2. ABCDE's
a. **A**irway: If the patient is alert and answers the questions with a clear voice, the airway is intact. If the patient's airway is not secure, rapid sequence endotracheal intubation or a definitive surgical airway should be established. Special considerations include:

(1) Mental status: Glasgow Coma Scale score of less than 8 requires intubation. Agitation or combativeness may be signs of hypoxia (see Chapter 68).

(2) Facial trauma: Upper airway landmarks can be distorted by soft-tissue damage or blood.

(3) Continue cervical spine protection.

(4) Large hemothorax or pneumothorax can cause breathlessness or hypoxia.

b. **B**reathing: Assess oxygen saturation via pulse oximetry. Anemia, hypotension, and hypothermia can affect the reliability of the pulse oximeter. Palpation, percussion, auscultation, and inspection of chest cavity should be performed.

c. **C**irculation and hemorrhage control: Shock is defined as inadequate tissue perfusion to support metabolic demands. The trauma patient can present with hypovolemic, cardiogenic, or neurogenic shock, or a combination of all three. Two large-bore (16–18 gauge) peripheral intravenous lines should be established.

(1) Vital signs: Tachycardia can be the first sign of hypovolemic shock. Blood pressure can be misleading, because in hypovolemic shock, hypotension is not seen until 30% to 40% of the blood volume is lost. Absence of tachycardia may be present in patients taking beta-blockers, taking digoxin, or in spinal shock (see Chapter 10).

(2) Physical examination: Mental status, capillary refill, and peripheral pulses in all extremities must be assessed.

(3) Hypovolemic shock: This is caused by loss of blood volume (see Table 63-1 for classes of shock). Two liters of isotonic fluids are given initially. If the patient still has signs of shock (decreased end-organ perfusion, tachycardia, hypotension), blood products should be given.

(4) Cardiogenic shock: This is caused by blunt or penetrating cardiac injury; can also be caused by tension pneumothorax. Patients in cardiogenic shock may have cardiac tamponade, which is associated with *Beck's triad:* hypotension, muffled heart sounds, and

| TABLE 63-1 | | | | |
|---|---|---|---|---|
| CLASSIFICATION OF HEMORRHAGE | | | | |
| Parameter | I | II | III | IV |
| Blood loss (ml) | <750 | 750–1500 | 1500–2000 | >2000 |
| Blood loss (%) | <15 | 15–30 | 30–40 | >40 |
| Pulse rate | <100 | >100 | >120 | >140 |
| Blood pressure | Normal | Normal | Decreased | Deceased |
| Respiratory rate | 14–20 | 20–30 | 30–40 | >35 |
| Urine output (ml/hr) | >30 | 20–30 | 5–15 | Negligible |
| Central nervous system symptoms | Normal | Anxious | Confused | Lethargic |

distended neck veins. Cardiac tamponade is treated with pericardiocentesis or thoracotomy.

(5) Neurogenic shock: This is caused by injuries to the spinal cord that result in loss of sympathetic tone, vasodilatation, and inability to mount a tachycardic response. Neurogenic shock is treated with fluid resuscitation and pressors.

d. **D**isability: After the airway, breathing, and circulation are assessed, the mental status and neurologic function are evaluated. The Glasgow Coma Scale is a standardized method of classifying head trauma (see Chapter 68).

e. **E**xposure: All clothing should be completely removed to perform a thorough assessment. Warm blankets and warmed fluid should be used to decrease hypothermia.

## B. FURTHER EVALUATION AND TRANSFER

1. Transfer of trauma patients: Some trauma facilities do not have the resources to deal with certain injuries. The patient should be stabilized as much as possible and transferred by air or ground depending on the distance and injury severity.

2. Additional studies/diagnostics

a. Foley catheter to monitor urine output. Contraindicated if blood is present at urethral meatus, scrotal or penile hematoma, or high riding prostate on rectal examination. If any contraindications, perform retrograde urethrogram to determine whether urethral injury is present. If no extravasation, a Foley catheter may be safely inserted (see Chapter 69).

b. Nasogastric tubes can be helpful for decompression. Massive gastric distension can contribute to nausea, vomiting, tachycardia, and hypotension. Intubated patients should receive a nasogastric tube. Orogastric tubes are preferred over nasogastric tubes in patients with midface trauma.

c. Radiographic studies: In patients who are critically ill, it is important to obtain only studies that will affect management. A portable chest and pelvic radiograph can provide valuable information on the unstable patient. Patients being transported for studies or procedures must have a stable airway, be hemodynamically stable, and be on a cardiopulmonary monitor.

d. Laboratory evaluation: Draw a standard laboratory panel while establishing intravenous access. Recommend: Type and screen, complete blood cell count, and electrolyte panel. Lactic acid and base deficit are helpful to monitor the degree of shock.

## C. SECONDARY SURVEY

Survey consists of a complete history and physical examination. It is not done until all the ABCDE's have been addressed and the patient's hemodynamics are beginning to improve. Often the secondary survey is delayed until a definitive operation has been done.

63

TRAUMA OVERVIEW

1. History: Includes complete questioning of the patient, prehospital personnel, and the family. The important aspects of history are in the pneumonic AMPLE:

   **A**—Allergies

   **M**—Medications

   **P**—Past illness and operations

   **L**—Last meal

   **E**—Events and environment related to the injury

2. Specific considerations

a. Firearms: It is important to know type of weapon, number of shots heard, and distance of victim from gun.

b. MVCs: Important questions include position of victim in car, extrication time, type of accident (head on, side impact, rear ended), speed of vehicle, loss of consciousness, restraint use (seatbelts, air bags), and outcome of others passengers in the car.

c. Fall: Important questions include height of fall, landing surface, position body landed on, and loss of consciousness.

3. Physical examination: Complete and thorough physical examination looking for missed injuries. Special attention should be paid to the back, axilla, and perineum, where injuries can be missed.

## III. PEDIATRIC TRAUMA

Children have different mechanisms of injury, hemodynamic responses to stress, communication barriers, relatively small total blood volume, increased metabolic requirements for growth, and problems with thermoregulation.

### A. MECHANISMS OF INJURY

1. Fifty percent of trauma deaths are MVC related.
2. Accidents in the home account for 35% of trauma injuries.
3. Bicycles account for a large percentage of accidents.

### B. PRIMARY SURVEY

The ABCDE's are followed; however, there are some specific considerations:

1. Airway: Children have a shorter neck, short trachea, large tongue, and floppy epiglottis. The proper size endotracheal tube (ET) should be placed.

a. An oversized ET tube can cause future tracheal stenosis.

b. Undersized ET tube will not allow for adequate ventilation.

c. ET size is determined by diameter of child's fifth digit or calculated as follows: (age in years + 16)/4.

d. A cuffless ET tube should be used in children younger than 8 years or lighter than 60 lbs.

2. Breathing: Children are primarily diaphragmatic breathers, and any interference with diaphragm excursion will interfere with breathing.

a. Children swallow air when crying, which can cause gastric distension and decrease left hemidiaphragm movement. Gastric decompression should be accomplished early.

b. Tension pneumothorax can progress quickly to ventilatory failure.
3. **Circulation:** Tachycardia is usually the first sign of hypovolemia. Table 63-2 details the normal vital signs of children. Other signs of hypovolemic shock are changes in mentation, decreased capillary refill, skin pallor, and hypothermia.
4. **Intravenous access:** Antecubital lines are the first location but can be challenging in children. Other sites include:
a. Femoral line
b. Saphenous vein cutdown at the ankle
c. Intraosseous infusion in tibia or sternum

## IV. TRAUMA AND PREGNANCY

**63**

Trauma is the leading cause of death during pregnancy. It is important for the trauma surgeon to be aware of the unique set of physiologic variables of gravid women.

### A. EPIDEMIOLOGY
1. MVCs, falls, and assaults are the leading causes of trauma.
2. MVCs, falls, and firearms are the leading causes of fetal death.
3. Maternal deaths are responsible for 11% of fetal deaths.

### B. ANATOMIC AND PHYSIOLOGIC CHANGES DURING PREGNANCY
(See Table 63-3)

### C. MATERNAL EVALUATION
The mother is always the priority in care and treatment because the most common cause of fetal demise is maternal death.
1. **Primary survey**
a. ABC: Securing the airway and providing adequate oxygenation is important to decrease maternal catecholamines, which can cause vasoconstriction and maternal/placental insufficiency.
b. Supine hypotensive syndrome
    (1) Caused by aortocaval compression by the uterus
    (2) Place mother in left lateral decubitus position while keeping the spine neutral.
c. Signs of shock can be delayed because of physiologic hypervolemia.

**TRAUMA OVERVIEW**

---

**TABLE 63-2**

**VITAL PARAMETERS BY AGE**

| Age Group | Respiratory Rate | Heart Rate (beats/min) | Systolic Blood Pressure (mm Hg) |
|---|---|---|---|
| Newborn | 30–50 | 120–160 | 50–70 |
| 1–12 months | 20–30 | 80–140 | 70–100 |
| 13–36 months | 20–30 | 80–130 | 80–110 |
| 3–5 years | 20–30 | 80–120 | 80–110 |
| 6–12 years | 20–30 | 70–110 | 80–120 |
| 13+ years | 12–20 | 55–105 | 110–120 |

| TABLE 63-3 | | |
|---|---|---|
| **ANATOMIC AND PHYSIOLOGIC CHANGES DURING PREGNANCY** | | |
| System | Change | Implication |
| Cardiovascular | ↓ Peripheral vascular resistance, ↓ venous return, ↓ blood pressure (10–15 mm Hg) | Supine hypotensive syndrome (10–15 mm Hg) |
| Blood volume | ↑ Plasma and blood volume, ↑ white blood cell count to 20,000/L | Physiologic hypervolemia |
| Coagulation | Hypercoagulable, ↑ clotting factors, ↓ fibrinolysis | ↑ Venous thromboembolism |
| Respiratory | ↑ Diaphragm excursion, ↑ tidal volume, ↑ minute ventilation, ↓ $Pco_2$, | Chronic compensated respiratory alkalosis |
| Gastrointestinal | ↓ Motility, ↓ gastroesophageal sphincter competency | ↑ Risk for aspiration |
| Renal | ↑ Glomerular filtration rate, ↑ creatinine, ↓ blood urea nitrogen | Hydronephrosis and hydroureter |
| Endocrine | ↑ Parathormone, ↑ calcitonin | ↑ Calcium absorption |

## D. FETAL ASSESSMENT
The fetus is viable after 24 weeks of gestation.
1. **Heart rate: Reference range is 120 to 160 beats/min.**
a. Heard by a Doppler instrument by 12 weeks of gestation
b. Initial response to stress is tachycardia followed by bradycardia in severe distress.
c. Cardiotechnographic monitors assess fetal heart rate and uterine contractions.
2. **Fetal exposure to radiation: All necessary radiographic tests should be done if they will benefit the mother.**
a. Death of embryo can result in implantation (<3 weeks).
b. Three to 16 weeks: Radiation can affect organogenesis.
c. More than 16 weeks: Neurologic deficits are most common.
d. X-ray exposure: Ten rads is safe for the embryo/fetus.
   (1) X-ray of abdomen, pelvis, or lumbar spine delivers about 1 rad.
   (2) X-ray of skull, chest, or extremities delivers about 0.1 rad.
   (3) CT scan delivers 0.2 to 0.5 rad.
e. When possible, shield the uterus with a lead apron when taking radiographs.

## V. PENETRATING NECK TRAUMA
Penetrating neck trauma is usually caused by firearms or stabbings. The neck has been divided into three anatomic zones (Fig. 63-1). After the ABCDE's are evaluated, neck trauma should be managed based on the anatomic zone (Fig. 63-2). Refractory shock warrants immediate exploration. Injuries to zone I require immediate exploration. Injuries in zones I and III can be difficult to expose. Preoperative imaging in theses zones can be helpful to guide operative management.

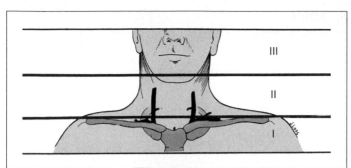

**FIG. 63-1**

Zones of the neck.

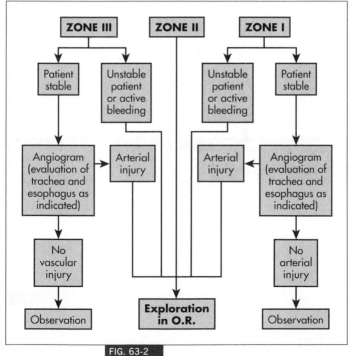

**FIG. 63-2**

Penetrating neck trauma algorithm.

### A. ZONE I
1. Horizontal between clavicles and cricoid cartilage

### B. ZONE II
1. Cricoid cartilage to angle of mandible

### C. ZONE III
1. Angle of mandible to base of skull

### D. NECK EXPLORATION
1. Make longitudinal incision along the anterior boarder of the sternocleidomastoid.
2. Retract the sternocleidomastoid laterally.
3. Dissect cervical fascia, and identify and examine the internal jugular vein.
a. Most commonly injured vascular structure in the neck is the internal jugular vein.
b. Repair injury with 5–0 polypropylene suture or ligation if necessary.
4. Ligate the facial vein along the anterior border of the neck.
5. Identify and open carotid sheath.
6. Examine the carotid artery for injuries.
a. Identify the vagus nerve.
b. Gain proximal and distal control of the carotid.
c. Carotid artery injuries should be repaired. Carotid ligation, if necessary, is generally tolerated. (Specify when this is indicated—when patient in extremis or has complete neurologic deficit before surgical intervention.)

### RECOMMENDED READING
Hirshberg A, Mattox KL: *Top Knife: The Art and Craft of Trauma Surgery.* Shropshire, United Kingdom, TFM Publishing Co. 2005.
Moore EE, Feliciano DV, Mattox KL: *Trauma.* 5th ed. New York, McGraw-Hill; 2004.

# Abdominal Trauma

*Nathan L. Huber, MD*

## I. EPIDEMIOLOGY

Epidemiology information is based on National Trauma Data Bank 2006 report (not necessarily reflecting an urban trauma center distribution).

### A. BLUNT TRAUMA

1. Motor vehicle collisions—41% of cases, 45% of mortalities, most hospital and intensive care unit (ICU) days, peak incidence occurs at age 19 years.
2. Falls—27% of cases, 22% of mortalities, peak incidence occurs at around age 85.
3. Assault—6.4% of cases

### B. PENETRATING TRAUMA

1. Gunshot wounds (GSWs)—5.6% of cases, 22% of mortalities, peak incidence occurs at age 19.

### C. ORGANS INJURED (IN ORDER OF FREQUENCY)

1. Blunt—spleen, liver, retroperitoneal hematoma, small bowel
2. Penetrating
   a. GSWs—small bowel, colon, liver, abdominal vessels
   b. Stab wounds—liver, small bowel, diaphragm, colon

### D. TRAUMA MORTALITY HAS A TRIMODAL DISTRIBUTION.

1. First peak: occurs seconds to minutes after trauma event—because of overwhelming injury involving brain, high spinal cord, heart, airway, and great vessels (aortic transection).
2. Second peak: the "golden hour" after trauma event where intervention has greatest impact—deaths in this period result from intracranial hemorrhage, hemothorax, tension pneumothorax, ruptured spleen, severe liver lacerations, open and/or femur fractures, and other multiorgan injuries.
3. Third peak: occurs several days to weeks after trauma event—sepsis and multiorgan failure.

## II. PATHOPHYSIOLOGY

### A. BLUNT TRAUMA

1. Direct blow (rupture of organs) versus deceleration injury (including tear at attaching ligaments)
2. Key questions—speed of vehicle, angle of impact, fate of other passengers, wearing seat belt, airbag deployed, extraction time, height of fall

### B. PENETRATING—STAB WOUND OR GSW

1. Key questions—timing of injury, caliber/size of weapon used, distance from gun barrel, number of wounds
2. High-velocity GSW (uncommon in urban setting) impart more kinetic injury to abdominal organs and create a larger cavitation (remember, $KE = 1/2\ mv^2$, where $KE$ represents kinetic energy, $m$ represents mass of the moving particle, and $v^2$ represents volume of the particle squared).

## III. DIAGNOSIS

Diagnosis is based on the standard Advanced Trauma Life Support (ATLS) primary approach that includes a structured primary and secondary survey (see Chapter 63).

### A. SECONDARY SURVEY ADJUNCTS—OPERATIVE DECISION MAKING.

1. Plain film radiographs—urgent chest, abdominal, and pelvic (anteroposterior view)
   a. Evaluate for associated thoracic injury (diaphragm injury, hemo/pneumothorax).
   b. Place paper clip markers at penetrating injuries; assess missile trajectory.
   c. Evaluate for free intraabdominal air.
2. Focused Assessment Sonography in Trauma (FAST)—ultrasound probe placed over four interfaces to look for free fluid: pericardium, hepatorenal fossa, splenorenal fossa, pelvis/pouch of Douglas.
   a. Advantages over diagnostic peritoneal lavage (DPL)—rapid (2–3 minutes to complete), some localization of injury, noninvasive, inexpensive, includes evaluation of pericardium
      (1) Skilled users can appreciate hemothorax, pneumothorax, inferior vena cava (IVC) fullness.
   b. Limitations—sensitivity anywhere from 44% to 91% in ruling out solid organ injury, does not examine retroperitoneum, is less sensitive than DPL for small amounts of intraperitoneal blood. The minimum amount of fluid required for a positive examination is at least 200 to 400 ml.
      (1) Most stable patients with abdominal pain or unreliable examination will get computed tomographic (CT) scan to look for missed solid organ or retroperitoneal injury.
   c. Think of FAST as a tool to help determine when and where to make incision. It is sensitive in determining need for laparotomy in trauma patient with hypotension.
3. DPL—largely replaced by FAST; indications include evaluation for small-bowel injury when fluid seen on CT is not explained by solid organ injury bleeding, when CT is not available, and for stab wounds with uncertain depth.
   a. See Chapter 79 for details and interpretation of results.

b. Decompress stomach and bladder first (Salem sump tube and Foley catheter).

**4.** Abdomen/pelvis CT scan with intravenous (IV) contrast

a. Only for hemodynamically stabilized patients

b. Useful because many injuries can be missed with DPL and FAST, including solid organ hematomas; diaphragmatic, pancreatic, and retroperitoneal injuries; and because many injuries can be managed without surgery (observation or embolization)

c. Oral contrast is not typically given—no definite improvement in detecting small bowel injury, increases delay in obtaining CT scan, aspiration risk.

d. Early pancreas and small-bowel injuries are the most commonly missed diagnoses on CT scanning.

**64**

## B.  BLUNT TRAUMA INDICATIONS FOR LAPAROTOMY

**1.** Hypotension that is suspected to be secondary to intra-abdominal injury (do not waste time in the emergency department with more than a radiograph and type and cross-match if hypotension persists)

**2.** Positive DPL or FAST if hemodynamically unstable

**3.** Evisceration or diaphragmatic rupture

**4.** Peritonitis (can be difficult to determine in the bruised blunt trauma patient)

**5.** CT scan showing extravasation from liver or spleen injury, renal pedicle injury, pancreatic hematoma, mesenteric hematoma, large amount of free fluid in pelvis not explained by solid organ injury (suggests small-bowel injury)

## C.  PENETRATING TRAUMA INDICATIONS FOR LAPAROTOMY

(In addition to indications above)

**1.** GSW penetrating "the box" bordered by nipple line superiorly, perineum and gluteal folds inferiorly, flank (posterior axillary line) laterally

**2.** Stab wounds that penetrate the anterior abdominal wall fascia

a. This can be verified with local wound exploration (although the false-negative rate is nearly 30%) or positive DPL.

b. A safer diagnostic step is to take the patient to the operating room, place a single umbilical port, and do diagnostic laparoscopy.

## D.  INDICATIONS FOR ANGIOGRAPHY/EMBOLIZATION

**1.** Pelvic fracture with active arterial extravasation

**2.** Selected use for extravasation from liver and spleen laceration

### IV. TREATMENT

Continue with initial resuscitation measures (see Chapter 63). When diagnostic steps are complete, triage nonoperative patients (discharge, floor, ICU). When indications for laparotomy are met, proceed as outlined in the following sections.

ABDOMINAL TRAUMA

## A. BASIC OPERATIVE MANEUVERS

1. Request special equipment as needed (Cell Saver, vascular tray, rigid sigmoidoscope, etc.).
2. Broad-spectrum IV antibiotics before incision—usually cefazolin at the University of Cincinnati
3. Wide prep—sternal notch to anterior thighs (access to the chest if needed and access to proximal greater saphenous vein for graft if needed)
4. Midline laparotomy—goals are stopping bleeding, then controlling contamination, followed by definitive repair. Rapidly inspect all four quadrants and pack if bleeding. Apply pressure to bleeding areas or ligate bleeding vessels. Use clamps or single sutures to control contamination.

a. Clot often represents the site of injury.
b. Right upper quadrant—palpate liver, visualize diaphragm and kidney (usually dividing the falciform ligament for better visualization and avoidance of traction).
c. Left upper quadrant—palpate/visualize spleen, visualize diaphragm.
d. Lower quadrants—look for obvious bladder or bowel injury, retroperitoneal hematomas.
e. Eviscerate and run small bowel from ligament of Treitz to ileocecal valve, examining both sides and the mesentery.
f. Run colon from cecum to peritoneal reflection.
g. Inspect the retroperitoneum for hematomas.

5. Special considerations

a. Kocher maneuver—mobilization of first and second portion of duodenum by dissection through lateral attachments. Indications include bile staining or bruising of second portion of duodenum, concern for pancreas injury on CT scanning.
b. Catell–Braasch maneuver (right medial visceral rotation)—continuation of Kocher maneuver, taking down lateral attachments of ascending colon along right paracolic gutter, reflect colon medial with dissection anterior to Gerota's fascia. Indicated for exposure of right colon injuries, and aortic and IVC injures below the superior mesenteric artery.
c. Splenic mobilization if concern about left upper quadrant bleeding or injury or distal pancreas injury (see section V)
d. Mattox maneuver—left medial visceral rotation: take down splenorenal ligament and left peritoneal reflection along white line of Toldt down to distal sigmoid colon. Indicated for exposure of entire aorta including origin of celiac axis, superior mesenteric artery, and left iliac, left renal arteries.

6. Abdominal closure options

a. Primary fascial closure if negative or injuries definitively treated
b. There are many temporary closure options in setting of large-volume resuscitation or planned take back for second look.
   (1) Towel clips to skin or blue towels covered with loban dressing—very quick but tendency to leak, least durable

(2) Silastic mesh—more durable but takes time to suture in place

(3) Bogota bag closure is similar to this and popular at many institutions.

(4) "Kentucky Patch" made from two pieces of slush basin plastic (popular at the University of Cincinnati)

    (a) Plastic lines the peritoneal surface of abdominal cavity, preventing adhesion to bowel, and provides water-tight closure.

    (b) Can be sequentially tightened in the ICU to avoid loss of abdominal domain

c. Vicryl mesh closure is used if fascia cannot be reapproximated after above temporary closures—provides absorbable covering of omentum and bowel that will eventually granulate and can be skin grafted.

## B. DAMAGE CONTROL LAPAROTOMY

1. Standard of care for the patient who presents in extremis and/or develops the triad of death during the operation (acidosis, coagulopathy, hypothermia)

2. Stage 1: operative control of hemorrhage and contamination

a. Solid organ injury tamponade (packing)

b. Repair/ligate accessible blood vessels

c. Perforated bowel occlusion/resection

d. External tube drainage (bile/pancreatic ducts and ureters)

e. Rapid temporary closure of abdominal cavity

3. Stage 2: ongoing resuscitation in the ICU setting

4. Stage 3: reexploration and definitive treatment

5. Stage 4: definitive abdominal wall closure

## V. ORGAN-SPECIFIC INJURY MANAGEMENT

Table 64-1 lists injury staging that often guides therapy.

## A. DIAPHRAGM

1. Usually (75%) occurs on the left because of the blocking effect of the liver on the right and usually involves the central tendon. On x-ray film, look for blurring of the diaphragm, nasogastric tube coursing up into the chest, or hemothorax. Ultrasound can also be helpful to detect bowel in the chest.

2. Can usually be repaired via laparotomy with horizontal mattress permanent sutures. If there is no rim to sew to on the thoracic wall or if delayed diagnosis and subsequent scarring, this may require thoracotomy and repair from above.

3. Grade V injury may require Alloderm patch or Marlex (polypropylene) mesh to span defect. The diaphragm can also be reattached more cephalad in the thoracic cavity.

## B. STOMACH

1. Suspect injury when CT scanning shows unexplained intraperitoneal fluid, pneumoperitoneum, stomach wall thickening or surrounding

**64**

**ABDOMINAL TRAUMA**

**TABLE 64-1**

ORGAN INJURY GRADING SCALE

| Organ | Grade | | | | |
|---|---|---|---|---|---|
| | I | II | III | IV | V |
| Diaphragm | Contusion | L <2 cm | L = 2–10 cm | L >10 cm or tissue loss <25 cm² | Tissue loss <25 cm² |
| Liver | H <10% surface area, L <1 cm depth | H 10–50% surface area, L = 1–3 cm depth, <10 cm length | H >50% surface area, expanding or ruptured, L >3 cm depth | H with active bleeding, L involving 25–75% parenchyma or ≤3 segments | L >75% of lobe or >3 segments in single lobe, vena caval, or central hepatic vein injury (Note: grade VI = hepatic avulsion) |
| Spleen | H <10% surface area, L <1cm depth | H 10–50% surface area or <5 cm diameter, L = 1–3 cm depth not involving trabecular vessels | H >50% surface area or >5 cm diameter, expanding or ruptured, L >3 cm depth or involving trabecular vessels | H with active bleeding, L involving segmental/hilar vessels devascularizing >25% of spleen | Completely devascularize or shattered spleen |
| Stomach | H <3 cm, partial thickness L | H >3 cm, L <3 cm | L >3 cm | L involving vessels on greater or lesser curvature | Extensive rupture (>50%), devascularization |
| Pancreas | Small H/L without duct injury | Large H/L without duct injury or tissue loss | Distal transection or L with duct injury | Proximal transection/ parenchymal L involving ampulla | Massive head disruption |

| | | | | | |
|---|---|---|---|---|---|
| Duodenum | H in one segment, partial-thickness L without perforation | H in multiple segments, small L <50% circumference | Large L (50–75% circumference D2, 50–100% circumference other segments) | Very large L of D2 (75–100% circumference), rupture of ampulla or distal common bile duct (CBD) | Massive duodenopancreatic injury or devascularization of duodenum |
| Jejunum/Ileum | H without devascularization, partial-thickness L without transection | Small L <50% circumference | Large L (>50 circumference without transection) | Transection | Segmental tissue loss, devascularization |
| Colon | Contusion, H, partial-thickness L | Small L (<50% circumference) | Large L (>50% circumference) | Transection | Transection with devascularized segment, tissue loss |
| Rectum | Contusion, H, partial-thickness L | Small L (<50% circumference) | Large L (>50% circumference) | Full-thickness L with perineal extension | Devascularized segment |
| Kidney | Contusion, hematuria | Nonexpanding perirenal H, L <1 cm, no urine extravasation | L >1 cm but without collecting system rupture or urine extravasation | L through renal cortex to collecting system, injury to main renal artery | Shattered, devascularized |

H = hematoma; L = laceration.

**ABDOMINAL TRAUMA**

64

stranding, or extravasation of oral contrast. Intraoperatively, visualize anterior gastric surface from the gastroesophageal junction to the pylorus; if injury seen or suspected, open gastrocolic ligament to enter lesser sac and visualize posterior surface.

2. Grade I: Unroof and evacuate hematoma because this may be hiding a deeper injury; perform seromuscular closure with interrupted sutures.
3. Grade II-III: Repair primarily in a two layer fashion.
4. Grade IV-V: Perform partial gastrectomy and gastroduodenostomy or gastrojejunostomy to reestablish enteric drainage.

## C. LIVER

1. Many low-grade liver lacerations or hematomas diagnosed with CT without active extravasation of contrast can be managed nonoperatively in the stable patient. They require close monitoring, serial (every 4–6 hours) hematocrits until stable, and a high index of suspicion for postinjury complications including infected hematoma and biloma. Hypotension and ongoing transfusion requirements are indications for operative exploration and repair. If injury is discovered intraoperatively, attempt to control bleeding with packing first, then proceed based on grade of the injury.
2. Basic maneuvers for profuse bleeding from right upper quadrant
a. First-line therapy is to pack the liver well (above and below). Many liver injuries will not need direct repair but will tamponade and clot because of the low-pressure system. If bleeding persists, proceed as follows.
b. Exposure: Take down the falciform ligament, then triangular and coronary ligaments as needed to palpate and inspect for liver fractures, using your hands first, then folded laparotomy pads (four at a time) to compress bleeding parenchyma.
c. Pringle maneuver: Bluntly tear open the lesser omentum/gastrohepatic ligament and guide a vascular clamp through the foramen of Winslow and the hole in the lesser omentum and clamp; this includes portal vein, hepatic arteries (even if they are replaced), and common bile duct. Limit duration of continuous clamping, but you can clamp up to an hour without irreversible injury.
3. Grade I-II injuries—Bovie or argon beam electrocautery, apply topical clotting agents (Surgicel or FloSeal) or pack with omentum; do not place drains; close abdomen after other injuries treated.
4. Grade III-V injuries when Pringle maneuver controls bleeding—treat topical bleeding as in grade I or II above, ligate parenchymal bleeding vessels with silk sutures, and reapproximate liver parenchyma with 0 chromic catgut sutures.
a. There is unclear evidence on the benefit of closed suction drainage of liver injuries.
b. If packs are left in, remove during take-back laparotomy in 1 to 2 days.
5. Grade III-V injuries when Pringle maneuver does not control bleeding— significant ongoing bleeding indicates injury to hepatic vein or vena

cava. Get better exposure by taking down additional attaching coronary and triangular ligaments, extend laparotomy to median sternotomy to gain exposure above and below diaphragm, stop bleeding with one of the methods below, then definitively repair the bleeding vessels either at that time or during take-back laparotomy after patient is stabilized.

a. Hemostasis adjuncts

    (1) Place additional packing, especially if the right lobe is injured. The goal is to use the anterior chest wall, the diaphragm, and the retroperitoneum to circumferentially compress the liver parenchyma for an extended period.

    (2) Intrahepatic balloon tamponade: This is basically a hand-crafted expandable cylinder constructed with a hollow catheter (Foley or red rubber) and an overlying 2.5-cm Penrose drain sutured distally and proximally. This is filled with contrast for follow-up on imaging and removed on take back within 2 days. It will temporarily control venous, not arterial, bleeding.

    (3) Atrial-caval (Schrock) shunt—premade bypass tubing kits are used for this at University of Cincinnati; otherwise, use 9-mm endotracheal tube with side holes created proximally or chest tube to bypass liver.

        (a) Make hole in right atrium, insert proximally clamped tube, and guide inferiorly through IVC to level below injury (preferably above renal veins).

        (b) Inflate balloon (or suture there with umbilical tape if chest tube used).

        (c) Purse-string suture hole in right atrium—blood will flow within tube from below level of hepatic veins to right atrium via side holes.

    (4) Moore–Pilcher balloon—endovascular hollow device placed via femoral vein with balloon inflated at level of hepatic veins to form temporary covered stent.

    (5) Complete vascular isolation—cross-clamp aorta at the diaphragm, then the suprahepatic and infrahepatic vena cava as in a liver transplant.

        (a) This reduction in preload is usually not tolerated well in a bleeding trauma patient. If needed, do venovenous bypass (see Chapter 50).

b. Definitive repair

    (1) Hepatic parenchymal sutures—chromic catgut horizontal mattress placed with large, curved, blunt-tipped needle to avoid tearing through Glisson's capsule (with or without pledgets). If it works, this is far less invasive than other methods.

        (a) Criticized as a source of hepatic necrosis (ischemia)

        (b) Can be used to close entrance and exit wounds of penetrating injuries, but this risks future infected intrahepatic hematoma

    (2) Hepatotomy with selective ligation of bleeding vessels

**64**

**ABDOMINAL TRAUMA**

      (a) Can use finger fracture or Kelley crush/clamp methods, LigaSure, or white load (vascular) reticulating laparoscopic staplers to extend laceration tract until actual bleeding vessel is visualized

      (b) Can be extended to anatomic liver resection if needed, that is, large left lobe injuries not amenable to successful packing compression or when large segment of liver is deemed nonviable. Anatomic hepatic resection is associated with high mortality rate (50%) in the setting of trauma.

    (3) Hepatic artery ligation or angioembolization for deep arterial bleeding

    (4) Nonviable hepatic tissue should be debrided bluntly after patient is stable and can tolerate the unavoidable blood loss.

**6.** Postoperative management—overall mortality rate of patients with hepatic injuries is nearly 10%. Mortality rate is greater as grade of injury increases and is greater in blunt trauma. Infection rates are greater in penetrating injuries.

a. Delayed hemorrhage—usually from missed vascular injury, return to operating room, or angiography for attempted embolization if patient is coagulopathic.

b. Perihepatic infection—fever or increased white blood cell count 3 to 4 days after injury, rule out common things such as pneumonia, infected line, urinary tract infection first, then get CT scan with oral and IV contrast, and do CT-guided percutaneous drainage as needed.

c. Biliary leak—suspect with increasing bilirubin level and persistent or worsening right upper quadrant pain. Usually resolves with time and NPO (nothing by mouth). If no resolution, do endoscopic retrograde cholangiopancreatography with stent placement to ensure that enteric route is least resistant path of bile drainage.

    (1) Biloma—sterile ones will be resorbed (discovered incidentally on CT), infected ones should be treated like abscesses (percutaneous drainage).

    (2) Biliary ascites—explore, washout, attempt definitive repair over T-tube if necessary.

d. Hepatic artery pseudoaneurysm—result of untreated arterial injury, embolize if hemobilia (rupture into bile duct) or portal hypertension (rupture into portal vein) occurs.

## D. SPLEEN

**1.** Concern for the rare but often fatal overwhelming postsplenectomy infection from encapsulated bacteria has led to an increase in nonoperative management of splenic injuries, especially in pediatric trauma. Injury is easily graded on CT scan with IV contrast. If discovered operatively, decide between splenic repair (splenorrhaphy) or splenectomy. Practically speaking, the indication for partial splenectomy in this setting is rare.

2. Splenectomy—dissection is often done bluntly with fingers in the unstable patient with brisk bleeding from the left upper quadrant. Ideally, the sequence of dissection is as follows:

a. Divided splenocolic ligament

b. Lateral to the spleen, incise the peritoneum 1 to 2 cm lateral to the spleen starting inferiorly and extend posterior and superior to the esophagus.

c. Rotate spleen medially and dissect between the spleen and Gerota's fascia and the pancreas.

d. Ligate short gastrics and splenic hilar vessels (avoid the tail of the pancreas).

3. Splenic artery embolization—selective versus complete, area embolized will infarct and may result in chronic pain

4. Postoperative management—pneumococcal vaccine within 2 weeks of injury or immediately before patient is discharged

## E. PANCREAS AND DUODENUM

1. The key determinants of outcome include delay in diagnosis and the integrity of the pancreatic duct. Have a high index of suspicion based on mechanism (steering wheel, handlebar, or GSW to epigastrium). CT is only 70% to 80% sensitive and specific; look for subtle findings including fluid between splenic vein and the pancreatic body, fluid in the lesser sac, thickened left anterior renal fascia, or retroperitoneal blood or air. Amylase levels are unreliable for diagnosis within first 3 hours. Explore all patients operatively if pancreas injury suspected.

2. Duodenal hematoma (grade I)—main issue is bowel obstruction, if diagnosed on imaging: NPO, nasogastric tube decompression, repeat gastric emptying studies (small-bowel follow-through) every 5 days, use total parenteral nutrition if obstructed longer than 5 days, explore if remains obstructed longer than 14 days. If diagnosed with laparotomy, evacuate.

3. Duodenal laceration

a. Grades I-II—primary sutured closure in two layers. Consider pyloric exclusion if there is associated pancreas injury.

b. Grade III—primary suture repair when possible; when not possible, treatment based on location of injury.

   (1) Proximal to ampulla—antrectomy, gastrojejunostomy, stump closure

   (2) Distal to ampulla—Roux-en-Y duodenojejunostomy to proximal end of injury, oversew distal end

c. Grades IV-V—trauma Whipple

4. Pancreas injury

a. Exposure—open the lesser sac through the gastrocolic ligament just outside the gastroepiploic vessels, Kocher maneuver (see earlier), expose splenic hilum to see pancreatic tail. If needed, bluntly take down lateral splenic attachments with finger dissection and mobilize the spleen laterally, allowing bimanual palpation.

b. Grades I and II—goal is hemostasis and adequate drainage. If no duct injury seen, place JP drains and get out. Remove JP drains when drain amylase is less than serum amylase. Pancreatic fistula is defined by drain output persisting more than 3 days and amylase content $\geq 3\times$ serum amylase (see management of pancreatic fistula below).

c. Grade III—distal pancreatectomy
   (1) Perform stapled or with mattress sutures, but not both, because this increases ischemia. Some buttress the stump with an omental patch.
   (2) U-stitch the transected duct (absorbable vs. nonabsorbable sutures is controversial).
   (3) Place feeding jejunostomy for injuries with grade $\geq$ III; begin elemental tube feeds early.

d. Grade IV—if duct injury is indeterminate on local exploration, consider intraoperative pancreatic ductography either via needle into gallbladder or duodenotomy and ampulla cannulation.
   (1) Stable patient—oversew salvageable portion of proximal pancreas stump, Roux-en-Y anastomosis of distal pancreas to jejunal limb.
   (2) Unstable patient—get hemostasis, drain widely, get out. Postoperative endoscopic retrograde cholangiopancreatography to define injury and possibly place duct stent.
   (3) Consider pyloric exclusion.

e. Grade V—trauma Whipple; high morbidity and mortality rates

f. Postoperative management—complication rate for injuries to this organ are high (20–40%).
   (1) Fistula—minor (<200 ml/day) usually resolve, high-output fistulas (>700 ml/day) need endoscopic retrograde cholangiopancreatography to guide operative treatment or stenting. Octreotide decreases volume of output but not time to closure.
   (2) Pancreatitis/secondary hemorrhage—rare, may require reoperation or embolization.
   (3) Abscess—percutaneous drainage versus surgical debridement
   (4) Pseudocyst—results when duct injuries are missed or treated with external drains only; if persistent or painful, fenestrate into gastrointestinal tract (cystgastrostomy or cystojejunostomy)

## F. SMALL BOWEL (JEJUNUM AND ILEUM)

1. Suspect when CT shows significant intraperitoneal fluid without liver or splenic injury, or Chance fracture (thoracic or lumbar fracture dislocation)
2. Fix simple (grades I-II) injuries—single-layer Lembert sutures for serosal tears/hematomas, two-layer closure for injuries up to 50% of circumference if the closure will not significantly narrow the bowel lumen.
3. Resect complex injuries (grades III-V).
a. Usually stapled, functional side-to-side anastomosis for the sake of time
b. May need to create ostomy if delayed diagnosis, unstable patient

c. Preserve ileocecal valve if possible if significant length of bowel is being resected.

   (1) Less than 200-cm jejunum and ileum at risk for short-bowel syndrome

## G. COLON

1. Repair and resection with primary anastomosis have replaced resection and diversion as the treatment of choice for the majority of colon injuries. Diagnosis is straightforward at the time of laparotomy; other signs include stool from wound, blood from rectum.
2. Partial thickness (grade I)—seromuscular closure with silk sutures
3. Full thickness nondestructive (grades II-III)—repair by primary closure.
4. Destructive injury in stable patient (grades IV-V)—resect destroyed segment, do primary anastomosis (usually side-to-side stapled).
5. Destructive injury in unstable patient (transfusion of more than six units packed red blood cells, delayed diagnosis with fecal peritonitis, in shock)—resect with end colostomy (Hartmann's procedure) or resection with anastomosis and proximal diversion.
6. Postoperative management

a. Consider delayed primary closure of abdominal wound in the setting of gross stool spillage. The ideal time for delayed closure of these wounds is postoperative days 3 to 5, when wound bacterial counts have been found to be lowest. Secondary skin closure is also an option to avoid the risk for wound infection and subsequent hernia risk.

b. Colostomy takedown—usually wait until at least 3 months after injury to allow dense adhesions to thin, study distal end with contrast enema; first rule out distal strictures and fistulas.

## H. RECTUM

1. Most common mechanisms of injury include penetration with foreign object and GSW to the pelvis/buttocks or perineum. Digital rectal examination is mandatory looking for gross blood and palpating for rectal wall defect or hematoma. This should be followed by rigid sigmoidoscopy (easier done in the operating room than the emergency department) if injury is suspected.
2. Rectal injuries to peritonealized surfaces (anterior or lateral side walls of upper two thirds of rectum) should be treated just as colon injuries.
3. Rectal injuries to extraperitoneal surfaces (lower third and entire posterior rectum) are treated based on accessibility.

a. Most injuries can be accessed and repaired primarily—effectively, these become intraperitonealized from the dissection.

b. Perform diverting loop colostomy.

c. Distal rectal washout performed by lavaging distal limb of loop colostomy with liters of saline was popularized in Vietnam War injuries, but need for this is questionable based on current literature.

64

ABDOMINAL TRAUMA

d. If injury could not be accessed during exploratory laparotomy (narrow pelvis, excessive mesorectal fat, too low, etc.), place in lithotomy position and place presacral drains to prevent retroperitoneal abscess.
   (1) Curvilinear incision between anus and coccyx
   (2) Blunt dissection with finger in presacral space placing Penrose drains

## I. KIDNEY, URETERS, BLADDER (SEE CHAPTER 69)

1. Urology service is usually called for injuries to the genitourinary system.
2. Diagnosis: Suspect injury in the setting of hematuria, CT is the gold standard—get portal venous phase to see arterial bleeding and 10-minute delayed cuts to look for urinary extravasation.
3. Kidney: Consider the status of the contralateral kidney (Is it present? Does it enhance on contrast imaging?).
a. Grades I-II—observe, low risk for rebleeding.
b. Grades II-IV—observe stable patients with serial hematocrits. If active arterial bleeding but isolated injury, angiography and embolization.
c. Grades V and VI renovascular injuries
   (1) Operative exploration—gain renal artery control before opening Gerota's fascia.
   (2) Repair if possible, 4–0 absorbable sutures for collecting system defects, sharp debridement of injured cortex, hemostasis with topical agents if needed, closure of capsule, closed suction drainage of renal fossa, do not close Gerota's fascia.
   (3) Nephrectomy if not repairable
4. Ureter
a. Primary repair
   (1) Debride devitalized tissue.
   (2) Reapproximate watertight with full-thickness, spatulated, tension-free anastomosis over double J stent.
   (3) Cover repair with omentum pedicle when possible.
b. Transureteroureterostomy for proximal ureter injuries that cannot be repaired tension free
   (1) Injured ureter is passed behind the mesocolon to the contralateral side and anastomosed to a 1- to 2-cm opening in the medial side of the normal ureter with double J stent spanning anastomosis.
c. Bladder reimplantation
   (1) Ligate distal stump of injured ureter.
   (2) Bring the proximal end of the ureter through a new hiatus on the back wall of the bladder.
   (3) Spatulate ureter and approximate to the bladder mucosa with interrupted chromic sutures over a double J stent.
   (4) Place closed-suction retroperitoneal drain and leave Foley.
5. Bladder
a. Extraperitoneal injury—treat with Foley, no repair needed unless internal fixation of coexistent pelvic fracture planned.

b. Intraperitoneal injury repaired with 3–0 absorbable suture to close detrusor and mucosa in one layer. Place 20 Fr Foley for 7 days.

6. **Complications**

a. Kidney pseudoaneurysm with delayed hemorrhage—angiography and embolization

b. Urinoma—treat with percutaneous drainage.

## J. RETROPERITONEAL HEMATOMAS AND MAJOR VESSEL INJURIES

1. **Zone I (midline along aorta)—management for blunt and penetrating is the same.**

a. Superior to the transverse mesocolon

   (1) Exposure via left medial visceral rotation, divide left crus of diaphragm if needed for more superior exposure, clamp aorta proximally or use aorta compression device.

   (2) Small aorta injuries—repair with 3–0 Prolene or polytetrafluoroethylene graft.

   (3) Proximal left gastric, splenic, and common hepatic artery injuries can be ligated.

   (4) Superior mesenteric artery injuries—reimplant in distal aorta away from likely injured pancreas.

   (5) Proximal renal artery injuries—repair/reimplant if less than 4 hours from injury, otherwise ligate.

   (6) Superior mesenteric vein—repair with 5–0 Prolene if possible, leave abdomen open if superior mesenteric vein ligated.

b. Inferior to transverse mesocolon—aorta injury

   (1) Expose via retracting transverse colon superiorly, eviscerating small bowel to the right, opening midline retroperitoneum over distal aorta, and extending superiorly to left renal vein.

   (2) Repair primarily or with graft, cover with a viable omental pedicle to prevent aortoenteric fistula.

c. Inferior to mesocolon: IVC injury—suspect when bleeding from base of the mesentery of hepatic flexure or ascending colon or asymmetric hematoma (R > L).

   (1) Perform Cattell–Brasch maneuver to expose IVC, control hemorrhage with Satinsky clamp or gauze sponges.

   (2) Repair primarily with 4–0 Prolene or bovine pericardial patch.

   (3) Infrarenal IVC can be ligated in destructive injuries, but watch for leg compartment syndrome.

2. **Zone II (laterally including the kidneys)**

a. Blunt injury: The only reason to open a hematoma in this setting is if it is ruptured, pulsatile, or rapidly expanding, even if CT shows an injured kidney. Repair as in penetrating injury below.

b. Penetrating injury: Obtain proximal control of renal vessel with vessel loop first, then open hematoma and repair according to renal injury section above.

**64**

**ABDOMINAL TRAUMA**

**3.** Zone III (pelvis)

a. Blunt injury: Open hematoma only if ruptured, pulsatile, or rapidly expanding, or if there is loss of ipsilateral iliac or femoral pulse. Repair as in penetrating injury below.

b. Penetrating injury: Expose bifurcation of aorta and IVC. Control proximal iliac distal external iliac vessels with vessel loops, clamp internal iliac vessels, open hematoma, and attempt to repair.

(1) Ligation is simplest, quickest maneuver in setting of exsanguination, but it is associated with 50% amputation rate. This can be reduced by fem-fem crossover graft within 6 hours (see Chapter 33).

(2) Stable patients: Options based on extent of destruction include lateral arteriorrhaphy, bovine pericardium patch angioplasty, complete transection, and primary end-to-end anastomosis versus polytetrafluoroethylene graft.

(3) Unstable patient: Consider temporary intraluminal shunt (Argyle or Javid shunt), then definitive repair within 6 hours.

## VI. SPECIAL CIRCUMSTANCES

### A. ABDOMINAL COMPARTMENT SYNDROME

**1.** Adverse physiologic consequences of increased intraabdominal pressure (>25 mm Hg)

**2.** Risk factors include packing remaining in the abdomen after initial laparotomy, bowel edema caused by massive crystalloid resuscitation and/or reperfusion injury, ongoing intraabdominal bleeding, and primary fascial closure.

**3.** Diagnosis

a. Hypotension—impaired venous return (IVC kinking), impaired cardiac compliance, reduced cardiac output

b. Hypoxia and increased airway pressures—lung compression from elevated diaphragms decreases ventilation.

c. Oliguria—renal vein and parenchymal compression impairs renal function.

d. Monitor abdominal examination and intraabdominal pressures (transduced bladder pressure).

**4.** Treatment

a. Open the abdomen—at bedside if patient crashing or in the operating room urgently.

### B. PREGNANCY

**1.** These patients are hypervolumic at baseline, which thus can mask more significant blood loss before showing signs of shock. Their pelvic veins are enlarged, making them at greater risk in the setting of pelvic fractures. The fetus cannot survive without the mother—treat her first.

**2.** Initial assessment/diagnosis—place patient on left side or just elevate right hip as soon as safely possible from spinal standpoint to avoid caval compression by gravid uterus.

a. Volume status—liberal crystalloid and blood resuscitation for the sake of the fetus
b. Assess fundal height, uterine tenderness, vaginal bleeding, or amniotic fluid in vagina.
c. Look for fetal heartbeat and fetal movement during FAST examination.
d. Use radiography as indicated in nonpregnant patients; if DPL done, use open technique above the uterus.

**3. Operative treatment**

a. Uterine rupture—explore (with potential for emergency C-section) unstable patients or if imaging shows extended fetal extremities, abnormal fetal position, free intraperitoneal air.
b. Perimortem C-section—for more than 24 weeks' gestation, ideally perform starting 4 minutes after mother's cardiac arrest while cardiopulmonary resuscitation continues during and after C-section. Do not perform in unstable patient because of anticipated cardiac arrest.
   (1) One-pass midline incision from xiphoid to pubic symphysis
   (2) One-pass incision over uterus—get the baby out, clamp, and cut the cord (the neonatologist should already be there).

**4. Management**

a. Consult obstetrician on all pregnant trauma patients, although they may not monitor nonviable (<20 week) pregnancies.
b. If more than 20 weeks' gestation, cardiotocographic monitoring for minimum of 6 hours, longer if anything concerning such as contractions, nonreassuring heartbeat, or if mother is seriously injured. Watch for signs of placental abruption and disseminated intravascular coagulopathy.
c. Kleihauer–Betke test—blood test that measures fetal hemoglobin in mother's blood.
   (1) Used to dose of Rh immunoglobulin to inhibit formation of Rh antibodies in the Rh-negative mother

## C. RECENT DEVELOPMENTS

### 1. Hemostatic agents

a. Recombinant activated factor VII 60 to 90 $\mu$g/kg
   (1) Currently FDA approved to treat bleeding in hemophiliacs (not for trauma)
   (2) Anecdotal reports of miraculous cessation of bleeding with limiting nonconfirming prospective data, being used by U.S. military and in many civilian trauma centers
   (3) Extremely expensive (cost is about $4,500 for one-time dose for 80-kg patient) and should be used in salvageable patients (as defined by the trauma surgery attending) with ongoing medical bleeding despite aggressive conventional blood and blood product resuscitation
b. Quikclot—zeolite granules that absorb water, concentrate blood clotting factors, create exothermic reaction that can instantly stop audible bleeding (mainly used in the military but has been used successfully at the University of Cincinnati).

2. Permissive hypotension—new paradigm of titrating initial fluid resuscitation to mental status and tolerating systolic blood pressure in the 80 to 89 mm Hg range in penetrating trauma until source of hemorrhage is controlled in operating room.

## RECOMMENDED READING

American College of Surgeons: *ATLS Advanced Trauma Life Support Program for Doctors,* 7th ed.

Eastern Association for the Surgery of Trauma on line: Available at: east.org

Shilling AT, Gay SB, Wurth RJ: *Abdominal trauma.* Available at: http://www.med-ed.virginia.edu/courses/rad/abdtrauma. Accessed April 10, 2008.

Trauma.org online: Available at: Trauma.org

# Thoracic Trauma

*Steven R. Allen, MD*

## I. BRIEF HISTORY

### A. EGYPT (6000–3500 BC)
1. Surgeons performed various procedures including cataracts, amputations, and general wound care.

### B. EDWIN SMITH PAPYRUS (3000–1600 BC)
1. Surgical treatise of 48 cases of trauma to the entire body including thoracic injuries

### C. THE *ILIAD* (950 BC)
1. Homer described thoracic wounds.

### D. CLAUDE GALEN
1. Noted that left ventricular wounds were the most rapidly fatal of all cardiac wounds

### E. OTTO HOCHE
1. Noted that thoracic wounds comprised 6% of all injuries in World War I, with a 56% mortality rate

### F. RESUSCITATIVE THORACOTOMY
1. Developed by Schiff together with his promotion of open cardiac massage in 1874

### G. BLOCK
1. Suggested that thoracotomy may be applied to the repair of cardiac lacerations

### H. KOUWENHOVEN
1. Described closed cardiac compression in 1960, and afterwards, more selective approach to emergency thoracotomy was applied.

### I. EMERGENCY THORACOTOMY
1. Revisited by Beall in 1967 for "moribund" patients with penetrating chest trauma

## II. EPIDEMIOLOGY OF THORACIC TRAUMA

### A. THORACIC TRAUMA
1. Ranks third behind head and extremity trauma, with motor vehicle crashes being the most common causative factor in the United States

### B. BLACK MALE INDIVIDUALS
1. Have a 1 in 20 chance of being shot or stabbed before the age of 30 in urban America.

### C. MOTORCYCLE ACCIDENTS
1. 75% of fatally injured riders had a thoracic injury.

## III. PHYSICAL EXAMINATION OF THE CHEST
### A. POINT TENDERNESS
1. Clinical evidence of rib fractures
2. May not see rib fractures on plain chest radiograph

### B. FLAIL CHEST
1. Paradoxical breathing
2. Two or more segments of the same rib or more ribs that are fractured
3. Judicious fluid management
4. Patients may have an underlying pulmonary contusion.
5. Excellent candidates for an epidural block

### C. SUBCUTANEOUS EMPHYSEMA
1. Check for tracheal or esophageal injury and pneumothorax.

### D. DULL VERSUS RESONANT PERCUSSION
1. Hemothorax versus pneumothorax

### E. SEATBELT SIGNS
1. Seen across the chest, but pathology could be elsewhere

## IV. THE WIDENED MEDIASTINUM
### A. MAY SUGGEST AORTIC INJURY
1. 8 cm is the "textbook definition"

### B. CHEST RADIOGRAPHS
1. Largely unreliable if they are negative

### C. CT SCAN OF THE CHEST WITH IV CONTRAST
1. Should have a relatively low threshold to obtain in the appropriate patient
2. Appropriate to repeat the chest radiograph as an upright film if possible
3. The initial chest radiograph can be inadequate secondary to being an anteroposterior film while the patient is lying supine.

## V. PATHOPHYSIOLOGY OF THORACIC TRAUMA
### A. CONSEQUENCES SECONDARY TO THE RESULT OF EFFECTS ON RESPIRATORY AND HEMODYNAMIC FUNCTIONS
### B. DEATH SECONDARY TO IMPAIRMENT OF OXYGEN DELIVERY, TRANSPORT, OR BOTH

1. Pulmonary gas exchange
2. Cardiac output
3. Hemoglobin concentration
4. Oxygen-hemoglobin affinity

## C. THE TWO MAJOR INTERVENTIONS DURING RESUSCITATION ARE:
1. Ventilatory support
2. Control of hemorrhage

## D. BLUNT CARDIAC INJURIES
1. Obtain electrocardiogram because cardiac isoenzymes may not be diagnostic.
2. Observe for 24 hours in monitored setting if arrhythmias; most common are tachyarrhythmias.
3. Echocardiogram is diagnostic study of choice.

## E. BLUNT AORTIC INJURIES
1. Majority of aortic transections occur just distal to the take-off of the left subclavian artery.
2. Most (85%) people with blunt aortic injuries exsanguinate at the scene, and those who make it to the hospital have a significant risk for rupture.
a. Must have aggressive blood pressure and heart rate control with agents such as esmolol to keep systolic blood pressure less than 110 mm Hg and heart rate ~60 beats/min
3. Computed tomographic scan is thought to be the best way to make the diagnosis of blunt aortic injury.
4. Aortic disruption may be also be diagnosed by several radiographic clues.
a. Tracheoesophageal deviation
b. Left mainstem bronchial depression
c. Left apical capping
d. Wide mediastinum
e. Mediastinal hematoma with contrast extravasation
5. Contraindications to immediate repair
a. Unstable patients with intraabdominal injuries requiring emergent laparotomy
b. Severe closed head injuries requiring craniotomy
c. Patients who cannot withstand single lung ventilation
d. Patients who are unable to systemically anticoagulate while on cardiopulmonary bypass
e. Those who cannot tolerate intracranial pressure because of cross-clamping
f. Inability to reposition the patient because of other associated injuries
6. Traditional management involves emergent posterolateral thoracotomy and replacement of the injured segment of aorta with a prosthetic graft.

**65**

**THORACIC TRAUMA**

7. A few small studies and case series have reported endovascular repair of the injured aorta as a safe, viable option.
   a. Does not require systemic anticoagulation
   b. The need for single lung ventilation is avoided.
   c. Positioning of the patient is also less of an issue in patients with multiple injuries.
   d. Early and delayed type I endoleaks have been reported.
   e. Long-term data are not available.

## F. DIAPHRAGM INJURIES
1. Presentation
   a. Occurs in ~2% to 4% of all abdominal injuries
   b. Likely occurs with equal frequency between blunt and penetrating injuries, although historical reports would favor blunt injuries over penetrating trauma
   c. Requires high index of suspicion to diagnose
   d. Dyspnea, orthopnea, chest pain—can have referred pain to scapula.
   e. Gastric distention with ipsilateral lung collapse in extreme situations
   f. Diagnosis can be difficult; however, several studies may be used.
      (1) Look for nasogastric tube in left hemithorax on chest radiograph.
      (2) Computed tomographic scan
      (3) Fluoroscopy—mobility of left hemidiaphragm (most commonly injured)
      (4) Bowel sounds in the chest on auscultation
      (5) Cardiac displacement
2. Repair
   a. Early diagnosis—repair via laparotomy with horizontal mattress sutures; recommend nonabsorbable monofilament, but almost any permanent suture will suffice.
   b. Late diagnosis—repair via thoracotomy, laparoscopic or open; less scar tissue to deal with.

## G. DECELERATION INJURY
1. Hemothorax, great vessel injury, and lung contusion
2. Severity of injury related to impact velocity, type of impact, and adequacy of restraint.
3. Profound deceleration causes the heart to swing on the aorta, tearing the great vessels.
4. Most commonly just distal to the ligamentous attachment of the descending aorta to the left pulmonary artery
5. May disrupt bronchi, leading to pneumothorax

## H. CRUSH INJURY
1. Compression of the myocardium between sternum and vertebrae
   a. Contusion, rupture, or possible great vessel disruption
   b. Cardiac valve injuries caused by shearing or crushing forces

## I. PENETRATING TRAUMA

1. Results in localized anatomic disruption to blood vessels
a. Injuries within "the box"—heart and great vessel involvement likely

**Pearl:** *"The box" anatomically is medial to the nipples and between the costal margin and clavicles.*

2. Track of projectile may be difficult to predict despite entry and exit wounds.
3. High-velocity projectiles (>1000 feet/sec) produce profound tissue damage.
4. Hemorrhage
a. Arterial bleeding may stop by arterial retraction and vasoconstriction.
b. Venous bleeding may arrest by tamponade as intravenous pressure decreases.
c. Identified and treated most often with tube thoracostomy
   (1) Surgical exploration warranted if initial output exceeds 1500 ml blood or if drainage is more than 250 ml/hr for 3 consecutive hours.
5. Pericardial tamponade may occur secondary to myocardial laceration or injury to the coronary vessels.
a. Results in decreased right atrioventricular filling, which leads to decreased cardiac output
b. Systemic hypotension, tachycardia, distended neck veins, and muffled heart tones are all pathognomonic
c. Early stage: Filling pressures maintained by aggressive fluid resuscitation maintaining blood pressure and overcoming the effect of the tamponade
d. Late stage: Precipitous and profound hypotension because patient is no longer able to compensate
6. Pneumothorax
a. If entry is smaller than glottis, the pneumothorax is usually small and ventilation is preserved.
b. However, if larger than the glottis, the air will pass preferentially through the injury site, leading to a large pneumothorax.
7. Air embolism (estimated incidence rate of 4–14%) caused by direct communication between blood vessels and airways or parenchyma.
a. Catastrophic if air embolizes to the cerebral arteries, coronaries, or heart chambers
b. May lead to sudden circulatory collapse after tracheal intubation and initiation of positive pressure ventilation
c. Unexplained neurologic deficits or seizures may indicate a cerebral air embolism.
d. If associated with unilateral lung injury, treat with immediate thoracotomy and placement of clamp around the hilum to prevent further passage of air into the systemic circulation.
e. Selective ventilation of the uninjured lung may also be life saving.

**65**

**THORACIC TRAUMA**

8. Emergent thoracotomy: Considered only if loss of vital signs and induction of cardiopulmonary resuscitation for less than 5 minutes in nonintubated patients and less than 10 minutes in intubated patients.

a. Major review of the literature by the American College of Surgeons Committee on Trauma revealed a survival rate of 11.2% with penetrating trauma and only 1.6% for blunt trauma.

  (1) Overall survival rate of 13% in penetrating trauma in a series of 2400 patients, which is an optimistic figure that excludes those with neurologic catastrophes; gunshot wounds have 7% survival rate; stab wounds have 18% survival rate

  (2) Survival in the pediatric population—stab wounds, 9%; gunshot wounds, 4%; blunt trauma, 2%

b. Stab wounds have a much better prognosis than gunshot wounds.

  (1) Pericardial tamponade is a protective mechanism, especially with stab wounds.

c. Most helpful in those with penetrating cardiac injuries who have physiologic collapse caused by pericardial tamponade

d. Technique of emergency department thoracotomy

  (1) Patient in supine position with side to be operated on elevated with a towel roll by 15 degrees

    (a) Left-sided thoracotomy for resuscitation

  (2) Both arms at right angles to the torso

  (3) Anterolateral incision at fifth intercostal space is made with a scalpel from sternum to the table (inframammary fold). The intercostal muscles are incised with curved Mayo scissors.

  (4) The rib spreader is inserted spreading the rib interspace (handle toward the axilla).

  (5) Grasp the pericardium with toothed pickups and incise the pericardium anterior to the phrenic nerve; incise cranial and caudad.

    (a) This relieves tamponade, allows direct cardiac massage, and allows access to the heart for any direct injuries.

      (1) Internal cardiac massage: Hinged clapping motion of the hands with wrists apposed

      (2) Internal defibrillation: 15 to 30 J

      (3) Sutures or staples may be used to close cardiac injuries.

  (6) The descending aorta may be cross-clamped and the pulmonary hilum may also be cross-clamped or the lung twisted to stem hemorrhage.

    (a) Aortic cross-clamping should not exceed 30 minutes.

    (b) Aortic declamping is associated with sudden reperfusion.

      (1) Release of inflammatory mediators into the cardiopulmonary system

  (7) The thoracotomy may be extended across the sternum to the right side (clam shell), allowing better access to the heart and the opposite chest cavity.

(8) Factors leading to discontinuation of resuscitation during thoracotomy; that is, "when to stop"
  (a) Systolic blood pressure less than 70 mm Hg after 15 minutes despite fluid resuscitation.
  (b) Self-sustaining rhythm is not achieved within 15 minutes of thoracotomy.
  (c) Aortic cross-clamping results in increased blood pressure proximal to cross-clamp to restore coronary and cerebral perfusion.
  (d) Absence of pericardial effusion without cardiac activity on entering the chest.
  (e) Evidence of other devastating injuries (such as massive head injury) with independently poor prognoses.

## VI. OTHER THORACIC PROCEDURES IN THE FACE OF TRAUMA

### A. FAST (FOCUSED ASSESSMENT WITH SONOGRAPHY FOR TRAUMA) EXAMINATION
1. Able to detect pericardial or peritoneal fluid
2. Allows expeditious surgical intervention
3. No ionizing radiation, so may repeat as many times as necessary

### B. PERICARDIOCENTESIS
1. Useful in a stable patient
2. Beck's triad—distended neck veins, muffled heart sounds, hypotension
3. Take off the cervical collar to examine the neck; muffled heart sounds may be difficult to appreciate in the trauma bay.
4. If pericardial effusion or tamponade, the patient likely requires a pericardial window (Trinkle procedure) or pericardial exploration.
5. Able to transport to the operating room for urgent thoracotomy
6. May benefit from at least partial relief of an acute pericardial tamponade

### C. SUBXIPHOID PERICARDIOTOMY
1. Also suitable in the stable patient with suspected pericardial tamponade
2. More easily able to evacuate clotted pericardial blood
3. Downside may be that it releases the tamponade without adequate control of the injury.

### D. BOTH PROCEDURES BELIEVED TO BE OBSOLETE BY SOME BECAUSE OF THE USE OF ULTRASOUND (FAST).
1. May be useful in the face of delayed or septic pericardial effusion after trauma
2. Also appropriate diagnostic tools for suspected cardiac injury with questionable signs and symptoms

### E. THORACOSCOPY
1. Assessment and examination of thoracic structures in elective procedures

a. Evacuation of clotted hemothoraces
b. Assessment of injuries to the diaphragm
c. Examination of the pericardium
d. Control of chest wall or intrathoracic bleeding

## VII. POSTOPERATIVE CARE OF THE PATIENT WITH A CHEST INJURY

### A. CONDITIONS OF PATIENTS WITH PULMONARY CONTUSIONS

1. Likely will worsen over 48 to 72 hours before they improve clinically because the contusion tends to evolve over that time
2. Aggressive ventilator support may be required with conversion to a pressure control mode and greater positive end-expiratory pressure to maintain adequate oxygenation and ventilation, and reduce long-term injury to the lungs.

### B. CHEST TUBE MANAGEMENT
(See Chapter 76, "Placement of Chest Tubes")

1. Chest tubes remain on suction ($-10$ to $-20$ cm $H_2O$) until the resultant air leak has resolved. This may take hours to days.
a. Dependent on the nature of the injury such as a simple pneumothorax versus large parenchymal injury
2. Chest tubes to water seal once air leak has resolved
3. Chest radiograph is obtained 4 hours after water seal to identify recurrent pneumothorax; if a pneumothorax recurs, then the chest tube is placed back on suction.
4. Chest tube output should be less than 100 ml/shift for 24 hours.
5. If these criteria are met, then it is usually safe to remove the chest tube.
6. Typically, a chest radiograph is not obtained after the chest tube is removed, unless the patient decompensates clinically.

## VIII. COMPLICATIONS OF THORACIC TRAUMA

### A. POSSIBLE COMPLICATIONS
Of blunt and penetrating thoracic trauma

1. Persistent air leak
a. May require video-assisted thoracoscopic surgery to staple off the injured portion of lung to seal the air leak
2. Bronchopleural fistula
3. Empyema
a. Often a result of the gross contamination from an open chest wound.
b. May also be a result of chest tubes placed in an emergent situation where the sterile technique may have been broken
4. Retained hemothorax
a. Results from inadequate chest tube drainage
b. May be treated with tissue plasminogen activator infusion via the chest tube to fibrinolyse the retained clot

(1) A protocol of 4 doses of tissue plasminogen activator over a 48-hour period has been shown to produce good results.

(2) If tissue plasminogen activator fails, then video-assisted thoracoscopic surgery versus open thoracotomy for drainage and decortication may be necessary.

5. **Acute respiratory distress syndrome—patchy bilateral infiltrates on chest radiograph, $P(Pao_2):F(Fio_2)$ ratio less than 200, noncardiogenic**

a. May result from the systemic response to significant injury

b. Significant pulmonary contusions may also evolve into acute respiratory distress syndrome.

c. Results in significantly reduced compliance of the lungs

(1) May require increased positive end-expiratory pressure and $Fio_2$ to maintain oxygenation

(2) Pressure control ventilation to minimize/optimize peak airway pressures, which often increase significantly in the face of decreased lung compliance

(3) Placing the patient in a prone position may also be beneficial.

## RECOMMENDED READING

Esme H, Solak O, Sahin DA, Sezer M: Blunt and penetrating traumatic ruptures of the diaphragm. *Thorac Cardiovasc Surg* 54:324–327, 2005.

Hirschberg A, Mattox KL: *Top knife: the art and craft of trauma surgery.* Shropshire, United Kingdom, TFM Publishing Co. 2005.

Hoornweg LL, Dinkelman MK, Goslings JC, et al: Endovascular management of traumatic ruptures of the thoracic aorta: A retrospective multicenter analysis of 28 cases in the Netherlands. *J Vasc Surg* 43:1096–1102, 2006.

Hunt PA, Greaves I, Owens WA: Emergency thoracotomy in thoracic trauma—a review. *Injury* 37:1–19, 2006.

Simeone A, Freitas M, Frankel HL: Management options in blunt aortic injury: A case series and literature review. *Am Surg* 72:25–30, 2006.

65

THORACIC TRAUMA

# Orthopedic Emergencies

*R. Michael Greiwe, MD*

The evaluation of a trauma patient involves attention to all body systems including the musculoskeletal system. Careful evaluation of fractures, dislocations, injuries to the neural and vascular systems, and intraarticular wounds are important parts of the orthopedic examination. A complete and systematic evaluation of every body part and joint must be performed. This chapter outlines how to evaluate orthopedic injuries/emergencies that may arise during the evaluation of a trauma patient.

## I. EVALUATION OF THE FRACTURED LIMB

Each identified fracture can be classified by the following scheme. The following descriptors determine the prognosis of a given fracture and are extremely useful when orthopedic consultation is required.

### A. OPEN VERSUS CLOSED FRACTURE
### B. NAME OF FRACTURED BONE
### C. LOCATION OF THE FRACTURE (FIG. 66-1)
1. Diaphyseal (shaft) versus metaphyseal (near the articular surface)
2. Intraarticular versus extraarticular

### D. STATUS OF THE SOFT TISSUE
1. Bullae present?
2. Ecchymosis
3. Laceration
4. Multiple excoriations ("road rash")
5. Degloving injury
6. Swelling (wrinkles present or absent in skin)

### E. DESCRIPTORS (TELL ABOUT THE ENERGY OF INJURY)
1. Pattern (transverse, oblique, spiral, comminuted; Fig. 66-2)
a. Helps determine mechanism of force transmission
2. Displacement
3. Angulation
4. Rotation
5. Length
6. Presence of comminution (multiple fragments)

## II. OPEN FRACTURES

Open fractures are a true orthopedic emergency. They require immediate attention and can have devastating sequelae in the otherwise healthy patient.

### A. DEFINITION
1. Fracture in which a breach in the skin communicates directly with a fracture or its hematoma. An archaic synonym is a "compound fracture."

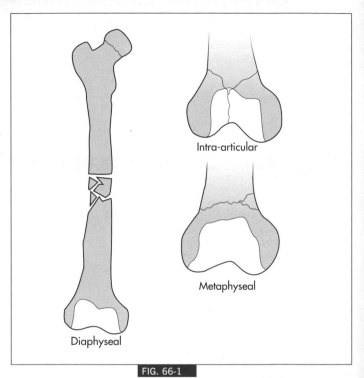

**FIG. 66-1**

Location of fractures.

## B. COMPLICATIONS OF OPEN FRACTURES INCLUDE:

1. Delayed healing or nonhealing of fractures
2. Infection (soft tissue or osteomyelitis)
3. Multiple surgeries
4. Longer recovery time
5. Injuries to nerves and vascular structures

## C. CLASSIFICATION SYSTEM

1. A useful classification system for open fractures is the Gustilo–
   Anderson classification system (Table 66-1). This system is used
   worldwide to assist with the management and prognosis of open
   fractures.

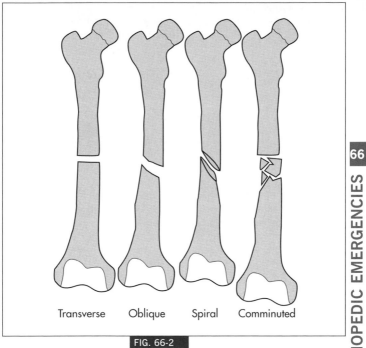

Transverse    Oblique    Spiral    Comminuted

FIG. 66-2

Patterns of fractures.

66

ORTHOPEDIC EMERGENCIES

## D. EMERGENCY DEPARTMENT MANAGEMENT OF OPEN FRACTURES

**1.** History—mechanism of trauma and geographic location of open injury

a. Barnyard

b. Asphalt

c. Athletic field

TABLE 66-1

GUSTILO-ANDERSON CLASSIFICATION SYSTEM

| Open Fracture Grade | Wound Defect |
| --- | --- |
| Grade I | <1-cm laceration |
| Grade II | >1-cm, <10-cm laceration |
| Grade IIIa | >10-cm laceration, no soft-tissue defect |
| Grade IIIb | Soft-tissue defect requiring flap coverage |
| Grade IIIc | Any open injury with vascular compromise |

**2. Clinical evaluation**

a. Other injuries—caused by the high energy required for an open fracture, one must be vigilant for other fractures/injuries. Smaller injuries are easy to miss.

b. Size of laceration

c. Neurovascular evaluation—evaluate always when patient is awake.

**3. Acute treatment**

a. Hemorrhage control (point pressure only, no tourniquet)

b. Tetanus

    (1) Tetanus toxoid should be given to anyone who has not received a booster in 5 years.

    (2) No immunizations suspected? Must give tetanus immunoglobulin.

c. Antibiotics

    (1) Gustilo I and II—first-generation cephalosporins

    (2) Gustilo III and severely contaminated wounds—first-generation cephalosporin and aminoglycoside

    (3) Barnyard-type contamination—first-generation cephalosporin, aminoglycoside, and penicillin G

    (4) Suggested dosages:

        (a) Cefazolin—1 g every 6 hours

        (b) Gentamicin—2.5 mg/kg every 12 hours

        (c) Penicillin G—2 million units every 4 hours; used for barnyard injury for Clostridial coverage.

d. Irrigation and debridement

    (1) All visible debris should be removed from the wound.

    (2) Irrigation with 3 L normal saline should be performed.

    (3) Provisional stabilization with splints or traction should be administered.

e. Formal irrigation and debridement in operating room—should be performed within 8 hours of injury, and sooner if vascular compromise is present.

f. Relative indications for primary amputation in open fractures

    (1) Complete disruption of posterior tibial nerve in adults

    (2) Crush injuries with warm ischemia time longer than 6 hours

    (3) Severe ipsilateral foot trauma

    (4) Anticipated protracted course in soft-tissue coverage and bony reconstruction, which patient will not tolerate

    (5) Crush injury to muscles and skin with complete neurovascular injury

    (6) Insensate limb with intact vascular system but limited motor function

## III. COMPARTMENT SYNDROME

**A. DEFINITION**

**1.** Compartment syndrome is characterized by increased pressure within a closed space that potentially causes irreversible damage to the contents of that space (i.e., nerves, muscles).

## B. MECHANISM
1. Anything that can increase external pressures on a closed space or diminishes the volume of the space.

## C. CAUSES OF COMPARTMENT SYNDROME
1. Extracompartmental hematoma
2. Cast or external compressive dressings
3. Intracompartmental hematoma
4. Fractures
5. Military antishock trousers
6. Reperfusion injury secondary to ischemia
7. Burns—increased capillary permeability

## D. PATHOPHYSIOLOGY
1. Increased tissue pressure leads to decreased or absent capillary perfusion pressure, which causes ischemia to muscles and nerves within the fascial compartment.
2. Amount of tissue damage is proportional to the amount of *pressure* and the amount of *time* exposed to a certain pressure.

## E. SEQUELAE
1. Can be devastating—permanent loss of motor/sensation
2. One should always be suspicious of compartment syndrome because of its devastating consequences.

## F. EARLIEST HISTORY/PHYSICAL EXAMINATION FINDINGS
1. Pain increases steadily throughout process until nerves begin to die.
2. Tense swollen compartment—when palpated, reproduces pain
a. Possible to miss a deep compartment syndrome with this test
3. Passive stretch test
a. Stretch muscle bellies inside compartment by moving the joints they move.
b. Clinical example—compartment syndrome of deep posterior compartment of leg. Passively flex and extend toes. If painful, consideration is made for compartment syndrome because these muscle bellies originate from the deep posterior compartment.
4. Late findings (disastrous implications to muscles/nerves)
a. Absent sensation/motor from a nerve traversing the compartment
b. Absent or weak motor function
c. Pulselessness

*Clinical Pearls:*

1. Palpable pulses are present even in face of compartment syndrome and should not be relied on for diagnosis of compartment syndrome.

66

ORTHOPEDIC EMERGENCIES

2. Distinguish between compartment syndrome and injury to nerves or vessels.
3. Fasciotomy is the only cure for compartment syndrome; one should have a high index of suspicion and act accordingly if this diagnosis is considered.

## G. COMPARTMENT MONITORING
### 1. Indications
a. Unconscious patient with suspicions for compartment syndrome
b. Equivocal findings on physical examination
### 2. Types of monitoring systems
a. Solid-state transducer intracompartmental catheter (Stryker, Ace)—handheld device that allows quick and simple measurement of compartment pressure
b. Arterial line setup—easily accessible in all surgical intensive care units and most emergency departments.
c. Pressures within 30 mm Hg of diastolic blood pressure or pressures greater than 25 mm Hg are reasons for fasciotomies.
### 3. Indication for fasciotomy

**Clinical Scenario:** *A 59-year-old man is involved in a motorcycle crash. He was combative and intubated at the scene. His blood pressure is 100/60 mm Hg, pulse is 120. Among other orthopedic injuries, you note a comminuted, right bicondylar tibial plateau fracture. You are concerned for compartment syndrome. His right lower leg compartments are swollen, but you cannot obtain an examination. You use an arterial line and note a pressure of 35 mm Hg in the deep posterior compartment. What should you do?*

**Answer:** *Take the patient for emergent fasciotomy of the right leg and external fixation of his bicondylar tibial plateau fracture.*

**Reasoning:** *Compartment syndrome can occur when the intracompartmental pressure reaches within 30 mm Hg of the diastolic pressure. In this scenario, the pressure was within 25 mm Hg of the diastolic pressure.*

## H. MOST COMMON LOCATION FOR COMPARTMENT SYNDROME—LOWER LEG, DEEP POSTERIOR COMPARTMENT
### 1. Must open all four compartments of the lower leg:
a. Anterior compartment
b. Posterior compartment
c. Anterolateral compartment
d. Deep posterior compartment
### 2. Two-incision technique (Fig. 66-3)
a. Uses two vertical incisions separated by skin bridge of at least 7 cm

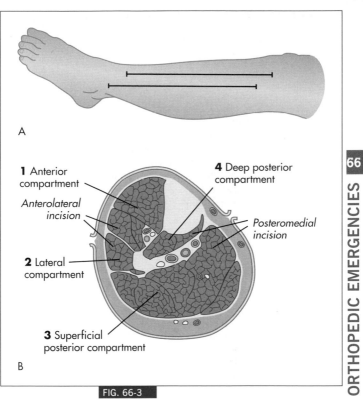

**1** Anterior compartment

*Anterolateral incision*

**2** Lateral compartment

**4** Deep posterior compartment

*Posteromedial incision*

**3** Superficial posterior compartment

A

B

**FIG. 66-3**

Compartments of the lower extremity.

b. Center lateral incision over anterior and anterolateral compartments.
c. Medial incision is located 2 cm posterior to posteromedial border of tibia.
d. Release underlying fascia.

### IV. PELVIC FRACTURES

A frequent situation seen in the emergency department is a patient with hypotension with multiple injuries and pelvic fractures on the typical anteroposterior pelvis radiograph taken as part of the trauma series. This situation is also an orthopedic emergency with dire consequences if the patient's pelvis is not stabilized and bleeding controlled.

## A. EVALUATION OF PELVIC RING FRACTURES

### 1. History

a. Frequently result from high-energy trauma
  (1) Motor vehicle collision—57% of cases
  (2) Pedestrian struck—18% of cases
  (3) Motorcycle collision—9% of cases
  (4) Falls—9% of cases
  (5) Crush—4% of cases

### 2. Physical examination

a. Rule out open fracture (rectal and vaginal examination on all patients).
b. Inspect for hematoma, hemorrhage, contusions.
c. Leg length or rotational discrepancies
d. Rotational stability test—pelvic compression across anterior iliac spines; do not repeat if positive findings.
e. Vertical stability test—push/pull evaluation to determine vertical stability

### 3. Radiographs

a. Anteroposterior pelvis—recommended as an ASTLS diagnostic adjunct for use in resuscitation of patients with blunt trauma.
b. Inlet view—used to assess posterior displacement of sacroiliac joints, sacrum, iliac wing, and rotational deformities of the sacrum and ilium.
c. Outlet view—used to assess vertical displacement and evaluate the sacral foramina.
d. Judet views—used to evaluate acetabular fractures.
  (1) Obturator oblique—evaluates anterior column and posterior wall.
  (2) Iliac oblique—visualizes the posterior column and anterior wall.
e. CT scan pelvis—obtained in conjunction with abdominal CT scan evaluates posterior pelvis and acetabulum.

### 4. Associated injuries

a. Urologic injuries (15%)—20% bladder rupture, 10% urethral injury
  (1) Physical examination findings
    (a) Blood at meatus
    (b) "Floating" or "high-riding" prostate
  (2) Diagnostic test—retrograde urethrogram before Foley insertion in all male patients with anterior pelvic ring fractures
  (3) Note: Female patients have a shorter urethra, and it is less commonly injured; therefore, no urethrogram is necessary.
b. Hemorrhage—frequently results in massive blood loss into retroperitoneal space
  (1) Signs
    (a) Gray–Turner sign—flank ecchymosis
    (b) Cullen sign—periumbilical ecchymosis
    (c) "Vervet monkey" sign—sign of hemorrhage into scrotal sac
  (2) Most common major vessels injured—internal iliac system (venous)

c. Gastrointestinal injury—open fractures and parenchymal injuries are common because of the close anatomic nature of these structures. Open fractures with gastrointestinal contamination require diverting colostomy. Mortality rate is close to 50%.
   (1) Infrequently, intestinal obstruction can occur from entrapment within the fracture.
d. Neurologic injury—associated with injury to sciatic and sacral nerves as they exit the lumbosacral plexus

# Burn Care

*Brian S. Pan, MD*

In the United States, approximately 1 million people annually seek care for burn injuries. Sadly, more than 90% of these injuries are preventable, the majority of which are related to smoking and substance abuse. Since the 1970s, the number of burn deaths has decreased yearly, as well as the mortality associated with larger burns. The advent of large trauma and burn centers has not only improved survival but also the cosmetic and functional outcome because of a multidisciplinary, multispecialty team approach to patient care.

## I. CAUSATIVE FACTORS

### A. SCALDS
1. Most common type of burn injury
2. Usually from hot water
a. Exacerbated by overlying garments that prolong contact
3. Common burn injury seen in child abuse
a. *Distribution exhibits a "dip" line pattern.*

### B. FLAME
1. Second most common type of burn injury
2. Full-thickness burns are common given the flammability of overlying garments.

### C. FLASH
1. Related to the explosion of flammable liquids and gases

### D. CONTACT
1. Result from contact with heated or cooled objects.
2. Seen frequently in industrial and trauma-related accidents

## II. INDICATIONS FOR HOSPITAL ADMISSION

### A. OUTPATIENT SETTING
1. Select burn cases can be managed as outpatients.
2. Must be seen and examined by an experienced practitioner
3. Availability of close follow-up care
4. Adequate social support for wound care
5. Burn wounds greater than 5% to 10% total body surface area (TBSA) should be referred to a burn center for evaluation.

### B. BURN UNIT SETTING
Admission to a burn unit is indicated in the following situations based on the guidelines of the American Burn Association injury severity grading system:
1. Partial- and full-thickness burns of more than 10% TBSA in patients younger than 10 or older than 50 years

2. Partial- and full-thickness burns of more than 20% TBSA in any other age group
3. Full-thickness burns greater than 5% in any age group
4. Involvement of the face, hands, feet, or perineum
5. Presence of electrical, chemical, or inhalation injury
6. High-risk factors—age older than 65 years, younger than 3 years; preexisting medical problems; multitrauma
7. Suspicion of abuse or neglect

## III. INITIAL MANAGEMENT

Initial management is immediately directed toward resuscitation, stabilization, and a thorough evaluation of all potential injuries. This process should be conducted in a systematic fashion according to the Advanced Trauma and Life Support protocols.

### A. HISTORY

1. Ascertain the circumstances associated with the injury.
a. History of unconsciousness, arrest, and the report given by the first responders
    (1) Avoid immediate concentration on the burn injuries alone.
2. Burn agent—flame, scald, chemical, electrical
3. Open versus closed space—to assess the possibility of inhalation injury
4. Time of burn—important for calculating adequate resuscitation
5. Prehospital treatment administered and vital signs during transport—patients are often found to be overresuscitated or underresuscitated.
6. Medical history—allergies, immunizations, current medications, and concomitant medical problems

### B. AIRWAY/BREATHING

1. Ensure adequacy of the airway
a. Prophylactic intubation/tracheostomy indicated for the following conditions:
    (1) Significant inhalation injury
    (2) Extensive (>60%) burns
    (3) Deep facial burns
    (4) Supraglottic obstruction
    (5) Extensive facial fractures
    (6) Closed head injury with unconsciousness
2. Inhalation injury—major contributor to mortality
a. Carbon monoxide (CO) poisoning—CO displaces oxygen and binds hemoglobin, forming carboxyhemoglobin.
b. Poor oxygen delivery is the result.
    (1) Diagnosis—signs and symptoms of hypoxia and/or serum carboxyhemoglobin level greater than 10% (nonsmokers) or greater than 20% (smokers) are diagnostic.

(2) Levels of 40% to 50% are not uncommon in survivors with aggressive care.
(3) *Oxygen saturation levels are normal despite high levels of carboxyhemoglobin.*
(4) Treatment—100% $O_2$ reduces half-life of CO.
   (a) Follow with carboxyhemoglobin levels and continue to treat until levels are 10% to 15%.
   (b) Persistent metabolic acidosis despite adequate volume resuscitation implies CO poisoning of cellular respiration.
(5) Treatment with hyperbaric oxygen may be of theoretical advantage but is often logistically difficult.
(6) Carboxyhemoglobin levels greater than 50% are potentially lethal.
(7) *CO has a 200 times greater affinity for hemoglobin and cytochromes than oxygen.*

c. Results from exposure to carbon monoxide, chemical irritants, and toxic gases
   (1) Rarely is inhalation injury caused by thermal injury (exception is superheated steam).
   (2) Suspect inhalation injury if the following are present:
      (a) Closed-space injury (e.g., house fire)
      (b) Presence of facial burns, singed nasal hairs, bronchorrhea, carbonaceous sputum, wheezing and rales, tachypnea, progressive hoarseness, and difficulty clearing secretions

d. Upper airway—obstruction may occur within the ensuing 48 hours (maximal edema ~24 hours).

e. Lower airway—pulmonary edema and chemical tracheobronchitis caused by noxious gases.

f. Diagnostic modalities—any concern for inhalation injury should mandate intubation.
   (1) Upper airway—perform direct laryngoscopy looking for carbon deposits, airway edema, and oropharyngeal burns.
   (2) Lower airway—perform fiberoptic bronchoscopy looking for gross airway edema, carbon deposits in tracheobronchial tree, and mucosal erythema and necrosis.

g. Treatment—implement immediate $O_2$ supplementation, ventilatory assistance, aggressive pulmonary toilet, $O_2$ saturation monitor, placement of an arterial line for serial arterial blood gases, bronchodilators, and bronchioalveolar lavage to remove debris.
   (1) *Corticosteroids and antibiotics have not been shown to decrease morbidity or mortality.*

## C. BURN EVALUATION

The patient should be totally exposed, and any burned clothing and constricting jewelry removed.

### 1. Depth of the burn wound

a. First degree—only the epidermal layer is involved.

67

BURN CARE

(1) Painful to palpation

(2) Pink in appearance without blistering

b. Second degree (partial thickness)—the dermal layer is only partially involved.

(1) Painful to palpation

(2) White to pink in appearance; blebs and blisters may be present.

(3) Deeper burns result in the destruction of epidermal appendages.

(a) Spontaneous reepithelialization is markedly delayed (similar to third-degree injury).

c. Third degree (full thickness)—entire dermal layer affected

(1) All dermal appendages destroyed.

(2) The area is insensate.

(3) White, black, or red in appearance with a dry and leathery (inelastic) texture

d. Fourth degree—the underlying fascia, muscle, and/or bone is involved.

**2.** *The estimate of the TBSA of the burn injury is the sum of second- and third-degree burns only.*

**3.** *Epithelialization occurs in partial-thickness burns from epithelial cells surrounding hair follicles or sweat glands (skin appendages) and from the wound edges.*

**4.** Size estimation (Fig. 67-1).

a. The "rule of 9s" approximates the size of the affected area.

(1) 9% head and neck

(2) 9% each upper extremity

(3) 18% each lower extremity

(4) 18% anterior trunk

(5) 18% posterior trunk

(6) 1% perineum

b. Children have a proportionally larger head and trunk with a smaller lower body (refer to Fig. 67-1 for percentages).

c. Calculate TBSA (71.84 × weight [kg] × height [cm]) or use a standard nomogram.

## D.  FLUID RESUSCITATION

**1.** Access

a. Initially, two large-bore (>18-gauge) peripheral catheters can be used even if the access site has been burned.

b. Central venous access—more suitable than peripheral catheters for long-term use and if vasopressors are needed for hemodynamic instability

c. Central venous pressure or pulmonary catheters are used in patients with cardiac or pulmonary disease, questionable fluid status, or hemodynamic instability.

(1) Catheters are routinely changed via a Seldinger technique every 48 hours, and a new site is established every 96 hours at our institution.

d. In children, femoral or jugular insertion sites are preferred given the risk for pneumothorax with a subclavian approach.

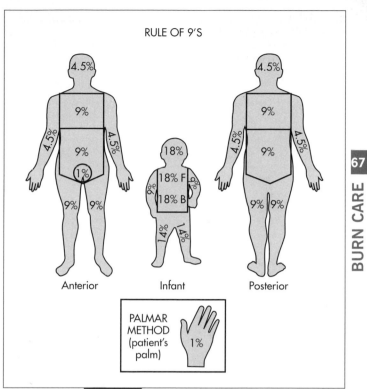

**FIG. 67-1**

Estimation of burn surface area by Rule of 9's.

2. Formulas for fluid resuscitation—multiple formulas and resuscitation schemes have been devised; however, the Parkland formula is the most widely used.

a. *Parkland formula:* This resuscitation scheme uses lactated Ringer's (LR) solution at 4 ml/kg/% burn, with half the total volume given over the first 8 hours (calculated from the time of burn), and the other half over the following 16 hours.

b. Maintenance fluid requirements should also be added to the resuscitation requirement (refer to sample calculation in Table 67-1).

c. Initial $K^+$ supplementation is not required, although large amounts are needed in the anabolic phase of healing.

| TABLE 67-1 |
| --- |

**RESUSCITATION CALCULATIONS**

Parkland Formula: 4 ml × ___ kg × ___ % burn = ___ ml
*Half of this volume is given over the first 8 hours and half is given over the next 16 hours; however, basal fluid requirements must also be considered during this time.
Calculated resuscitation:
(4 ml × ___ kg × ___ % burn) + basal requirements (1500 ml × BSA [$cm^2$]) = _ ___ ml/24 hours
Resuscitation fluid per 8 hours:
1st half is given over 8 hours = ___ ml/8 hours = ___ ml/hr
2nd half is given over the next 16 hours = ___ ml/16 hours = ___ ml/hr

| **Maintenance:** | |
| --- | --- |
| Basal fluid requirement: | Total BSA = ___ $m^2$ |
| | 24 hours = ___ ml |
| | 1 hour = ___ ml/h |
| Evaporative water loss: | Adults: (25 + ___ % burn) $m^2$ = ___ ml/hr |
| | Children: (35 + ___ % burn) $m^2$ = ___ ml/hr |
| | Calculated evaporative loss: (___ + ___ % burn) ___ $m^2$ = ml/hr; ___ ml/24 hours |
| Total maintenance fluids: | Basal requirement and evaporative loss |
| | 24 hours = ___ ml |
| | 1 hour = ___ ml |

BSA = body surface area.

---

d. Colloid may be given as early as 12 hours after injury in large burns and usually consists of albumin infused at a constant rate. Fresh frozen plasma may be given if coagulation deficits are present.
e. Hypertonic saline appears to replenish intravascular fluid (from intracellular source) more quickly and improves cardiac contractility while decreasing total intravenous (IV) fluid volume and edema.
   (1) Its use remains controversial, and it is not used in some burn centers.
f. Blood should not be used for initial resuscitation (unless the patient is anemic secondary to other injuries).
g. Fluid boluses are generally avoided, but IV rate can be adjusted as needed.
h. Resuscitation formulas serve only as a guideline for initial IV fluid administration.
   (1) Adjust the IV rate based on physiologic response.
3. **Goals of resuscitation**—the end point of resuscitation is to maintain adequate tissue perfusion, which is difficult to quantify; however, the following parameters can be used:
a. Adequate urine output—adults, 0.5 ml/kg/hr; children, 1 to 2 ml/kg/hr
b. Normal mentation
c. Well-perfused extremities (warm, good capillary refill)
d. Normal arterial pH, lactate levels, and base excess
e. Mixed venous $O_2$ saturations greater than 70%

f. Inadequate volume restoration is manifested by oliguria, tachycardia, and persistent or worsening base deficit.

## E. INITIAL PROCEDURES

1. Foley catheterization—required for accurate urine output measurements during resuscitation in patients with more than 20% TBSA burns.
2. Nasogastric tube—gastric ileus occurs frequently after burns; also a useful route for oral medications.
3. Nasojejunal feeding tube—placed under fluoroscopy beyond the ligament of Treitz, with immediate initiation of enteral feedings.
a. *Early enteral feeding has been shown to decrease sepsis-related complications.*
4. Escharotomies—may be required for burns to extremities and chest to prevent compartment syndrome and respiratory compromise.
a. Compartment syndrome—the symptoms are the 5 P's *(pain, pallor, poikilothermia, pulselessness, and paresthesias)* exhibited by loss of motor and sensory nerve function, diminished peripheral pulses, decreased capillary refill, *pressure greater than 30 mm Hg by direct measurement (causes collapse of the capillary beds).*
   (1) Decompression achieved by incising the lateral and medial aspects of the extremity.
   (2) If symptoms are unrelieved, then fasciotomy may be required to relieve compartment syndrome.
   (3) If the hand is involved, a carpal tunnel release is included.
   (4) Especially important in electrical burns
b. Circumferential chest burns—reduce compliance of chest wall, but escharotomies are rarely needed.
   (1) Escharotomies should be performed in the presence of increased peak pressures, increased partial pressure of carbon dioxide ($P_{CO_2}$), and decreased compliance.

## F. INITIAL TESTS

1. Baseline weight
2. Laboratory tests—complete blood cell count, electrolytes, arterial blood gas with carboxyhemoglobin (for large burns or suspected inhalation injury), coagulation studies
3. Chest radiograph and electrocardiogram (history of cardiac problems or electrical burns)
4. Urinalysis

## G. MEDICATIONS

1. Tetanus prophylaxis—unless received booster within last 5 years
2. Ulcer prophylaxis—may use sucralfate (Carafate) 1 g orally four times daily or H2 blocker (ranitidine 50 mg IV every 8 hours), with antacids 30 ml every 2 to 4 hours per nasogastric tube to titrate gastric pH greater than 5.0

67

BURN CARE

3. Fungal prophylaxis—Nystatin 15 ml swish and expectorate, and 15 ml per nasogastric tube three times daily
4. Multivitamins (particularly vitamin C and the other antioxidants) in tube feedings
5. Hemoglobinuria/myoglobinuria—treat myoglobinuria based on urine color. If tea colored or reddish, increase urine output to more than 1 ml/kg/hr by increasing IV rates. If there is no improvement, may give mannitol 12.5 g IV, and alkalinize urine with 1 ampule $NaHCO_3$ in IV fluids to keep urine pH greater than 7.0. If not adequately treated, renal failure can occur. Watch $K^+$ levels as well.
6. *Prophylactic antibiotics are contraindicated.*

## IV. PATHOPHYSIOLOGIC CHANGES ASSOCIATED WITH BURN INJURIES

### A. EDEMA
1. Maximal at 18 to 24 hours after the burn for the following reasons:
a. Generalized increase in microvascular permeability secondary to release of inflammatory mediators in affected tissue (histamine)—involves nonburned tissue if burns more than 20% TBSA
b. Generalized impairment in cell membrane function—increased intracellular volume drawn in by increased intracellular $Na^+$ with concomitant loss of $K^+$.

### B. HEMODYNAMICS
1. Relatively predictable pattern seen in large burn injuries
2. Initial hypodynamic state with decreased cardiac output/contractility and increased vascular resistance
a. This usually resolves with adequate resuscitation.
3. By days 2 to 3, a hyperdynamic state exists with increased cardiac function and decreased vascular resistance.
4. Metabolism—there is a state of wound–, central nervous system–, and stress hormone–induced hypermetabolism.
a. Begins at 48 hours after burn
b. Caloric needs increased 1.3 to 2 times normal.
c. Characterized by increased oxygen consumption, heat production, increased body temperature, hypoproteinemia caused by catabolism and wound exudate, gluconeogenesis, and hyperglycemia
d. Gradually returns to normal after wound is closed and the inflammation is resolved
5. Immunocompromised
a. All aspects of the immune function are initially depressed including:
   (1) Cellular-mediated immunity (T cells), humoral-mediated immunity (B cells), opsonization caused by decreased complement and antibodies, decreased phagocytosis and bactericidal activity by macrophages and neutrophils, and loss of natural barrier function of the skin
b. Predisposes the patient to infections and multiorgan failure

## V. BURN WOUND CARE

### A. GOALS OF BURN WOUND CARE

1. Cover wound.
2. Decrease infection.
3. Allow for optimal reepithelialization of partial-thickness burns.
4. Burns (second or third degree) that do not heal by 2 to 3 weeks produce more scarring; thus, these wounds require early excision and grafting for best cosmetic and functional results.
5. The mortality of large burns has been reduced by the early excision of the burn wound followed by coverage with autograft or allograft.

### B. TOPICAL AGENTS

Goal is to decrease wound sepsis, not prevent colonization of eschar.

1. Bacitracin ointment—useful for partial-thickness burns and facial burns; apply twice daily.
2. Silver sulfadiazine (Silvadene)—broad spectrum, includes *Candida* coverage.
   a. Intermediate eschar penetration but less than mafenide acetate; best used for dirty wounds
   b. Nonpainful on application; apply twice daily.
   c. *Contraindicated in patients with glucose-6-phosphate dehydrogenase deficiency*
3. Mafenide acetate (Sulfamylon)—not used frequently in initial burn care.
   a. Broad spectrum, but less fungicidal activity; apply twice daily.
   b. Penetrates eschar well but causes pain on application
   c. *Carbonic anhydrase inhibitor and absorption can cause hyperchloremic metabolic acidosis.*
4. Silver nitrate 0.5%—applied as a wet dressing with poor eschar penetration.
   a. *May result in electrolyte leaching and can cause methemoglobinemia.*

### C. LOCAL CARE

1. First-degree burns—minor care, symptomatic pain control
2. Partial-thickness burns—initially wash with antiseptic soap (e.g., chlorhexidine gluconate), remove debris, unroof vesicles.
   a. Apply topical agents (bacitracin) wrapped with a nonadherent dressing.
3. Deep partial-thickness, full-thickness burns—initially treat as for partial-thickness burns.
   a. If there is no healing after 2 weeks, grafting is required.

### D. EARLY EXCISION AND GRAFTING

1. Excise eschar in layered fashion to the point of capillary bleeding.
2. Perform within 2 to 7 days of admission for obvious deep second- and third-degree burns.
3. Graft immediately or cover temporarily with homograft or biologic dressing.

67

BURN CARE

4. Can perform staged excision and grafting the next day (decreases operative blood loss).

a. Advantages include early removal of eschar and coverage, improved joint function, shortened hospitalization, earlier mobilization and rehabilitation, improved immune status, and decreased wound sepsis.

## E. GRAFTING

1. Decreases evaporation, desiccation, pain; protects neurovascular tissue and tendons
2. Superficial partial-thickness wounds should heal spontaneously by day 14.
3. Without immediate physiologic coverage, fascial desiccation and subsequent infection may occur.
4. Sheet versus mesh graft
a. Sheet grafts are optimal for cosmetic appearance but do not expand to cover a large surface area.
b. Mesh grafts are better for nonoptimal recipient beds.
c. Sheet grafts are preferred for hands, feet, and face.
5. Grafts are usually 0.010 to 0.014 inches thick (split thickness).
a. Thicker grafts have less scarring but slightly increased risk for graft failure and increased scarring of donor sites.
b. Full-thickness grafts include the entire dermis.
6. Types of grafting material
a. Autograft (from self)—optimal; split thickness versus full thickness, sheet versus mesh.
b. Allograft (same species, i.e., cadaver). The following are indications for use of allograft:
   (1) Insufficient autologous skin available
   (2) Temporary wound coverage before autologous grafting
   (3) Speeds epithelialization
   (4) Prevents infection
c. Xenograft (different species, i.e., porcine)—infrequently used because of the establishment of skin banks
d. Skin substitutes
   (1) Cultured keratinocytes—infrequently used
      (a) For use in large burns when little donor skin available (needs a viable dermis)
      (b) Poor resistance to infection
      (c) Fragile, easily scars
      (d) Variable take
      (e) Place on dermal allografts.
      (f) Products include Epicel.
   (2) Dermal substitutes—cover wound until autograft is available.
      (a) Dermal allograft
      (b) Collagen glycosaminoglycan
      (c) Polyglactic acid (Vicryl) mesh

(d) Products include Biobrane, TransCyte, Dermagraft, Integra, Alloderm, and Dermatrix.

(3) Skin substitutes (bilayer material)
  (a) Both dermal and epidermal components
  (b) Improved take in recent reports
  (c) Still not as good as split-thickness autologous graft
  (d) Products include Apligraf and Laserskin.

7. Priority of sites to be grafted—hands, feet, joints, extremities, and face first, then trunk
8. Graft care

a. Donor site—covered with topical antimicrobial (bacitracin, silver sulfadiazine) and biologic dressing such as calcium alginate (Kaltostat) or an occlusive dressing (Adaptic).

b. Graft site
  (1) Wet—dressings irrigated with antibiotic solution to be kept constantly damp
    (a) Mixture of Sulfamylon with double antibiotics alternating every 2 hours.
  (2) Dry—nonstick gauze (Adaptic) with a pressure dressing over graft
  (3) Nonadherence of graft is due to avascular or infected graft bed, hematoma, seroma, or graft movement.

## VI. SUPPORTIVE CARE
### A. NUTRITION
The importance of starting early nutritional support cannot be emphasized enough given the hypermetabolic state that exists secondary to a burn injury and the risk for sepsis.

1. The metabolic rate is proportional to burn size up to 40% to 50% TBSA burns.
2. Total body $O_2$ consumption and water loss are proportional to burn size.
3. Nutrient requirements need to be determined.
a. Caloric needs based on Harris–Benedict equation using a multiplier
b. Indirect calorimetry is often used.
4. Route
a. Enteral (nasoduodenal) preferred, start during first 12 hours after injury.
  (1) Leads to decreased infection, complication rates, and decreased cost
b. Total parenteral nutrition is associated with an increased rate of sepsis in burn patients.

### B. PHYSICAL AND OCCUPATIONAL THERAPY
1. Aggressive physical therapy and occupational therapy are necessary to prevent contracture and maintain joint function.
2. Positioning of limbs and joints begins on day 1.
3. Splinting is required to prevent contractures after grafts are applied.

4. Active exercise program with stretching is greatly superior to passive range of motion.
5. Involve occupational therapy early for long-term rehabilitation planning.

## C. ANALGESIA
1. Use methadone for long-term baseline pain management, with IV morphine for acute pain.

## VII. MANAGEMENT OF INFECTION IN THE BURN PATIENT

### A. THE MOST COMMON INFECTION IN BURN PATIENTS IS PNEUMONIA.
1. Early pneumonia—commonly the result of gram-positive organisms
2. Later pneumonia (>7 days after hospitalization)—typically the result of gram-negative organisms
3. More common in intubated patients, although can occur in nonintubated patients

### B. PATHOGENESIS OF WOUND SEPSIS IN AN UNTREATED BURN WOUND
1. Surface bacteria proliferate, migrate through nonviable tissue, pause at the subeschar space, and when microbial invasiveness "outweighs" host defense capability, invade viable tissue with microvascular involvement and systemic dissemination.
2. Avascularity and ischemia of full-thickness burn wound allow microbial proliferation and prevent delivery of systemic antibiotics and cellular components of host defense.

### C. CLINICAL SIGNS
1. Conversion of a partial- to full-thickness injury
2. Rapidly spreading ischemic necrosis

### D. DIAGNOSIS OF INVASIVE BURN WOUND SEPSIS
1. Cultures of burn wound surface do not accurately predict progressive bacterial colonization or incipient burn wound sepsis.
2. Bacterial growth is best monitored by semiquantitative burn wound biopsy.
a. Calculate the precise number of organisms per gram of tissue.
b. If biopsy cultures reveal more than $10^5$ organisms per gram of tissue, or if there is a 100-fold increase in the concentration of organisms per gram of tissue within a 48-hour period, then the organisms have escaped effective control by the topical chemotherapeutic agent.
c. Wound colonization of dead tissue must be differentiated from invasion of viable tissue.
    (1) Best evaluated by clinical diagnosis

    (2) Biopsy will find organisms in viable subeschar tissue on histologic examination.

    (3) Microvascular invasion connotes possible hematogenous dissemination and mandates systemic antibiotic therapy.

  d. Wound—often dry, crusted, black or violaceous color, or may be unchanged

  e. Clinical picture of sepsis—fever, hypoxia, mental status changes, leukocytosis, new-onset ileus, tachypnea, thrombocytopenia, hypotension, oliguria, acidosis, tachycardia, hyperglycemia

## E. BACTERIOLOGY OF NOSOCOMIAL BURN INFECTION

1. Know your hospital's flora and antibiotic sensitivities of species.
2. Most common pathogens—*Staphylococcus aureus, group A streptococci (less common), Pseudomonas aeruginosa, other gram-negative rods, Enterococcus spp, Candida albicans*

## F. PREVENTION OF BURN INFECTION

1. Dressing changes twice daily and application of topical agents
2. Use strict hand washing.

## G. TREATMENT OF BURN INFECTION

1. Remove all devitalized tissue.
2. Surgically drain closed-space abscesses.
3. Apply diffusible topical agent.
4. Empiric antibiotic therapy—broad spectrum
  a. Always cover initially for *Pseudomonas* spp; rarely need anaerobic coverage.
  b. Our routine triple-antibiotic therapy is vancomycin, piperacillin, and an aminoglycoside.

## H. NONBACTERIAL INFECTION

1. Viral infection—usually improves with time
  a. Virucidal agent recommended for systemic involvement.
2. Fungal infection—topical application of nystatin effectively clears fungi and yeast, and may be used prophylactically before eschar excision.
  a. Amphotericin B is used for systemic involvement.

## VIII. ELECTRICAL INJURIES

## A. TISSUE DESTRUCTION

1. Most severe at the points of entry and exit (the points at which the electrical current is most concentrated)
2. *Deep tissue damage often greatly exceeds skin injury.*
  a. Not obvious at the time of initial injury
  b. Electrical resistance of tissues—(from least to most) is nerve, blood, blood vessel, muscle, skin, tendon, fat, and bone.

67

BURN CARE

## B. TREATMENT

1. Cardiopulmonary resuscitation—high-voltage currents usually cause cardiac arrest, whereas low-voltage (<440 volts) currents usually produce ventricular fibrillation.
2. Protection against neurologic damage caused by fractures of the spine
a. Place in cervical spine collar and on a long backboard to immobilize the entire spine.
b. Tetanic contraction of muscle may cause fractures of the cervical and lumbosacral spine and long bones.
   (1) Perform screening radiographs.

## C. FLUID RESUSCITATION

1. Cannot be calculated from percentage of skin burns
2. Give sufficient volume to establish urine output of 1.5 ml/kg/hr.
3. High incidence of muscular and blood injury causes hemoglobinuria/myoglobinuria.
a. May need mannitol (25 g/hr) and $NaHCO_3$ to prevent precipitation of myoglobin/hemoglobin in the renal tubules
4. Progressively severe metabolic acidosis occurs with electrical injuries and massive tissue destruction.
a. Use IV sodium bicarbonate to temporarily correct base deficit.

## D. EARLY DEBRIDEMENT

1. Of grossly necrotic tissue; amputation may be needed if unable to control acidosis.

## E. IMMEDIATE EXTREMITY FASCIOTOMY

1. Frequently required; check compartment pressures.

## IX. CHEMICAL INJURIES

A significant problem in the management of chemical injuries is the failure to recognize ongoing destruction of tissue.

## A. MANAGEMENT

1. Initially dilution with copious amounts of water
2. *Do not neutralize a chemical burn because the heat of neutralization can extend the injury.*
3. Avoid hypothermia.
4. Special precautions
a. Lithium—remove particles before irrigation.
b. Hydrofluoric acids—apply 10% calcium gluconate cream in most cases; can inject calcium gluconate subcutaneously for severe burns.
c. Phenol—irrigation must be vigorous (shower) because absorption increases when spread over a large area.
d. Tar/asphalt—use bacitracin or other petroleum-based product.

## X. OUTPATIENT AND CLINIC TREATMENT

### A. SELECTION

1. If the patient does not meet admission criteria, he or she can be treated as an outpatient.

### B. TREATMENT

1. Tetanus prophylaxis
2. Wounds washed with mild soap
3. Debris and blisters should be debrided.
4. Apply antibiotic ointment (bacitracin, Neosporin, Polysporin) and nonstick porous gauze (Adaptic), and wrap with gauze.
5. Pain management

### C. FOLLOW-UP CARE

1. Dressing care twice daily—wash with mild soap (to remove debris and fibrinous exudate) and reapply dressing.
2. Vigorous range-of-motion exercises and massage of postburn scar
3. Return to clinic and/or physical therapy as needed.

### D. WOUNDS

If the wounds are deep partial- or full-thickness burns, the patient may be treated as an outpatient until excision and grafting are required.

1. If the wound is not reepithelialized by 2 weeks, it should undergo excision and grafting.
2. Longer healing time increases scarring.
3. If hypertrophic scarring is a problem, the patient should be fitted for pressure garments and wear them 23 hours a day until wounds no longer blanch.
4. Use moisturizing cream on healing skin.
5. As long as the healed wound is hyperemic and blanches, the patient should vigorously put pressure on the wound daily to help prevent scarring.
6. Avoid sun exposure to graft or burn because it may cause hyperpigmentation.
7. Pruritus is treated with moisturizing cream and oral diphenhydramine (Benadryl) or hydroxyzine (Vistaril) as needed.

## XI. COMPLICATIONS OF BURN INJURIES

### A. GI

1. Adynamic ileus—gastric and colonic involvement
a. Generally resolves within 24 hours with IV hydration and nasogastric suction
2. Ulcers—"Curling's ulcer" generally involves stomach, duodenum, and jejunum.
a. Cause is unknown, but may be due to hypovolemia or hypoperfusion.

**67**

**BURN CARE**

b. Incidence is rare now with early antacids and H2 blockers, and with early enteral feeding.

3. Acalculous cholecystitis—uncommon, but diagnosed with a hydroxy iminodiacetic acid (HIDA) scan or ultrasound

a. Treat with antibiotics and either percutaneous drainage or cholecystectomy.

## B. OCULAR
1. Keep eyes moist using artificial tears or ointments.
2. Corneal abrasions—associated with facial burns
a. Treatment includes topical antibiotics, and release and grafting of ectropion.
3. Cataracts (especially with electrical injury)

## C. CUTANEOUS
1. Wound contracture—may result in cosmetic or functional problems, limiting range of motion.
a. Contractures may be released surgically with grafting or Z-plasty.
2. Hypertrophic scar
a. Occurs with wounds that take more than 2 weeks to heal
b. Increased incidence with deep burns and extended exposure of ungrafted burn wound
c. Treatment
   (1) Pressure-fitted masks, garments, and massage are used for the first year to reduce scar formation.
   (2) Resurface with graft later.
   (3) Cosmetic treatment is often disappointing.
3. Keloids—variant of hypertrophic scarring that extends beyond the original wound
a. Difficult to treat, but steroid injections have been used. Often recur after excision.

## D. MISCELLANEOUS
1. Heterotopic calcification
a. Elbow is the most common joint affected.
b. May be related to vigorous occupational/physical therapy and frequent microtrauma to the affected joint
2. Chondritis—secondary to *S. aureus* and *Pseudomonas* spp, involving the ear and joint
3. Hyperpigmentation—avoid sun exposure for at least 1 year. Use sun-blocking agents (>15 sun protection factor).

# Neurosurgical Emergencies

*Bradford A. Curt, MD, and Ondrej Choutka, MD*

Neurosurgical emergencies represent both cranial and spinal pathologies that require rapid evaluation and appropriate intervention to significantly reduce morbidity and mortality. Early assessment of altered level of consciousness and focal neurological deficits, as well as prompt initial management, ensures the best possible outcome. It must be stressed that conditions leading to central, uncal, upward cerebellar, and tonsillar herniation syndromes can be fatal within a few minutes. This chapter provides the basic principles necessary for the care of the patient with an acute neurosurgical problem.

**68**

## I. APPROACH TO THE UNCONSCIOUS PATIENT

### A. UNCONSCIOUSNESS

The state of "unconsciousness" implies bilateral hemispheric dysfunction, depression of the reticular activating system in the upper brainstem, or both.

### B. CAUSATIVE FACTORS

1. Structural causes of coma: Coma may originate for multiple reasons including traumatic, vascular (both ischemic and hemorrhagic), neoplastic, infectious, congenital, and inflammatory factors.
   a. Supratentorial mass
      (1) Compression of brain and eventually brainstem
      (2) Progressive loss of consciousness
      (3) Symmetric deterioration suggests central herniation, whereas asymmetric decline suggests uncal herniation.
   b. Infratentorial mass
      (1) Direct compression of the reticular activating system causes sudden onset of coma.
2. Toxic and metabolic causes of coma: Onset of coma is gradual, with a symmetric neurologic examination and preserved pupillary responses. Look for asterixis, tremor, myoclonus, and acid-base disturbances that are characteristic of toxic and metabolic causes.
   a. Electrolyte or endocrine imbalance
   b. Intoxication (self-induced, accidental, or iatrogenic)
   c. Central nervous system or systemic infection
   d. Nutritional deficiencies
   e. Inherited metabolic disorders
   f. Global hypoxia or ischemia
   g. Seizure (may include status epilepticus)
   h. Organ failure (e.g., uremic and hepatic encephalopathy)

### C. HISTORY

1. Important features include abrupt versus subacute versus insidious onset, presence of lucid interval, recent neurologic complaints, and spatial progression of neurological deficit.

2. Look for factors in medical and surgical histories, allergies, social and sexual habits, occupational exposure, and travel that could explain decline, including recent use of alcohol or drug abuse.
3. A medication history, especially history of psychotropic, sedative, and opiate use

## D. PHYSICAL EXAMINATION

1. General
a. Vital signs
b. Respiratory pattern
c. External evidence of trauma or intravenous drug abuse
d. Nuchal rigidity
2. Level of consciousness
a. Awake and alert—eyes open, responsiveness to verbal stimuli
b. Lethargic—sleepy, but arouses easily to full awake state
c. Obtunded—sleeps unless continually stimulated but can be fully aroused with effort
d. Stupor—responds to vigorous physical stimuli but cannot be fully aroused to waking state
e. Coma—totally unarousable
3. Glasgow Coma Scale (GCS) (Table 68-1)
a. Score ranges from 3 to 15.
b. Not a replacement for a complete neurological examination but is a reproducible measure of level of consciousness in the setting of trauma
c. Rates head injury into three categories: mild—GCS score 14 to 15; moderate—9 to 13; and severe—≤8
4. Children's Coma Scale—age 4 or younger (Table 68-2)

## E. COMPREHENSIVE NEUROLOGIC EXAMINATION

1. Assess level of consciousness; perform Mini-Mental State Examination if appropriate.
2. Cranial nerve examination

### TABLE 68-1

GLASGOW COMA SCALE

| Points | Best Eye Opening | Best Verbal | Best Motor |
|--------|------------------|------------------|-------------------|
| 6 | — | — | Follows commands |
| 5 | — | Oriented | Localizes pain |
| 4 | Spontaneous | Confused | Withdraws to pain |
| 3 | To speech | Inappropriate | Flexor posturing |
| 2 | To pain | Incomprehensible | Extensor posturing |
| 1 | None | None | None |

**TABLE 68-2**

CHILDREN'S COMA SCALE

| Points | Best Eye Opening | Best Verbal | | Best Motor |
|---|---|---|---|---|
| 6 | — | — | | Follows commands |
| 5 | — | Smiles, oriented to sound, follows objects, interacts | | Localizes pain |
| 4 | Spontaneous | Crying Consolable | Interaction Inappropriate | Withdraws to pain |
| 3 | To speech | Inconsistently consolable | Moaning | Flexor posturing |
| 2 | To pain | Inconsolable | Restless | Extensor posturing |
| 1 | None | None | None | None |

68

NEUROSURGICAL EMERGENCIES

a. Response to visual threat—cranial nerves (CNs) II, VII
b. Pupillary response—CNs II, III
c. Corneal reflexes—CNs V, VII
d. Extraocular movement—CNs III, IV, VI. Assess conjugate versus dysconjugate gaze, gaze deviation, and roving eye movements
e. Oculocephalic reflex—CNs VI, VIII. Doll's eyes reflex
f. Oculovestibular reflex—CNs VI, VIII. Cold calorics test
g. Gag reflex—CNs IX, X
h. Response to central pain using supraorbital, sternal, or temporomandibular joint pressure. Tests general integrity of motor and sensory tracts in the brainstem. Use only if the patient is not obeying commands.

**3.** Motor examination
a. Check tone and bulk.
b. Formal strength testing if possible
c. Decorticate (flexor) posturing—indicates level of lesion above red nucleus
d. Decerebrate (extensor) posturing—indicates level of lesion above lateral vestibular nucleus but below the red nucleus

**4.** Sensory examination
a. Evaluation of pain, light touch, vibration, and temperature
b. Difficult to assess in an unconscious patient
c. Check response to pain—localizes, withdraws, or postures.

**5.** Reflex examination
a. Check superficial and deep-tendon reflexes.
b. Check the presence or absence of pathologic reflexes—Hoffman's, Babinski's, sustained clonus, frontal release signs.
c. Check sphincter tone.

**6.** Cerebellar examination
a. Assess stability of finger to nose.
b. Rapid alternating movements

**7.** Gait examination

a. Assess stance and gait. Pathologic gaits include festering gait, wide-based gait, antalgic gait, slapping gait.
b. Tandem walking

## F. INITIAL MANAGEMENT OF COMA—GCS SCORE ≤8.

The evaluation and treatment of coma is a series of steps that occur simultaneously.

**1.** Airway: Intubate for airway protection.
**2.** Breathing: Ventilate to prevent hypoxemia.
**3.** Circulation: Optimize hemodynamic status with fluids and vasopressors if necessary.
**4.** Disability: Stabilize cervical spine.
**5.** Treatment of reversible causes of coma
a. Hypoglycemia: Administer glucose (50 ml of 50% glucose).
b. Opiate/benzodiazepine overdose: Administer naloxone or flumazenil.
c. Thiamine deficiency: Administer 100 mg thiamine to prevent Wernicke's encephalopathy (give thiamine before glucose).
d. Seizure: For active seizure activity, administer lorazepam 1 to 2 mg intravenously (IV), load with phenytoin 10 to 15 mg/kg loading dose, 100 mg IV/orally three times daily (alternative antiepileptic used at our institution is levetiracetam [Keppra] 1000 mg orally/IV twice daily).
**6.** Laboratory studies
a. Complete blood cell count, renal profile, Ca, Mg, PO4, arterial blood gas, coagulation profile, toxicology screen for ethyl alcohol, narcotics, barbiturates, acetaminophen, type and screen, and urinalysis
**7.** If suspected head injury with increased intracranial pressure (ICP), perform the following while arranging head computed tomography (CT) scanning.
a. Head of bed at 30 degrees
b. Neutral head position to promote venous outflow, loosen C-collar
c. Hypertonic therapy (bolus of mannitol 1 g/kg IV or 250 ml of 3% saline)
d. Short-term hyperventilation to reduce partial arterial pressure of carbon dioxide ($Paco_2$) to 25 to 30 mm Hg

## II. CRANIAL EMERGENCIES

### A. HEAD INJURY

**1.** Mild head injury—GCS score 15 to 14
a. Can be asymptomatic
b. Clinical findings may include headache, dizziness, memory loss, scalp laceration, or bruising.
c. Cranial imaging may be normal or may demonstrate a small contusion, subdural hematoma (SDH), or traumatic subarachnoid hemorrhage (SAH).
d. In patients with abnormal imaging:
(1) Monitor for neurologic changes.
(2) Repeat imaging in 6 to 24 hours to confirm stability of head injury.

(3) Urgent repeat imaging with deterioration in level of consciousness.

(4) May be discharged home with stable imaging and examination

## 2. Moderate head injury—GCS score of 12 to 9

a. Depressed level of consciousness and patients are usually amnesic to the event.

b. Associated with skull fractures and multiple traumatic injuries

c. Full traumatic evaluation is necessary to rule out other traumatic abnormalities.

d. Admission is necessary due to likely progression of injury.

## 3. Severe head injury—GCS score ≤8

a. Patients are comatose by definition.

b. Focal neurologic deficit is more likely.

c. CT scan may demonstrate mass lesion such as:

(1) Hemorrhagic contusions or hematomas

(2) Diffuse cerebral edema

(3) Diffuse axonal injury

(4) Depressed skull fracture

(5) Penetrating head injury

d. Fifty percent to 60% of patients have multisystem trauma.

e. Five percent of patients will have simultaneous spinal injury.

f. Sustained GCS score ≤8 warrants ICP monitoring and directed ICP therapy.

g. Antiseizure prophylaxis decreases early posttraumatic seizures.

## B.  INCREASED ICP

### 1. Clinical manifestations

a. Classic signs are headache, oculomotor palsies, and Cushing's triad (hypertension, bradycardia, and respiratory irregularities).

b. Suspect increased ICP if there is deterioration in neurologic examination, decline in GCS score to ≤8, or progression of focal neurologic deficit.

c. Upper limits of normal ICP = 20 mm Hg

d. Treatment is indicated if ICP greater than 20 to 25 mm Hg for sustained period (physiologic spikes may occur). Sustained elevated ICP increases mortality.

### 2. Indications for ICP monitoring (intraventricular or intraparenchymal monitor)

a. GCS score ≤8 without other factors that can account for depressed level of consciousness such as ethyl alcohol, drugs, or seizures (after resuscitation) *and* an abnormal CT head (hematomas, contusions, swelling, herniation, or compressed basal cisterns).

b. GCS score ≤8, normal CT head, and two or more of the following:

(1) Age older than 40 years

(2) Unilateral or bilateral motor posturing

(3) Systolic blood pressure less than 90 mm Hg

   c. Relative—multisystem trauma in which other therapies may have adverse effect on the ICP or ability to follow neurologic examination (e.g., paralytics, heavy sedations) in the presence of head injury.

   d. Ventriculostomy is superior to parenchymal, subarachnoid, and epidural or subdural monitors. Parenchymal monitors cannot be calibrated in situ.

**3. Other modes of monitoring of head injured patients may include:**

   a. Brain temperature and oxygenation monitor—Licox ($Pbo_2$)

   b. Cerebral blood flow monitor

   c. Jugular venous oxygen saturation ($SjVo_2$)

**4. Management of increased ICP. This process can be divided into three tiers of therapy.**

   a. Tier I

     (1) Maintain head of bed at 30 degrees (elevating head of bed >30 degrees negatively affects cerebral perfusion pressure [CPP]).

     (2) Head in a neutral position (promotes optimal venous outflow)

     (3) Adequate sedation with short-acting agents that allow frequent neurologic examination (e.g., propofol)

     (4) Keep cervical collar on loosely to promote venous outflow.

     (5) Keep patient normothermic and treat fevers (hypothermia may be beneficial in traumatic brain injury).

     (6) Avoid hypotension (systolic blood pressure <90 mm Hg) and hypoxia ($Sao_2$ <90%).

   b. Tier II

     (1) Osmotic therapy

       (a) Mannitol—1-g/kg bolus (avoid hypotension) with signs of increasing pressure and herniation. Prolonged use is not backed by evidence.

       (b) Hypertonic saline (3% saline)—protocol used at our institution. Infuse to increase serum sodium to 150 to 155 mmol/L or rescue bolus (150–250 ml).

     (2) Cerebrospinal fluid (CSF) diversion as needed to decompress ventricular system

     (3) Maintain CPP greater than ~50 to 60 mm Hg.

       (a) Aggressive attempts to keep CPP greater than 70 mm Hg associated with acute respiratory distress syndrome.

     (4) Hyperventilation

       (a) Causes vasoconstriction, thus decreasing cerebral perfusion

       (b) Used as a temporizing measure to reduce ICP while preparing for operative intervention or other Tier III treatments

     **(5) Steroids are contraindicated.**

       (a) Do not reduce ICP or improve outcome.

       (b) Associated with increased mortality in moderate and severe head injury (Level I evidence, CRASH Trial 2004)

   c. Tier III

     (1) Barbituate coma—avoid hypotension

     (2) Paralytics

     (3) Hemicraniectomy

## C. SPECIFIC TRAUMATIC CRANIAL INJURIES

### 1. Epidural hematoma

a. Seen in 1% of patients with head trauma

b. Classic presentation is brief loss of consciousness, followed by a lucid interval, then progressive obtundation, ipsilateral pupillary dilation, and contralateral hemiparesis (seen in 60% of cases). Other presentations include headache, nausea, vomiting, seizure, unilateral hyperreflexia, and Babinski's sign.

c. Usual causative factor is laceration of the middle meningeal artery by fracture of squamous portion of the temporal bone, but it can also be produced by a dural sinus tear.

d. On CT scan, seen as lenticular, biconcave hyperdense, or isodense mass overlying brain. Mass will not generally cross suture lines.

e. Optimally treated with surgical evacuation

f. Isolated epidural hematoma carries a low mortality rate with optimal treatment.

### 2. SDH

a. Twice as common as epidural hematoma

b. Source of bleeding is usually venous but can also be arterial.

c. Classified as acute from 0 to 48 hours, subacute from 2 days to 3 weeks, and chronic if more than 3 weeks

d. Acute SDH resulting from cortical arterial or parenchymal injury

e. Chronic SDH may be asymptomatic in acute stage with subsequent, gradual accumulation of fluid resulting in slow progressive deterioration

f. Chronic SDH—confusion, incontinence, ataxia, weakness

g. On CT scan, seen as crescent-shaped mass overlying convexity. It appears hyperdense if acute, hypodense if chronic, or has mixed density if combined.

h. Surgical management is dependent on type of SDH.

   (1) Acute SDH—craniotomy (thick blood clot)

   (2) Chronic SDH—burr hole or trephine evacuation of fluid. This can be done even under local anesthetic.

### 3. Hemorrhagic contusions

a. Most commonly found in temporal, frontal, and occipital lobes where bone ridges can damage brain during acceleration and deceleration

b. Will typically "blossom" for 24 to 72 hours after presentation

c. Generally managed nonoperatively with observation and ICP-lowering therapy if indicated

d. Surgical intervention when medical measures fail (e.g., decompressive craniectomy with or without resection of damaged brain)

e. Patients with an isolated temporal lobe contusion can proceed to brain herniation and die without evidence of increased ICP because of local temporal swelling (uncal herniation).

f. Diffuse axonal injury

(1) Results from shearing of the white matter tracts from rotational forces at the time of impact
(2) Can be visualized on magnetic resonance imaging (MRI) or CT scan as punctate hemorrhages in centrum semiovale, corpus callosum, or brainstem
(3) Generally not associated with increases in ICP
(4) If brainstem is affected, the prognosis for functional recovery is extremely poor.

g. Skull fractures
(1) Can be open, closed, linear, compound, or depressed
(2) Raccoon's eyes diagnostic of fracture of the floor of the anterior fossa
(3) Basilar skull fracture usually diagnosed clinically without benefit of CT, in presence of Battle's sign (retroauricular hematoma), CSF otorrhea, or CSF rhinorrhea.
(4) Look for "ring" sign if CSF leak suspected and fluid is blood-tinged.
(5) Criteria to elevate skull fracture
   (a) More than 8 to 10 mm of depression; generally if the outer table of the skull is depressed below the inner table
   (b) Deficit related to compression of the underlying brain
   (c) CSF leaking from the wound secondary to dural laceration
   (d) Open, depressed skull fracture

## D.  TRAUMATIC BRAIN INJURY PROGNOSIS

1. Approximately 20% of patients with admission GCS score of 3 will survive and only 8% to 10% will have a functional recovery (Glasgow Outcome Scale scores 4 and 5).
2. Age is a strong independent predictor of outcome, with a significant increase in poor outcome in patients older than 60 years.
3. A single episode of hypotension (systolic blood pressure <90 mm Hg) during the acute care of a patient with head injury doubles the mortality rate.
4. A strong correlation exists between the severity of abnormal findings on initial CT scan and outcome.

## III. SPINAL EMERGENCIES
## A.  GENERAL

"Spinal emergencies" encompass multiple clinical situations but mostly include injuries involving the spinal cord, vertebrae, or soft tissues (ligaments, discs). Nerve roots are occasionally affected as well. The level and degree of involvement of each one of the elements determines the clinical picture associated with a particular injury. It is important for all surgeons to be familiar with presentation and basic early management of spinal injuries as they commonly occur in the polytrauma patient (particularly with loss of consciousness).

1. Prehospital stabilization (collar, backboard) is essential in trauma patient.
a. Ten percent of quadriplegics used to become so not at impact but some time thereafter (1957).

2. Patients with history of unconsciousness or injury above the clavicle must be considered to have an associated cervical spine injury, unless proven otherwise—BOTH clinically and radiographically.
3. If in doubt, maintain immobilization (collar) and neutral spine position (flat) until full spinal assessment, clearance, or specialist consult.
4. The majority of patients with spinal injuries have normal peripheral neurologic findings.

## B. ASSESSMENT

Clinical assessment follows a standard approach to any patient; however, the patient's level of consciousness will determine how much cooperation will be provided and what films may be needed for spinal clearance or spinal injury. The following usually occurs simultaneously and should be done in concordance with Advanced Trauma Life Support guidelines.

1. History
a. Mechanism (e.g., high velocity, seatbelt, ejection, gunshot, fall)
b. Symptoms (e.g., pain, numbness, tingling, weakness, or paralysis)
c. Onset, duration, and progression of symptoms

2. Examination
a. ABC principle applies to all patients, including those with spinal injury. Spinal shock may be the cause in hypotensive patient (see later).
b. Maintain spinal precautions during the assessment.
c. Mechanical assessment involves log-roll of patient for visualization of the entire spine.
   (1) LOOK for any obvious deformities, open wounds, or so-called step-offs (prominent, unequal spinous processes).
   (2) FEEL for tenderness, deformities, and step-offs.
d. Neurologic examination is guided by the level of consciousness; however, a detailed assessment helps guide treatment and prognosis. It must include motor, sensory, and sphincter function assessment. The following questions should be answered in a timely manner:
   (1) Is there a neurologic deficit (weakness, paralysis)?
   (2) If so, what is the level of injury?
   (3) Is the injury complete or partial? This determines the urgency of subsequent intervention.
e. Incomplete spinal cord injury is an emergency. It includes patients with the following conditions:
   (1) Any motor or sensory function below the level of injury
   (2) Sacral sparing of sensation (to pinprick)
   (3) Preservation of voluntary sphincter function

**Pearl:** *Presence of anal wink or bulbocavernosus reflex does not represent sacral sparing.*

f. The level of spinal cord injury is determined by sensory and motor examinations (Fig. 68-1).

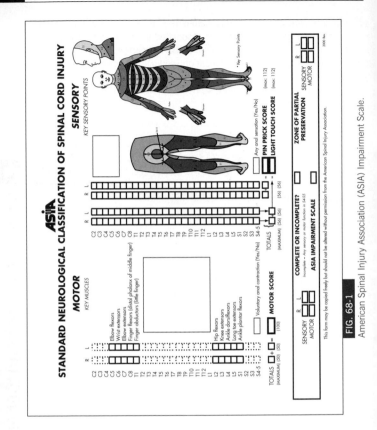

This form may be copied freely but should not be altered without permission from the American Spinal Injury Association.

**FIG. 68-1**
American Spinal Injury Association (ASIA) Impairment Scale.

g. Higher cervical injuries may be accompanied by respiratory compromise.

**Pearl:** *C3/4/5 keeps the diaphragm alive.*

h. Assess and document anal tone, presence of pathologic or absence of normal deep tendon reflexes.

i. Spinal shock—abrupt loss of sympathetic tone
   (1) Usually occurs in complete spinal cord injuries
   (2) Hypotension, bradycardia, warm peripheries (dilated peripheral vessels), loss of reflexes, and flaccid paralysis

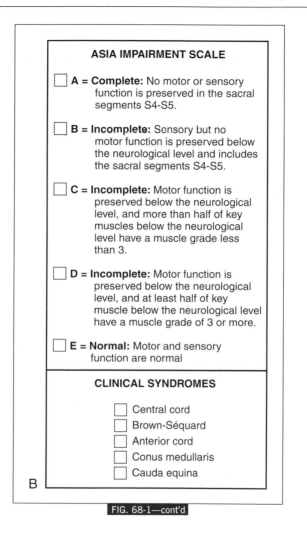

**ASIA IMPAIRMENT SCALE**

☐ **A = Complete:** No motor or sensory function is preserved in the sacral segments S4-S5.

☐ **B = Incomplete:** Sensory but no motor function is preserved below the neurological level and includes the sacral segments S4-S5.

☐ **C = Incomplete:** Motor function is preserved below the neurological level, and more than half of key muscles below the neurological level have a muscle grade less than 3.

☐ **D = Incomplete:** Motor function is preserved below the neurological level, and at least half of key muscle below the neurological level have a muscle grade of 3 or more.

☐ **E = Normal:** Motor and sensory function are normal

**CLINICAL SYNDROMES**

☐ Central cord
☐ Brown-Séquard
☐ Anterior cord
☐ Conus medullaris
☐ Cauda equina

B

FIG. 68-1—cont'd

68

NEUROSURGICAL EMERGENCIES

j. The absence of bulbocavernosus reflex (anal sphincter contraction in response to glans penis pinch or Foley catheter tug) in a patient with spinal shock carries a prognostic value, and its return may indicate resolution of shock period.
3. Radiographic assessment

a. May include one or combination of plain films (multiple static and dynamic flexion/extension), CT, and/or MRI
b. Review of any imaging modality should assess alignment, presence of fractures, and soft-tissue abnormalities (swelling, hematoma, etc.).
c. Urgent MRI in all patients with incomplete spinal cord injury whose findings are not explained by plain radiographs, CT, or both
   (1) Epidural hematoma or traumatic herniated disc requires emergent surgical intervention.
d. Decreased level of consciousness or history of loss of consciousness
   (1) Adequate plain films of C/T and L spine
   (2) C-spine films should include anteroposterior, lateral, and transoral views.
   (3) If unable to visualize cervicothoracic or craniocervical junction on plain films, obtain CT scan (Eastern Association for the Surgery of Trauma [EAST] guidelines).

**Pearl:** *CT of C-spine is commonly obtained together with CT head scan in trauma patients with altered mental status; T+L spine can be reconstructed from CT of chest and abdomen if already obtained.*

e. No history of loss of consciousness and GCS score of 15
   (1) Mechanism of injury and clinical examination should guide radiographic evaluation.
   (2) Patients with no spinal tenderness or pain on movement are unlikely to have sustained significant spinal injuries and may not require any imaging.
   (3) Obtain films through areas of abnormal examination findings.
f. If a fracture is identified, the rest of the spinal axis must be imaged (plain radiographs or CT) because there is ~20% chance of a second, occult fracture.

**4. Spinal clearance**
a. "Clearance" of spine in a trauma patient involves clinical and/or radiographic assessment depending on mechanism of injury, altered mental status, or history of unconsciousness.
b. Clinical criteria for cervical spine stability (NEXUS—5 *N*'s):
   (1) No mental status change
   (2) No intoxication (drugs, alcohol)
   (3) No neck pain or tenderness
   (4) No distracting injury/pain
   (5) No neurologic deficits

**Pearl:** *Canadian C-spine rules can be used, or a combination of both.*

c. If one of the above is present, the patient cannot be clinically cleared and should remain immobilized and undergo imaging studies.

d. Radiographic assessment involves plain films and/or CT through poorly visualized or suspicious areas (see earlier).

e. Interval assessment (2 weeks), dynamic plain films, or MRI with fat-suppression images to exclude ligamentous injury during the acute phase of injury may be required in patients with negative imaging but clinically not cleared (institution dependent, evidence not clear).

f. Unconscious patients, therefore, should not have their collar removed at the initial assessment, even with negative imaging.

g. Absence of thoracolumbar tenderness and neurologic symptoms renders those regions clinically clear.

h. Remove backboard as soon as possible to prevent unnecessary pressure ulcers.

**Pearl:** *If in doubt, keep patient safe with full spinal precautions and ask for help.*

## C.  SPECIFIC SPINAL INJURIES
### 1. Spinal cord injury

a. More frequent in men and result of road accidents (40%) and violence (25%)

b. Urgent assessment necessary to avoid delay in treatment

c. High cervical cord injuries may require intubation (or tracheostomy).

d. Spinal shock may require intravenous fluids and the use of vasopressors (sympathomimetics).
   (1) Dopamine preferred historically.
   (2) Phenylephrine (Neo-Synephrine) used despite theoretical risk for reflexive bradycardia. Alternative agent if it occurs.

e. Determine whether neurologic deficit is complete or incomplete (see Fig. 68-1).

f. Incomplete spinal cord injury requires an urgent MRI and treatment.

g. The use of methylprednisolone infusion remains controversial.
   (1) May be associated with increased morbidity (polytrauma, elderly)
   (2) National Acute Spinal Cord Injury Study (NASCIS) trials with only mild motor improvement, never reproduced
   (3) Use 24-hour protocol in isolated, blunt spinal cord injury presenting within 8 hours of injury (30-mg/kg bolus followed by 5.4-mg/kg/hr infusion × 23 hours).

h. Spine team consultation required in all spinal cord injuries.

i. Immobilization and/or realignment of obvious deformities may be achieved through the use of Gardner–Wells tongs (maximum of 10 lb/each cervical level).

j. Postoperative care requires appropriate skin care, bowel and bladder training, and involvement of rehabilitation units as soon as possible.

68

NEUROSURGICAL EMERGENCIES

**2.** Cauda equina syndrome

a. Cauda equina compression/injury results in areflexic paraparesis with alternating or bilateral radiculopathy (early), combined with saddle anesthesia and disturbance of bowel or bladder function (late).

b. Suspected cauda equina syndrome requires an urgent MRI and, in presence of a surgical lesion (disc/abscess/fracture/dislocation/tumor), emergent treatment (surgery or radiation).

c. Spine team consultation is mandatory.

**3.** Cervical fractures

a. Suspect cervical fracture with any injury above clavicle.

b. Immobilize until clearance or diagnosis possible.

c. Gardner–Wells tongs for immobilization and/or reduction of certain cervical fractures or dislocations

d. Fractures treated conservatively may require the use of a hard collar (subaxial spine) or halo-vest (craniocervical junction).

e. Bracing of cervicothoracic junction fractures requires extension of bracing to the thorax (e.g., Minerva brace).

f. Consider vertebral artery injury (dissection) in fractures involving transverse foramina of cervical vertebrae (angiogram, computed tomographic angiography, or magnetic resonance angiography).

g. Be familiar with some cervical pathologies.

   (1) Atlanto-occipital dislocation is usually fatal but commonly missed in survivors.

   (2) Jefferson fracture is fracture of atlas and stable if transverse ligament intact as assessed by lateral mass overhang—"rule of Spence."

   (3) Odontoid fractures

      (a) Type I: tip—stable, external immobilization

      (b) Type II: shaft of the dens—prone to malunion, treat surgically

      (c) Type III: body—stable, external immobilization

   (4) Hangman's fracture

      (a) Bilateral pars interarticularis of atlas, thus disrupting C2-3 junction

      (b) Historically, judicial hanging (hyperextension with distraction)

      (c) Treatment: C2-3 anterior cervical discectomy and fusion

   (5) Perched or jumped facets

      (a) Closed reduction in tongs (awake and with fluoroscopy) or open posterior reduction, followed by fixation and fusion

      (b) Beware of possible vertebral artery injury and disc disruption.

**4.** Thoracolumbar fractures

a. Thoracolumbar fractures can be classified as shown in Figure 68-2 and Table 68-3.

b. Stability determines treatment.

c. Nonsurgical treatment may require the use of external braces, for example:

   (1) Minerva brace above T6

   (2) Thoracolumbosacral orthosis below T6

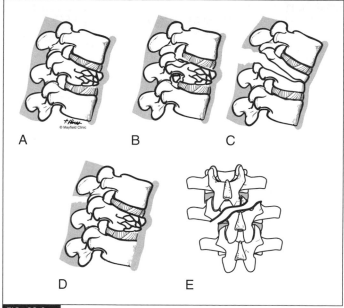

**FIG. 68-2**

Classification of thoracolumbar fractures: *(A)* compression; *(B)* burst; *(C)* chance; *(D)* flexion-distraction; *(E)* translational/fracture dislocation.

d. Open reduction and internal fixation for unstable fractures
e. Spine team must be consulted.

**Pearl:** *Isolated lumbar transverse process fractures do not require any intervention or spine team involvement but are indicative of the severity of forces involved; thus, intraabdominal or retroperitoneal organ injuries must be suspected.*

## IV. OTHER NEUROSURGICAL EMERGENCIES

### A.  SAH

**1. Causative factors**

a. Trauma—most common overall cause of SAH
b. Aneurysm—75% to 80% of spontaneous SAH cases
c. Arteriovenous malformation—5% of spontaneous SAH cases
d. Unknown cause—15% of spontaneous SAH cases

**2. Clinical**

a. Symptoms—"Worst headache of my life," neck stiffness, photophobia, loss of consciousness

**TABLE 68-3**

**MCAFEE CLASSIFICATION OF THORACOLUMBAR SPINE FRACTURES**

| Fracture Type | Pathology |
|---|---|
| Wedge compression* | Isolated anterior column failure; flexion injury |
| Stable burst* | Anterior and middle-column compression failure, posterior column intact |
| Unstable burst I | As above but anterior vertebral height <50%, spinal canal compromise >50%, or kyphosis >20 degrees; spinal cord injury requires decompression |
| Chance fracture | Horizontal vertebral avulsion injury with center of rotation anterior to vertebral body (seatbelt) |
| Flexion-distraction injury | Compressive failure of anterior column, tensile failure of posterior column; the center of rotation is posterior to anterior longitudinal ligament |
| Translational injuries/ fracture dislocation | Disruption of spinal canal alignment in transverse plane, shear mechanism common |

*Stable fractures.

  b. Examination—determine patient's level of consciousness
  c. Tests
    (1) Noncontrast head CT scan shows hyperdense subarachnoid spaces and detects SAH in 90% of cases if performed within 48 hours.
    (2) Hydrocephalus may be present.
    (3) Lumbar puncture if CT inconclusive in high suspicion scenarios
      (a) Large number of red blood cells (thousands) failing to clear between tubes
      (b) Differentiation from traumatic tap may be difficult.
      (c) Xanthochromia (yellow CSF) present approximately 4 hours after rupture of aneurysm and persists for 3 to 4 weeks
    (4) Vascular studies
      (a) Cerebral angiography—gold standard, invasive, 1% of stroke cases
      (b) Computed tomographic angiography—noninvasive, fast, becoming popular
      (c) MRI/magnetic resonance angiography—sensitive for blood detection, misses small aneurysms
      (d) In patients with an aneurysm, 20% will have multiple ones.
 **3. Initial management of aneurysmal SAH**
  a. Keep systolic blood pressure less than 140 mm Hg because hypertension may lead to rerupture.
  b. Seizure prophylaxis (phenytoin [Dilantin] or Keppra)
  c. Start nimodipine (calcium channel blocker) at 60 mg every 4 hours orally for 21 days—improves outcome without radiographic improvement of spasm (neuroprotection rather than vasodilatation).
  d. CSF diversion with ventriculostomy if needed to treat acute hydrocephalus
  e. Intubation if necessary

f. Treat ICP increases.

g. Obtain a vascular study (see earlier).

**4. Surgical management**

a. For aneurysmal SAH, evaluation and management by the neurosurgical team is necessary to determine the best treatment.

b. Craniotomy with aneurysm clipping and endovascular coiling available

c. Early intervention (within 48–72 hours) allows for the following results:

    (1) Protection from rerupture

    (2) Safe treatment of potential vasospasm (hypertension, hypervolemia, hemodilution—"triple H")

## B. INTRACEREBRAL HEMORRHAGE

Intracerebral hemorrhage is a hemorrhage within the brain parenchyma. It accounts for ~10% of all strokes and is easily seen in noncontrast CT as a region of high density within the brain parenchyma. The location of the hemorrhage of CT often suggests a cause for the bleed. Basal ganglia, thalamic, pontine, and cerebellar intracerebral hemorrhage are likely related to hypertension.

**1. Causative factors**

a. Hypertension

b. Arteriovenous malformation

c. Aneurysm

d. Neoplasm (hemorrhage into and around a cranial tumor)

e. Arteriopathies (amyloid angiopathy, fibrinoid necrosis, or lipohyalinosis)

f. Coagulation or clotting disorders

    (1) Primary (e.g., thrombotic thrombocytopenic purpura [TTP], leukemia, aplastic anemia)

    (2) Iatrogenic (e.g., warfarin, aspirin, thrombolysis)

g. Thrombosis of venous sinuses

h. Trauma

i. Hemorrhagic conversion of an infarct

j. Drugs (e.g., cocaine)

k. Other vascular malformation—venous angioma, cavernous malformation, or capillary telangiectasia

**2. Central nervous system infection (fungal, granulomas, herpes simplex encephalitis)**

**3. Initial management**

a. Blood pressure control

b. Correct coagulopathy

c. Evaluate possible underlying lesion (e.g., MRI/magnetic resonance angiography, angiogram).

d. Ventriculostomy for CSF diversion if associated with intraventricular hemorrhage and ICP monitoring

e. Further treatment depends on the cause of the hemorrhage, the patient's neurologic condition, and the location of the hemorrhage.

**68**

**NEUROSURGICAL EMERGENCIES**

f. Hypertensive intracerebral hemorrhages can be controlled medically, but if a patient's condition deteriorates, the hemorrhage can be evacuated stereotactically, endoscopically, or through an open procedure.

## C. CAROTID DISSECTION

1. Traumatic versus spontaneous
2. High suspicion in patients with a lateralizing sign that cannot be explained by an intracranial finding on CT.
3. Diagnosed by angiography, computed tomographic angiography, or magnetic resonance angiography. Characterized by a "string sign" or "double-lumen sign."
4. Most dissections heal with recanalization and are treated with anticoagulation (intravenous heparin followed by warfarin [Coumadin]) to prevent clot propagation and emboli.
5. Clinically significant dissections with luminal narrowing and flap may require endovascular stenting or vessel occlusion.

## D. STATUS EPILEPTICUS

1. Defined as a recurrent seizure occurring too frequently for consciousness to be fully regained between seizures, or any seizure activity that lasts longer than 30 minutes
2. Most common scenario is a patient with known seizure disorder with low anticonvulsant levels for any reason.
3. Permanent central nervous system injury or death can occur if seizures are not controlled.
4. Management involves:
a. Intubate if airway compromised or if seizures persist.
b. Lorazepam 1 to 2 mg IV every 5 to 10 minutes, repeat if ineffective. Alternatively, may use diazepam 10 mg IV every 20 minutes if necessary for three doses. Prehospital rectal diazepam may also be given.
c. Load patient with phenytoin 15 to 20 mg/kg, then maintain with 100 mg every 8 hours. Check a phenytoin level and optimize.
d. If seizure activity persists, consider lorazepam drip or phenobarbital drip.
e. If seizures still continue, initiate general anesthesia.

## E. BRAIN DEATH

The criteria used at our institution are listed below; however, these vary across the country.

1. Absence of brainstem function
a. Pupils nonreactive
b. Corneal reflexes absent
c. Oculocephalic reflex absent (doll's eyes)
d. Oculovestibular reflex absent (cold calorics)

e. Gag reflex absent

f. Cough reflex absent

2. No response to central stimulation at three different locations: sternal rub, supraorbital pressure, temporomandibular joint pressure

3. Apnea test: No spontaneous respirations observed during an increase of $Paco_2$ to more than 60 or more than 20 mm Hg from baseline at the start of the apnea test (in patients with chronically increased $Paco_2$, e.g., chronic obstructive pulmonary disease).

4. During the test, the patient must have a temperature of more than 96.5°F, a systolic blood pressure greater than 90 mm Hg, and be absent of paralytics or sedation medication or toxins.

5. Two separate physicians must confirm brain death.

6. At our institution, no further laboratory testing or confirmatory testing such as electroencephalography, angiography, or cerebral blood studies are necessary or required.

**68**

## V. USEFUL WEB SITES, TRIALS, AND GUIDELINES

Traumatic Brain Injury Guidelines (include surgical and pediatric guidelines): *www.braintrauma.org*

CRASH (Corticosteroid Randomisation after Significant Head Injury) Trial (*Lancet* 2004 and 2005)

ASIA (American Spinal Injury Association) Impairment Scale: *www.asia-spinalinjury.org/publications/2006_Classif_worksheet.pdf*

EAST (Eastern Association for the Surgery of Trauma) Cervical Spine Guidelines: *www.east.org/tpg/chap3u.pdf*

NASCIS (National Acute Spinal Cord Injury Study) I-III (1990s)

NEXUS (National Emergency X-ray Utilization Study; *Annals of Emergency Medicine 1998, New England Journal of Medicine 2000*)

Canadian C-Spine Rules (*Journal of the American Medical Association* 2001)

ISAT (International Subarachnoid Aneurysm Trial; *Lancet* 2002 and 2005)

# Urologic Trauma

*Benjamin L. Dehner, MD*

**Case Scenario:** *A 28-year-old man is brought to the emergency department after losing control of his motorcycle and colliding with a guardrail at 50 miles/hr. He was thrown 10 feet before landing on gravel. Fortunately, he wore a helmet and was given a Glasgow Coma Scale score of 15 at the scene and on presentation to the emergency department. His vital signs are stable. However, he describes diffuse abdominal pain and, on examination, has blood at the urethral meatus. Computed tomography (CT) scan shows a widened pubic symphysis and a grade II left renal laceration. Should you place a Foley catheter now? What imaging procedure do you want next? What is your plan concerning the renal laceration?*

**69**

## I. OVERVIEW
### A.  U'S AFTER ABC'S
1. For all trauma cases, the ABC's (airway, breathing, circulation) should be followed (see Chapter 63).
2. After ABC clearance, attention can be turned to other injuries.
3. Ten percent of injuries involve the genitourinary tract.
4. Evaluate mechanisms of injury—blunt versus penetrating injury; kidneys versus bladder versus urethra.

## II. PROCEDURES
### A.  RETROGRADE URETHROGRAM (RUG)
1. RUG: Insert 14-Fr Foley catheter into fossa navicularis.
2. Inflate balloon with 1 to 2 ml normal saline.
3. Inject 10 ml of contrast and obtain radiograph.

### B.  CYSTOGRAM
1. Fill bladder via Foley catheter with 350 ml of contrast material to distend bladder and image; drainage film is necessary to evaluate for extraperitoneal extravasation (contrast in pelvis).
2. Intraperitoneal extravasation will appear as free contrast in abdomen surrounding bowel loops.

## III. RENAL TRAUMA
### A.  GENERAL
#### 1. Blunt versus penetrating injury
a. Eighty-five percent of injury is blunt trauma to abdomen, back, or flank.
b. If blunt injury, was this a rapid deceleration injury (i.e., car accident, fall)? Associated with damaged renal vessels, intimal flap, and subsequent thrombosis or avulsion injury
c. Penetrating injury—assume renal injury with any gunshot or stabbing to flank. Eighty percent of cases are associated with gastrointestinal injuries.

## 2. Hematuria
a. Best indicator of trauma to genitourinary system; however, does not correlate to severity. Thirty-six percent of patients with blunt trauma do not have hematuria.
b. If systolic blood pressure is less than 90 mm Hg and microscopic hematuria is present (<5 red blood cells/high-power field), the risk for significant renal injury is increased.

## B. WORKUP (TABLE 69-1 AND FIG. 69-1)
1. Blunt trauma: Recommend CT with intravenous contrast if blunt trauma with gross hematuria or patients with microhematuria (<5 red blood cells/high-power field) with systolic blood pressure less than 90 mm Hg.
2. *All penetrating injuries with hematuria necessitate imaging.*
3. Initial complete blood cell count may have normal hematocrit; may decrease if serial complete blood cell counts are performed.
a. Decrease in hematocrit seen with enlarging retroperitoneal hematoma.
b. Hematocrit decrease ceases spontaneously in 85% of cases.

## C. MANAGEMENT
1. Nonoperative versus operative management
a. Approximately 98% of renal injuries are nonoperative.
b. Admit for bedrest and hydration with Foley placement. Once urine clears, patient may be ambulatory. If patient tolerates ambulation, can discharge home with close follow-up.
c. Grade I to III renal lacerations are usually monitored without operation; newer recommendations show that even grade IV lacerations may not require surgery in all cases.
2. Operative management
a. Blunt injury—indications are persistent retroperitoneal hematoma expansion, urinary extravasation, renal pedicle injuries, and renal parenchyma necrosis.

### TABLE 69-1

**GRADING OF RENAL LACERATION BY COMPUTED TOMOGRAPHY SCAN**

| Grade | Injury |
| --- | --- |
| I | Contusion with hematuria or subcapsular hematoma without expansion |
| II | Nonexpanding perirenal hematoma or renal cortex laceration <1 cm without urine extravasation |
| III | >1-cm laceration of renal cortex without urine extravasation; collecting system not involved |
| IV | Laceration extends through cortex, medulla, and collecting system; renal artery/vein injury with contained hemorrhage; renal artery thrombosis or intimal flap |
| V | Shattered kidney or devascularized kidney through avulsion of renal hilum |

Adapted from Walsh P, Retik A, Vaughan E, Wein A: *Campbell's Urology*, 8th ed. Philadelphia, Saunders, 2002.

b. Penetrating injury
   (1) Usually associated with visceral organ injury; therefore, renal exploration is usually an extension of ongoing management.
   (2) Unnecessary if imaging shows only minor parenchymal injury without extravasation of urine

## D. SURGICAL APPROACH
1. Transabdominal approach allows inspection of visceral organs.
2. *Early control of vessels is key.*
   *Pearl: Anatomy from anterior to posterior of renal hilum? Renal vein, renal artery, ureter*
a. In 1982, McAnich and Carroll showed early vessel control decreased nephrectomy rate from 56% to 18%.
3. Renal reconstruction
a. Goal is good exposure with vascular control, debridement, hemostasis, a watertight collecting system reconstruction, and coverage of parenchymal defect.
b. If polar injury exists and inability to reconstruct, a partial nephrectomy with omental pedicle flap coverage may be performed.

## E. RENAL ARTERY THROMBOSIS
1. Caused by rapid deceleration during blunt trauma.
2. Renal artery stretches caused by kidney mobility; results in arterial intima disruption, thrombosis, occlusion, and ischemia
3. Salvage is possible with prompt treatment (<8 hours), with success ranging from 70% to 86%.
4. Long-term potential for hypertension

## F. COMPLICATIONS
1. Urinoma, perinephric abscess, and infection
a. Treatment is antibiotics and follow-up.
b. May require ureteral stenting or interventional radiology drainage
2. Delayed bleeding
a. Treatment is bedrest and hydration.
b. Potential need for embolization
3. Hypertension—activation of renin-angiotensin axis caused by stenosis of renal artery, compressed renal parenchyma, or arteriovenous malformation

## IV. URETERAL TRAUMA
### A. GENERAL
1. Usually iatrogenic trauma during abdominal surgery
2. Less than 1% of patients with blunt trauma; less than 4% of patients with penetrating trauma
3. Most common site of penetrating injury is midportion of the ureter.

69

UROLOGIC TRAUMA

## B. SYMPTOMS
1. Flank/abdominal pain, nausea, vomiting associated with ureteral ligation and acute hydronephrosis
2. Hematuria—no hematuria is present in 25% to 45% of cases.
3. If from penetrating trauma, 90% will have only microhematuria.

## C. WORKUP
1. KUB (kidneys, ureter, bladder)—may show area of increased density in pelvis; however, extremely nonspecific.
2. CT with intravenous contrast with delayed images to show extravasation is the preferred imaging modality.

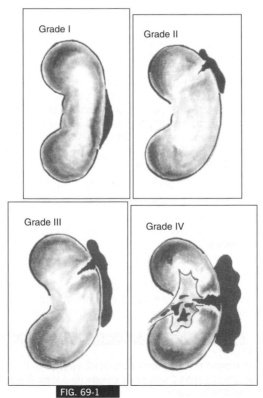

Grade I

Grade II

Grade III

Grade IV

**FIG. 69-1**

Depiction of grades of renal laceration.

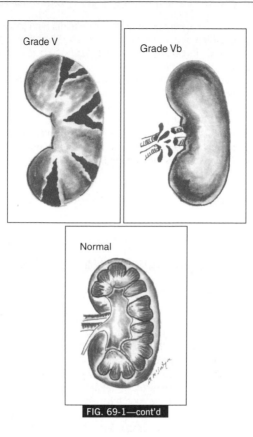

Grade V

Grade Vb

Normal

FIG. 69-1—cont'd

a. If iatrogenic causative factor, recommend intraoperative intravenous pyelogram and excretory urogram.
b. Intraoperative cystoscopy with retrograde pyelograms can also be performed.

## D. MANAGEMENT
1. Goals—debridement, tension-free and watertight anastomosis, and retroperitoneal drainage
2. Depends on location of trauma
a. Upper third of ureter—direct ureteroureterostomy or transureteroureterostomy (ureteral reimplantation into contralateral ureter)
b. Middle third of ureter—direct ureteroureterostomy or transureteroureterostomy

c. Lower third of ureter—reimplant ureter into bladder with psoas hitching to minimize tension of the ureteral anastomosis. Alternative is to perform Boari flap (from bladder) to bridge defect.

**3. Stenting**
a. Stenting of ureter for 3 to 4 weeks after surgery with double-J stents
b. Minimizes stenosis and urinary extravasation

## E. DELAYED REPAIR
Option if immediate surgery not feasible because of patient instability
1. Tie off ureter and place percutaneous nephrostomy tube.
2. Return with repair as described earlier.

## F. COMPLICATIONS
1. Urine leak—comprises 10% to 24% of repairs.
2. Abscess
3. Fistula
4. Stenosis—occurs in 5% to 12% of patients.

## V. BLADDER TRAUMA

### A. GENERAL
1. Eighty-three percent to 100% of cases has associated pelvic fracture.
2. Blunt trauma source more common than penetrating source. Usually associated with full bladder with direct blow causing increased intravesical pressure and rupturing of bladder wall.
   (1) Laplace's law—change in pressure = wall tension/radius
   (2) Dome of bladder rupture results in intraperitoneal urine leakage.
   (3) Pelvic fracture usually results in retroperitoneal urine leakage because of laceration by bone fragments.
3. Fifteen percent of cases are associated with urethral injury.
   *Pearl: What fracture is most associated with bladder rupture?*
   *Fracture of pubic arch.*

### B. SYMPTOMS
1. Pelvic or lower abdominal pain, usually associated with pain because of pelvic fracture
2. May have inability to void
3. Usually gross hematuria with voiding
4. If intraperitoneal rupture, may present with peritonitis, acute abdomen, fever, or shock

### C. WORKUP
1. Catheterization is needed with pelvic trauma. However, if blood at meatus, an RUG is needed to rule out urethral injury in all patients.
a. If RUG is normal, proceed with Foley catheterization.
b. Gross hematuria usually present.

**2.** Imaging

a. A ruptured bladder may not be seen on focused assessment with sonography for trauma (FAST) ultrasound examination.

b. CT cystogram with delayed images is recommended method of imaging; if unable to be performed with CT, have cystogram performed separately. Urethrogram should be performed first if indicated by examination.

    (1) Allows visualization of kidneys, ureters, and abdominal viscera

    (2) Cystogram allows for differentiation between extraperitoneal (urine enters into perivesical and fascial planes) and intraperitoneal bladder rupture (urine surrounds abdominal organs and pelvic gutters). One hundred percent accurate according to Carroll and McAninch (1984).

**D. CLASSIFICATION**

**1.** Contusion

a. About 67% of bladder injuries are from blunt trauma.

b. No therapy needed; hematuria will clear without complication.

**2. Extraperitoneal bladder rupture**

a. Managed with indwelling Foley catheterization (10 days) and antibiotics (e.g., ciprofloxacin) for 14 days

b. Follow up with repeat cystogram at 10 to 14 days. If no urine extravasation, catheter can be discontinued; if leak seen, repeat cystogram in 1 week.

c. Contraindications—bone fragments within bladder, open pelvic fracture, or rectal perforation (increases infection risk of extravasated urine)

d. *Exception: If patient is to go to the operating room with orthopedic surgery to plate the pubic symphysis*

    (1) Allows bladder inspection and suprapubic catheter placement

    (2) Decreases urine extravasation onto orthopedic hardware and minimizes infection risk

**3. Intraperitoneal bladder rupture**

a. Twenty-five percent of bladder injuries are solely intraperitoneal; 12% are associated with extraperitoneal rupture.

b. Usually involves bladder dome caused by increased intravesical pressure with blunt trauma

c. Requires two-layered closure to create water-tight seal and prevent peritonitis. Place Foley catheter and suprapubic tube to decompress bladder. Remove after repeat cystogram lacks contrast extravasation

d. Treat with 3 days of perioperative antibiotics and repeat cystogram in 1 week.

**E. COMPLICATIONS**

**1.** Infection

**2.** Abscess

**3.** Pelvic hematoma

a. Caused by pelvic vessel rupture with trauma

b. May require packing of pelvis during exploration or angiographic embolization

**69**

**UROLOGIC TRAUMA**

4. Incontinence—associated with bladder neck laceration. Should be repaired if bladder is explored to minimize long-term sequelae.

## VI. URETHRAL INJURY

### A. GENERAL

1. *PIMP: What are the five anatomic divisions of the urethra from distal to proximal? Fossa navicularis, bulbous urethra, pendulous urethra, membranous urethra, and prostatic urethra*
2. Functionally, the urethra can be divided into two portions:
   a. Anterior urethra—fossa navicularis, bulbous, and pendulous urethra
   b. Posterior urethra—membranous and prostatic urethra
3. *If blood is present at the meatus of the penis, RUG before Foley placement.*

### B. ANTERIOR URETHRAL INJURY

1. Rare injury
2. Straddle injury to bulbar urethra is most common.
   a. Caused by falling astride an object or direct perineal trauma
   b. Results in bulbous urethra being crushed against the pubic symphysis.
   c. Blood and urine will be enclosed within Colles' fascia.
      (1) Present in scrotum and penile shaft
      (2) Does not cross abdominal wall
      (3) Prostate within normal position

### C. POSTERIOR URETHRAL INJURIES

1. Most commonly caused by blunt trauma with bilateral pubic rami fractures
   a. Shears the membranous urethra from the prostatic urethra at the prostatomembranous junction
   b. Blood and urine extravasate above the triangular ligament around the prostate and bladder. Hematoma is seen along the perineum.
   c. Distraction injury more common in male than female individuals.
2. Signs—*TRIAD: blood at meatus, inability to urinate, palpable bladder*
   a. Present in 50% of cases
   b. Amount of blood at meatus does not correlate to degree of injury.
   c. High-riding prostate is an unreliable sign.

### D. MANAGEMENT

1. RUG—to evaluate for extravasation. A contusion will show no signs of extravasation.
2. Contusion
   a. If patient able to void without pain or hematuria, no treatment is necessary.
   b. If hematuria, urethral catheterization is needed.

3. Laceration

a. Place suprapubic cystotomy tube for urinary diversion for 1 to 3 weeks. Urethral Foley placement risks further urethral injury and hematoma rupture

b. May require secondary repair if extensive laceration or transaction

  (1) Will reconstruct in 6 weeks to 3 months by anastomotic urethroplasty

  (2) Allows fibrosis and scar tissue to develop, allowing for reconstruction

4. Anastomotic urethroplasty

a. Perform RUG and cystogram before surgery.

  (1) Allows visualization of length of resultant stricture

  (2) Excise stricture with primary anastomosis. May require grafting if stricture smaller than 2 cm.

b. Complications

  (1) Stricture—develops in less than 5% of cases; usually does not require surgical correction.

  (2) Impotency—occurs in 6% of cases. Caused by transected parasympathetic fibers or damaged bilateral deep corporal arteries.

## VII. PENILE INJURY

### A. PENILE FRACTURE

1. General

a. Results from sexual intercourse (partner on top)

b. Caused by disruption of tunica albuginea with ruptured corpus cavernosum

c. Tumescence thins the protective tunica albuginea, increasing fracture risk.

2. Signs

a. During intercourse, "popping sound" with immediate pain and detumescence

b. Ecchymosis is present (eggplant deformity).

c. If Buck's fascia is disrupted, hematuria is present.

3. Management—*Surgical: Immediate repair with hematoma evacuation.* If not managed with surgery, patient with increased deformity, pain, and hospital stay.

4. Complications

a. Impotency—caused by veno-occlusive dysfunction

b. Infection

c. Hematoma

### B. AMPUTATION

1. General—increased association with psychiatric history and self-mutilation

2. Treatment—surgical reapproximation of dorsal artery, vein, and nerve. Place suprapubic tube.

3. Obtain psychiatric consultation.

69

UROLOGIC TRAUMA

### C. PENETRATING INJURY TO CORPORA
1. Treatment—perform RUG. Primary repair with anastomosis versus staged repair with grafting if extensive damage.

## VIII. TESTICULAR TRAUMA

### A. GENERAL
1. More commonly blunt trauma than penetrating. Penetrating injury usually occurs with other injuries.

### B. SIGNS
1. Blunt injury—pain, nausea, vomiting
a. Hematoma may be present.
b. Increased risk for testicular torsion
2. Penetrating injury
a. As described earlier, with wound exposure
b. Increased risk for testicular rupture

### C. IMAGING
1. Ultrasound is useful to image the testis and determine rupture and testicular torsion. Should not delay surgical management if severe dislocation or trauma is present.

### D. MANAGEMENT
Transverse scrotal incision allows for hematoma evacuation to decrease intrascrotal pressure.
1. All devitalized tissue should be debrided with tunica albuginea reapproximation. Results in decreased orchiectomy rate.
2. Torsed testicle should be detorsed and watched to ensure blood flow resumes.
a. Will appear as a change in testicle coloration from blue/black to pink
b. If testicle does not recover, perform orchiectomy.
c. If testicular blood flow resumes, perform orchiopexy.
d. Controversy exists regarding contralateral testicle orchiopexy if viable.

## RECOMMENDED READING

Altman A, Haas C, Dinchman K, Spirnak P: Selective nonoperative management of blunt grade 5 renal injuries. *J Urol* 164:27–31, 2000.

Basta A, Blackmore C, Wessells H: Predicting urethral injury from pelvic fracture patterns in male patients with blunt trauma. *J Urol* 177:571–575, 2007.

Carroll PR, McAninch JW: Major bladder trauma: Mechanisms of injury and a unified method of diagnosis and repair. *J Urol* 132:254–257, 1984.

Mydlo J, Harris C, Brown J: Blunt, penetrating, and ischemic injuries to the penis. *J Urol* 168:1433–1435, 2002.

Santucci R, Wessells H, Bartschm G, et al: Evaluation and management of renal injuries: Consensus Statement of the Renal Trauma Subcommittee. *BJU Int* 93:937–954, 2004.

Tanagho EA, McAninch J: *Smith's General Urology,* 16th ed. New York, Lange Medical Books/McGraw Hill, 2004.

Walsh P, Retik A, Vaughan E, Wein A: *Campbell's Urology,* 8th ed. Philadelphia, Saunders, 2002.

Wessells H, Suh D, Porter J, et al: Renal injury and operative management in the United States: Results of a population-based study. *J Trauma* 54:423–430, 2003.

Wright J, Nathens A, Frederick R, Wessells H: Renal and extrarenal predictors of nephrectomy from the National Trauma Data Bank. *J Urol* 175:970–975, 2006.

# PART XIV

# Pediatric
# Surgery

PART XIV

# Pediatric Surgery

# Pediatric Surgery: Abdomen and General

*Marcus D. Jarboe, MD*

## I. GASTROINTESTINAL TRACT

### A. HYPERTROPHIC PYLORIC STENOSIS

1. Gastric outlet obstruction caused by hypertrophied pyloric muscle
2. Affects 1 in 150 live births; male-to-female ratio is 4:1.
3. Occurs in first 2 months of life, with average age of clinical presentation 2 to 8 weeks. Nonbilious, postprandial that increases in volume and frequency is seen. Often emesis is projectile and infant is hungry after emesis. Presents classic electrolyte picture of "contraction" alkalosis (hypokalemia, hypochloremia, metabolic alkalosis, "paradoxical aciduria"). Unconjugated hyperbilirubinemia may also be present.
4. Ninety percent of patients have palpable pyloric tumor ("olive") in the midepigastrium to right upper quadrant; examination is facilitated by nasogastric decompression and calming with dextrose/water solution.
5. Ultrasound is study of choice for confirming diagnosis (>3 mm thick, >14 mm long) when pyloric tumor is not palpable or equivocal.

**Pearl:** *'Py'lorus* − $\pi$ = 3.14

6. Preoperative management
   a. Operation is never an emergency, and adequate preoperative preparation is necessary for low morbidity.
   b. Nasogastric decompression may be needed if continued emesis.
   c. Fluid resuscitation and electrolyte correction including potassium repletion (once urine output ensured) are mandatory before operative repair. Correct $HCO_3$ to less than 30.
   d. D5 1/2 normal saline at 125% to 150% maintenance for minor electrolyte disturbances, D5 normal saline bolus of 10 to 20 ml/kg for severe disturbances
7. Surgical treatment—classic operation is Fredet–Ramstedt pyloromyotomy via right upper quadrant, periumbilical, or laparoscopic approach.
   a. One to 2 mm proximal to pyloric vein (vein of Mayo) to 1.5 cm onto stomach past hypertrophy
   b. Blunt spread of the muscle fibers; do not enter mucosa.
8. Postoperative management
   a. Nasogastric tube removed in operating room
   b. Continued intravenous hydration if necessary
   c. Emesis common after procedure
   d. Oral fluids (electrolyte solution) begun 4 to 6 hours after surgery, gradually advanced over 1 to 2 days to full-volume formula feeds

## B. INTESTINAL OBSTRUCTION IN THE NEONATE

1. Should suspect with history of maternal polyhydramnios, bilious emesis, abdominal distention, or failure to pass meconium within first 24 hours of life
2. Bilious vomiting in an infant is a surgical emergency and requires emergent evaluation to rule out malrotation and midgut volvulus.

**Pearl:** *If it's yellow, call the fellow; if it's green, call the team.*

3. Intrinsic duodenal obstruction
   a. Frequent association with other anomalies
   b. May be caused by duodenal web, atresia, or stenosis
   c. Presents with bilious vomiting, minimal abdominal distention, only proximal bowel and stomach
   d. Abdominal radiographs reveal "double-bubble" sign.
   e. Surgical treatment includes excision of webs or duodenostomy for atresia and evaluation of distal bowel for other atresias.
4. Extrinsic duodenal obstruction—malrotation
   a. Malrotation of the midgut results in a narrow base and lack of fixation for the midgut mesentery, with predisposition to volvulus and intestinal infarction.
   b. Presents with sudden onset of bilious vomiting as newborn (bilious emesis in child younger than 1 year is volvulus until proven otherwise)
   c. Volvulus frequently results in significant vascular compromise and intestinal necrosis.
   d. Most reliably diagnosed by upper gastrointestinal to visualize malpositioned ligament of Treitz
   e. Treatment includes emergent laparotomy and Ladd's procedure. This consists of evisceration, reduction of volvulus by counterclockwise rotation (Pearl: "Turning back the hands of time."), division of "Ladd's bands," thereby widening the mesenteric base between the duodenum and the colon, appendectomy, and placement of the small bowel in the right side and the colon in the left side of the peritoneal cavity.
   f. Nonviable bowel should be resected; questionably viable bowel should remain with a planned 24-hour second-look laparotomy.
   g. Delay in diagnosis can lead to significant loss of bowel length resulting in short gut syndrome.
5. Jejunoileal obstruction—atresia and stenosis
   a. Result of late mesenteric vascular accidents in utero
   b. Abdominal radiographs show dilated loops of small bowel; contrast enema usually demonstrates small, unused "microcolon," although it may be normal.
   c. Classification of jejunoileal atresia:
      **Type I**—single mucosal atresia, bowel wall and mesentery in continuity, and normal bowel length
      **Type II**—single atresia with discontinuity of bowel and gap in mesentery (blind ends joined by fibrous cord running on intact mesentery)

**Type IIIa**—disconnected blind ends as in type II but no cord connecting and a mesenteric gap

**Type IIIb**—"apple peel" or "Christmas tree" deformity with markedly decreased bowel length

**Type IV**—multiple atresias resulting in short bowel length

d. Operative management is individualized, depending on number and length of atresias; includes resection with anastomosis, tapering enteroplasty, and exteriorization in the presence of compromised bowel; resection of proximal dilated bowel with end-to-end anastomosis.

e. Contrast barium enema to rule out colonic atresia

### 6. Meconium ileus

a. Obstruction of the distal ileum from inspissated meconium—associated with cystic fibrosis

b. Simple meconium ileus—bowel is impacted with pellets of meconium, with proximally dilated ileum packed with thick, tarlike meconium.

c. Complicated meconium ileus—associated with meconium cysts, atresia, perforation, meconium peritonitis, volvulus, or intestinal necrosis

d. Simple meconium ileus presents with progressive abdominal distention and failure to pass meconium; abdominal radiograph obstruction shows no air–fluid levels; "soap bubble" appearance in proximal colon; contrast enema shows microcolon with inspissated plugs of meconium.

e. Complicated type presents with sepsis, distention, often respiratory distress.

f. May respond to nonoperative therapy with Gastrografin enemas after hydration, nasogastric decompression, empiric antibiotics, and vitamin K to correct any coagulopathies

g. Operative intervention indicated for complicated cases and where nonoperative therapy fails; ranges from simple enterotomy and irrigation of bowel with *N*-acetylcysteine (Mucomyst) to bowel resection with primary anastomosis or temporary diverting colostomy or distal chimney enterostomy.

h. Short-term survival rate approximately 100% for simple and 85% for complicated meconium ileus.

### 7. Hirschsprung's disease

a. Absence of parasympathetic ganglion cells in the affected segment of intestine; rectum and rectosigmoid most common.

b. Familial forms of Hirschsprung's disease associated with mutations in RET protooncogene, endothelin receptor B, and endothelin-3 genes.

c. Cardinal symptoms—failure to pass meconium in first 24 hours, abdominal distension, and vomiting. Also suspected in any infant who has chronic constipation during the first year of life.

d. Diagnosis suggested by transition point on barium enema (rectum of small to normal size with proximal colorectal dilation) and confirmed with suction rectal biopsy (absence of ganglion cells in Meissner's [submucosal] and Auerbach's [intermuscular] plexus; increase in acetylcholinesterase staining).

e. Currently, most infants with a new diagnosis of Hirschsprung's disease are treated with a one-stage pull-through operation. Previously, the standard was a multistage approach starting with diverting colostomy proximal to the aganglionic segment, followed by a definitive pull-through procedure at 9 to 12 months of age.

f. Laparoscopic one-stage pull-through procedures are becoming more frequently used.

g. Complications include enterocolitis (10–30%), anastomotic leak (1–5%), and stricture (3–5%).

## C. INTESTINAL OBSTRUCTION IN THE INFANT (2 MONTHS TO 2 YEARS)

**1. Intussusception**

a. Most common cause of bowel obstruction in 2 months to 2 years age range; more than 50% have documented recent viral infection.

b. Caused by telescoping of one segment of bowel (intussusceptum) into another (intussuscipiens). Ileocecal occurs most commonly.

c. Sudden onset of recurring severe, cramping abdominal pain; vomiting; drawing up of legs; 60% have bloody ("currant jelly") stools. An elongated mass may be palpable in right upper quadrant with an "empty" right lower quadrant.

d. Diagnosis by air or barium enema—"coiled spring" appearance

e. Initial treatment by attempted hydrostatic/pneumatic reduction during air/contrast enema if peritonitis or free air has been ruled out first (50–90% success rate).

f. Requires surgical exploration if air enema reduction is unsuccessful or if peritonitis is present; manual reduction is performed distal to proximal, followed by appendectomy if bowel remains viable. If manual reduction is not possible or if lead point is identified, resection is indicated.

**2. Incarcerated hernia (see Chapter 21)**

## D. NECROTIZING ENTEROCOLITIS

**1.** Most common gastrointestinal emergency in the premature neonate

**2.** More than 90% of cases are found in premature or low-birth-weight infants; occurs in 5% of neonatal intensive care admissions.

**3.** Unknown cause—appears to be related to ischemic intestinal damage, bacterial colonization, and intraluminal substrate (feedings).

**4.** Early clinical findings—ileus, gastric retention, bilious vomiting, and bloody stools. Progressive findings include lethargy, apnea, bradycardia, hypothermia, shock, acidosis, and neutropenia.

**5.** Radiographic findings—pneumatosis intestinalis (air in bowel wall). Late findings include "fixed" loop of bowel (suggests gangrenous changes) and portal vein air or free air. Pneumatosis with portal venous air is pathognomonic for necrotizing enterocolitis.

**6. Medical management**

a. Gastric decompression, nothing by mouth

b. Systemic antibiotics

c. Fluid resuscitation, correction of acidosis, parenteral nutrition

d. Close monitoring—serial complete blood cell count, platelet count, and upright abdominal films (every 6 hours)

**7.** Indications for surgery

a. Free air or portal vein air on radiograph (absolute indication)

b. Clinical deterioration—persistent acidosis, thrombocytopenia, leukopenia

c. Diffuse peritonitis, abdominal wall erythema, or induration

d. Paracentesis suggestive of nonviable bowel if fluid brown and cloudy, extracellular bacteria on Gram stain, large number of white blood cells with differential more than 80% neutrophils

e. Goal of surgical management is maximum bowel preservation. Leave questionable bowel intact and come back for second look to assess viability.

## E. MECKEL'S DIVERTICULUM

**1.** Meckel's diverticulum is the most common form of congenital malformation of small bowel. Persistent vitelline duct remnant; less commonly persistent vitelline duct with sinus, persistent omphalomesenteric band, and vitelline duct cyst.

**2.** Occurs on antimesenteric border of ileum within 60 cm of ileocecal valve

**3.** Complications

a. Bleeding—40% to 60% of cases; usually painless, caused by ulceration of adjacent tissue from ectopic gastric mucosa; usually stops spontaneously but can be massive.

b. Obstruction—25% of cases; intussusception or secondary to internal hernia around persistent omphalomesenteric band

c. Diverticulitis—10% to 20% of cases; mimics acute appendicitis.

**4.** Diagnosis—high degree of suspicion, confirmed by 99m technetium-pertechnate scan; can have false-positive results with enteric duplications or false-negative results with small amounts of gastric mucosa, recent barium study, or pelvic Meckel's hidden behind the bladder

**5.** Treatment by laparoscopic diverticulectomy, wedge resection of diverticulum, or segmental ileal resection with primary anastomosis; includes appendectomy

**6.** Incidental Meckel's diverticulum—generally recommend resection in patient younger than 18 years, particularly if heterotopic tissue present; not indicated in asymptomatic adults

**7.** Remember the "rule of 2s"—occurs in 2% of the population, symptomatic in 2% of cases, approximately 2 feet from the ileocecal valve, 2 inches in length, 2 types of mucosa (gastric/pancreatic), twice as many male as female cases, 2 presentations (bleeding, obstruction)

## F. APPENDICITIS (SEE CHAPTER 19)

**1.** Most common emergent abdominal operation in children

**2.** Ruptured in 20% to 76% of children at presentation (approximately 100% in <1 year old, 82% in <5 years old)

70

PEDIATRIC SURGERY: ABDOMEN AND GENERAL

### G. GASTROESOPHAGEAL REFLUX

**1.** See Adult reflux, Chapter 24

**2.** Differs from adult gastroesophageal reflux

a. Emesis is the most common presentation; malnutrition and failure to thrive; aspiration pneumonia and asthma; esophagitis; laryngospasm.

b. Frequently associated with mental retardation

c. Preoperative evaluation

    (1) Upper gastrointestinal to exclude gastric outlet obstruction and malrotation

    (2) Esophagogastroduodenoscopy to rule out Barrett's and to grade esophagitis (not necessary in young children)

    (3) pH probe is most sensitive and specific for pathologic reflux (pH <4 for >4% of the time), although may not be needed with good clinical picture.

    (4) Obtain technetium gastric emptying scan to rule out delayed gastric emptying or outlet obstruction.

d. Initial treatment is nonoperative for 6 to 8 weeks—has a 80% response rate.

    (1) Upright position, thickened feedings, metoclopramide, H2 blockers

    (2) Frequently resolves spontaneously

    (3) Contraindicated in patients with esophageal stricture or near-miss sudden infant death syndrome

e. Operative therapy

    (1) Usually not performed in children younger than 6 months

    (2) Indications—failed medical therapy, severe esophagitis, Barrett's metaplasia, stricture, bleeding, neurologically impaired patient who needs a gastrostomy tube

    (3) Two most common repairs: Nissen (360 degree) and Thal (270 degree)—10% and 20% recurrence rates, respectively. Laparoscopic approach is frequently used.

    (4) Pyloroplasty in patients with delayed gastric emptying

## II. ABDOMINAL WALL DEFECTS

### A. OMPHALOCELE

**1.** A covered defect of the umbilical ring into which abdominal contents herniate; sac composed of an outer layer of amnion and an inner layer of peritoneum

**2.** More than 50% of infants have serious associated congenital defects (genitourinary, cardiac, gastrointestinal); always associated with malrotation.

**3.** Sac may contain only intestine but usually contains liver as well; may be associated with loss of abdominal domain, with contracted abdominal cavity.

**4.** Management includes covering sac with sterile dressing, protection from hypothermia, gastric decompression, parenteral nutrition, and broad-spectrum antibiotics.

5. Surgical treatment: Small defects can be closed primarily; moderate defects can have the skin closed with the subsequent hernia being repaired later; larger defects require staged closure using Silastic silo.
6. Overall survival depends on the size of the defect and the severity of associated congenital defects; mortality rate averages 30% to 35% (almost exclusively because of associated abnormalities).

## B. GASTROSCHISIS
1. Defect of the anterior abdominal wall just lateral and usually to the right of the umbilicus
2. No peritoneal sac, with resulting antenatal evisceration of bowel through the defect
3. Always associated with nonrotation; 15% associated with intestinal atresias; other congenital defects unusual.
4. Management
   a. Prevention of excessive insensible fluid and heat loss through exposed bowel; gastric decompression
   b. Large amounts of intravenous fluids needed to maintain perfusion; initiation of total parenteral nutrition; broad-spectrum antibiotics.
   c. Primary repair successful in 70% of cases; if not possible, it is treated with gradual decompression using a Silastic silo.

## C. UMBILICAL HERNIA
1. Defect of the umbilical ring; more common in premature and black infants, incarceration is rare in general population.
2. Spontaneous closure in 80% to 90% of patients, usually if 2 cm in diameter or smaller; if larger than 2 cm, less chance of spontaneous closure
3. Observation recommended until child is 2 to 3 years of age; if larger than 2 cm, undergo elective repair; large defects are repaired earlier.

## D. INGUINAL HERNIA
1. Caused by persistence of the embryonic processus vaginalis
2. Incidence varies with gestational age (preterm > term, male/female ratio is 8:1, overall incidence rate of 1–5%).
3. Approximately 10% bilateral; contralateral exploration indicated if patient is younger than 1 year (60% bilateral). Laparoscopy through the hernia sac can be used to perform exploration of contralateral side.
4. Most are indirect.
5. Examination reveals reducible mass in groin extending along spermatic cord up to the internal ring if not incarcerated or strangulated.
6. Major complication is bowel incarceration with strangulation and possible infarction; significantly higher in preterm infant and in infants in first year of life. Premature infants with hernia are repaired before discharge from hospital.

70

PEDIATRIC SURGERY: ABDOMEN AND GENERAL

7. Examination in face of incarceration or strangulation reveals an immobile, tender mass in groin, with mass extending along spermatic cord up to the internal ring.

8. High ligation of sac is adequate repair; may repair bilateral hernias simultaneously.

9. Incarcerated hernia: In the absence of signs of compromised bowel (fever, peritonitis, leukocytosis) or obstruction, attempt reduction when diagnosed; achieved by placing firm pressure in the direction of the inguinal canal; facilitated by sedation and elevation of the legs and torso. If irreducible, or if strangulation is suspected, urgent repair is indicated.

## H. SHORT-BOWEL SYNDROME

1. Disorder resulting from removal of large portion of small bowel resulting in insufficient absorptive surface area.

a. Length of bowel needed at time of resection to avoid short-bowel syndrome depends on many factors such as age of patient and presence or absence of ileocecal valve. Overall, patients with 30 cm or more of small bowel are more likely to survive on enteral nutrition, whereas with less than 30 cm, they are more likely to need parenteral nutrition.

2. Causative factors—necrotizing enterocolitis (most common), atresias, volvulus, gastroschisis, others

3. Overall survival rate is 78% to 94%.

4. Clinical syndrome—malnutrition, weight loss, steatorrhea, and diarrhea

a. Initial stage is severe fluid and electrolyte loss (1–2 weeks).

b. Second stage is intestinal adaptation (starting at 48 hours and up to 1 year).

c. Last stage is plateau stage when adaptive process is maximized (reached 1–2 years after resection).

5. Treatment is hydration, total parenteral nutrition, and enteral feeds as tolerated for 1 year, then consider surgical therapy if no further progress.

a. Medical management includes H2 blockers (treats hypersecretion), glutamine, cholestyramine (improve diarrhea), and opioids (slows transit time).

b. Complications include line sepsis, total parenteral nutrition–induced liver disease, and intestinal bacterial overgrowth.

6. Surgical approaches target three anatomic/physiologic abnormalities seen. Surgery goals are as follows:

a. Slow transit—intestinal valves, reverse segments, recirculating loops, colon interposition, intestinal pacing

b. Improve function—tapering enteroplasty, stricturoplasty

c. Increase mucosal surface area—intestinal lengthening, neomucosa, Iowa model, transplantation

## I. ANORECTAL MALFORMATIONS

1. Anorectal malformations encompass a large spectrum of defects ranging from mild anal anomalies to complex cloacal malformations.
   a. Most common malformations in male patients are imperforate anus with rectourethral fistula followed by rectoperineal fistula.
   b. Most common malformations in female patients are rectovestibular fistula, perineal fistula, followed by persistent cloaca.
   c. Incidence of malformations—1 in 4000 to 5000 newborns.
2. Diagnosis made by careful physical examination and, in some cases, prone cross-table plain films.
3. Two questions in first 48 hours of life:
   a. Other associated defects endangering patient's life—VATER symptom complex:
      **V**—vertebral
      **A**—anorectal
      **T**—tracheal
      **E**—esophageal
      **R**—renal
   b. Whether patient needs colostomy before perineal repair
4. No colostomy needed in perineal fistula or anal stenosis.
5. Operative procedure is posterior sagittal anorectoplasty.
6. Outcomes depend on the preoperative malformation. Functional sequelae:
   a. Constipation—bowel regimen
   b. Fecal incontinence—bowel management programs
   c. Urinary incontinence—intermittent catheterization

## III. NEOPLASMS

### A. NEUROBLASTOMA

1. Usually in children younger than 4 years (approximately 80%)
2. Origin—neural crest tissue, pathologically classified as a small, round, blue cell tumor of childhood
3. Metabolically active—catecholamines (90%)
4. Wide range of biologic behavior from highly malignant to benign ganglioneuroma or spontaneous regression
5. Presentation—70% disseminated at presentation
   a. Abdominal mass—retroperitoneal, adrenal medulla, or paraspinal ganglia
   b. A large thoracic primary may present with respiratory distress, spinal cord compression, symptoms of catecholamine, or vasoactive intestinal polypeptide excess.
   c. Horner syndrome may result from a cervical primary tumor.
6. Diagnosis
   a. Urinary catecholamine breakdown products.
   b. Computed tomography or magnetic resonance imaging—may demonstrate spinal involvement more accurately.

70

PEDIATRIC SURGERY: ABDOMEN AND GENERAL

   c. Bone scan and bone marrow aspiration

   d. MIBG (metaiodobenzylguanidine I123) nuclear scan shows bone involvement and primary tumor.

**7. Treatment—based on assessment of biologic features (karyotype, *N-myc* amplification) and clinical stage.**

   a. Stage 1 or 2 (localized with no metastasis, crossing of midline or contralateral nodal involvement)—operative resection with node removal

   b. Stage 3 or 4 (disseminated tumor, contralateral nodal involvement)— primary or delayed operative resection, chemotherapy and radiation therapy

**8. Prognosis—inversely related to age**

   a. Tumor stage and location

   b. *N-myc* gene amplification, stroma-poor or nodular-rich pathology, increased serum ferritin or lactate dehydrogenase associated with poor prognosis

## B. NEPHROBLASTOMA (WILMS' TUMOR)

**1. Embryonal renal neoplasm—mesenchymal origin. Two related but separate tumors are clear cell sarcoma and malignant rhabdoid tumor.**

**2. *WT1* and *WT2* are tumor suppressor genes in sporadic cases, whereas *FWT1* and *FWT2* are involved with inherited forms of Wilms' tumors.**

**3. Presentation**

   a. Maximal incidence—1 to 3 years of age (90% of cases present before age 7 years)

   b. Ten percent of cases are associated with congenital abnormalities— WAGR (*W*ilms' tumor, *a*niridia (no iris), *g*enitourinary malformations, mental *r*etardation) syndrome, Beckwith–Wiedemann syndrome, Denys–Dash syndrome.

   c. Symptoms—fever; abdominal pain; firm, irregular, painless abdominal mass; hematuria; hypertension

   d. Diagnosis—ultrasound (cystic vs. solid, invasion of vena cava), computed tomography or magnetic resonance imaging, chest radiograph to screen for pulmonary metastases

**4. Treatment**

   a. Operative—tumor removal even with distant metastases; 5% to 8% of cases have bilateral involvement.

   b. Solitary lung metastases may be excised.

   c. Adjuvant chemotherapy and radiation therapy are beneficial. Preoperative chemotherapy and radiation therapy may enable operative therapy for tumors initially too large for resection, those with intravascular extension of tumor thrombus proximal to intrahepatic vena cava, and those with bilateral Wilms' tumors.

**5.** Prognosis—worse with anaplasia, sarcomatous changes, positive nodes, higher staging, older age

a. Five- to 7-year survival rate of approximately 90% for all cases

**RECOMMENDED READING**

Ashcraft KW, Holcomb GW, Murphy JP (eds): *Pediatric Surgery*, 4th ed. Philadelphia, Elsevier, 2005.

Ziegler MM, Azizkhan RG, Weber TR (eds): *Operative Pediatric Surgery*. New York, McGraw-Hill, 2003.

# Pediatric Surgery: Thoracic and Neck

*Grace Z. Mak, MD*

Children are not simply little adults. Rather, the physiology and pathology are unique to the pediatric population.

## I. GENERAL CONSIDERATIONS

### A. THERMOREGULATION

1. Extremely thermolabile so careful regulation of ambient environment is crucial.

2. Premature infants are particularly susceptible because of inability to shiver, lack of fat stores, impaired thermogenesis, and lack of adaptive mechanisms to cope with surrounding environment.
3. Great care must be taken to conserve heat during transport and intraoperatively (heating lamps, warming blankets, warming of inspired gases, coverage of extremities and head, warm irrigation fluids).
4. Hypothermia can result in cardiac arrhythmias or coagulopathy.

### B. VENOUS ACCESS

1. Infants—cutdown approach in antecubital fossa, external jugular vein, facial vein, or proximal saphenous vein
2. Children more than 2 kg—percutaneous access of subclavian, internal jugular, or femoral veins
3. Complication rate in children is high.
a. Catheter-related sepsis or infection approaches 10%.
b. Superior or inferior vena caval occlusion is a significant risk, especially in small premature infants.

## II. FLUID AND ELECTROLYTE REQUIREMENTS

### A. MAINTENANCE FLUIDS

1. Infants born with body water surplus normally excreted by end of first week of life
a. Birth—fluid requirements of 65 ml/kg (750 ml/m$^2$) over 24 hours
b. End of first week—fluid requirements increase to 100 ml/kg (1000 ml/m$^2$) over 24 hours.
2. Maintenance fluids can be calculated by a variety of methods.
a. Maintenance fluid—D5 1/4 normal saline
b. Body weight method
   (1) 100 ml/kg/24 hours (4 ml/kg/hr) for first 10 kg PLUS
   (2) 50 ml/kg/24 hours (2 ml/kg/hr) for 11 to 20 kg PLUS
   (3) 25 ml/kg/24 hours (1 ml/kg/hr) for each additional kilogram more than 20 kg

(4) Example—25-kg child:
    (a) First 10 kg—200 ml/24 hours (40 ml/hr)
    (b) Next 10 kg—100 ml/24 hours (20 ml/hr)
    (c) Final 5 kg—25 ml/24 hours (5 ml/hr)
    (d) Total—325 ml/24 hr (65 ml/hr)
c. Body surface area method
  (1) 2000 $ml/m^2$/24 hours
  (2) Not accurate for infants with less than 10 kg body weight
  (3) Calculation of body surface area from nomogram using height and weight

## B. MAINTENANCE ELECTROLYTES
1. $Na^+$—3 to 5 mEq/kg/24 hours
2. $K^+$—2 to 3 mEq/kg/24 hours
3. $Ca^{2+}$—2 mEq/kg/24 hours
4. $Mg^{2+}$—0.15 to 1 mEq/kg/24 hours

## C. RESUSCITATION FLUIDS
1. Crystalloid—lactated Ringer's or normal saline, 10- to 20-ml/kg bolus
2. For ongoing fluid loss (i.e., nasogastric tube output, protracted vomiting or diarrhea), replace fluid 1 ml per 1 ml every 4 hours using D5 1/2 normal saline + 20 mEq KCl/L.
3. Colloid
a. 5% albumin—10- to 20-ml/kg bolus
b. 25% albumin—2- to 4-ml/kg bolus
4. Blood product replacement
a. Estimated blood volume for infant—85 ml/kg
b. Whole blood—10 to 20 ml/kg
c. Packed red blood cells—5 to 10 ml/kg
d. Plasma—10 to 20 ml/kg
e. Platelets—1 unit/5 kg
f. Caused by coagulation deficiencies that may develop with extensive blood transfusion; plasma and platelets should be available with transfusion of more than 30 ml/kg

## D. FLUID BALANCE
1. Distinction between dehydration and fluid overload is very fine.
a. Clinical signs of dehydration
  (1) Tachycardia
  (2) Reduced urine output
  (3) Depressed fontanelle
  (4) Lethargy
  (5) Poor feeding
b. Clinical signs of fluid overload
  (1) New or increased oxygen requirements
  (2) Respiratory distress

    (3) Tachypnea
    (4) Tachycardia

## E. ACID-BASE BALANCE
1. Metabolic acidosis
a. Caused by inadequate tissue perfusion
b. Causes
    (1) Intestinal ischemia caused by necrotizing enterocolitis in newborns, midgut volvulus, or incarcerated hernia.
    (2) Chronic bicarbonate loss from gastrointestinal (GI) tract caused by diarrhea.
    (3) Chronic renal failure with acid accumulation
c. Treatment
    (1) If serum pH less than 7.25, sodium bicarbonate should be replaced.
        (a) Replacement = base deficit × weight (kg) × correction factor
            (1) Correction factor:
                (a) 0.5 in newborns
                (b) 0.4 in smaller children
                (c) 0.3 in older children
        (b) Dose should be administered at concentration of 0.5 mEq/ml.
        (c) Half of calculated replacement administered, then pH measured.
        (d) During cardiopulmonary resuscitation, administer half corrective dose as intravenous bolus followed by slow intravenous infusion of remaining half.
2. Metabolic alkalosis—most commonly caused by gastric acid loss due to pyloric stenosis or overaggressive diuresis.
3. Respiratory acidosis—caused by hypoventilation.
4. Respiratory alkalosis—caused by hyperventilation.

## III. TOTAL PARENTERAL NUTRITION
### A. GENERAL
1. Indicated for prolonged ileus, GI fistulas, gastroschisis, intestinal atresia, supplementation of oral feeds (short-bowel syndrome, malabsorption states), catabolic wasting states (malignancy or sepsis), and in treatment of necrotizing enterocolitis.
2. Children, particularly neonates, have little nutritional reserve, so must consider total parenteral nutrition early to allow for normal growth and healing of surgical wounds.
a. Inadequate protein and carbohydrate calories can lead to growth failure and impaired central nervous system development.
3. Total maintenance rates for intravenous fluids are calculated first; then the concentration of nutrients in the total parenteral nutrition is gradually increased daily.

4. Enteral nutrition preferred whenever possible.
a. Promotes growth and function of GI tract and allows infant to learn to feed
5. Estimate maintenance water requirements as in section I.A.

## B. SPECIFIC REQUIREMENTS
1. Caloric requirements (include allowance for stress, growth):
a. Zero to 6 months—100 to 120 kcal/kg/day
b. Six months to 1 year—100 kcal/kg/day
c. One to 7 years—90 to 100 kcal/kg/day
d. Seven to 12 years—60 to 70 kcal/kg/day
e. Twelve to 18 years—45 to 60 kcal/kg/day
2. Protein calories (15% of total calories)
a. Zero to 6 months—2 g/kg/day
b. Six months to 1 year—1.5 g/kg/day
c. One to 7 years—1 to 1.2 g/kg/day
d. Seven to 12 years—1 g/kg/day
e. Twelve to 18 years—1 g/kg/day
3. Lipid calories (30–40% total calories, should not exceed 50%)
a. Lipid formulations
   (1) 10% = 10 g/100 ml = 1.1 kcal/ml
   (2) 20% = 20 g/100 ml = 2.0 kcal/ml
b. Begin with 0.5 g lipid/kg/day and increase by 0.5 g/kg/day to a maximum of 3 g/kg/day.
4. Carbohydrate calories (50% total calories)—minimum glucose infusion rate of 4 to 6 mg/kg/min for neonates
5. Supplemental copper, zinc, and iron

## C. COMPLICATIONS
1. Liver failure
a. Cholestasis with progression to end-stage hepatic fibrosis
b. Can be prevented by administration of enteral feeds, meticulous catheter care minimizing infections, aggressive treatment of all infections, and early cycling of total parenteral nutrition

## IV. LESIONS OF THE HEAD AND NECK
### A. GENERAL
1. Must determine duration and location of lesion.
a. Midline location
   (1) Thyroglossal duct remnants, thyroid masses, thymic cysts, dermoid cysts
b. Lateral location
   (1) Branchial cleft remnants, cystic hygromas, vascular malformations, salivary gland tumors, torticollis
   (2) Lipoblastoma—rare benign mesenchymal tumor of embryonal fat

   c. Nonspecific
     (1) Lymphadenopathy
     (2) Rhabdomyosarcoma

## B.  LYMPHADENOPATHY
1. Most common neck mass in children
2. Can be found in midline or lateral neck
3. Tender lymphadenopathy often caused by bacterial infection with *Staphylococcus* or *Streptococcus*
   a. Treatment of primary cause should suffice
   b. Fluctuant lymph nodes may require incision and drainage.
4. Chronic lymphadenitis caused by tuberculosis, atypical mycobacteria, cat-scratch fever
   a. Diagnosed by serology and excisional biopsy
   b. Infectious mononucleosis can be diagnosed by serology.
5. Firm, fixed neck lymph nodes with associated axillary and inguinal lymphadenopathy (also firm and fixed).
   a. Excisional biopsy indicated to evaluate for hematologic malignancy.
   b. Chest radiograph to check for mediastinal mass

## C.  THYROGLOSSAL DUCT REMNANTS
1. Causative factors
   a. Thyroid develops from evagination in base of tongue (foramen cecum) at 3 weeks of gestation.
   b. Thyroid tissue becomes more anterior and caudal as the fetal neck continues to develop.
   c. Descent of the thyroid connected to formation of hyoid bone.
   d. Residual thyroid tissue from descent may persist in midline as thyroglossal duct cyst, which may become enlarged and symptomatic.
2. Presentation
   a. Two- to 4-year-old child
   b. Most frequently occurs as rounded, cystic mass of varying size in midline of neck at or below level of the hyoid bone that moves with swallowing and tongue protrusion
   c. Occasionally presents as intrathyroid mass
   d. Most are asymptomatic.
   e. Symptoms can include dysphagia, pain, infected mass (if duct retains connection to pharynx).
   f. Symptoms of hypothyroidism may be present.
   g. Rarely is a site for adult carcinoma (<1% of patients)
     (1) Should be suspected with rapid growth of cyst or ultrasound showing complex anechoic pattern or calcifications
3. Differential diagnosis
   a. Submental lymphadenopathy, midline dermoid cyst
   b. Midline ectopic thyroid tissue

**71**

PEDIATRIC SURGERY: THORACIC AND NECK

(1) If diagnosis unclear or normal thyroid gland not palpable, document presence of normal thyroid tissue separate from cyst via nuclear medicine scan.

4. **Treatment**
a. Abscess should be incised and drained with administration of antibiotics.
   (1) After resolution of inflammation, definitive resection can be performed.
b. Sistrunk procedure
   (1) Total excision of cyst en bloc with central body of hyoid bone and tract to pharynx with ligation at foramen cecum
   (2) Curative
c. Recurrence more common after infection (more than two infections before surgery), age younger than 2 years, and inadequate initial operation.
d. If total excision of thyroid tissue unavoidable, thyroxine supplementation will be required.

## D. BRANCHIAL CLEFT ANOMALIES

1. **Causative factors**
a. Paired branchial clefts and arches develop during week 4 of gestation.
b. First cleft and first, second, third, and fourth pouches develop into adult organs.
c. Branchial sinuses and cysts are remnants of these embryologic structures (may contain small pieces of cartilage and cysts).
d. Persistent embryologic communication between pharynx and skin results in fistula.
   (1) Most common anomaly arises from second branchial cleft (fistula from tonsillar fossa to anterior border of sternocleidomastoid muscle).

2. **Presentation**
a. Fistulae are usually discovered in childhood.
   (1) Second branchial cleft sinus presents with clear fluid draining from anterior border of lower third of sternocleidomastoid muscle.
b. Cysts frequently present along the anterior border of the sternocleidomastoid and are not seen until adulthood.
   (1) Present as mass anterior and deep to upper third of sternocleidomastoid
   (2) May become infected
   (3) Ten percent of cases are bilateral.
   (4) Risk for in situ carcinoma in adults
c. Goldenhar's complex
   (1) Rare
   (2) Branchial cleft anomalies with associated biliary atresia and congenital cardiac anomalies

3. **Diagnosis—ultrasound to identify cystic nature of mass if not apparent by physical examination**

4. Treatment
a. If infected, incision and drainage with antibiotics (coverage for *Staphylococcus* and *Streptococcus*) and formal resection once inflammation has resolved
b. Total excision of cyst and tract during formal neck dissection under general anesthesia
   (1) Can pass fine lacrimal duct probe from external tract opening to facilitate dissection of distal sinus tract
   (2) Injection of methylene blue dye into tract is also helpful.
   (3) Multiple small transverse incisions in "stepladder" fashion preferred to long oblique neck incision

## E.  CYSTIC HYGROMA (LYMPHANGIOMA)

1. Causative factors
a. Caused by sequestration or obstruction of developing lymphatics
b. Benign tumor of lymphatic origin
c. Cysts lined by endothelium and filled with lymph
d. Occurs in 1 in 12,000 births

2. Presentation
a. Most often located in posterior triangle of neck with predilection to the left side, axilla, groin, and mediastinum
b. Can also involve tongue, floor of mouth, and structures deep in neck
c. Mass may be diagnosed at birth or may appear and enlarge rapidly during first weeks to months of life with accumulation of lymph.
d. Ninety percent of cases are diagnosed by second year of life.
e. Can cause respiratory insufficiency in infancy or when glottic structures are involved
f. Extension into axilla or mediastinum (10%)
g. Usually presents as multiple cysts infiltrating surrounding structures and distorting normal anatomy
   (1) Adjacent connective tissue shows extensive lymphocytic infiltration.
h. Sudden enlargement and discoloration usually caused by hemorrhage into lesion.
   (1) Occasionally, nests of vascular tissue found within hygroma may bleed.
i. Infections can develop due to *Staphylococcus* and *Streptococcus.*

3. Diagnosis
a. Chest radiograph
b. Ultrasound
c. Computed tomography (CT) scan
d. Transillumination can help distinguish cystic hygroma from solid masses.
e. Prenatal ultrasound before 30 weeks of gestation
   (1) Can diagnose extremely large lesions causing airway compromise and distortion with polyhydramnios

     (2) To secure airway at time of delivery, orotracheal intubation or urgent tracheostomy performed while infant remains attached to placenta in the ex utero intrapartum technique (EXIT procedure)

**4. Treatment**

a. Conservative excision with unroofing of remaining cysts is treatment of choice.

     (1) Radical surgery, that is, excising involved blood vessels and nerves, is contraindicated.

     (2) Repeated partial excisions of residual hygroma may be necessary.

b. Postoperative wound drainage is important.

c. Sclerotherapy with multiple agents such as bleomycin, doxycycline, and fibrin glue has been used with mixed results.

**F. TORTICOLLIS**

**1. Lateral neck mass in infant with rotation of head to opposite side of mass**

a. Palpable in two thirds of cases

**2. Caused by fibrosis of sternocleidomastoid muscle**

a. Histologically, collagen and fibroblasts present around atrophied muscle cells

**3. Physical therapy often beneficial**

**4. Surgical transection of muscle can be curative in rare cases.**

## V. THORACIC DISORDERS

**A. PULMONARY SEQUESTRATION**

**1. Pathophysiology**

a. Lung tissue with absent or abnormal bronchial communication to the normal tracheobronchial tree

b. Blood supply not from pulmonary artery, rather from systemic artery from aorta

c. Theorized to result from abnormal budding of developing lung with systemic blood supply without forming a connection to bronchus or pulmonary vessels

d. Usually in left lower chest

e. Uncommon

**2. Types**

a. Extralobar—66% of cases diagnosed in infancy.

     (1) Small area of nonaerated lung separate from main lung mass but invested in visceral pleura

     (2) Arterial supply usually low thoracic aorta immediately above left diaphragm; venous drainage can be systemic or pulmonary.

     (3) Ninety percent located in left posterior costophrenic sulcus.

     (4) Most frequently is asymptomatic and found incidentally on chest radiograph

     (5) Rarely manifests as respiratory insufficiency

(6) May become infected by hematogenous spread of bacteria despite lack of communication with airway or lung tissue

(7) Commonly have coexisting congenital anomalies (15–40%), especially diaphragmatic hernia

b. Intralobar—majority diagnosed after age 1 year, often in adulthood

(1) Communicates with normal lung only via the pores of Kohn or secondary connection to tracheobronchial tree caused by infection or intrapulmonary shunts

(2) Arterial supply systemic, often with multiple vessels frequently originating below diaphragm; venous drainage systemic or pulmonary

(3) Sixty percent in left hemithorax (most commonly within parenchyma of left lower lobe)

(4) Should suspect in patients with recurrent pneumonias within same bronchopulmonary segment

## 3. Diagnosis

a. Chest radiograph—findings vary from opacification to cystic parenchymal lesions with air-fluid levels.

b. Color ultrasonography with Doppler-flow analysis is highly sensitive and specific.

c. Chest CT scan with three-dimensional reconstruction also valuable for diagnosis; angiography infrequently used

## 4. Treatment

a. Symptomatic sequestrations require resection.

(1) Extralobar by simple excision

(2) Intralobar frequently requires formal lobectomy because of late diagnosis after multiple infections.

b. Life-threatening hemorrhage possible if systemic vascular supply not recognized and controlled intraoperatively

c. Extralobar resection not necessary if asymptomatic and diagnosis confirmed

## 5. Prognosis—excellent

## B. BRONCHIECTASIS

### 1. Pathophysiology

a. Abnormal and irreversible dilation of bronchi and bronchioles with subsequent chronic infection

b. Can also be due to prolonged bronchial foreign body

c. Usually with associated congenital pulmonary anomaly, cystic fibrosis, or immune deficiency

### 2. Presentation—chronic cough, recurrent pneumonias, hemoptysis

### 3. Diagnosis—chest radiograph

a. Increased bronchovascular markings in affected lobe

b. Chest CT scanning

### 4. Treatment

a. Medical—antibiotics, postural drainage, bronchodilator therapy

b. Surgical

(1) Indicated for localized disease refractory to maximal medical therapy

(2) Lobectomy or segmental resection

## C. BRONCHOGENIC CYSTS

### 1. Pathophysiology

a. Derived from abnormal budding of primitive tracheobronchial tube

b. Hamartomatous histology

    (1) Mucoid central core surrounded by wall of cartilage and smooth muscle

    (2) Cyst lined with ciliated columnar respiratory epithelium

c. Can occur anywhere along respiratory tract from neck to lung parenchyma

d. Seventy percent of cysts within lung tissue

e. Thirty percent of cysts within mediastinum, extrinsic to lung

### 2. Presentation

a. Symptoms vary based on anatomic location of cyst.

    (1) Tracheal, bronchial, or esophageal obstruction

    (2) Pneumonia

    (3) Mediastinal compression

    (4) Rarely, cystic rupture

b. May be asymptomatic with incidental discovery on chest radiograph

c. Can present at any age

### 3. Diagnosis

a. Chest radiograph showing dense mass

b. CT or magnetic resonance imaging can delineate exact anatomic location.

### 4. Treatment

a. Cyst excision regardless of symptoms

    (1) Usually by simple excision, although formal lobectomy may be required

b. Can be done open or thoracoscopically

## D. CONGENITAL CYSTIC ADENOMATOID MALFORMATION

### 1. Pathophysiology

a. Cystic proliferation of terminal airways forming cysts consisting of mucus-producing respiratory epithelium and elastic tissue in cyst wall without cartilage

b. Results from focal pulmonary dysplasia rather than hamartomatous change

c. Most commonly in left lower lobe

d. Can occur bilaterally simultaneously

### 2. Classification

a. Large and multiple cysts (type I)

b. Smaller and more numerous cysts (type II)

c. Resemble fetal lung without macroscopic cysts (type III)

3. Presentation
a. Variable from no symptoms to severe respiratory failure
b. Most common presentation is respiratory distress in newborn.
c. Can present in later life because of recurrent pulmonary infection
d. Symptoms produced by progressive air trapping with enlargement of mass and compression of normal lung and airways; may have associated pulmonary hypoplasia and pulmonary hypertension.

4. Diagnosis
a. Chest radiograph
b. CT chest scan
c. Ultrasound—can aid in distinguishing congenital cystic adenomatoid malformation and congenital diaphragmatic hernia.

5. Differential diagnosis
a. Type I in left lower lobe can be confused with left congenital diaphragmatic hernia.
b. Congenital lobar emphysema
c. Pulmonary sequestration

6. Treatment—lobectomy
a. Rarely, systemic arterial supply may be present as in pulmonary sequestration.
b. May be performed urgently if severe respiratory distress

7. Prognosis
a. Resection curative
b. Excellent

## E.  CONGENITAL LOBAR EMPHYSEMA

1. Pathophysiology
a. Progressive obstructive emphysema of one or more lobes of lung leading to massive distension of involved lobe(s)
   (1) Inspired air trapped in lobe leads to progressive overexpansion of lobe causing atelectasis of adjacent lobe(s).
b. Further overexpansion can cause mediastinal shift and compromise of contralateral lung.
c. Caused by intrinsic bronchial obstruction from poor bronchial cartilage development or extrinsic compression (ball-valve effect)
d. Occurs, in order of frequency, in left upper, right upper, right middle, and lastly lower lobes

2. Epidemiology
a. Two thirds of patients are male.
b. Rare in blacks and premature infants
c. Fourteen percent of patients have associated cardiac defects.
   (1) Enlarged left atrium or major vessel compressing ipsilateral bronchus

3. Presentation
a. Variable
   (1) Range from mild respiratory distress to respiratory failure (tachypnea, dyspnea, cough, cyanosis)

(2) Symptoms may be stable or progress rapidly.

(3) Can be life-threatening in newborn period

(4) Less respiratory distress in older infants

b. Symptoms may mimic tension pneumothorax.

c. More than 50% of patients experience development of symptoms within first few days of life

d. Neonates often trap fetal lung fluid in lobe, so chest radiograph may look like pneumonia until fluid clears.

e. May present with recurrent pneumonia, failure to thrive (increased work of breathing caused by overexpanded lung)

**4. Diagnosis**

a. Chest radiograph

(1) Hyperlucency of affected lobe with adjacent lobar compression and atelectasis

(2) Varying degrees of mediastinal shift with contralateral lung compression

b. CT chest scan may be helpful.

c. Bronchoscopy not advisable unless foreign body or mucous plug suspected

(1) Can cause more air trapping and lead to respiratory distress in an otherwise stable infant

**5. Treatment—lobectomy**

a. Usually performed several months after birth unless necessitated earlier by symptoms

**6. Prognosis—excellent**

## F. CONGENITAL DIAPHRAGMATIC HERNIA (BOCHDALEK HERNIA)

**1. Pathophysiology**

a. Occurs as result of failure of fusion of the transverse septum and the pleuroperitoneal folds during the 8th week of fetal development

b. Posterolateral portion of diaphragm is last to complete development—Bochdalek hernia.

c. Development of ipsilateral (and to varying degrees contralateral) pulmonary hypoplasia caused by abdominal contents within pleural cavity.

(1) Decreased bronchial and pulmonary arterial branching

(2) Decreased lung weight, volume, and DNA content

(3) Decreased surfactant present that further compounds respiratory insufficiency.

d. Persistent fetal circulation (persistent pulmonary hypertension of the newborn) results in right-to-left shunting with failure of oxygenation and ventilation.

e. Prognosis depends on severity of pulmonary hypoplasia.

**2. Epidemiology**

a. Occurs in up to 1 in 2000 live births

b. Posterolateral defects (75–85%)

(1) Left side (80–90%)

c. Associated congenital defects (40%)
   (1) Trisomies 18 and 21
   (2) Cardiac malformations (60% of associated anomalies)

### 3. Presentation

a. Respiratory distress (dyspnea, cyanosis, hypoxemia, hypercarbia, metabolic acidosis, decreased breath sounds)
   (1) Caused by intrathoracic bowel compressing mediastinum causing shift to contralateral chest that further hinders air exchange in contralateral lung
   (2) Persistent fetal circulation
   (3) Ipsilateral pulmonary hypoplasia, essentially nonfunctional lung
b. Scaphoid abdomen with underdeveloped small abdominal cavity
c. Symptoms may develop immediately (more common) or several hours after birth ("honeymoon period," associated with better prognosis).

### 4. Diagnosis

a. Prenatal
   (1) Ultrasound diagnosis as early as 15 gestational weeks
      (a) Herniated abdominal viscera, abnormal intraabdominal anatomy, mediastinal shift away from viscera
   (2) Lung-to-head ratio predictor of severity of left congenital diaphragmatic hernia
      (a) Product of right lung length and width at level of cardiac atria divided by head circumference
      (b) Lung-to-head ratio less than 1—poor prognosis
      (c) Lung-to-head ratio greater than 1.4—more favorable outcome
b. Chest radiograph
   (1) Usually confirms diagnosis
   (2) Gas-filled bowel loops seen within chest (may be confused with cystic adenomatoid malformation); may require GI contrast study in the stable patient to confirm diagnosis.

### 5. Treatment

a. Cardiorespiratory stabilization
   (1) Goals
      (a) Prevention or reversal of pulmonary hypertension
      (b) Minimize barotrauma whereas optimizing oxygen delivery
   (2) Mechanical ventilation
      (a) Conventional ventilator with "gentle" settings—low airway pressures, volumes
      (b) Permissive hypercapnia tolerated with arterial partial pressure of carbon dioxide ($Paco_2$) 50 to 60 mm Hg if pH greater than 7.25.
      (c) High-frequency oscillatory ventilator can be used if conventional tidal volume ventilation unsuccessful.
      (d) Avoid mask ventilation.

**71**

PEDIATRIC SURGERY: THORACIC AND NECK

        (3) Echocardiography to assess pulmonary hypertension, associated cardiac anomalies

           (a) Inhaled nitric oxide (up to 40 parts per million in ventilatory circuit) to minimize pulmonary hypertension

        (4) Administration of bicarbonate solution can correct metabolic acidosis and minimize degree of pulmonary hypertension.

        (5) Be careful not to administer excess fluids because this can worsen right-sided heart failure.

        (6) May need to administer inotropic agent such as epinephrine to optimize cardiac contractility and maintain mean arterial pressure.

        (7) Patients who do not improve with maximal ventilatory support may be candidates for extracorporeal membrane oxygenation (ECMO).

           (a) Venovenous or venoarterial bypass can be used.

           (b) Eligibility criteria

               (1) Normal cardiac anatomy by echo

               (2) Absence of fatal chromosomal abnormalities

               (3) Weight more than 2.5 kg

               (4) Gestational age more than 34 weeks

           (c) ECMO continued until pulmonary hypertension reversed and lung function (compliance) improved (generally within 7–10 days)

           (d) ECMO complications

               (1) Bleeding most significant

                  (a) Caused by systemic anticoagulation

                  (b) Can occur intracranially or at cannulation sites

               (2) Sepsis—may necessitate decannulation.

  b. Monitoring catheters—postductal arterial line, adequate venous access

  c. Stomach decompression with 10-French Replogle tube

  d. Surgery

      (1) Once infant stabilized medically

      (2) Can be performed with patient still on ECMO

      (3) Transabdominal approach using subcostal incision

      (4) Reduction of herniated abdominal contents

      (5) Often attenuated posterior margin of defect

      (6) Primary closure of diaphragmatic defect or patch closure with prosthetic material

      (7) Chest tube often left in place in patients on ECMO to minimize hemothorax

      (8) Prosthetic patch may be needed to close abdomen after reduction of abdominal viscera (can be removed later with repair of ventral hernia).

      (9) After surgery, infants must be weaned slowly from ventilator to prevent recurrent pulmonary hypertension.

**6. Prognosis—overall mortality rate in most series is 60% to 70%.**

## G. MEDIASTINAL MASSES

1. Superior—thymoma, thymic cyst, lymphoma, thyroid mass, parathyroid mass
2. Anterior—thymoma, thymic cyst, teratoma, dermoid, lymphangioma, hemangioma, lipoma, fibroma
3. Middle—pericardial cyst, bronchogenic cyst, lymphoma, granuloma
4. Posterior—neurogenic tumors (neuroblastoma, ganglioneuroma), foregut duplications and cysts

## VI. FOREIGN BODIES

### A. AIRWAY

1. Most common in toddlers
2. Peanuts most commonly aspirated
   a. Oil from peanut can be irritating and lead to pneumonitis or pneumonia.
3. Most common location for aspirated foreign body—right mainstem bronchus or right lower lobe
4. Solid foreign body can lead to air trapping, atelectasis, and pneumonia.
5. Diagnosis
   a. Chest radiograph
      (1) Radiopaque foreign bodies can be visualized.
      (2) Nuts, seeds, or plastic items cannot be seen—evidence of hyperlucency in affected lobe on expiration.
   b. Rigid bronchoscopy—both diagnostic and therapeutic

### B. ESOPHAGUS

1. Most common in toddlers
2. Most common foreign body is coin, then small toy parts.
3. Esophageal locations of retention (areas of normal anatomic narrowing)
   a. Cricopharyngeus
   b. Area of aortic arch
   c. Gastroesophageal junction
4. Symptoms depend on area involved and degree of obstruction.
   a. Initially, GI symptoms (dysphagia, drooling, vomiting)
   b. Respiratory symptoms (cough, stridor, wheezing) develop with prolonged presence of foreign body.
5. Diagnosis
   a. Chest radiograph can visualize radiopaque items such as coins.
   b. Contrast swallow necessary for nonradiopaque items.
6. Treatment
   a. For coins in upper esophagus for less than 24 hours, Magill forceps can be used.
   b. Esophagoscopy (rigid or flexible)
   c. Esophagotomy rarely required for removal of particularly sharp objects.
7. Follow-up
   a. Diligent follow-up required particularly for batteries (can cause strictures due to alkali) and sharp objects (can damage esophagus).

b. Magnets pose a dangerous situation if swallowed because of adhesions between adjacent bowel loops.

## VII. ESOPHAGUS

### A. ESOPHAGEAL ATRESIA AND TRACHEOESOPHAGEAL FISTULA (TEF)

1. Pathophysiology
a. Embryonic failure of separation of the trachea from the esophagus (normally occurs by 36 days of gestation)
b. May be related to deficiency in Sonic-hedgehog signaling pathway
c. Associated congenital anomalies
   (1) Twenty percent of infants with esophageal atresia also have congenital heart disease.
   (2) VATER or VACTERRL syndrome
      (a) Vertebral (missing vertebra)
      (b) Anorectal (imperforate anus)
      (c) Cardiac (severe congenital cardiac disease)
      (d) TEF
      (e) Renal (renal agenesis)
      (f) Radial limb hyperplasia

2. Anatomic variations (Fig. 71-1)
a. Type A (8–10%)—isolated esophageal atresia without fistula; gasless abdomen on radiograph
b. Type B (1%)—esophageal atresia with proximal TEF
c. Type C (75–85%)—esophageal atresia with distal TEF, abdominal gas seen on radiograph
d. Type D (1–2%)—esophageal atresia with proximal and distal TEFs
e. Type E (5–8%)—TEF without atresia (H type)
f. Type F (1%)—esophageal stenosis without fistula

3. Presentation
a. Variable depending on specific anatomic variant present
b. With blind-ending esophagus or proximal TEF (types A, B, C, or D), infants have excessive salivation, feeding intolerance (choking or coughing immediately after feeding), or gagging.
   (1) Aspiration via fistulous tract after feeding
   (2) With coughing or crying in types C or D, air passes from the fistula into the stomach, causing abdominal distension leading to respiratory difficulty. This leads to further atelectasis. These patients are also more susceptible to chemical pneumonitis from refluxed gastric contents via fistula into tracheobronchial tree.
c. H-type fistula (type E) may present at later age with recurrent pneumonias, bronchospasm, and failure to thrive.

4. Diagnosis
a. Prenatal ultrasound
   (1) Failure to visualize stomach, maternal polyhydramnios caused by inability of fetus to swallow amniotic fluid

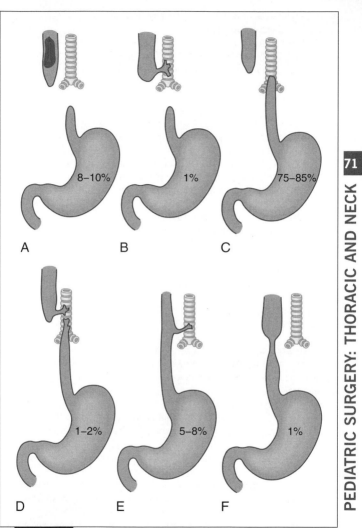

FIG. 71-1

Types of tracheoesophageal fistulas. See VII.A.2 for descriptions of each type.

b. Inability to pass orogastric catheter beyond esophagus
c. Chest radiograph (upright)
   (1) Dilated proximal pouch may be visible.
   (2) Coiled orogastric catheter in proximal pouch
   (3) Absence or presence of gas in stomach and GI tract (delineates anatomical variant)
d. Contrast esophagram
   (1) Confirms diagnosis of atresia and often TEF
   (2) Also may aid in differentiating esophageal perforation at piriform sinus from traumatic insertion of orogastric or nasogastric tube
e. Associated anomalies
   (1) Echo to examine heart for cardiac anomalies, great vessels, position of aortic arch (left or right sided)
   (2) Plain vertebral radiographs, spinal ultrasound if abnormal radiographs
   (3) Clinical confirmation of patent anus
   (4) Abdominal ultrasound to evaluate kidneys
   (5) Plain radiographs of anomalous extremities

5. **Initial management**
a. Infant warmer with head elevation at least 30 degrees
b. 10-French Replogle catheter into proximal segment to prevent aspiration
c. Intravenous broad-spectrum antibiotics
d. Warmed supportive fluid, electrolyte, and nutritional intravenous solutions
e. Avoid right upper extremity if possible for intravenous access (may interfere with patient positioning during surgery).
f. Avoid mask or pressure ventilation.

6. **Surgery**
a. Rarely an emergency
b. Repair can be performed once infant is hemodynamically stable with good oxygenation after complete evaluation for associated congenital anomalies.
c. Ventilated, premature infant with hyaline membrane disease (unique case)
   (1) TEF can worsen pulmonary status because of recurrent aspiration and increased abdominal distension impairing lung expansion.
   (2) Degree of positive pressure ventilation must be minimized to decrease amount of air passing into stomach—often requiring high-frequency oscillatory ventilator.
   (3) If gastric distension is severe, gastrostomy tube can be placed. Tube should be placed to water seal, elevated, or intermittently clamped because ventilated gas may preferentially pass through the fistula into gastrostomy tube, further worsening hypoxemia.
   (4) If above therapy is unsuccessful, TEF can be ligated at the bedside.

     (5) Once underlying hyaline membrane disease improves and infant is stable, definitive repair can be performed.

  d. Isolated atresia without fistula
     (1) Lower esophageal segment frequently too short for primary repair
     (2) Initial cervical esophagostomy with gastrostomy tube
     (3) Serial bougienage to lengthen proximal pouch
     (4) If primary repair unable to be performed, esophageal replacement with stomach, colon, or small-bowel interposition can be performed (usually around 1 year of age).

  e. Definitive repair
     (1) Left lateral decubitus positioning with right posterolateral thoracotomy
     (2) Bronchoscopy to identify additional fistulas and identify laryngotracheoesophageal cleft.
     (3) Retropleural approach
     (4) TEF ligation
     (5) Oversewing of tracheal defect
     (6) Primary esophagoesophagostomy under no tension
     (7) Transanastomotic feeding tube
     (8) Retropleural chest drainage

  f. H-type fistulas—can generally be repaired via cervical approach with TEF ligation.

**7. Complications**

  a. Anastomotic leak (10–15%)
     (1) Early—new pleural effusion, pneumothorax, sepsis
       (a) Immediate exploration—likely complete disruption of anastomosis
       (b) If possible, revise anastomosis.
       (c) Otherwise, cervical esophagostomy with gastrostomy tube and later reconstruction of esophagus
     (2) Late
       (a) Often heals with conservative management (broad-spectrum antibiotics, pulmonary toilet, nutritional optimization).
       (b) Repeat esophagram after 1 week to assess healing of leak.

  b. Anastomotic stricture (10–20%)
     (1) More common after leaks
     (2) May present at any time with choking, gagging, or failure to thrive
     (3) Often apparent when transitioning to solid foods
     (4) Contrast swallow or esophagoscopy are diagnostic.
     (5) Treatment with dilation (may need to be repeated)

  c. "Recurrent" TEF
     (1) Missed proximal pouch fistula or true recurrence because of anastomotic disruption
     (2) May heal spontaneously, with the use of fibrin glue, or require reoperation

  d. Gastroesophageal reflux (44%)

8. Prognosis
a. Nearly normal esophageal function in most patients after surgical repair
b. Survival largely dependent on preoperative ventilator dependence and associated congenital defects, particularly birth weight less than 1500 g and major congenital cardiac disease.
   (1) Birth weight more than 1500 g without major cardiac disease—survival rate of 97%
   (2) Birth weight less than 1500 g *or* major cardiac disease—survival rate of 54%
   (3) Birth weight less than 1500 g *and* major cardiac disease—survival rate of 22%

## B. CAUSTIC ESOPHAGEAL INJURY
1. Most common in toddlers
2. After ingestion of corrosive substances such as lye, antifreeze
3. Both strong acids and strong alkalis can cause liquefaction or coagulation necrosis
4. Children often drool and are unable to swallow saliva without complaints of pain.
5. Diagnosis
a. Examination of oropharynx
b. Endoscopy (rigid or flexible) only to level of initial burn to avoid perforation
c. Barium swallow may delineate extent of mucosal injury.
6. Initial treatment
a. Antibiotics during acute phase
b. Steroids have not been shown to modify extent of injury or alter stricture formation.
c. Dependent on extent of injury
   (1) Circumferential injury with necrosis
      (a) High likelihood of later stricture formation
      (b) Gastrostomy tube placement
      (c) Endoscopic insertion of string from mouth through esophagus to gastrostomy tube for later retrograde dilations
7. Subsequent strictures occur at normal areas of anatomic narrowing (cricopharyngeus, midesophagus, gastroesophageal junction).
a. If severe strictures unresponsive to dilation, esophageal replacement may be necessary
   (1) Colon (right or transverse), stomach
   (2) Feeding jejunostomy placed at time of surgery
8. Close follow-up into adulthood mandatory because late ulcers and strictures can develop.

# PART XV

# Future of Surgery

# New Surgical Technologies

*Julian Guitron, MD, and Lynn C. Huffman, MD*

We are living at the beginning of a new age in surgery. Though not universally recognized, there has been a paradigm shift with new scientific disciplines and technologies. Ready or not, these innovations are taking us forward. Clear examples of such advances are shown in this chapter.

## I. MODERN BIOLOGY
The age of modern biology has brought recombinant DNA technology, polymerase chain reaction techniques, and completion of the Human Genome Project.

## 72

## II. GENOMIC INFORMATION
BRCA and RET-protooconogene, to name a few, are used to direct prophylactic procedures by removing tissues that will develop malignancies.

## III. BIOMEDICAL ENGINEERING
Biomedical engineering brings surgery, medicine, engineering, and a variety of other disciplines together to develop new technologies, procedures, and processes.

## IV. SURGICAL EDUCATION
With the emergence of robotics, information systems, telecommunications, and simulators, the surgical field is rapidly moving toward reality simulators, much as pilots are trained before ever flying a new aircraft. The *Center for Surgical Innovation (CSI)* at the University of Cincinnati bridges the College of Medicine, College of Engineering, and several industrial partners with expertise in surgical robotics, medical simulation, telecommunications, and medical/health informatics. It promotes and expedites the generation and transformation of knowledge and technology.

## V. BIOTECHNOLOGY AND SURGERY
Now more than ever, surgery is bound intimately to biotechnology. The following surgical technologies that promise to impact the way surgery is practiced the most are reviewed in this chapter.

### A. MEMS (MICROELECTROMECHANICAL SYSTEMS) SURGERY
1. Novel technology that integrates sensors, actuators, and electronics on a silicone plate
2. Produced through microfabrication technology
3. They are complete systems-on-a-chip. That is, traditional microelectric circuits, which function as the "brain" of the system, now have the decision-making ability through "eyes" and "arms" (MEMS), enabling these microsystems to sense and control the environment.

4. Sensors can gather different types of impulses such as mechanical, thermal, biological, chemical, optical, and magnetic phenomena, allowing the electric circuit ("brain") to react by moving, positioning, or regulating among many other functions, achieving a desired effect in its environment.

5. This technology promises to revolutionize almost all technology categories. In medicine, there are significant MEMS applications under development; in some instances, these applications are already being used in human subjects.

6. CardioMEMS, Inc., specializes in surgical MEMS applications.

a. The *EndoSure Wireless AAA Pressure Measurement System* was cleared by the FDA for the measuring of intrasac pressure during endovascular abdominal aortic aneurysm (AAA) repair and during endovascular thoracic aneurysm repair.

b. It serves as an adjunctive tool in the detection of intraoperative leaks of the stent graft during AAA repair.

c. More than 2000 patients have been treated with the EndoSure system.

d. This device is about 4 by 1 cm in size and is placed through a 14-French delivery system during the same procedure as the graft placement.

e. This microsystem, roughly the size of a paperclip, is powered by an external source (no batteries required) using radiofrequency technology. The external module powers the devise, which beams back the information.

7. Several more applications are under investigation.

a. Pulmonary artery MEMS device

   (1) It is floated like a Swan–Ganz catheter and deployed (the device embolizes into the pulmonary artery surrounded by loops of wire that allows for minimal blood flow impairment).

   (2) Once in place, the patient can go home and obtain cardiovascular parameters several times a day, allowing the physician to customize therapy.

   (3) Congestive heart failure exacerbations are the number one cause of hospitalizations among Medicare users in the United States, accounting for more than 2 million admissions each year, with an average hospital stay of 6 days.

   (4) This technology promises to detect exacerbations early on, allowing the physician to adjust the dose of medications, thus preventing the need to admit the patient to the hospital late during decompensation, and potentially saving the health system a significant amount of resources.

b. Future potential applications of MEMS technology

   (1) The natural history of AAA has allowed technicians to determine the size of the aneurysm that requires surgical repair; however, some patients present with acute rupture even at smaller sizes.

(2) MEMS devices could be used on patients with known AAA to trace the pressures of the sac, allowing for timely intervention and perhaps even setting new cutoff parameters for surgical intervention in selected groups.

c. Further information is available at the following Web sites:

(1) http://www.memsnet.org/mems

(2) http://www.cardiomems.com

(3) http://www.unloadstudy.com/faqs.html

## B.  GENE SURGERY

1. Precise molecular "plasties" of protein production

2. Conventional genetic techniques modify the target genes at their location in the DNA before transcription.

3. More recently, a new technique aims at those genes after transcription, right before translation out of the nucleus. This technique is also known as gene surgery.

4. Even though not ready for clinical trials yet, successful intervention has been achieved not only in laboratory cells but in laboratory animals and blood samples from patients.

5. One of the first therapeutic targets has been sickle cell anemia. Through gene surgery, faulty hemoglobin genes are corrected, markedly improving signs and symptoms. A target of 10% to 20% of corrected circulating hemoglobin would suffice to have a significant impact on the patients.

6. Several ongoing experiments are aimed at developing treatments of infections and cancer, all through the use of ribozymes, key instruments in this novel technique.

7. Another form of gene surgery involves injecting antisense oligoribonucleotides designed to cause the messenger RNA splicing machinery to skip faulty exons, allowing the production of better quality proteins.

8. Significant success has been achieved treating mice with Duchenne muscular dystrophy, in which this technique produced an astonishing increase in dystrophin concentrations, resulting in improved muscle function and decreased pathology.

9. *Chimeraplasty* is yet another novel technique that actually modifies specific DNA sequences.

a. This method has curative potential given that the DNA alteration is permanent.

b. Chimeric molecules of DNA and RNA are used to specifically correct point mutations or to induce alternative splicing, thus correcting the genomic defect.

c. Currently under intense investigation is the impact of chimeraplasty on Hemophilia A and B.

d. Gene surgery has proved efficacious and reproducible in animal subjects, soon to be used in human trials.

10. Further information is available from the following sources:
a. http://news.bbc.co.uk/2/hi/health/106827.stm
b. http://www.hdlighthouse.org/see/genetherapy/chimeraplasty.htm
c. Tidball JG, Spencer MJ: Skipping to new gene therapies for muscular dystrophy. *Nat Med* 9:997–998, 2003

## C. ROBOTIC SURGERY

1. Robotics—beyond laparoscopy or thoracoscopy
2. Much debate has been generated over the efficacy of traditional open surgical procedures compared with minimally invasive operations, particularly using laparoscopic or thoracoscopic technology.
3. One step further has been the development of robotic technology. Originally designed for telesurgical procedures in the U.S. Army, robotics uses laparoscopic methods, adding a "wrist" function to the tip of the instruments, enabling the surgeon to perform more complex tasks.
4. The evolution of robotic surgery can by traced through the FDA approval of specific procedures (Table 72-1).
5. Intuitive Surgical suggests the following benefits might play a significant role in the recovery of robotic patients:
a. Reduced trauma to the body
b. Reduced blood loss and need for transfusions
c. Magnification
d. Less postoperative pain and discomfort
e. Less risk for infection
f. Shorter hospital stay
g. Faster recovery and return to daily activities
h. Less scarring and improved cosmesis
6. Robotic assisted surgery offers three-dimensional view through its goggles whereas standard laparoscopy presents two-dimensional images through a monitor.
7. Haptics (the sense of touch) is, on the other hand, a feature lost at the console of the da Vinci system, whereas it is maintained in laparoscopy. Current research focuses on bringing tactile feedback to the robotic controls in the future.

**TABLE 72-1**

**FDA APPROVAL OF SPECIFIC PROCEDURES**

| Date of FDA Approval | Procedure |
| --- | --- |
| January 1997 | Surgical assistance |
| July 2000 | General laparoscopic surgery |
| March 2001 | Internal mammary artery harvesting for coronary bypass and lung surgery |
| May 2001 | Laparoscopic radical prostatectomy |
| November 2002 | 1. Laparoscopic assisted cardiotomy procedures |
| | 2. Mitral valve repair |
| January 2003 | Totally endoscopic atrial septal defect repair |
| April 2005 | Gynecologic procedures |

8. Robotic surgery is an evolving field, and only time and experience will determine which procedures are best completed with such technology as opposed to standard laparoscopic or thoracoscopic procedures.
9. Further information is available at the following Web sites:
   a. http://biomed.brown.edu/Courses/BI108/BI108_2005_Groups/04/davinci.html
   b. http://www.intuitivesurgical.com/products/index.aspx

## D.  BIOSURGERY

1. The new importance of larvae in the advent of poliresistent bacteria
2. Chronic wounds continue to pose a significant challenge to the health system.
3. One of the fundamental principles of wound healing is the frequent debridement of devitalized tissue to decrease the rate of infection and promote healing.
4. Biosurgery refers to the use of maggot (larvae) therapy to achieve such debridement.
5. Ambrose Parè is credited with the first description of the benefits of myiasis in suppurative wounds of soldiers.
6. The first clinical use of fly larvae was documented during the American Civil War by the surgeon J. F. Zacharias.
7. Its popularity peaked in the 1930s in the United States, Canada, and Europe, but later experienced a sharp decline with the tremendous success of antibiotics.
8. Renewed interest in biosurgery has emerged with the advent of multi-resistant bacteria, particularly methicillin-resistant *Staphylococcus aureus* infections.
9. Flies in biosurgery include mainly blowflies *(Calliphoridae)* and green-bottle flies *(Lucilia sericata)*. Some facts about the larvae include:
   a. Eggs hatch in 12 to 24 hours and the larvae are then used in the wounds.
   b. About 200 maggots will consume 15 g necrotic tissue per day.
   c. They reach maturity in about 4 to 5 days (10 mm long) and stop feeding.
   d. The metamorphosis into adult flies varies from days to months.
10. Maggot secretions are a subject of considerable research. Although there are still multiple unknown substances, the presence of several growth factors has been confirmed. They have a direct prohealing effect on fibroblast.
11. Management of biosurgery aims mainly at the following tasks:
    a. Keeping maggots in the wound
    b. Providing sufficient oxygen
    c. Keeping the wound moist but not swamped
    d. Multiple devices and mediums to accomplish the above objectives exist, and their optimal use is institution-dependent.
    e. After 3 to 5 days, the maggots are removed by a simple shower.

f. Typically one or two sessions are needed; however, in cases of osteomyelitis, up to 10 biosurgical treatments can be used.

12. Further information is available at the following sources:

a. Wollina U, Karte K, Herold C, Looks A: Biosurgery in wound healing—the renaissance of maggot therapy. *J Eur Acad Dermatol Venereol* 14:285–289, 2000.

b. Beasley WD, Hirst G: Making a meal of MRSA: The role of biosurgery in hospital-acquired infection. *J Hosp Infect* 56:6–9, 2004.

### E. NOTES (NATURAL ORIFICE TRANSLUMINAL ENDOSCOPIC SURGERY)

1. New incisionless surgical technique that is still at the experimental stage but is gaining wide recognition.

2. The proposed benefits of NOTES procedures are:

a. Reduced recovery time

b. Reduced pain or physical discomfort

c. Virtually no visible scars

3. Several reports of successful procedures completed in humans exist.

4. Current protocols are being established to perform cholecystectomy, gastric bypass, fallopian tube ligation, oophorectomy, diagnostic exploration, and appendectomy.

5. Procedures can be performed through the rectum, vagina, bladder, and urethra.

6. NOSCAR (Natural Orifice Surgery Consortium for Assessment and Research) is a joint venture of the Society for American Gastrointestinal and Endoscopic Surgeons and the American Society for Gastrointestinal Endoscopy. In October 2006, NOSCAR announced its partnership with Ethicon Endo-Surgery.

7. Further information is available at the following sources:

a. http://www.noscar.org/faq.php

b. Rattner D, Kalloo A; ASGE/SAGES Working Group. ASGE/SAGES Working Group on Natural Orifice Translumenal Endoscopic Surgery. October 2005. *Surg Endosc* 20:329–333, 2006.

### SUGGESTED READING

Broderick TJL: *NASA and the emergence of new surgical technologies.* Presented at Association of Academic Surgery, November 12, 2004, Houston, TX.

Feng X-H, Matthews JB, Lin X, Brunicardi FC. Cell, genomics, and molecular surgery. In: Brunicardi FC, Andersen DK, Billiar TR, et al, eds. *Schwartz's Principles of Surgery,* 8th ed. New York, McGraw-Hill, 2005, pp 403–452.

Satava RM: The future of surgical simulation and surgical robotics. *Bull Am Coll Surg* 92:13–19, 2007.

Wolf RK: A perspicacious view. *Innovations* 1:1–2, 2005.

# PART XVI

# Procedures

# External Ventricular Drain (Ventriculostomy)

*Ondrej Choutka, MD, and Bradford A. Curt, MD*

Placement of an external ventricular drain is an important and effective tool in the treatment of acute hydrocephalus and in the management of increased intracranial pressure (ICP) in the comatose or head injured patient. At our institution, this skill may be taught not only to neurosurgery residents but also to residents rotating through a neurosurgery clerkship, neuro-intensive care unit fellows, and trauma surgeons.

**73**

## I. INDICATIONS

A. **ACUTE HYDROCEPHALUS—EMERGENT DECOMPRESSION OF OBSTRUCTED VENTRICULAR SYSTEM (SUBARACHNOID HEMORRHAGE, INTRACRANIAL HEMORRHAGE INTO THE VENTRICLES, OR TUMOR)**
B. **SEVERE HEAD INJURY—ICP MONITORING FOR GOAL-DIRECTED THERAPY AND TREATMENT WITH EGRESS OF CEREBROSPINAL FLUID (CSF)**
C. **SHUNT INFECTION—EXTERNAL DRAINAGE OF INFECTED CSF DURING ANTIBIOTIC TREATMENT**

## II. CONTRAINDICATIONS

Contraindications may be relative in life-threatening situations.

A. **COAGULOPATHY (INTERNATIONAL NORMALIZED RATIO >1.3)**
B. **THROMBOCYTOPENIA (PLATELET COUNT <75 × 10⁹/L)**
C. **LESION (E.G., TUMOR) IN THE PROPOSED TRAJECTORY (CHOOSE OPPOSITE SIDE)**

## III. MATERIALS

A. **INTRACRANIAL ACCESS KIT (SINGLE USE OR REUSABLE) THAT CONTAINS:**
   1. Prep—DuraPrep, Chloraprep, Betadine
   2. Marking pen and ruler
   3. Sterile drapes
   4. Scalpel—#10 blade
   5. Hand drill and bit
   6. Forceps, needle drivers, curette, scissors
   7. Ventricular drainage catheter
   8. Suture materials
   9. External drainage collection system
   10. Sterile dressing kit

## IV. PROCEDURE

### A. REVIEW COMPUTED TOMOGRAPHY OR MAGNETIC RESONANCE IMAGING.

Review the intracranial pathology to determine the most appropriate entrance site. Either an anterior frontal or posterior site may be chosen. Most commonly, a right frontal site is chosen to reduce the risk for damage to the dominant hemisphere.

### B. POSITION AND PREP

1. Patient should be placed supine with the head of the bed elevated to approximately 15 to 20 degrees with the neck in a neutral position.
2. Shave the head using electrical clippers.
3. Mark entry site (Kocher's point)—lies 1 cm anterior to the coronal suture in the midpupillary line (~3.5 cm from midline and 10 cm behind glabella). This avoids the motor cortex and the superior sagittal sinus (Fig. 73-1*A*).
4. Prep and drape the area in standard fashion.
5. Infiltrate the area with 1% lidocaine and epinephrine.

### C. TECHNIQUE

1. Make a 0.5-cm stab incision down to bone at marked site.
2. Holding the twist drill perpendicular to the skull, apply firm pressure and drill carefully through the cortex, then softer cancellous bone, and finally inner table of the skull. Avoid *plunging* into the brain parenchyma.
3. Remove bone debris, and gently probe the hole and feel for an intact dura.
4. Carefully puncture the dura using a needle or the sharp tunneling catheter.
5. If you pass the ventricular catheter (with a stylet) perpendicular to the skull to a depth of 5 cm (less in presence of hydrocephalus), you will reach the frontal horn of the lateral ventricle. There are 5- and 10-cm markings on the catheter. To ensure perpendicular trajectory of the catheter, check it in coronal and sagittal planes. It should be pointing to the ipsilateral medial canthus in the coronal (see Fig. 73-1*B*) and to or in front of the external auditory meatus in the sagittal plane (see Fig. 73-1*C*).
6. Remove the stylet and confirm good flow of CSF.
7. Advance catheter without the stylet to reach the foramen of Monro (~6–7-cm depth at the skin level).
8. Tunnel the catheter and secure with sutures.
9. Connect the catheter to the collection system and pressure transducer.
10. Confirm the presence of appropriate waveform.
11. Apply sterile dressing.

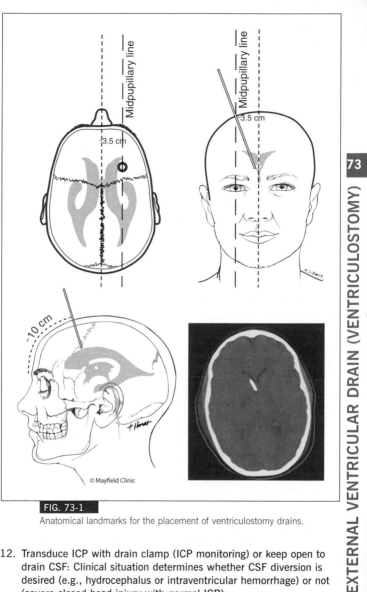

© Mayfield Clinic

**FIG. 73-1**

Anatomical landmarks for the placement of ventriculostomy drains.

12. Transduce ICP with drain clamp (ICP monitoring) or keep open to drain CSF: Clinical situation determines whether CSF diversion is desired (e.g., hydrocephalus or intraventricular hemorrhage) or not (severe closed head injury with normal ICP).

13. Finally, confirm adequate placement on follow-up imaging (CT head; see Fig. 73-1*D*).

73

EXTERNAL VENTRICULAR DRAIN (VENTRICULOSTOMY)

## D. PITFALLS AND PEARLS

1. Appropriate placement of the catheter is at the foramen of Monro on CT scan. Mass lesions causing midline shift must be taken into account to adjust trajectory.
2. Resist the urge to attempt multiple passes because this can cause hemorrhage along the tract or damage to critical structures.
3. Parenchymal ICP monitor can be used as a rescue option if ventriculostomy is not successful (thus losing the benefit of CSF diversion).
4. CSF sampling regimen to monitor for infection should be performed, given the risk for ventriculitis with indwelling catheters.

# Airway

*Ryan M. Thomas, MD*

## I. INDICATIONS FOR AN ARTIFICIAL AIRWAY

### A. ABSOLUTE

1. Hypoxia—inadequate oxygenation (partial pressure of oxygen [$Po_2$] <55 mm Hg), unresponsive to supplemental $O_2$; demands a secure airway to ensure proper tissue oxygenation
2. Hypoventilation—increasing partial pressure of carbon dioxide ($Pco_2$; >50 mm Hg) indicates inability to clear $CO_2$ waste and respiratory compromise, such as a patient who has tired from increased work of breathing
3. Acute airway obstruction—refractory to oropharyngeal "finger sweep" or Heimlich maneuver
4. Penetrating neck trauma
   a. Direct tracheal injury mandates an artificial airway.
   b. Lateral neck injuries that cause an expanding hematoma require an artificial airway to prevent impending airway compromise.
5. Central nervous system disorder—accompanying Glasgow Coma Scale score ≤ 8

### B. RELATIVE

1. Central nervous system disorders
   a. Status epilepticus/seizure disorder
   b. Severe alcohol/drug intoxication, combative patient
   c. Severe head injury
2. Chest wall injury
   a. Flail chest
   b. Multiple rib fractures with inadequate pain control ("splinting")
   c. Open pneumothorax
3. Inadequate pulmonary toilet
   a. Assists with airway suctioning and clearing of secretions
   b. Allows for diagnostic procedures (i.e., bronchoscopic alveolar lavage)
4. Shock
5. Trauma
   a. Burns with documented inhalational injury
   b. Maxillofacial

## II. NONSURGICAL AIRWAY OPTIONS AND METHODS

### A. INITIAL/TEMPORIZING MANEUVERS

1. Foreign body removal
   a. For acute airway obstruction and choking
   b. Performed via "finger sweep," Heimlich maneuver, or under direct visualization (i.e., bronchoscopy)
2. Supplemental oxygen
   a. Via nasal cannula or face mask

b. Continuous positive airway pressure mask may decrease patient's work of breathing and circumvent need for invasive airway.

c. For every 1 L/min oxygen delivered via nasal cannula, the fraction of inspired oxygen ($Fio_2$) increases by 4% up to 6 L/min (~45%), limited by the turbulence in the tubing and airway.

### 3. Chin-lift/jaw thrust

a. Maintain inline cervical immobilization for trauma patients.

b. Helps to relieve partial airway obstructions

### 4. Oropharyngeal

a. Useful in obtunded patient, but not tolerated in an alert individual

b. Moves tongue away from pharyngeal wall and relieves partial obstructions

c. Correct size chosen by measuring from oral commissure to earlobe. Insert with curve aimed toward oral palate and rotate 180 degrees into anatomic position to rest along base of the tongue.

### 5. Nasopharyngeal (nasal "trumpet")

a. Useful in awake patient because it is better tolerated than oropharyngeal and as adjunct for nasal suctioning.

b. Also relieves partial obstruction by moving soft palate away from pharyngeal wall

c. Lubricate well and insert into nare with bevel toward septum, and rotate 90 degrees so that it lies in anatomic position.

## B. OROTRACHEAL INTUBATION

### 1. Basics

a. Most common definitive airway, used in unconscious or anesthetized patients

b. Performed under direct visualization or fibroscopic guidance

c. Advantages—rapid; variety of tube types and sizes can be inserted.

d. Disadvantages—patient discomfort; tube can be dislodged or moved.

### 2. Procedure

a. Preparation

   (1) Obtain consent if possible and/or notify family.

   (2) Obtain and position necessary equipment—Ambu bag, $O_2$ saturation monitor, suction setup, laryngoscope (straight or curved blade depending on preference) with functioning light, and a variety of endotracheal tubes (ETTs); stylet is placed in tube of choice, 10-ml syringe to inflate balloon at the end of the procedure.

   (3) Tube choice—diameter of ring finger approximates ETT size in adults; male individuals = 8, female individuals = 7 to 7.5; ETT size ≥8 allows for bronchoscopy; for children, ETT size estimated by fifth digit or ETT size = (16 + age in years)/4.

   (4) Prepare induction medications (see Chapters 16 and 17).

b. Technique

   (1) Position equipment and head of the patient at comfortable height to perform intubation (if location permits).

(2) Preoxygenate patient with 100% oxygen via Ambu bag and monitor $O_2$ saturation; this ensures optimal tissue delivery of oxygen during the procedure.

(3) Time permitting and in conscious patient, sedate and induce anesthesia (short- and quick-acting agents such as midazolam and succinylcholine are ideal).

(4) Unless contraindicated (neck injury), place patient in "sniffing" position with neck gently extended and crown of head touching the bed.

(5) Open mouth widely with right hand using cross-finger or "scissor" technique (thumb pushes down on lower incisors and index finger presses up on upper incisors).

(6) With the left hand holding the laryngoscope, place it in the right side of the mouth moving to the left and posterior to sweep the tongue out of the way and visualize the epiglottis.

(7) For curved (Macintosh) blades, the tip of the blade is placed anterior to the epiglottis and should not touch the epiglottis itself. For straight (Miller) blades, the tip of the blade will be placed gently below (posterior) the epiglottis to retract it. Special attention should be made not to traumatize the epiglottis, especially when using a straight blade.

(8) Once blade is in correct position, lift handle toward the ceiling to visual cords. Special attention should be made not to use the teeth as a fulcrum, which may cause injury to the teeth and possibly dislodge a loose tooth, leading to aspiration.

(9) An assistant should apply cricoid pressure (Sellick maneuver) during the process to help visualize the vocal cords and to decrease aspiration risk via esophageal compression.

(10) Once cords are visualized, the assistant places the previously chosen ETT into the operator's right hand so that the cords remain visualized by the operator at all times.

(11) The ETT is placed through the vocal cords, timed with the patient's breathing to limit vocal cord damage. The tube is placed so that the cuff is just distal to the cords (typically 20–22 cm at the teeth). The balloon is then inflated to an appropriate level to prevent air leakage during ventilation (usually 3–5 ml of air or a cuff pressure of ≤20 mm Hg).

c. After intubation

(1) Correct positioning is initially confirmed with an end-tidal $CO_2$ monitor, moisture within the ETT, equal chest rise, and equal, bilateral breath sounds.

(2) Secure tube into place with adhesive tape or tracheostomy tie and document tube position at the incisors.

(3) Chest radiograph to confirm and document tube position

(4) Arterial blood gas 30 minutes after intubation and ventilator adjustment as necessary

74

AIRWAY

## C. NASOTRACHEAL INTUBATION

### 1. Basics

a. Placed via nasopharynx blindly, via laryngoscope, or with fiberoptic guidance

b. Method of choice in patients with possible neck trauma

c. Patient must be breathing spontaneously for a blind placement.

d. Contraindicated in patients with suspected basilar skull fractures—intubation of the cranium has occurred with catastrophic consequences.

e. Advantages—more comfortable for patient than orotracheal, easier oral care by nursing staff.

f. Disadvantages—more difficult to place; can take more time to place appropriately; smaller tube size needed, and thus may preclude future bronchoscopy.

### 2. Technique

a. Preprocedure setup and patient positioning are identical to the orotracheal route of intubation.

b. For patient comfort, anesthetize oropharynx and nasal mucosa (benzocaine/butamben/tetracaine [Cetacaine spray] or viscous lidocaine work well).

c. Preoxygenate patient as for orotracheal intubation.

d. With well-lubricated tube, gently advance appropriate-sized tube cephalad into nostril (this avoids the large inferior nasal turbinate) and then posterior and caudad into nasopharynx. Slight rotation of the tube will facilitate passage, and the natural curve of the nasopharynx will aid the passage of the ETT.

e. Look for moisture collecting in the ETT during the patient's exhalation, and time the passage of the tube into the trachea during inhalation, when the patient's vocal cords will be open.

f. If unable to pass the ETT blindly, use a laryngoscope and McGill forceps to visualize the tube position and guide the tube into the trachea.

### 3. After intubation—identical to orotracheal intubation

## D. COMPLICATIONS

1. Aspiration during attempted intubation

2. Airway trauma from multiple failed attempts or malposition of the laryngoscope that prevents placement of a nonsurgical airway

3. Malposition—esophageal intubation, right mainstem bronchial intubation

4. Trauma to teeth

5. Tube obstruction—mucous plug, tube kinking, or compression

6. Tracheoesophageal fistula—caused by excessive ETT cuff pressure, which causes tracheal necrosis and erosion into innominate artery

## III. SURGICAL AIRWAY OPTIONS AND METHODS

### A. CRICOTHYROIDOTOMY

### 1. Basics

a. Surgical airway through the cricothyroid membrane

b. Used in emergent situations when orotracheal or nasotracheal intubation cannot be performed

## 2. Technique

a. Ensure presence of all necessary equipment as for endotracheal intubation, including size 6 or 7 tracheostomy (in truly emergent setting, ETT can be used and trimmed at the end of the procedure).

b. Assistant should ventilate patient as much as possible with Ambu bag.

c. Position head with the neck extended and palpate thyroid cartilage and cricothyroid membrane.

d. If time permits, quickly prep neck with Betadine or chlorhexidine, but this should never take precedence to securing an airway.

e. Make a vertical midline incision over the cricothyroid membrane with a #15 blade scalpel that is large enough to allow palpation of the membrane with a fingertip (vertical incision reduces the chance of transecting the anterior jugular vein).

f. Visualize cricothyroid membrane, incise membrane in a horizontal direction, insert handle through the incised membrane, and turn 90 degrees to enlarge the ostomy. Alternatively, a tracheal spreader can be used to enlarge the ostomy. Ensure that the ostomy is large enough to accommodate tracheostomy.

g. Insert appropriate tracheostomy, following the curve of the tracheostomy in a caudad direction. Inflate tracheostomy cuff, attach to oxygen supply, and confirm appropriate placement with auscultation and end-tidal $CO_2$ monitor as before. Secure airway with sutures, adhesive tape, or tracheostomy tape.

h. If appropriate placement cannot be confirmed, remove tracheostomy and ensure ostomy is large enough. On occasion, the tracheostomy/ETT can track anterior to the trachea in the subcutaneous tissue (especially in obese individuals).

i. If a tracheostomy tube is not available, an ETT can be used—insert ETT through ostomy just past the balloon, inflate the balloon, and gently pull the ETT back so that the balloon abuts the ostomy. This will prevent placement of the ETT in the right mainstem bronchus.

## 3. After the procedure

a. Obtain radiograph to confirm and document tube position.

b. Convert cricothyrotomy to formal tracheostomy or orotracheal intubation when the patient's condition allows.

## B. TRACHEOSTOMY

### 1. Basics

a. Surgical airway placed through the second or third tracheal rings

b. Performed as an elective procedure—emergent airway needs are better served by a cricothyrotomy.

c. Performed for those with prolonged or anticipated prolonged intubation

d. Often used before elective head/neck operations when airway compromise may occur during the procedure

74

AIRWAY

e. Less dead space, better patient comfort, and easier for nursing staff to care for the airway than endotracheal intubation

**2. Technique**

a. Explain risks/benefits/alternatives to family and/or patient, then obtain consent.

b. Place towel rolls under patient's shoulders to allow neck to be hyperextended.

c. Palpate thyroid cartilage, cricothyroid membrane, and mark landmarks with a surgical pen, such as thyroid notch, suprasternal notch, and borders of trachea.

d. Sterilely prep and drape patient from chin to upper chest.

e. Ensure tracheostomy of appropriate size is available, inner cannula is in place, cuff functions appropriately, and tracheostomy is lubricated.

f. A horizontal or vertical incision, approximately 3 to 5 cm, is made over the second to third tracheal rings and continued through platysmas.

g. Strap muscles can be bluntly separated at the midline along their vertical plane.

h. The thyroid, thyroid isthmus, or both are encountered and can be retracted cranially with gentle dissection.

i. Tracheal rings are encountered and must be counted exactly to ensure preservation of the first tracheal cartilage, so that the tracheostomy tube does not erode into the first tracheal ring or cricothyroid cartilage.

j. Stay sutures with 3–0 or 4–0 monofilament placed laterally at the level where the tracheostomy will be created; these can be used for traction during the procedure as well if the tracheostomy tube becomes inadvertently dislodged after the procedure to relocate the tracheostomy site. A tracheal hook can be used at this time to elevate the trachea into the operative field to facilitate placement of the sutures and creation of the ostomy site (this is especially useful in obese patients).

k. The midline trachea is incised at the second and third tracheal rings. Care should be taken not to puncture the cuff of the ETT. A small portion may be excised or a simple incision can be created. Care should be taken not to excise too large a portion of trachea or create too large of a "flap" because this will increase the risk for tracheal stenosis when the opening scars and heals.

l. The ETT will now be seen through the ostomy, and the anesthesia team can deflate the cuff and withdraw the ETT just proximal to the ostomy.

m. Use tracheal spreader to gently enlarge the ostomy to accommodate the tube and place the previously lubricated tube into the ostomy following the curve of the tube into the trachea. Ensure that the tube enters the ostomy and does not track anterior to the trachea.

n. Remove inner tracheostomy cannula, attach tracheostomy to ventilator circuit, and confirm proper position with end-tidal $CO_2$ monitor, symmetric chest rise, and auscultation.

o. Only after intratracheal position is confirmed should the anesthesia team remove the previously placed ETT.

3. After the procedure

a. Suture tracheostomy to the skin with 2–0 silk suture and attach tracheostomy tape. Label previously placed stay sutures with "right" and "left" labels to ensure orientation in case the tracheostomy tube is accidentally dislodged in the first week after surgery and needs to be reinserted blindly.

b. Postprocedure radiograph to confirm and document tube position

## C. PERCUTANEOUS TRACHEOSTOMY

1. Basics

a. Minimally invasive tracheostomy that can be done at the bedside

b. Uses Seldinger technique to gain access to the trachea and, via a series of dilatations of the soft tissue and ostomy site, the tracheostomy is performed.

c. Used with bronchoscopy to ensure safest procedure to visualize location of the needle used to access the airway

d. Complications similar to open tracheostomy

e. Contraindicated in emergency airway situations, pediatrics, midline neck mass, and nonintubated patients

2. After the procedure

a. Wean ventilator back to preprocedure settings once paralytics have worn off.

b. Postprocedure radiograph to confirm and document tube position

## D. COMPLICATIONS

1. Bleeding
2. Wound infection
3. Tube dislodgement or malposition
4. Pneumothorax, pneumomediastinum, subcutaneous emphysema
5. Esophageal perforation
6. Tracheal malacia
7. Tracheal stenosis
8. Fistulas—tracheoesophageal, tracheoinnominate artery (surgical emergency)

## IV. ALTERNATE AIRWAY METHODS

## A. COMBITUBE

1. Dual lumen tube inserted blindly into oropharynx in which the distal lumen usually intubates the esophagus. This distal lumen is occluded and ventilation of the second lumen is undertaken to ventilate the lungs. If the distal lumen enters the trachea, then this lumen is used to ventilate the patient.

## B. FIBEROPTIC BRONCHOSCOPY

1. ETT of choice is placed over a bronchoscope and the patient is scoped. Once the tube is in correct position, the bronchoscope is

74

AIRWAY

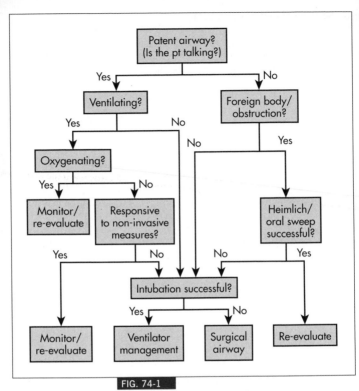

**FIG. 74-1**

Algorithm for airway management.

withdrawn while leaving the ETT in position. This technique is useful for difficult intubations or those with airway trauma.

## C.  JET VENTILATION

1. Insertion of a 12- or 14-gauge (16- or 18-gauge in children) needle catheter through the cricothyroid membrane that provides oxygen on a short-term basis and may enable enough time to relieve an obstruction or obtain a permanent airway. The catheter should be attached to wall $O_2$ at 15 l/min (40–50 pounds per square inch [PSI]) with a y-connecter or hole cut into the side of the tubing. This allows exhalation to occur (intermittently occlude the hole for 1 second to oxygenate, and leave open 4 seconds to allow exhalation). This process provides oxygenation for only 30 to 40 minutes in patients with normal pulmonary function, and $CO_2$ will accumulate because of inadequate exhalation.

## D.  LARYNGEAL MASK AIRWAY

1. Mask ventilation in which a seal is made against the glottis to ventilate and oxygenate. A laryngeal mask airway does not protect the patient from aspiration, but a small ETT can be placed through the laryngeal mask airway via bronchoscopy to provide a more secure airway.

## V. FLOW CHART/DECISION TREE (SEE FIG. 74-1)

# Wound Closure

Rian A. Maercks, MD

When treating traumatic wounds, remember to obtain a thorough history to assess for more severe injuries. Ask about a history of head trauma and loss of consciousness. Evaluate all extremities, joints, and abdomen for pain and bruising. Wound closure should not delay diagnostic studies such as computed tomography scans or operative exploration if indicated. Do not let a scalp laceration delay the diagnosis of a ruptured spleen! (See Chapter 63 for an overview of trauma.)

## 75

## I. EVALUATION AND CLOSURE OF THE TRAUMATIC WOUND

### A. BASIC PRINCIPLES

1. Examination—complete and document a thorough physical examination including sensory and motor examination. This is especially important in the hand and face.
2. Radiography—obtain radiographs and assess for fractures and foreign bodies before treating wound, when possible. Facial lacerations should be closed promptly, and treatment should not be delayed significantly for imaging.
3. Tetanus—check status.
   a. Tetanus is caused by the toxin of Clostridium tetani.
   b. Tetanus-prone wounds are old (>6 hours), deep (>1 cm), devitalized, and contaminated, especially those involving rusty metal, feces, or soil.
   c. Immunization in children younger than 7 years—requires four injections of diphtheria-pertussis-tetanus vaccine. A fifth dose may be given at 4 to 6 years of age. Thereafter, adult type (Td) is recommended for routine or wound boosters.
   d. Administration
      (1) Fully immunized patients and the last dose of toxoid was given within 10 years: For non–tetanus-prone wounds, no booster of toxoid is indicated. For tetanus-prone wounds and if more than 5 years have elapsed since the last dose, 0.5 ml adsorbed toxoid should be given intramuscularly.
      (2) Incompletely immunized patients: When the patient has had two or more prior injections of toxoid and received the last dose more than 10 years previously, 0.5 ml adsorbed toxoid should be given for both tetanus-prone and non–tetanus-prone wounds. Passive immunization is not required.
      (3) Nonimmunized patients with non–tetanus-prone wounds should be given 0.5 ml adsorbed toxoid. For tetanus-prone wounds, 0.5 ml adsorbed toxoid and ≥250 units of human tetanus immune globulin should be given using different needles, syringes, and sites of injection. Administration of antibiotics should be considered, although effectiveness in prophylaxis is unproven.

4. Rabies is a potentially fatal disease caused by the rabies virus, a single-stranded RNA virus of the rhabdovirus group. Generally less than five cases are reported in the United States each year.

a. Prophylaxis is indicated for bites by carnivorous wild animals (especially skunks, raccoons, foxes, coyotes, and bats). Prophylaxis is not indicated for bites by domestic animals (unless they are thought to be rabid or are unable to be supervised for the emergence of rabid characteristics) or rodents (e.g., mice, rats, or squirrels).

b. Previously nonimmunized persons should receive one 1-ml dose of human diploid cell vaccine by intramuscular injection on days 0, 3, 7, 14, and 28 (a total of five doses). Rabies immunoglobulin 20 IU/kg (preferable) or equine antirabies serum 40 IU/kg should be given before day 8, with half the dose infiltrated in the area of the wound and the remainder given intramuscularly. Rabies immunoglobulin or antirabies serum is not indicated after day 8.

5. Complexity: Determine whether the wound can be treated in the emergency department or necessitates the operating room. Ischemic extremities or digits require operative exploration. Extensive hand injuries that require visualization and protection or repair of neurovascular structures must be completed in the operating room with proper lighting magnification and instrumentation. Injuries in which local anesthesia control is difficult should also be taken to the operating room.

## B. TECHNIQUE

1. Anesthesia: After thorough examination, local anesthesia should be applied as indicated for the anatomic area (see Chapter 15 for principles and guidelines).

2. Irrigation and debridement: Once examination is completed and anesthesia is provided, the wound should be thoroughly irrigated with pressure irrigation.

a. Use the largest syringe available (60 ml) with a 20- to 22-gauge Angiocath or a splash-guard irrigation tip.

b. Wear eye protection. If you are wondering why you are wearing eye protection, you are not irrigating with enough pressure. Irrigation should be messy, and the tissue should change appearance. Most wounds require at least 1 to 2 L saline irrigation.

c. All clearly nonviable tissue should be sharply debrided. Be conservative on aesthetically sensitive areas such as the face. This is the most essential part of closure—irrigation and debridement are the most important early treatment.

3. Create a sterile field.

a. Use a wide field, especially on the face. This allows you to monitor the patient and restore landmarks.

b. Use plenty of sterile towels to ensure a sterile workspace.

c. Chlorhexidine—toxic to the cornea and should be avoided around the eyes or face.

4. Assess the defect. What is missing? What is viable? Areas of tension can be deceiving, especially when swollen. Careful evaluation of the clean site will reveal the true defect. Debride ragged tissue that is clearly nonviable. Do not aggressively debride questionable areas. Be conservative on the face. The scalp can tolerate more aggressive debridement and closure. Note obvious structures in the wound, but do not explore the hand, arm, or face in the emergency department to look for injured structures! The answers to these questions are gained from a good physical examination.

5. Bleeding—can almost always be addressed with direct local pressure.
a. Do not look for or tie off vessels in the emergency department. You will likely damage other structures (i.e., nerves).
b. Use one or two fingers firmly placed on gauze on top of the exact site for 15 minutes by the clock and repeat if necessary.
c. If the injury requires the operating room, get to the operating room!
d. Tourniquets can be helpful for fingertip injuries and some extensor tendons. A Penrose drain can be wrapped from distal to proximal, clamped proximally with a hemostat, and unwound distally to provide an exsanguinated fingertip for repair.
e. A midhumeral blood pressure cuff can also be used to provide a dry field for extensor tendon repairs.
f. Tourniquets, however, should not be used to control focal bleeding and should be used for short durations only while operating, less than an hour on the arm.

6. Use anatomic landmarks or artificial landmarks to guide closure.
a. Tattoos, scars, and defined structures such as the white roll of the lip or helical rim should be approximated first to guide closure.
b. It is sometimes helpful to mark structures with methylene blue for ease of accurate approximation.

7. Muscles—should be reapproximated using a limited number of absorbable sutures. This is particularly important in perioral injuries, because failure to reapproximate the orbicularis oris will result in contour defects, especially on facial animation.

8. Fascia—should not be tightly closed. Underlying injured muscle is likely to swell further. Do not create a compartment syndrome.

9. Tension—deep buried dermal sutures should carry the tension of the closure resulting in a gentle apposition and eversion of the epidermis. Monofilament suture should then gently oppose the skin with minimal tension. More tension equates to more scarring.

## C. CLASSIFICATIONS OF CLOSURE

1. Primary intention—direct closure of the wound. This is the goal when possible. Primarily close wounds when possible without undue tension in clean wounds. Do not close wounds that result from human bites! Dog bites of the face may often be loosely closed primarily if seen in a timely manner, and appropriately irrigated and debrided.

Consider leaving wounds open that have been open for more than 8 hours, are obviously infected, or occur in dirty environments such as farm injuries.

2. Secondary intention—wound closure by contraction and reepithelialization. This should be the initial treatment of small wounds that cannot be closed without deforming surrounding structures. Most wounds smaller than 2 cm can reepithelialize within approximately 1 to 2 weeks. Larger wounds take longer to heal, and contraction plays a significant part in their closure. Bacitracin and Adaptec or similar products are appropriate for managing these wounds. Wet to dry dressings aid in declaring wounds or those needing mild debridement.

3. Tertiary intention—definitive closure that is delayed. The process of secondary intention is disrupted for definitive closure. Dirty wounds can be managed in this manner with wet to dry dressing changes until a clean bed is achieved.

## D. SUTURE SELECTION

1. Fast absorbing sutures—that is, chromic, "cat gut." Hydrolyzed quickly because of a robust inflammatory response. Lose tensile strength in less than 7 days. Chromization, that is, chromic prolongs suture life two to four times, approximately 3 weeks. Use only where scarring is not a major concern. Appropriate for mucosa and in pediatric hand injuries.

2. Intermediate absorbable sutures—Vicryl (polyglycolic acid) or other braided absorbables are useful for closing muscle and dermis. They handle nicely and hold knots well. Lose tensile strength in 2 weeks. Monocryl or other monofilament absorbables are useful in dirty wounds because they have less surface area to promote bacterial adherence. Poliglecaprone glycolide (Monocryl) loses tensile strength in 3 weeks.

3. Permanent sutures such as nylon are useful for skin closure because they are nonreactive and do not promote scarring. Use 5–0 in the hand and 6–0 or finer in the face. Fibroblast migration begins to peak at days 3 to 5; thus, sutures in the face should be removed by day 5 to prevent "train tracks." In other locations, 7 to 10 days is acceptable.

## E. SUTURING TECHNIQUES

1. Deep sutures—closing deep layers of the wound should be completed with buried interrupted sutures. The deep dermal layer should carry most of the tension of closure. Sew from deep to superficial, catching the deep layer of the dermis.

2. Skin sutures
   a. Simple interrupted sutures—allow precise alignment of skin edges in irregular wound closures and should be considered in facial repairs.
   b. Running subcuticular sutures—absorbable monofilaments are used to reapproximate skin underneath the epidermis. The presence of suture beyond day 5 does not increase scarring in this location.

c. Running skin suture—"baseball stitch" allows faster skin closure because only two knots are required.

d. Mattress sutures—achieve improved skin eversion and allow for tissue swelling without compressing the wound edge. Horizontal mattress sutures place the exposed suture parallel with the wound edge. Vertical mattress sutures place the exposed suture perpendicular to the wound edge.

3. Skin glues—that is, cyanoacrylates (Dermabond) offer strength of closure similar to most superficial skin closure techniques with the advantage of being a waterproof dressing. It is appropriate to close clean wounds with well-placed deep dermal sutures and Dermabond.

4. Staples—offer quick closure technique in nonaesthetically sensitive areas. Never use staples in non–hair-bearing scalp or the face. They are appropriate for complicated traumatic injuries of the trunk and extremities and the hair-bearing scalp. They are not precise, but allow rapid closure and hemostasis.

5. Vacuum-assisted closure—has simplified the closure of large traumatic wounds. The wound must be clean before vacuum-assisted closure dressings are used. This modality can reduce the size of defects and help a granulation bed develop in preparation for skin grafting.

## F. SPECIAL CONSIDERATIONS

1. Facial injuries—should be closed whenever possible.

a. Clean the wound and look carefully for clues to reapproximate (skin creases, anatomic landmarks).

b. Dirty wounds and dog bites should be thoroughly cleaned and loosely closed.

c. Try to close the wound aligning the resultant scar with natural skin folds and tension lines.

d. Document facial sensation, symmetry of brows, and smile before administration of local!

e. Remove staples by day 5. Steri-Strips can be placed after suture removal.

2. Fight bites—any wound near the dorsum of the hand near the metacarpophalangeal joint should be considered a human bite. These wounds are cleaned and left open. Antimicrobial coverage for Eikenella is essential (i.e., PCN).

3. Hand injuries—examine and document the sensory and motor examination of the hand before administering local anesthetic. Assess the neurovascular status of each digit. A digit with compromised vascular status is an indication for emergent evaluation and repair in the operating room. In the absence of vascular compromise, hand injuries can be acutely treated with copious irrigation and skin closure with splinting. Definitive tendon and nerve repair can be delayed.

# Thoracentesis

*Ryan A. LeVasseur, MD*

## I. GENERAL INFORMATION

### A. INDICATIONS

1. Diagnostic evaluation of pleural fluid
2. Therapeutic aspiration of fluid or air to return lung volume

### B. MATERIALS AND PREPARATION

1. Thoracentesis kit: Become familiar with the kit available. All are based on a catheter-over-needle design.
2. Create your own kit.

a. Sterile tray, sterile drapes, prep kit, sterile 4 × 4 gauze, sterile dressing, sterile gown, gloves, and mask
b. Anesthesia—10 to 20 ml Luer–Lock syringe; 25-gauge needles for infiltration; 1.5- to 2-inch, 22-gauge needle for infiltration; 10 ml 1% lidocaine with 1:1,000,000 epinephrine for local anesthetic
c. Needle insertion/collection—0- to 60 ml Luer–Lock syringe for aspiration, needle catheter (depending on technique chosen): 2-inch, 20- to 22-gauge needle, over-the-needle catheter (16- to 20-gauge needle); scalpel (used during needle catheter technique only); 3-way stopcock; 2 curved clamps, intravenous pressure tubing, collection container, 500- to 1000-ml vacuum bottle
d. Specimen tubes—one plain tube, one EDTA tube, iced blood gas syringe
e. Culture tubes—both aerobic and anaerobic, 50-ml plain tube for cytology; one heparin tube

### C. POSITION

1. Have the patient in a comfortable position, sitting erect, leaning forward, with extended arms resting on a table. If patient is critically ill, the lateral decubitus position may be used.
2. Locate the effusion and determine its extent, both clinically by percussion and auscultation, as well as by chest radiograph or ultrasound. Obtain both posteroanterior and lateral decubitus chest radiograph. Blunting of the costophrenic angle on posteroanterior view indicates more than 250 ml fluid is present. Free-flowing fluid versus loculated fluid can be assessed in the decubitus film. Do not attempt unguided thoracentesis on loculated fluid.
3. Ultrasound is ideal for locating proper needle insertion site in high-risk patients, as well as locating fluid in small effusions, assessing the depth of fluid from the skin to the pleura, and for needle guidance during the procedure (as in the setting of loculations).
4. Needle insertion site
a. Perform along midscapular line, or posterior axillary line from the back

b. Correct site is one or two interspaces below the fluid level and 5 to 10 cm lateral to the spine. Never insert the needle below the eighth posterior intercostal space.

## D. PROCEDURE

1. Explain the procedure to patient, family, or both. Obtain informed consent.
2. Using sterile technique and observing universal blood and body fluid precautions, prep and drape the previously chosen area.
3. Using a 25-gauge needle attached to a 5- to 10-ml syringe filled with 1% lidocaine with 1:1,000,000 epinephrine, infiltrate local anesthetic first as a skin wheal. Switch to a 1.5-inch, 22-gauge needle and, while angling the needle slightly downward, proceed to infiltrate anesthetic intradermally over the superior margin of the rib (to avoid the neurovascular bundle) below the chosen interspace. Continue through the subcutaneous tissue and down to the periosteum of the rib. After making contact with the superior boarder of the rib, "walk the needle" over the border and continue to inject into the intercostal muscle layer. Remember to aspirate and inject small aliquots of anesthetic as the needle is advanced. Continue until pleural fluid is aspirated, and note the depth of the needle by attaching a clamp at the level of the skin. At this point, withdraw the needle 0.5 cm and infiltrate the pleura, then remove the needle.
4. Complications during needle insertion
   a. "Dry tap"—when no fluid is encountered. Fluid may be loculated, viscous, needle too short, insertion site too high or too low.
   b. Air bubbles—lung parenchyma has been violated; try a lower insertion site.
   c. Take time to reassess the patient position and chosen insertion site. Consider using ultrasound.
5. Once the needle is removed, access the same site using a 16- to 18-gauge Angiocath and advance to the previously measured depth. When fluid returns, carefully slide the Angiocath over the needle and remove the needle. Quickly occlude the lumen of the Angiocath to prevent pneumothorax.
6. Fluid is collected in a closed system with one-way valves. Most systems have a 60-ml Luer–Lock syringe attached to a limb of tubing that allows aspiration of fluid from the Angiocath. Another limb of tubing in turn connects the Luer–Lock syringe to the collection bag. Aspiration and collection of fluid occurs by moving the piston on the Luer–Lock syringe in and out in a pumping motion. The valve in the tubing automatically directs fluid from the Angiocath into the collection bag. Note that most systems have a side port where chemotherapeutic or sclerosing agents may be instilled, such as in a chemical pleurodesis.

7. For diagnostic purposes, removal of between 50 ml and 100 ml of fluid is adequate. For therapeutic purposes, fluid removal is continued until patient reports relief of dyspnea, or until 1000 ml fluid has been withdrawn. Note that after removal of 1000 ml fluid, it becomes necessary to monitor pleural pressures because of the risk for reexpansion pulmonary edema; at this point, terminate the procedure when the pleural pressure exceeds $-20$ mm Hg.

8. Remove the angiocatheter and apply a sterile dressing.

9. Send pleural fluid for the following studies:

a. Hematology—cell count and differential

b. Chemistry—specific gravity, pH, lactate dehydrogenase, amylase, glucose, and protein

c. Microbiology—Gram stain, bacterial/fungal and acid fast bacillus cultures

d. Pathology—cell cytology

10. After the procedure: Obtain chest radiograph to confirm efficacy of aspiration and to rule out pneumothorax.

**E. CLINICAL PEARLS**

1. If the patient exhibits symptoms of chest pain, shortness of breath, severe cough during the procedure, or any significant change in hemodynamic parameters or symptoms, STOP the procedure.

2. If using ultrasound, note the depth of fluid collection through the entire respiratory cycle. When lung expands during inspiration, there is less fluid at a particular site than first appreciated.

3. Generous use of local anesthetic improves patient comfort and makes the procedure easier.

4. Be mindful to keep the needle or catheter sealed when it is within the pleural cavity. If the hub becomes open to air, a pneumothorax can develop.

5. Once the pleural space has been accessed, there is no difference in risk to the patient in performing a "dry" (therapeutic) tap versus a "diagnostic" tap; thus, the fluid should always be tapped as completely as possible.

**76**

**THORACENTESIS**

## II. INTERPRETATION AND COMPLICATIONS

**A. INTERPRETATION OF RESULTS: TABLE 76-1 SHOWS THE DIFFERENCE BETWEEN AN EXUDATIVE VERSUS TRANSUDATIVE PLEURAL EFFUSION.**

**B. DIFFERENTIAL DIAGNOSIS**

1. Transudative—cirrhosis, nephritic syndrome, congestive heart failure, lobar atelectasis, viral infection

2. Exudative—empyema, malignant effusion, intraabdominal infection, pancreatitis, tuberculosis, trauma, pulmonary infection, chylothorax

3. Grossly bloody—iatrogenic injury, pulmonary infection, trauma, tumor, hepatic or splenic puncture

4. Extremely low glucose is consistent with rheumatoid process

**TABLE 76-1**

DIAGNOSIS OF EXUDATE VERSUS TRANSUDATE

| Lab Studies | Transudate | Exudate |
|---|---|---|
| Protein | <3 g/dl | >3 g/dl |
| Protein ratio (effusion:serum) | <0.6 | >0.6 |
| Specific gravity | <1.016 g/ml | >1.016 g/ml |
| LDH | Low | High |
| LDH ratio | <0.6 | >0.6 |
| Glucose | 2/3 serum glucose | Low |
| Amylase | <200 IU/ml | >500 IU/ml |
| RBC | <10,000/mm3 | >100,000/mm3 |
| WBC | <1000/mm3 | >1000/mm3 |

LDH = lactate dehydrogenase, RBC = red blood cell, WBC = white blood cell

## C. COMPLICATIONS
1. Pneumothorax
2. Hemothorax
3. Hepatic or splenic puncture
4. Parenchymal tear
5. Empyema

# Bladder Catheterization

*Jonathan R. Thompson, MD*

## I. URETHRAL CATHETERIZATION

### A. INDICATIONS FOR INDWELLING CATHETER

1. Continuous urine output monitoring
2. Relief of bladder obstruction
a. Benign prostatic hypertrophy
b. Acute urinary retention
3. Use after genitourinary procedure—a stent to guide healing to reduce incidence of stricture.
4. To provide continuous decompression after bladder, urethral repair
5. To prevent contamination of perineal wounds
6. Short-term management of incontinence
7. Short-term management of neurogenic bladder
8. Used for urologic study of the lower urinary tract

### B. INDICATIONS FOR INTERMITTENT CATHETERIZATION (ALSO KNOWN AS "STRAIGHT CATH")

1. Postvoid residual measurement
2. To obtain sterile urine specimen—needed in female patients because of labial contamination during urination
3. Long-term management of neurogenic bladder—clean intermittent catheterization has much lower risk for bladder infection compared with indwelling catheterization.

### C. COMPLICATIONS OF INDWELLING URINARY CATHETER

1. Urinary tract infection
a. Most common nosocomial infection—occurs in 40% of hospital inpatients
   (1) Comprises 80% of all nosocomial infections
b. Incidence rate—30% to 40% if left in place more than 4 days; 70% to 80% if left in place more than 2 weeks
   (1) This includes the platinum, silver, and gold catheters.
2. False passage/urethral disruption
a. If suspected, urgent urologic consultation is indicated
b. Can be caused by balloon inflation in urethra
3. Hematuria—may be transient because of mucosal trauma of the procedure.
4. Traumatic discontinuation
a. Treatment is to place a new Foley to tamponade bleeding.
5. Erosion of bladder neck
6. Postcatheter stricture

### D. CONTRAINDICATIONS OF BLADDER CATHETERIZATION

1. Suspected urethral disruption in the setting of trauma

a. Signs
  (1) Blood at urethral meatus
  (2) Scrotal hematoma
  (3) High riding prostate on rectal examination
b. Management
  (1) Urologic consultation
  (2) Retrograde urethrogram (see Chapter 69)
2. Prostatitis

### E. MATERIALS (FIGS. 77-1 AND 77-2)
1. Robinson catheter (also known as "straight cath" or "red rubber")
a. Used for intermittent bladder catheterization
2. Coudé catheter
a. Available with and without balloon port

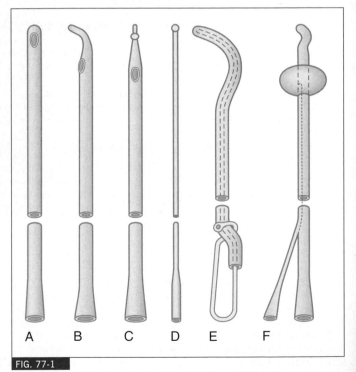

**FIG. 77-1**

Urethral catheters, including soft rubber *(A)*, coudé *(B)*, and Phillips *(C)*, which attaches to filiform *(D)*, which may be threaded over wire stylet *(E)*. *F,* Foley self-retaining urethral catheter.

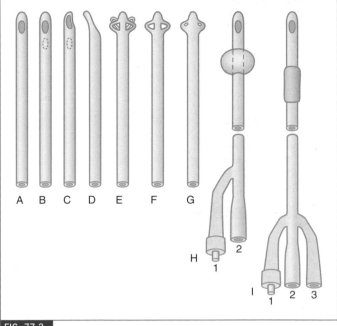

**FIG. 77-2**

Large-diameter catheters. *A,* Conical-tip urethral catheter. *B,* Robinson urethral catheter. *C,* Whistle-tip urethral catheter. *D,* Coudé hollow olive-tip catheter. *E,* Malecot self-retaining, four-wing urethral catheter. *F,* Malecot self-retaining, two-wing urethral catheter. *G,* Pezzer self-retaining drain, open-end head, used for cystostomy drainage. *H,* Foley-type balloon catheter. *I,* Foley-type, three-way balloon catheter, one limb of distal end for balloon inflation *(1)*, one for drainage *(2)*, and one to infuse irrigating solution to prevent clot formation within the bladder *(3)*.

b. Curved, firm rubber tip
c. Designed to bypass the S-shaped male bulbar urethra and often narrowed urethral angle of the prostatic urethra
d. Always insert with tip pointing up (12 o'clock position).
3. **Foley catheter**
a. Double-lumen catheter—small balloon lumen and large drainage lumen. Typically use 16 French (Fr). 1 Fr = 0.33 mm external diameter.
b. Use silicone Foley if patient is expected to leave in more than 1 week.
4. **Filiform catheter—serially inserted to find true urethral passage around stricture.**
5. **Phillips catheter—used to follow filiform to dilate urethral stricture.**

6. Malecot
a. Self-retaining catheter with wide outlet
b. Useful for draining clots
   (1) Malecot = Pezzer for practical purposes; cannot be placed transurethrally

7. Pezzer
a. Self-retaining catheter with wide outlet
b. Used for cystostomy drainage

8. **Three-way irrigation catheter**
a. Three-lumen design—small balloon lumen, small irrigation lumen, large drainage lumen

9. **Pediatric feeding tube**
a. 5 to 8 Fr may be used in infants. Catheter may be held in place with tape.
b. Do not use in adults because of coiling in the urethra.

## II. TECHNIQUE

### A. MALE PROCEDURE

1. Assemble all necessary equipment. Items usually in tray are sterile gloves, drapes, Foley catheter, 10 ml of sterile saline in syringe, collection bag, cotton swabs, povidone-iodine or chlorhexidine prep, prep forceps, sterile water, soluble lubricant or 2% viscous lidocaine.
2. Place patient in supine position. Open Foley tray in sterile fashion, then put on sterile gloves. Arrange all items so they are easily accessed and used with one hand. Test the Foley balloon. Drape the pelvic area.
3. Grasp the penis with nondominant hand. Retract the foreskin before preparation. Placing gauze over the retracted foreskin and then grasping will ensure that it remains retracted during the procedure. Prep the glans and meatus. After grasping penis, hand is no longer sterile and the remainder of the procedure is conducted with dominant operating hand.
4. Inject water-soluble lubricant or 10 to 15 ml of 2% viscous lidocaine into urethral meatus. Place penis on stretch angled toward the head to prevent folds from forming in the urethral mucosa (Fig. 77-3). Insert the catheter tip and advance with constant pressure. There may be resistance as the catheter encounters the external sphincter and prostatic urethra. Have the patient take slow, deep breaths and maintain constant pressure. Return of urine should be seen within catheter tubing. Remember, there are 3 cm of prostatic urethra beyond the external sphincter, so *do not inflate balloon until urine is seen and the catheter is "hubbed" to the balloon side port* (Fig. 77-4).
5. If urine is not seen with hubbed catheter, inject sterile saline into catheter and await return of urine. If no return, reposition catheter and repeat. If no return, upsize catheter or try Coudé catheter.

6. Inflate the balloon with 10 ml of sterile water. If there is any resistance, stop, aspirate injected saline, and reposition. Use only sterile water to inflate balloon in case of balloon failure. After inflation, seat the balloon at bladder neck.

7. Secure catheter to thigh with umbilical tape in correct position to prevent traumatic withdrawal. *Advance foreskin to prevent paraphimosis* (most common cause of paraphimosis is forgetting to replace after bladder catheterization).

## B.   FEMALE PROCEDURE (FIG. 77-5)

1. Prepare equipment as outlined in II.A.1 and II.A.2.
2. Patient is positioned supine and "frog-legged."

**77**

BLADDER CATHETERIZATION

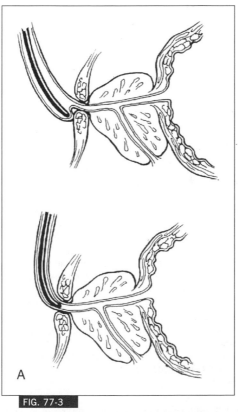

A

FIG. 77-3

The importance of stretch in male catheterization.

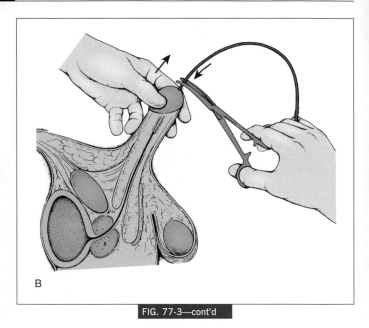

B

FIG. 77-3—cont'd

3. Retract labia with first finger and thumb of nondominant hand to expose urethra. Nondominant hand is now contaminated, and the remainder of the procedure must be done with sterile dominant hand. Urethra may be difficult to visualize at this point. Using povidone-iodine-(Betadine) or chlorhexidine-soaked cotton swabs, prep the urethra, superior vagina, and labia using downward swipes, one swipe per cotton swab. At this point, a difficult to visualize urethra may be seen with a slight pool of Betadine or a "wink" seen at urethral meatus.

4. Generously coat catheter tip with water-soluble lubricant or 10 to 15 ml of 2% viscous lidocaine. With dominant operating hand, insert catheter into urethral meatus and await return of urine.

5. Inflate balloon with 10 ml sterile water. Retract catheter to seat balloon at bladder neck.

6. Secure catheter to leg with umbilical tape to prevent traumatic withdrawal.

## C. DIFFICULT CATHETERIZATIONS
1. Male patients
a. Causes
   (1) Meatal stricture—balanitis xerotica obliterans, congenital narrowing, sexually transmitted disease

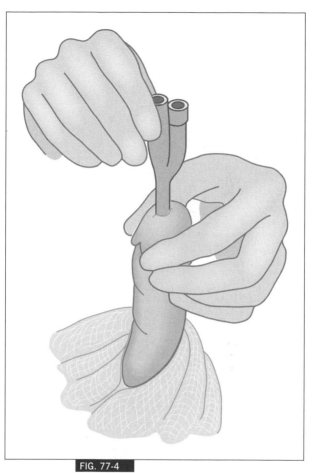

FIG. 77-4

Urethral catheterization in the male patient.

(2) Urethral stricture—fibrosis after trauma, instrumentation, sexually
transmitted disease
(3) Prostatic enlargement
    (a) Benign prostatic hypertrophy affects one third of men older than
        50 years, 90% of men older than 80 years.
    (b) Affects periurethral prostate tissue, causing impaired voiding
        symptoms and difficult catheterizations

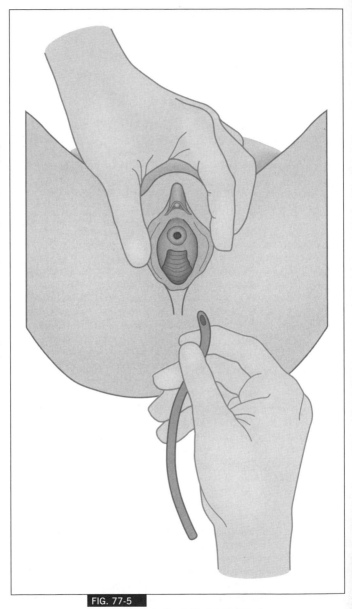

### FIG. 77-5

Urethral catheterization in the female patient.

    (4) Urethral false passage
        (a) Catheterization attempt with urethral trauma or rough catheter placement technique
        (b) Prevention is best solution.
            (1) Never catheterize with classic signs of urethral disruption.
            (2) Do not use unfamiliar instrumentation.
            (3) Any patient suspected of urethral disruption needs urologic consultation.
b. Solutions
    (1) Ensure adequate lubrication and traction on penis.
    (2) If patient is anxious, lorazepam or morphine can be used to facilitate sphincter relaxation.
    (3) If failure at first attempt, 10 to 15 ml of 2% viscous lidocaine should be injected into meatus and kept in place for 5 minutes before next attempt.
    (4) If resistance is still met, catheter should be upsized (yes, upsized) to 20 to 24 Fr to be able to maintain pressure and prevent coiling. If available, Coudé catheter should be used to help navigate prostatic urethra.
    (5) If failure after two attempts, a urologic consultation is warranted.
**2. Female patients—mostly stem from inability to locate urethral meatus.**
a. Causes
    (1) Obesity
    (2) Vulvar atrophy
b. Solutions
    (1) Assistant to retract
    (2) Vaginal speculum-assisted catheterization
    (3) Location and insertion of catheter by feel in vaginally located urethra

## III. CATHETER CARE
### A. CLOSED DRAINAGE SYSTEM
1. Should be considered sterile and should be treated as such when system violated. Use sterile gloves and prep if changing bags or injecting into the system.

### B. INDWELLING CATHETERS
Should be removed as soon as possible.

### C. INDWELLING CATHETERS
May be used for intraabdominal pressure measurement.
**1. Technique**
a. Clamp Foley tubing distal to access port.
b. Using sterile technique, inject 50 ml sterile saline into access port.
c. Using a transducer and pressure bag setup zeroed to the level of the bladder, transduce pressure.

77

BLADDER CATHETERIZATION

2. Use to monitor for abdominal compartment syndrome (pressure >25 mm Hg).

## D. CATHETER DISCONTINUATION
### 1. Urinary retention after catheterization
a. Void check—after discontinuation, void should be confirmed within 8 hours.
b. If no void after 8 hours, straight catheterization should be done. Void check should be repeated.
c. After straight catheterization and no void after 8 hours, Foley may be replaced. Alternatively, straight catheterization may be repeated until spontaneous void.
### 2. Failure to deflate balloon
a. Inject several milliliters of sterile water, then try to aspirate.
b. Cut balloon port.
c. Advance guidewire from a central line kit.
   (1) May dislodge occluding material
   (2) Central line catheter may be advanced over wire into balloon to deflate once guidewire is withdrawn.
     (a) Limited by length—male urethra is approximately 20 cm.
d. Balloon rupture (second choice)
   (1) Hyperinflation of balloon followed by firm end of guidewire insertion to pop balloon
   (2) External needle puncture with ultrasound guidance
   (3) Balloon must be inspected after removal to ensure all portions were removed.
     (a) If fragments are left in bladder, they must be removed with cystoscopy.

## IV. ALTERNATIVES
### A. SUPRAPUBIC CATHETER
### B. CONDOM (AKA TEXAS) CATHETER
1. Good alternative for immobilized male patients with normal voiding function
2. Often used in critically ill patients to avoid infectious risk of an indwelling catheter, but provide accurate output recording.

# Gastrointestinal Intubation

*Callisia N. Clarke, MD*

## I. NASOGASTRIC (NG) TUBES

When placing an NG tube, always pass the largest size tolerable.

### A. INDICATIONS

1. Decompression of stomach and small bowel
2. Analysis of gastric contents to aid in diagnosis
3. Gastric lavage
4. Introduction of fluids (e.g., oral contrast material)

### B. CONTRAINDICATIONS

1. Head trauma and/or maxillofacial fractures (risk for intracranial penetration)
2. Known presence of esophageal stricture or varices
3. Recent esophageal or gastric surgery (call your senior resident)
4. History of alkaline reflux (risk for perforation)
5. Unsecured airway in neurologically impaired (risk for aspiration)

### C. CAUTIONS AND COMPLICATIONS

1. C-spine precautions must be taken in patient with suspected cervical spine injury. Manual stabilization of the spine may be necessary to reduce the risk for spinal injury.
2. Aspiration pneumonia
3. Respiratory arrest or hypoxia caused by tracheal intubation

### D. TYPES OF TUBES

1. Salem sump tube—dual-lumen tube. The main lumen (white) should be placed to low continuous suction; the second port (blue) vents the tube to allow continuous sump suction without mucosal injury. The venting port should NEVER be flushed with fluid. Instead, flush with 15 ml of air every 3 to 4 hours to ensure patency. The main lumen may also be flushed with 30 ml saline as needed. The vent is patent when it "whistles" continuously.
2. Levin tube—a soft, single-lumen tube. Connect to low intermittent suction to prevent occlusion by gastric mucosa.

### E. METHOD OF INSERTION

1. Explain procedure to awake patient.
2. Position patient: If awake, patient should be sitting with neck flexed. If patient is unconscious, elevate the head of bed at least 30 degrees.
3. Most tubes are premarked by a series of four black marks on the main lumen. The proximal mark, at the nares, indicates insertion to the distal esophagus; the middle two marks indicate insertion to the body of the stomach; and the distal mark indicates insertion to the

pylorus/duodenum in the average person. However, you may estimate the distance required to reach the stomach by measuring the length from the nose to the earlobe and from the earlobe to the xiphoid process. Add the measurements together for the total distance.

4. Lubricate the tube with water-soluble lubricant or viscous lidocaine. Viscous lidocaine may also be inserted into the nostril with cotton-tip applicators or syringe.

5. Insert the tube into a nostril and pass it into the nasopharynx (a small bend in the tip of the tube aids passage).

6. Instruct the patient to swallow when the tube is felt in the back of the throat. Sips of water through a straw can help facilitate easy passage of the tube into the esophagus in an awake patient.

7. Advance into the stomach.

8. Ask the awake patient to say his/her name. Phonation is a good indicator that the vocal cords (and hence the trachea) are not occluded. Coughing, gasping for air, or inability to speak may be an early sign of tracheal intubation. Condensation may be visible in the tube. Immediately pull back the tube.

9. Confirm the tube position by instilling 20 to 30 ml of air while listening over the stomach with a stethoscope and by aspirating gastric contents. Aspiration of gastric contents is a more reliable method. Always confirm with a radiograph if the tube is to be used for feeding.

10. Secure the tube with tape. Tubes taped too tightly to the nostril or nasal septum may lead to pressure necrosis.

11. Patients with aberrant anatomy may require endoscopic guidance for safe insertion.

## II. OROGASTRIC TUBES

### A. INDICATIONS

1. NG intubation contraindicated (anterior basilar skull fracture, nasopharyngeal trauma)

### B. TYPES OF TUBES

1. Ewald tube—most commonly used. Especially suited for lavage of the stomach and emergency evacuation of blood, toxic agents, medications, or other substances. It is a large (18/36-Fr) double-lumen tube. The 36-Fr lumen is connected to continuous suction; the 18-Fr lumen is used for irrigation.

### C. METHOD OF INSERTION

1. Similar to NG tube insertion described earlier, except the tube is introduced into the mouth and down the esophagus into the stomach

2. In patients with loss of consciousness or loss of the gag reflex, insertion of a cuffed endotracheal tube before orogastric tube insertion is preferred.

3. Verify the position of the tube by aspiration of gastric contents and by auscultation.
4. Connect to suction; begin irrigation only after the stomach is empty. The amount of irrigant used should be monitored. The large bore of this tube may allow rapid overdistension of the stomach with the resultant risk for aspiration.

## III. FEEDING TUBES

### A. INDICATIONS

1. **Need for supplemental enteric feeding.** Indications include:
   a. Inadequate caloric intake (prematurity/failure to thrive)
   b. Central nervous system dysfunction
   c. Burns/trauma
   d. Esophageal anomalies/dysmotility
   e. Malignancy
   f. Eating disorders
2. **Short-term enteric feeding**
   a. These tubes are smaller in diameter, softer, and more flexible than NG tubes.
      (1) **Corpak**—nonweighted, has a bullet at the tip to prevent passage of the tube into regions of the tracheobronchial tree that lack cartilaginous support; a wire stylet may be used to pass the tube into the duodenum under fluoroscopic guidance.
      (2) **Frederick–Miller**—has a stylet that allows for improved manipulation; may be placed under fluoroscopic guidance to prevent inadvertent tracheobronchial placement; preferred when postpyloric placement is necessary.
      (3) **pH-guided nasointestinal feeding tubes**—rapid, easy placement of feeding tube with elimination of endoscopic/fluoroscopic requirement. Placement is similar to that for standard bedside feeding tube. The pH monitor allows for continuous readings. A pH of 3.5 to 5 confirms placement of tube in stomach. The tube is advanced until a sudden, rapid increase in pH readings is encountered, signifying transpyloric passage. If the rate of pH increase is gradual, the tube is likely to be curled in the stomach with the tip at the gastroesophageal junction.
   b. Tubes may be placed blindly in a similar fashion as outlined earlier for NG tubes or under fluoroscopic guidance.
   c. Placement must be confirmed radiographically before initiation of tube feedings.
   d. Placement of the tube past the ligament of Treitz eliminates most of the potential for aspiration.
3. **Long-term enteric feedings**
   a. Percutaneous endoscopic gastrostomy (PEG)—provides long-term enteric access (Fig. 78-1).
      (1) Advantages—fast, safe placement of gastrostomy tube. May be placed under sedation versus general anesthesia.

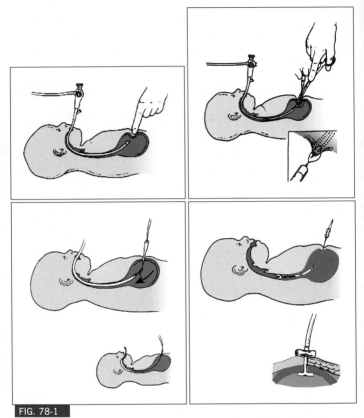

Placement of PEG tube. *(Reprinted from Texas Pediatric Surgical Associates: Tube feeding for children. Reprinted from:* http://www.pedisurg.com/PtEduc/Tube_Feeding .htm. *Accessed April 10, 2008.)*

(2) Contraindications are relative. Prior abdominal surgery makes this procedure higher risk.
(3) Technique (see Fig. 78-1): An endoscope is passed through the mouth and into the stomach. A site on the anterior gastric wall is identified and a needle introduced into the stomach percutaneously under direct visualization. A wire is then passed through the needle into the stomach and out through the oral pharynx. The gastrostomy

tube is then attached to the wire and guided through the stomach, exiting the skin at the site of the previous needle puncture. Care should be taken to prevent necrosis of the stomach wall by ensuring that the mucosa does not blanch because of excess pressure, and that the tube is able to spin easily against the stomach wall. The distance of the percutaneous endoscopic gastrostomy tube at the skin level should be noted and documented after surgery and on daily rounds. A distance of 1 to 3 cm at the skin in a person of normal habitus is within reference limits.

b. Open (Stamm) gastrostomy tube
   (1) Advantages: Allows for safe placement of gastrostomy tube even in the most difficult abdomen
   (2) Technique (Fig. 78-2): A small upper midline incision is made through the abdominal wall. Clamps are used to elevate the anterior gastric wall approximately 6 to 10 cm from the gastroduodenal junction. Two silk purse-string sutures are placed on the anterior wall of the stomach and a small incision made at the center of the purse-string sutures. A large-bore (18–22-Fr) Foley catheter is then passed into the stomach and the balloon inflated. The catheter is secured in place with the purse-string sutures and the open end passed through the anterior abdominal wall through a separate site. The anterior gastric wall is fixed to the anterior abdominal wall with silk sutures to minimize dead space; care should be taken to ensure that the balloon of the catheter is pulled up against the stomach and up to the abdominal wall. With time, the tract epithelializes to facilitate frequent exchanges of tubes as needed for optimal feeding.

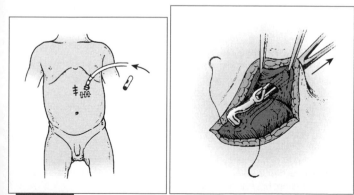

**FIG. 78-2**

*(Reprinted from Texas Pediatric Surgical Associates: Tube feeding for children. Reprinted from:* http://www.pedisurg.com/PtEduc/Tube_Feeding.htm.*)*

**78**

GASTROINTESTINAL INTUBATION

## IV. ESOPHAGEAL/GASTRIC TAMPONADE TUBES

1. The Sengstaken–Blakemore tube is an orogastric tube equipped with an esophageal and gastric balloon for tamponade and a distal suction port for aspiration. The Minnesota tube is similar but has an additional suction post above the esophageal balloon for proximal aspiration.
2. These tubes allow for nonoperative direct control of the bleeding from esophageal and gastric varices.
3. Causes immediate cessation of bleeding in approximately 85% of patients
4. Indications
   a. Bleeding esophageal varices refractory to sclerotherapy and medical management
5. Complications
   a. Frequent recurrence of hemorrhage after deflation of the balloon—25% to 55% of cases
   b. High incidence of complications—aspiration, asphyxiation
6. Insertion
   a. Before passing the tube, test each balloon for air leaks and proper inflation, and perform a gastric lavage to remove blood and clots.
   b. Endotracheal intubation is recommended to minimize aspiration. In unintubated patients, the pharynx should not be anesthetized so as to maintain the gag reflex.
   c. Lubricate the tube and pass it into the stomach via the mouth.
   d. Confirm the intragastric location of the gastric balloon by instilling a small amount of water-soluble contrast into the balloon and obtaining a radiograph before inflating the balloon fully.
   e. Inflate the gastric balloon with increments of 100 ml of air to a total of 450 to 500 ml. Stop air inflation immediately if the patient complains of epigastric pain or if insufflation of air is not audible over the epigastric region.
   f. Apply gentle traction on the tube until resistance indicates that the balloon is at the esophagogastric junction.
   g. Gastric lavage is performed through the gastric aspiration lumen using saline. The aspirate should clear if bleeding is controlled.
   h. If a Sengstaken–Blakemore tube is used, a second nasoesophageal tube must be passed into the proximal esophagus to check for continued bleeding above the gastric balloon and to aspirate salivary secretions. The Minnesota tube is a modification that has an esophageal port to obviate the need for this extra tube.
   i. If blood is detected continually in the gastric aspirate, the esophageal balloon should be inflated. Use the lowest pressure that stops bleeding. Do not inflate the esophageal balloon above 40 mm Hg.
   j. External traction is obtained by taping the tube to the face mask of a football helmet or attaching 1 to 2 pounds of traction.
   k. Both balloons are inflated for 24 hours, after which the esophageal balloon is slowly deflated and the patient is observed for signs of rebleeding. If rebleeding occurs, the esophageal balloon is reinflated.

l. If there is no rebleeding, the gastric balloon is deflated after 24 hours and the patient is observed.

m. If no further bleeding occurs 24 hours after the gastric balloon is deflated, mineral oil should be given before removal. The tube is completely transected with scissors and removed. This ensures that balloons are deflated completely and that the tube is not reused.

n. The esophageal balloon is always deflated first to prevent the risk for migration.

## V. NASOINTESTINAL TUBES FOR DECOMPRESSION OF THE SMALL BOWEL

### A. INDICATION

1. Rarely used, and if so, mainly for early postoperative bowel obstruction secondary to early adhesion formations or obstruction secondary to carcinomatosis

### B. TYPES OF TUBES

1. Cantor tube—single-lumen tube with a mercury-filled balloon at the distal end
2. Miller–Abbott tube—dual lumen with one lumen for intermittent suction and the other to attach a balloon that can be filled with mercury or water once the tube enters the stomach

### C. INSERTION

1. To prepare the balloon tip, inject 5 ml mercury into the middle of the balloon tangentially with a 21-gauge needle, then withdraw all air from the balloon.
2. Lubricate the tube and pass into the stomach.
3. Place the patient on the right side and advance the tube to the "P" position as marked on the outside of the tube. Tape the tube to the side of the face with a 4- to 6-inch loop. This permits the tube to advance by peristalsis. Have the patient remain in this position until the "D" mark is at the external naris, indicating passage into the duodenum.
4. Place the patient on the left side until the tube has advanced several inches. Allow the patient to resume activity and the tube to be drawn downward by peristalsis. Leave a 4-inch loop free. Pass the tube 3 inches every 4 hours. Irrigate with 15 ml saline before advancing the tube.
5. When the tube no longer advances by peristalsis, place the tube on low intermittent suction. Confirm position by radiograph.

78

GASTROINTESTINAL INTUBATION

# Diagnostic Peritoneal Lavage and the Focused Assessment with Sonography in Trauma

*Gerald R. Fortuna, Jr., MD*

The workup and evaluation of patients with potential intraabdominal pathology in the emergency department and after trauma is still a frequent task faced by general surgeons today. Despite newer technologies and advanced imaging, diagnostic peritoneal lavage (DPL) and the focused assessment with sonography in trauma (FAST) remain useful tools to the trauma surgeon in the evaluation of these patients. This chapter provides information on the indications, usefulness, advantages, and disadvantages of using both DPL and FAST in emergency situations in an attempt to provide a framework for surgeons to choose the appropriate workup in the trauma bay.

**79**

## I. GENERAL CONSIDERATIONS

1. Root and colleagues introduced DPL in 1965, and since that time it has been a mainstay in the evaluation of unstable patients with blunt abdominal trauma and selected cases of penetrating trauma.
2. It remains a rapid, inexpensive, and accurate test when performed in appropriately selected patients suspected to have intraperitoneal hemorrhage after abdominal trauma.
3. Ideally, DPL should be performed by the surgeon caring for the patient because it is a surgical procedure that alters subsequent examinations and potentially the treatment of the patient.
4. The use of DPL, focused abdominal examination with ultrasound and/ or computed tomography (CT), depends on the familiarity of the diagnosing physician with the use of ultrasound, the availability of CT, and the time available for patient evaluation (Table 79-1). CT scan should be performed with intravenous contrast material and only in hemodynamically stable patients.
5. Timing of these studies is critical. DPL is usually performed early in the evaluation of the trauma patient, typically during the secondary survey. Abdominal and pelvic films should be completed before performing DPL to rule out free air and significant pelvic fractures.
a. Free air or pelvic fractures can influence the decision to perform DPL, as well as whether a supraumbilical or infraumbilical approach is taken.
6. Limitations of each of the studies should constantly be kept in mind.
a. DPL is characteristically unreliable in assessing most retroperitoneal injuries.
b. Almost half of all patients with hemoperitoneum show no signs of peritonitis on examination.

TABLE 79-1

DIAGNOSTIC PERITONEAL LAVAGE VERSUS ULTRASOUND VERSUS COMPUTED TOMOGRAPHY IN BLUNT ABDOMINAL TRAUMA

| | DPL | Ultrasound | CT Scan |
|---|---|---|---|
| Indications | Document bleeding if decreased blood pressure | Document fluid if decreased blood pressure | Document organ injury if blood pressure stable |
| Advantages | Early diagnosis; sensitive; 98% accurate | Early diagnosis; noninvasive and repeatable; 86–97% accurate | Most specific for solid organ injury; 92–98% accurate |
| Disadvantages | Invasive; misses injury to diaphragm or retroperitoneum | Operator dependent; bowel gas and subcutaneous air distortion; misses diaphragm, bowel, and some pancreatic injuries | Cost and time; misses some diaphragm, bowel tract, and pancreatic injuries |

CT = computed tomographic; DPL = diagnostic peritoneal lavage.
From Advanced Trauma Life Support. Chicago, American College of Surgeons, 1997.

7. DPL is not just limited to trauma patients. It can also be a useful adjunct in the diagnosis and evaluation of the critically ill patient suspected of having intraabdominal processes.

## II. INDICATIONS FOR DIAGNOSTIC PERITONEAL LAVAGE

### A. MOST USEFUL
In blunt abdominal trauma and manifestations of hypovolemia—hypotension and tachycardia
1. Unconscious patients with concerns of a potential abdominal injury
2. Patients with high-energy injuries, suspected intraabdominal injury, and nonspecific abdominal physical findings
3. Presence of multiple injuries with unexplained shock
4. Patients with major noncontiguous or thoracoabdominal injuries
5. Patients with spinal cord injuries
6. Intoxicated patients with suspected intraabdominal injuries
7. Patients with suspected intraabdominal injuries but equivocal diagnostic testing who are being transferred to the operating room with general anesthesia where serial examinations and monitoring are not possible

### B. EQUIVOCAL ABDOMINAL FINDINGS
Often a result of lower rib fractures, pelvic fractures, and lumbar spine fractures
1. Abdominal findings such as localized tenderness and guarding
2. Low rib fractures, particularly on left side

## C. PENETRATING TRAUMA

With questionable involvement of the peritoneal cavity is controversial and has been debated extensively in the trauma literature

## D. CONTROVERSIAL INDICATIONS FOR DPL, CT, OR BOTH

1. Penetrating injury to surrounding areas
a. Lower chest—below nipples or fourth intercostal space
   (1) In this situation, the patient is at risk for thoracoabdominal injuries depending on the trajectory of the projectile. In an unstable patient, a positive DPL could help dictate which cavity is initially explored.
b. Flank
c. Buttocks and perineum
2. Stab wounds or low-caliber gunshot wounds with no significant physical findings. DPL in this setting may be helpful in identifying intraabdominal injury. Could also consider laparoscopy.

## III. CONTRAINDICATIONS

## A. ABSOLUTE CONTRAINDICATIONS TO PERFORMING DPL

1. Obvious indications for exploratory laparotomy
a. Presence of free air
b. Peritonitis
c. Isolated penetrating trauma from a gunshot wound
d. Pregnancy
e. Morbid obesity

## B. RELATIVE CONTRAINDICATIONS

1. Multiple abdominal operations or midline scars—appendectomy or Pfannenstiel's scar alone does not preclude DPL.
2. Inability to decompress bladder—use supraumbilical open technique.
3. Inability to decompress stomach—use infraumbilical open technique.
4. Pelvic fracture with possible hematoma—use supraumbilical open technique to avoid false-positive results obtained by entering retroperitoneal hematoma.

## IV. TECHNIQUES

## A. SEMI-OPEN TECHNIQUE

1. Insert nasogastric tube and urinary catheter—stomach and bladder must be decompressed to avoid injury.
2. Restrain patient and sedate if necessary.
3. Shave periumbilical region—above and below umbilicus.
4. Prep region widely with povidone-iodine (Betadine) and drape with sterile towels.
5. Use an infraumbilical incision except when the patient has pelvic fractures or suspected retroperitoneal hematoma.
6. Infiltrate proposed site (skin and subcutaneous tissue) with 1% lidocaine with epinephrine—enhances local hemostasis to minimize false-positive results; use even in comatose or anesthetized patient.

7. Incise skin (1–3 cm vertical incision needed depending on body habitus) and subcutaneous tissue down to midline fascia.
8. Place towel clips on both sides of the fascial incision for traction.
9. Using a #11 scalpel blade, make a 2- to 3-mm stab incision in fascia.
10. With strong upward traction on the towel clips by the assistant, place the trocar-catheter apparatus through the fascial opening and then push it through the posterior fascia and peritoneum. This initial push should be done perpendicular to the skin and must stop after one feels the "pop" of the peritoneum. At this point, the trocar-catheter apparatus is tilted down at a 45-degree angle, and the catheter alone is advanced into the pelvis and the trocar is removed.
11. Attach the aspirating device and aspirate using a 12-ml syringe.
    a. If more than 10 ml of gross blood is aspirated, the DPL is considered a positive test.
    b. If less than 10 ml of gross blood is aspirated, then the aspirate is returned to the abdomen with the lavage fluid. This will ensure the accuracy of DPL requirements once 1 L of fluid is instilled into the abdominal cavity.
12. If the aspirate is negative for blood, instill 1 L (10 ml/kg in children) lactated Ringer's solution or normal saline with the aid of a pressure bag. Shake the patient's abdomen periodically, or move the patient into and out of Trendelenburg. Be sure to use warm fluid in patients with hypothermia.
13. When only a small level of fluid remains in the bag, drop the near-empty bag to the floor to drain the fluid. The fluid drains by siphon action. If all the fluid is allowed to run in together with some air, the siphon will be lost and must be restarted by applying suction via a needle and syringe to a port in the tubing. Ensure the tubing used does not have a one-way filter device.
14. While the fluid is draining, keep a sponge packed into the wound for hemostasis and constantly hold the catheter in place.
15. After the fluid has returned (300–500 ml minimum), clamp the tubing and withdraw the catheter. This will avoid siphoning blood from the wound into bag.
16. Wound closure: A heavy suture may be placed to close the small fascial defect. The skin closure can be performed with skin staples.

## B. PERCUTANEOUS

1. The percutaneous approach is a closed Seldinger technique that uses a needle and trocar, guide wire, and advancing catheter.
2. Aspirating the pelvis, fluid insertion and recovery is performed as described earlier.

### C.  OPEN TECHNIQUE

1. Midline fascia is incised over 3 to 4 cm, the posterior fascia/
   peritoneum is held with hemostats and opened under direct
   vision, and a catheter without trocar is advanced into the peritoneal
   cavity.
2. Fascial closure is required at completion.

## V. SPECIFIC CONSIDERATIONS

### A.  TECHNICAL PROBLEMS

1. Poor fluid return: Adjust the catheter position, twist the catheter,
   place the patient in the reverse Trendelenburg position, apply manual
   pressure to the abdomen, instill an additional 500 ml fluid, have
   patient take deep breaths, and make sure there is not a one-way
   valve in the intravenous tubing (fluid may exit the chest tube or Foley
   catheter).
2. Air in tubing: Check all connections; make certain the catheter is
   advanced far enough to avoid exposed side holes, reestablish siphon
   as described earlier (see IV.A.13).
3. Infusion into abdominal wall: Recognize immediately and repeat
   the DPL.

### B.  COMPLICATIONS

1. Bowel injury
2. Bladder laceration
3. Injury to major blood vessels—aorta, inferior vena cava
4. Hematoma
5. Wound infection

### C.  INTERPRETATION

1. Grossly positive—more than 10 ml of blood on initial aspirate.
2. Microscopic/chemistry criteria—positive on lavage (blunt trauma).
   a. More than 100,000 red blood cells/mm$^3$—97% sensitivity, 99.6%
      specificity; more than 10,000 to 20,000 red blood cells/mm$^3$ for
      penetrating trauma (controversial)
   b. More than 500 white blood cells/mm$^3$
   c. Presence of particulate (fecal, vegetable) matter
   d. Presence of bacteria on Gram stain
   e. Increased amylase, bilirubin levels
   f. Fluid exiting the chest tube or Foley catheter
3. For penetrating abdominal trauma, the criteria are changed:
   a. More than 10,000 red blood cells/mm$^3$ or more than 1000 white blood
      cells/mm$^3$
      (1) This decreased threshold translates into a greater false-positive rate
          and more frequent nondiagnostic celiotomies and is one of the
          drawbacks to performing DPL in penetrating trauma.

**79**

**DPL AND FAST**

## VI. FAST

Sonography in trauma was first introduced by Kristensen and colleagues in 1971. It was popularized in the 1990s with several studies reported in the emergency medicine and surgery literature.

### A. INDICATIONS

1. Same as in DPL. Useful in all blunt abdominal traumas. Less useful in penetrating trauma. Currently, no literature exists to support its use in this setting; however, this is still dependent on operator and institutional preferences.
2. Sensitivity, specificity, and accuracy are comparable with CT and DPL in experienced hands. There is a steep learning curve and is very much operator dependent. Expertise is gained between 50 and 200 examinations.

### B. ADVANTAGES

1. Rapid, noninvasive means to diagnose intraabdominal injuries
2. May be repeated quickly at the bedside, allowing ongoing investigation
3. Not limited by contraindications of DPL
4. Useful in diagnosing cardiac injuries with pericardial fluid through the subxiphoid window
a. Could aid in deciding which organ cavity to explore first in a patient with multisystem injuries

### C. DISADVANTAGES

1. Not reliable in pediatric blunt trauma
2. Operator dependence and experience

### D. COMPLICATING FACTORS

1. Obesity
2. Subcutaneous air

### E. TECHNIQUE—SAME AS THAT FOR FORMAL ULTRASOUND

1. Includes subxiphoid pericardial window, hepatorenal fossa (Morison's pouch), splenorenal fossa, and the bladder/pelvis; some institutions add windows of both the right and left paracolic gutters.
2. Perform a second control scan after 30 minutes, used to detect progressive hemoperitoneum if there is initial doubt.

### F. CT SCAN

1. Should be used in hemodynamically stable patients only
a. Time consuming, used when no immediate need for celiotomy
b. Provides most specific information about individual organ injuries and their extent

    c. May diagnose retroperitoneal and pelvic organ injuries, which may be missed by DPL or physical examination

    d. Relative contraindications

       (1) Delay time to use scanner if not immediately available

       (2) Uncooperative patient who cannot adequately be sedated

       (3) Inability to give intravenous contrast agent because of allergy or renal insufficiency

2. CT may miss some gastrointestinal, diaphragmatic, and pancreatic injuries. Presence of free fluid in a patient with no liver or splenic injury mandates early exploration for suspected injury to the gastrointestinal tract or its mesentery.

# Principles of Abscess Drainage

*Eric M. Campion, MD*

## I. SUPERFICIAL ABSCESSES

Superficial or cutaneous abscesses often begin as cellulitis. They are in the subcutaneous tissue and are usually easily palpable.

### A. BACTERIOLOGY
1. Often polymicrobial
2. Most commonly isolated organism in superficial abscesses is *Staphylococcus* spp.
3. Perianal abscesses often contain anaerobic species.
4. Individuals with diabetes, intravenous (IV) drug users, dialysis patients, transplant patients, and any other immunocompromised individuals are prone to multiorganism infections.

## 80

### B. TECHNIQUE
1. Obtain full history and physical examination, including history of diabetes, immunosuppression, previous abscesses, trauma, IV drug use, and the possibility of foreign body.
2. Consider IV pain control (morphine, meperidine) and sedation (diazepam, midazolam) when possible because these abscess are often painful.
3. Localize the abscess. An abscess is clinically evidenced by a fluctuant mass in an area of induration, erythema, and tenderness.
4. Prep and drape the area in a sterile manner.
5. Use a local anesthetic to perform a field block of area (1% lidocaine with epinephrine). Local anesthesia in the abscess can be difficult to obtain secondary to the low pH of the abscess cavity, but anesthesia of the skin should not be affected. The addition of 8.4% sodium bicarbonate at a ratio of 1 ml bicarbonate to 5 ml of lidocaine may help offset the low pH and reduce burning caused by lidocaine injection.
6. Consider using an 18- or 20-gauge needle to collect a sample for Gram stain, aerobic, and anaerobic cultures. This may also help to localize the fluid collection.
7. Using a #11 or #15 scalpel blade, make an incision over the entire length of the abscess cavity. Use the skin creases when possible to minimize scarring. It is possible to use a smaller incision in cosmetically important areas, but it is essential that the abscess be fully drained. A linear incision is preferred, but some providers use an elliptical or cruciate incision to keep the wound from closing.
8. Break up any loculations using a finger or an instrument such as a hemostat. All loculations must be broken for adequate drainage.

9. Irrigate liberally with saline using high-pressure irrigation with a syringe and an angiocath or a splash guard.
10. Pack the cavity completely but loosely with thin-strip gauze. Then cover with a gauze dressing.
11. Have patient follow-up within 24 to 48 hours. Remove the packing at that time, then reevaluate. If it appears to be improving, the patient may be shown how to perform packing changes and instructed to return for regular follow-up.

## C. ANTIBIOTICS
1. Although commonly prescribed, no evidence exists for the need for antibiotics in otherwise healthy, immunocompetent individuals without valvular heart disease.
2. There is a transient bacteremia after incision and drainage of abscesses necessitating antibiotic coverage for patients with valvular heart disease. IV antibiotics covering the likely pathogens should be administered 1 hour before procedure. This is often followed by a second dose 6 to 8 hours after the initial one.
3. Therapeutic antibiotics should be given to immunocompromised, diabetic, or alcoholic patients. The first dose should be given intravenously before the incision and drainage. This should be followed by a 5- to 7-day course. These patients should be considered for admission to the hospital for IV antibiotics and monitoring of the wound.

## II. DEEP ABSCESSES
Deep abscesses include intraabdominal, intramuscular, deep breast, and perirectal types.

## A. DRAINAGE
1. These abscesses require drainage in the operating room to assure proper exposure and anesthesia.
2. Some abscesses (such as intraabdominal) may be amenable to drainage in interventional radiology using computed tomography or ultrasound guidance.

## B. ANTIBIOTICS
1. Antibiotics should be begun before surgery, then continued to complete a course of treatment appropriate to the patient's condition.
2. Treatment should be begun broadly and then narrowed based on culture results.

# Central Venous Lines

*Bryon J. Boulton, MD*

## I. BACKGROUND
### A. GENERAL PRINCIPLES
1. Indications
   a. Poor venous access
   b. Total parenteral nutrition infusion
   c. Requiring invasive monitoring (pulmonary artery catheters)
   d. Infusion of inotropic agents
   e. Hemodialysis
   f. Chemotherapy
   g. Large-volume resuscitation
2. **Contraindications (all are relative in a life-threatening situation)**
   a. Presence of a deep venous thrombosis in site of choice
   b. Presence of a coagulopathy or significantly depressed platelet count (i.e., $<60,000/mm^3$)
   c. Subclavian vein approach in a patient on hemodialysis or expected to require hemodialysis in the future because of the increased rate of subclavian vein stenosis after central venous catheter (CVC) placement
   d. Untreated sepsis/bloodstream infections
   e. Previous femoral vascular surgery (for femoral approach)
3. **Informed consent**
   a. Discuss with the patient the indications, risks, and benefits of this procedure.
   b. If patient is unable to provide consent, one should contact next of kin, medical power of attorney, or designated medical decision maker.
   c. In emergent medical situations, implied consent is presumed.
4. **Patient evaluation**
   a. Evaluate the patient's prothrombin time/international normalized ratio/ partial thromboplastin time (if clinically appropriate), platelet count, hemoglobin and hematocrit, and whether there is a history of bleeding disorders.
   b. History of deep venous thrombosis, locations, and whether they have resolved.
   c. Physical examination for deformities or scars from previous CVC placement
5. **Preparation/tips**
   a. Notification and/or presence of appropriate attending supervision
   b. Involvement and presence of assistance (i.e., nurse)
   c. Cardiac monitoring.
   d. Collection of necessary supplies
      (1) CVC kit
      (2) Obtaining ultrasound device if available

81

    (3) Sterile gown, sterile gloves, face mask, head protection, 0.9% normal saline for flush, sterile towels, sterile drape, sterilization/prepping agent (i.e., chlorhexidine), sterile dressing kit, 1% lidocaine, shoulder roll, sterile intravenous tubing, ultrasound with sterile covering and gel, sterile intravenous caps, and any missing components from standard triple-lumen catheter kit (i.e., wire, #11 blade, etc.)

  e. Correct patient positioning

    (1) Together with identification of landmarks, this is the most important step of the entire procedure; therefore, no time should be wasted getting the patient into the correct position and the surgeon in a comfortable position.

    (2) Rearrange the room to remove any obstacles to a less obstructive position (i.e., ventilators), move the bed away from the wall, and take down the bed rails.

    (3) Patient positioning

      (a) Subclavian/internal jugular (IJ): Place patient in supine Trendelenburg position (head down) with a shoulder roll placed under the patient (longitudinally for subclavian and transversely for IJ). Allow patient's ipsilateral shoulder and arm to fall to the side and be as relaxed as possible; gentle retraction may need to be applied by an assistant. Turn patient's head toward the contralateral shoulder for an IJ approach. For patients with large pendulous breasts, gentle retraction is beneficial in the subclavian approach.

      (b) Femoral: Place patient in supine reverse Trendelenburg position, retract any significant panus, and make sure leg is not maximally externally or internally rotated.

  f. Being comfortable inserting the needle with either hand is beneficial, making the surgeon less awkward and more comfortable regardless of the position or approach.

  g. The first time one uses a kit, it is beneficial to take time to familiarize oneself with the contents of the kit and how the equipment works.

  h. Once the patient has been draped, place the wire in an easily reached location.

  i. Flush the proximal and middle ports before insertion so they can be flushed if they do not withdraw after insertion to free them from attachment to the sidewall of the vein.

**6. Placement**

  a. Depth of CVC placement depends on patient body habitus, type of catheter used, and site of insertion

  b. Cordis, hemodialysis catheters, and other large-diameter CVC catheters should be placed up to the hub depending on the length of the CVC.

  c. On chest radiograph (CXR), the catheter tip of a CVC should at least make a bend into the superior vena cava; extension into the right atria is tolerable as long as it does not cause ectopy, but ideally should be pulled back into the superior vena cava.

d. Depth of insertion can be estimated by holding the tip of the TLC to the right of the patient's sternum in the third intercostal space and coursing it along the central venous system to the selected site of insertion.

e. On subclavian TLC placement in an obese individual with a large amount of chest fat, placing the catheter to the hub is suggested until CXR is obtained because once the patient sits upright, the catheter will be pulled out as the chest fat falls to its dependent position.

f. When in doubt, always err on the side of placing the TLC too deep because the catheter can always be withdrawn; however, once the line has been dressed, it should not be advanced farther into the patient because it is no longer sterile.

7. **Seldinger technique**

a. After insertion site is selected, create a weal with 1% lidocaine, as well as infusing some along the subcutaneous track in the direction of planned needle insertion.

b. Insert an 18-gauge needle according to the technique unique to the selected site, aspirating while probing.

c. If blood is encountered and it can be easily aspirated, remove the syringe; if blood does not flow out, quickly place thumb over hole to prevent air emboli. Unless the central venous pressure is extremely high, venous blood should slowly drip out.

d. Without the slightest movement of the needle, insert the J-wire, J-tip first; it should pass with little resistance. With the needle bevel facing the patient's feet, it is easier for the wire to be directed toward the heart. Advance the wire at least 20 cm into the patient; if cardiac ectopy on the cardiac monitor is encountered, this confirms that the wire is within the heart (for nonfemoral lines).

e. Once the wire has been passed, before removing the needle, make at least a 3-mm nick in the skin with the scalpel and then remove the needle.

f. Always keep a hand on the wire so as not to lose it in the patient.

g. Insert the dilator only 3 to 4 cm to dilate the subcutaneous tissues, and remove while maintaining control of the wire.

h. Slide the CVC over the wire down to the level of the skin, and back the wire up into the CVC until the tip appears at the end of the CVC. Then slide the CVC down the wire without advancing the wire any farther into the patient (keeping the wire still in space).

i. Advance the CVC to desired depth and then remove the wire. Once the wire is removed, immediately place thumb over the port to prevent air emboli until an airtight cap can be placed.

j. With normal saline in the syringe, withdraw on all three ports until blood is seen in the syringe. Flush saline down the CVC with the plunger upright so air is not flushed into the patient.

k. Suture the CVC onto the skin in at least three locations and place a sterile dressing. Obtain a stat CXR and check it yourself to verify correct placement in the superior vena cava and to rule out a pneumothorax.

**81**

**CENTRAL VENOUS LINES**

## II. TECHNIQUES

### A. INFRACLAVICULAR SUBCLAVIAN VEIN APPROACH

**1. Positioning**

a. Position patient as described earlier.

**2. Identify landmarks.**

a. Identify deltopectoral groove, sternal notch, and course of clavicle before draping patient.

**3. Prep**

a. Widely prep, including ipsilateral neck up to the jaw (in case conversion to an IJ approach is necessary), down to nipple, the lateral aspects of the shoulder, and to the contralateral side of the sternum.

**4. Technique**

a. Palpate the deltopectoral groove and infiltrate 1% lidocaine, two finger-breadths inferior to the clavicle along the deltopectoral groove, creating a weal. Place index finger of the nondominant hand in the sternal notch and the thumb between the weal of lidocaine and the clavicle along an imaginary line between the weal of lidocaine and the tip of the index finger in the sternal notch. While aspirating, advance the needle down to the clavicle, and infuse lidocaine onto the periosteum and inject lidocaine while withdrawing the needle.

b. With an 18-gauge needle, and the bevel facing either toward the ceiling or the patient's feet, advance the needle while aspirating toward the center of the sternal notch/tip of the index finder, always keeping it parallel to the floor, and sliding it under the clavicle. Transcutaneous pressure from the infraclavicular thumb assists driving the needle under the clavicle.

c. It is advised not to drive the needle into the clavicle and then "walk down" the clavicle until the needle is under the clavicle because this creates a downward trajectory of the needle as it slides under the clavicle.

d. If there is no blood return once the needle reaches the hub, withdraw the needle slowly until it is nearly out of the skin and repeat the above technique, this time aiming 0.5 to 1 cm more cranial than the previous target.

e. If arterial blood or air is encountered, stop and consult section III.

### B. SUPRACLAVICULAR SUBCLAVIAN VEIN APPROACH

**1. Positioning**

a. Position the patient as described earlier, with the head rotated to the contralateral side.

**2. Identify landmarks.**

a. Identify the clavicle, clavicular head of the sternocleidomastoid (SCM), anterior and middle scalene, and attempt to palpate the subclavian artery before it enters the chest.

**3. Prep**

a. A wide prep is beneficial, including the ipsilateral neck and subclavicular regions if an alternate approach is required.

4. **Technique**
a. This approach is technically easier for a right-handed surgeon to stand at the head of the bed for a right-sided approach or to the patient's side for a left-sided approach (vice versa for a left-handed surgeon).
b. Infuse lidocaine in an area one fingerbreadth superior to the midpoint of the clavicle. If given the option, select the right side to avoid placing the catheter into the thoracic duct.
c. With an 18-gauge needle, or 22-gauge finder needle if new to this approach, insert it one fingerbreadth superior to the clavicular midpoint and advance while aspirating, aiming at the underside of the sternal notch. Alternatively, the needle can be inserted at the lateral edge of the SCM-clavicular junction. The subclavian vein is encountered posterior to the sternal head/clavicular head insertion of the SCM muscle. If no blood is encountered, slowly withdraw back to the level of the skin. If arterial blood flow is encountered, stop and consult section III.
d. Once good venous blood flow is encountered, follow the Seldinger technique as described earlier.
e. If using a finder needle, once the location of the subclavian vein has been determined, remove the finder needle and insert the introducer needle through the same entrance point and along the same trajectory.

## C.  ANTERIOR IJ APPROACH
1. **Positioning**
a. Position the patient as described in section I.A., with the head rotated toward the contralateral side and in the Trendelenburg position.
2. **Identify landmarks.**
a. Identify the SCM muscle, the insertion of the sternal and clavicular heads, and trace them back to their point of convergence. This point forms the superior apex of a triangle formed by the clavicle and the sternal and clavicular heads of the SCM. Palpate the carotid pulse as it courses through the neck.
3. **Prep**
a. A wide prep is beneficial, prepping the ipsilateral chest for a possible subclavian approach and the posterior lateral neck for a possible posterior IJ approach.
4. **Technique**
a. Palpate the carotid pulse and infuse 1% lidocaine at the superior apex of the two heads of the SCM superficially.
b. Insert a 22-gauge finder needle at the superior apex of the two heads of the SCM and advance while aspirating at 45 to 60 degrees to the skin, directing the needle toward the ipsilateral nipple while palpating the carotid pulse with the opposite hand.
c. Withdraw the needle slowly if there is no blood return, and redirect the needle through the same entrance point, aiming lateral to the previous trajectory. If this is unsuccessful, continue redirecting laterally for 1 to

CENTRAL VENOUS LINES

3 cm before directing the needle medial to the original trajectory, always being mindful of the location of the carotid artery.

d. If there is still no blood return, attempt to aspirate the IJ without palpating the carotid because the IJ may have been compressed. If there is still no further blood return, reassess the landmarks and reattempt or consider a posterior approach.

e. Once blood return has been achieved, remove the finder needle, because it creates an obstacle if left in the skin, and have the 18-gauge introducer needle within reach to insert along the same trajectory without having to look away from the patient. If arterial blood is aspirated, stop immediately and consult section III.

f. At the same angle and trajectory, insert the 18-gauge introducer needle while aspirating. Once good blood return is demonstrated, remove the syringe and insert the CVC using the Seldinger technique as described in the previous section.

## D. POSTERIOR IJ VEIN APPROACH

### 1. Positioning

a. Position the patient as described in section I.A., with the head rotated to the contralateral side.

### 2. Identify landmarks.

a. Identify the SCM and external jugular vein, and palpate the carotid artery.

### 3. Prep

a. Once again, a wide prep is recommended to be able to change to either an anterior or subclavian approach without having to break sterile technique.

### 4. Technique

a. With 1% lidocaine, anesthetize the skin three fingerbreadths above the clavicle along the posterolateral border of the SCM, which is inferior to the external jugular.

b. Insert a 22-gauge finder needle, directing it just deep to the SCM and advancing, while aspirating, toward the cricoid-thyroid junction along the midline. Advance the needle while palpating the carotid artery, and pinching and slightly elevating, rather than depressing, the SCM with the opposite hand.

c. If no blood return is demonstrated, withdraw slowly and redirect the needle slightly inferior. If no blood return is again demonstrated, continue to palpate the carotid, but do not pinch the SCM because the IJ may be compressed by this maneuver.

d. Once good blood return is demonstrated, remove the 22-gauge finder needle and insert, while aspirating, the 18-gauge introducer needle with the bevel facing the patient's feet. If arterial blood is withdrawn, stop and consult section III.

e. Once good blood return is demonstrated, place the CVC using the Seldinger technique as described previously.

### E. FEMORAL VEIN APPROACH

1. Positioning

a. Position the patient on a flat bed in reverse Trendelenburg position with the leg slightly abducted. Avoid allowing the leg to be maximally rotated either internally or externally. Retract any panus up and away from the groin.

2. Identify landmarks.

a. Identify the pubic tubercle, anterior superior iliac spine, and inguinal ligament, and palpate the femoral pulse. Remember NAVEL (lateral to medial):

**N**—nerve, **A**—artery, **V**—vein, **E**—empty, **L**—lymph

3. Prep

a. After shaving any necessary hair, a wide prep is beneficial to visualize and palpate important bony landmarks.

4. Technique

a. Begin by palpating the femoral artery as it exits the femoral canal. If it cannot be palpated, it exits the femoral canal less than 1 cm medial to the midpoint of the inguinal ligament.

b. Administer 1% lidocaine in an area several centimeters inferior to the inguinal ligament, medial to the femoral pulse.

c. Retract the femoral artery laterally and insert the 18-gauge introducer needle, while aspirating, at a 45-degree angle to the skin in a direction parallel to the palpated pulse, 1 cm medial to the palpated femoral pulse. The needle direction tends to be at an angle aimed several centimeters inferior to the umbilicus.

d. If there is no blood return, slowly withdraw the needle to the level of the skin and redirect it just medially. If further attempts are unsuccessful, insert the introducer needle just medial to the palpated pulse.

e. Once good blood return has been demonstrated, place CVC via Seldinger technique as described earlier. If arterial blood is seen, stop and hold pressure for at least 5 minutes before reattempting to find the vein just medial to where the femoral artery is encountered.

### III. COMPLICATIONS

### A. ARTERIAL PUNCTURE

1. Subclavian

a. Withdraw needle and hold pressure for 10 minutes. Complete occlusion or near compression of the subclavian artery can be accomplished by placing one finger above the clavicle at the site of the artery exiting between the scalene muscles where a pulse can be palpated, and the other finger below the clavicle along the trajectory of the subclavian artery. This is typically done with the thumb and index finger pinching around the clavicle. Occlusion can be verified if an ipsilateral arterial line is in place.

b. Monitor vitals and breath sounds for possible hemothorax.

c. Catheterization can be resumed, assuming no signs of bleeding are present (hematoma).

**2. Carotid/femoral**

a. Withdraw the needle and hold pressure for 5 to 10 minutes.

b. Monitor vitals and breath sounds for possible hemothorax.

c. Catheterization can be resumed, assuming no signs of bleeding are present.

**3. Uncertain arterial versus venous puncture**

a. Obtain sterile intravenous extension tubing and attach on end to the needle; withdraw blood into the tubing and hold the tubing up toward the ceiling; arterial pressure will maintain the blood at the level to which it is withdrawn, whereas venous pressure is not sufficient to maintain the blood at the level to which it is withdrawn and will fall back down the intravenous tubing.

b. If the catheter has been placed, it can be hooked up to a pressure transducer, and if arterial pressure and waveform are seen, arterial placement is confirmed. Alternatively, an arterial blood gas can be sent.

**4. Arterial cannulization**

a. Once the artery is dilated with either the dilator or placement of CVC, the safest course of action is to place the CVC into the artery to control the bleeding by plugging the hole with the catheter. Notify upper-level resident and staff, and have the operating room available to be able to take patient emergently to the operating room if bleeding cannot be controlled by manual pressure when the catheter is pulled.

## B. PNEUMOTHORAX

**1. Tension pneumothorax**

a. If suspected, place a 16-gauge Angiocath needle in the second intercostal space along the midclavicular line, with subsequent chest tube placement.

**2. Simple pneumothorax**

a. If small (<10% or <2 rib spaces on CXR), nonexpanding, and asymptomatic, chest tube placement is not necessary. Follow the patient with serial examinations and place them on a cardiopulmonary monitor.

b. If more than 10%, expanding, or symptomatic, place a chest tube to evacuate the pneumothorax.

## C. AIR EMBOLUS

**1. Management**

a. Attempt to withdraw air through the CVC if possible. This can be aided by inserting the CVC as deep as possible into the patient.

b. Place patient into Trendelenburg position, rotated to the patient's left to trap the air in the apex of the right ventricle.

c. Maintain supportive care if the patient becomes symptomatic, and transfer patient to appropriate level of care (intensive care unit). Initiate Advanced Cardiac Life Support if cardiac or pulmonary arrest develops.

d. Air emboli can be demonstrated on CXR, which can be used for follow-up to demonstrate resolution, which will occur gradually as the air is absorbed.

### D. MALPOSITIONING
1. **Right atrial or ventricular placement**
a. Withdraw into superior vena cava.
2. **Contralateral subclavian vein**
a. Position change is not necessary, and the catheter can be used as placed. If adjustment is desired, placement of guidewire into superior vena cava may require guidance under fluoroscopy.
3. **IJ**
a. Place guidewire and withdraw TLC, maintaining a sterile procedure, and then advance the TLC far enough in to withdraw blood from the middle port. Remove and then reinsert the guidewire after turning the patient's head to the ipsilateral side and compressing on the IJ to close the IJ orifice.
b. If this maneuver is unsuccessful, placement under fluoroscopic guidance is required.
4. **Internal mammary/thoracic duct**
a. Place guidewire and perform the procedure described above for IJ.

### IV. ULTRASOUND
### A. BACKGROUND
1. Small bedside ultrasound machines have become commonplace in most hospitals to assist in placement of CVC.
2. Ultrasound guidance can assist in placement of both IJ and femoral lines with a theoretical decrease in complications.

### B. PROCEDURE
1. After turning on machine and adjusting the depth to an appropriate level, before prepping the patient, looking for the artery and vein can be beneficial to determine the patency of the vein before beginning the procedure.
2. Aside from an understanding of basic anatomy, the easiest way to determine the difference between the artery and vein, without using Doppler flow, is that the vein is easily compressible as compared with the artery.
3. After sliding the sterile sleeve over the ultrasound probe, the needle can be placed under direct, live visualization of the needle entering the vein. Some devices have a guiding cuff to further assist centering the needle in the middle of the visualized field.

81

CENTRAL VENOUS LINES

# Arterial Lines

*Rian A. Maercks, MD*

## I. INDICATIONS

### A. CONTINUOUS REAL-TIME BLOOD PRESSURE MONITORING
1. Predicted hemodynamic instability
2. Titration of vasopressors
3. Unreliable noninvasive measurements

## II. TECHNIQUES

### A. RADIAL ARTERY CATHETERIZATION
1. Perform Allen's test and document result in chart.

a. Exsanguinate the hand by squeezing the patient's hand in a fist. Hold firm digital pressure over the radial pulse and open the hand. Observe the hand. Rapid refill should be present throughout the hand.
b. If the Allen's test is abnormal, do not perform radial artery catheterization.
c. The test can also be completed using a pulse oximeter on the index finger or thumb and occluding the radial artery. A decreased reading suggests poor ulnar contribution and should deter the surgeon from catheterizing the radial artery.
2. Prepare the room.
a. Ensure nursing is aware and ready with pressure transduction setup and a sterile line to connect.
b. Prepare yourself with universal precautions (gown, gloves, mask, eye protection).
c. Place the patient's wrist in slight extension using a gauze roll and an armboard. It is helpful to tape the patient's hand over the roll and armboard to a Mayo stand or procedure table. Defer taping the proximal arm to the armboard until after the procedure. Prep along the radial pulse from the wrist crease to several centimeters proximal. Use sterile towels to create a large sterile field to prevent contaminating the wire.
3. Take your time. Feel the pulse and create a mental map of its location. Blind attempts at cannulation will cause spasm and increase difficulty of the procedure.
4. Choose the catheter. Several devices exist to assist with arterial access; become familiar with all of them and select the technique that works best for you.
a. Large-bore needle (size varies by kit): Inject local anesthesia adjacent to artery to help with vasodilatation. Before entering the skin, prepare the wire by advancing the guide over the J-bend and rest the needle next to the patient's arm. With two fingers of your nondominant hand, appreciate the point of maximal impulse at a proximal and distal point. Insert the needle between your fingers at about a 30-degree angle to the skin, bevel up. Aim just deep to your proximal fingertip and advance slowly. The artery is superficial and it is easy to go right through it. Pulsatile red blood will be produced on entry to the artery.

While stabilizing the needle, advance the wire through the needle. If there is good pulsatile blood return but the wire does not advance, lower the needle to a more acute angle (more parallel with the course of the artery) and try again. Once the wire is advanced, remove the needle while controlling the wire. Next guide the short catheter over the wire. Remove the wire and place your thumb over the catheter while you ask for the transduction tubing. Once connected, confirm an arterial tracing on the monitor. Secure your line at three points with the suture provided. Do not use Steri-Strips or less than three sutures—they will not last in the intensive care unit environment.

b. Self-contained device: These devices have the advantage of a needle, wire, and catheter in one unit. Holding the device like a pencil, enter the artery as described earlier. Once red blood begins filling the device, lower your hand to create a more acute angle between the skin and device. Advance the wire. The wire should meet little to no resistance. Once the wire is advanced, slide the catheter in over the wire. Remove the device, holding the catheter at the skin. Connect, confirm, and secure as explained earlier. If there is no return after the device is removed, slowly withdraw the catheter until pulsatile return is present. At this point the wire can be introduced and the catheter advanced again over the wire.

c. Needle with catheter (most central line kits have the short catheter preloaded onto this needle): Insert the needle and catheter as described earlier. On encountering arterial return, advance the needle and catheter a few millimeters. Blood return stops as you exit the lumen. Remove the needle. With the wire prepared for insertion in your dominant hand, slowly withdraw the catheter with your nondominant hand. When pulsatile return is encountered, again advance the wire. After the wire freely advances into the artery, the catheter can be advanced and the wire removed. Connect, confirm, and secure as described earlier.

## B. FEMORAL ARTERY CATHETERIZATION

1. Indications—the femoral artery is relatively easy to quickly and reliably access in patients with hypotension in trauma and shock situations.

2. Complications—infection, hematoma, arteriovenous fistula, thrombosis/embolus

3. Technique

a. Prepare by ensuring nursing team is aware and readying transduction tubing.

b. Prep widely, including visual or palpable access to anterior superior iliac spine.

c. The groin crease is an approximation of the inguinal ligament in a thin person; however, increased abdominal fat or pannus can be deceiving. In these patients, an assistant with sterile garb can assist by providing superior traction on the pannus. Try to appreciate the pulse below the groin crease. In a thin person, enter the skin 2 cm inferior to the groin crease. In a more robust body habitus, select an area near the crease that is clearly compressible against the femoral head.

d. A pulseless patient can be catheterized by noting the position of the lateral aspect of the pubis and the anterior superior iliac spine; the artery is exactly at the midpoint of these two structures.

e. Enter the artery with a large-bore needle from the arterial line kit with a readied wire and guide. When pulsatile flow is encountered, advance the wire. Lowering to a more acute angle assists with wire advancement. Remove the needle while controlling the wire and advance the long catheter over the wire. Connect, confirm, and secure the catheter as described earlier.

## C.  BRACHIAL ARTERY CATHETERIZATION

1. Indications—brachial artery catheterization can be used when attempts at radial artery have been unsuccessful.
2. Complications—the brachial artery is an end artery to the hand; both radial and ulnar arteries bifurcate from the brachial. A thrombosis of the brachial is an emergency that may require immediate intervention to save the hand.
3. Technique—the brachial artery courses from the lower border of the teres major to the apex of the antecubital fossa. The artery can be easily accessed with the patient's arm externally rotated and abducted to near 90 degrees. The pulse can be appreciated by gently retracting the flexor mass and palpating the groove between the flexor and extensor compartment. In this position, use a technique as described earlier for radial line placement. Use two fingers to appreciate the artery and insert your access needle between your fingers at approximately 45 degrees. Once accessed, insert the wire while dropping the needle to a more acute angle. Remove the needle and insert the long catheter over the needle. Remove the wire and check the pressure wave.

## D.  AXILLARY ARTERY CATHETERIZATION

1. Indications—as detailed earlier
2. Complications—emboli/thrombosis to brain. Left side is preferred because of less direct route to carotid. Risk for brachial plexus injury, thrombosis, and bleeding.
3. Technique—position the patient with the arm abducted 90 degrees and externally rotated. Wrist restraints help maintain positioning. Palpate the pulse in the anterior axilla. Cannulation techniques are as described for other locations. Use the long catheter in the axilla. Suture with three-point fixation to avoid unintended displacement.

## E.  DORSALIS PEDIS ARTERY CATHETERIZATION

1. Indications—as detailed earlier. Contraindicated in patients with diabetes and vasculopathy.

2. Complications—compromise to great toe blood supply, wound healing issues
3. Technique—begin by testing the collateral supply to the great toe. Squeeze the great toe to blanch it, then occlude the dorsalis pedis artery with digital pressure. While maintaining pressure over the artery, release the toe. Watch for complete return of blood to the nail bed in less than 6 seconds. Technique is otherwise similar to radial artery access. The vessel is superficial.

# Pulmonary Artery (Swan–Ganz) Catheter

*Grace Z. Mak, MD*

## I. INDICATIONS FOR INVASIVE CARDIAC MONITORING

1. Invasive cardiac monitoring
a. Provides more direct measurement and data from which other measurements can be calculated
b. Central venous catheter—central venous pressure (CVP)
c. Pulmonary artery catheter—CVP, pulmonary artery systolic and diastolic pressures, pulmonary capillary wedge pressure (PCWP), cardiac output, systemic venous resistance
2. Complex surgical procedures
a. Associated with large volume shifts
3. Hemodynamic instability
4. Difficulty with fluid management
5. Inappropriate response to volume challenge
6. Deteriorating cardiac function
7. Deteriorating pulmonary function
8. Unexplained hypoxemia
9. Severe head injury
10. Surgical procedures in patients with baseline poor cardiac, respiratory, or renal function

## II. CENTRAL VENOUS PRESSURE MONITORING

### A. ACCURATE METHOD OF ESTIMATING RIGHT VENTRICULAR (RV) FILLING PRESSURE
1. Relevant in interpreting RV function

### B. FUNCTION OF FOUR INDEPENDENT VARIABLES
1. Volume and blood flow in central veins
2. Venomotor tone of central veins
3. Compliance and contractility of the right side of the heart during diastole
4. Intrathoracic pressure

### C. CLINICAL USES OF CVP CATHETER
1. Infusion of total parenteral nutrition, vasoactive substances, hypertonic solutions, or chemically irritating medications for prolonged period
2. Monitoring of right atrial pressures and consequently intravascular volume status
3. Aspiration of venous samples for chemical analysis (not a substitute for true mixed venous blood)
4. Head injury—increasing right atrial pressure results in increased intracranial blood volume and may increase intracranial pressure.

83

5. Sensitive in reflecting increased transmyocardial pressure in pericardial tamponade

## D. PITFALLS OF USING CVP IN CRITICALLY ILL PATIENTS
1. Water manometer system cannot reliably represent RV filling pressure: Transducer-monitor system is necessary; transducer systems also need to be accurately zeroed; that is, it is critical that the position of the transducer is at the level of the heart.
2. Misinterpretation of CVP data when extrapolating information relative to left ventricular (LV) performance
a. In normal situations, RV filling pressure may correlate with LV filling pressures; this may not be true in critically ill patients.

## III. BALLOON-TIPPED PULMONARY ARTERY (SWAN–GANZ) CATHETERS

### A. DESIGN
1. Catheter tip with balloon (1.5-ml capacity) allowing placement of the tip into the pulmonary artery and measurement of pulmonary artery systolic and diastolic pressures, as well as capillary wedge pressures
2. Proximal port allowing measurement of CVP
3. Thermistor 4 cm from tip senses changes in temperature.
a. Measures the flow of cold fluid injected via the proximal port, allowing calculation of cardiac output/index

### B. ADVANTAGES OVER CVP MEASUREMENTS
1. Independent assessment of RV and LV function, which may be dissimilar during critical illness
2. Measurement of pulmonary arterial diastolic and wedge pressures, thus approximating left atrial filling pressure (preload)
3. Continuous monitoring of pulmonary artery systolic and mean pressures reflects changes in pulmonary vascular resistance secondary to hypoxemia, pulmonary edema, pulmonary emboli, and pulmonary insufficiency; helps distinguish cardiogenic from noncardiogenic pulmonary edema
4. Sampling of global mixed venous blood
a. Global mixed venous blood saturations ($Sv-O_2$) provide an index of tissue perfusion and oxygenation. Increasing $Sv-O_2$ correlates with increasing cardiac output and tissue perfusion or decreased oxygen extraction (in sepsis or liver failure). Decreasing $Sv-O_2$ signifies decreasing cardiac output or tissue perfusion with increased oxygen extraction. $Sv-O_2$ cannot, however, reflect the changes in regional perfusion, which are often present in critically ill patients.
b. Calculation of arteriovenous oxygen content difference ($AVDo_2$) and physiologic shunt (Qsp/Qt) is helpful in the management of respiratory failure (Table 83-1).

**TABLE 83-1**

## FORMULAS USED IN CARDIOPULMONARY CRITICAL CARE

1. Mean arterial pressure (MAP):

$MAP = DP + 1/3(SP - DP)$

DP: diastolic pressure; SP: systolic pressure

Reference range: 80–90 mm Hg

2. Stroke volume (SV):

$SV = CO/HR$

CO: cardiac output; HR: heart rate

Reference range: 1 ml/kg

3. Stroke volume index (SVI):

$SVI = SV/BSA$

SV: stroke volume; BSA: body surface area

Reference range: 35–40 in intensive care unit (ICU) population

4. Cardiac index (CI):

$CI = CO/BSA$

CO: cardiac output; BSA: body surface area

Reference range: 2.5–4 L/min/m$^2$ in ICU population

5. Right ventricular stroke work (RVSW):

$RVSW = SV \times (MAP - CVP) \times 0.0136$

SV: stroke volume; MAP: mean arterial pressure; CVP: central venous pressure

Reference range: 10–15 g/m

6. Left ventricular stroke work (LVSW):

$LVSW = SV \times (MAP - PCWP) \times 0.0136$

SV: stroke volume; MAP: mean arterial pressure; PCWP: pulmonary capillary wedge pressure

Reference range: 60–80 g/m

7. Systemic vascular resistance (SVR) (also referred to as total peripheral resistance):

$SVR = [(MAP - CVP) \times 80]/CO$

MAP: mean arterial pressure; CVP: central venous pressure; CO: cardiac output

Reference range: 800–1200 dynes 3 sec/cm$^5$

8. Pulmonary vascular resistance (PVR):

$PVR = [(MAP - PCWP) \times 80]/CO$

MAP: mean pulmonary arterial pressure; PCWP: pulmonary capillary wedge pressure; CO: cardiac output

Reference range: 20–130 dynes 3 sec/cm$^5$

9. Myocardial oxygen consumption–correlate ($MVo_2C$):

$MVo_2C = (SP \times HR)/100$

SP: systolic pressure; HR: heart rate; this term is a fair calculated measure of myocardial oxygen demand

greater values = greater consumption

10. Alveolar $Po_2$ ($PAo_2$):

$PAo_2 = (PB - PH_2o) \times Fio_2 - PEco_2/R$

PB: barometric pressure (760 mm Hg at sea level); $PH_2o$ (at body temperature): water pressure (47 mm Hg); $PEco_2 = PAco_2$; $R = 0.8$ (assumed).

Thus,

$PAo_2 = (760 - 47) \times Fio_2 - Paco_2/0.8$

$Fio_2$: fraction of inspired oxygen; $Paco_2$: partial pressure of carbon dioxide, arterial

*Continued*

**83**

PULMONARY ARTERY (SWAN–GANZ) CATHETER

---

**TABLE 83-1—cont'd**

## FORMULAS USED IN CARDIOPULMONARY CRITICAL CARE

11. Capillary $O_2$ content ($Cc'o_2$):
$Cc'o_2 = (Pao_2 \times 0.0031) + Hb \times 1.39 \times 1$
$PAo_2$: alveolar partial pressure; Hb: hemoglobin (assumes 100% Hb saturation)
Reference value: 18.3 ml/100 ml
12. Mixed venous $O_2$ content ($Cv-O_2$):
$Cv-O_2 = Pv-O_2 \times 0.0031 + (Hb \times 1.39 \times Ven\ Sat)$
$Pv-O_2$: partial pressure of mixed venous oxygen; Hb: hemoglobin; Ven Sat: venous
   saturation
Reference value: 13 ml/100 ml
13. Arterial $O_2$ content ($Cao_2$):
$Cao_2 = Pao_2 \times 0.0031 + (Hb \times 1.39 \times Art\ Sat)$
$Pao_2$: partial pressure of oxygen, arterial; Hb: hemoglobin; Art Sat: arterial saturation
Reference value: 18 ml/100 ml
14. $O_2$ delivery ($Do_2$):
$Do_2 = CI \times 13.4 \times Hb \times Art\ Sat$
CI: cardiac index; Hb: hemoglobin; Art Sat: arterial saturation
Reference range: 520–570 ml/min per $m^2$
15. Arteriovenous $O_2$ difference ($AVDo_2$):
$AVDo_2 = Ca - Cv$
Ca: arterial content; Cv: venous content
Reference range: 3.5–4.5 ml/100 ml
16. $O_2$ consumption ($O_2$ Cons):
$O_2\ Cons = (Ca - Cv) \times CO \times 10$
Ca: arterial content; Cv: venous content; CO: cardiac output
Reference value: 250 ml/min
17. $O_2$ utilization (% Util):
% Util = Ca − Cv/Ca
Ca: arterial content; Cv: venous content
Reference range: 0.2–0.25
18. Intrapulmonary shunt (Qsp/Qt):
$Qsp/Qt = (Cc'o_2 - Cao_2)/(Cc'o_2 - Cvo_2)$
$Cc'o_2$: capillary $O_2$ content; $Cao_2$: arterial $O_2$ content; $Cvo_2$: mixed venous $O_2$ content
Reference value: <0.10
19. Body surface area (BSA):
$BSA = (W + H - 60)/100$
W: weight(kg); H: height (cm)

---

5. Accurate, reproducible measurement of cardiac output by thermodilution technique
6. Monitoring of RV filling pressure through the CVP access port
7. Evaluation of myocardial function—preload, contractility, and afterload (Table 83-2)
a. Myocardial perfusion pressure can be estimated from the difference between systemic diastolic pressure and PCWP.
b. Heart rate and systolic pressure can be combined to provide a "time tension index."

c. Systemic vascular resistance as an estimate of aortic impedance (afterload) can be calculated.

d. Effect of therapeutic interventions can be quantified in terms of physiologic cost.

8. Specialized pulmonary artery catheters permit (1) atrial, ventricular, or sequential atrioventricular pacing simultaneously; (2) continuous measurement of mixed venous oxygen saturations; (3) continuous cardiac output measurements; or (4) measurement of end-diastolic volumes.

## C. CLINICAL INDICATIONS FOR PULMONARY ARTERY CATHETER

1. Myocardial infarction, congestive heart failure, hemodynamic instability, unclear intravascular volume status, acute respiratory failure, sepsis, peritonitis, multiple traumas, noncardiogenic pulmonary edema, near drowning, overdoses, pulmonary edema in pregnancy, fat emboli, and elderly or critically ill patients undergoing noncardiac surgical procedures

## D. PITFALLS

1. PCWP is at best an estimation of LV filling pressures. The gold standard for measuring preload is LV end-diastolic volume, which is not practical clinically. PCWP is an extrapolation of left atrial pressure, which, in turn, is an estimate of LV end-diastolic pressure. Thus, in cardiac disease states with changes in myocardial compliance or valvular function, PCWP may be an inaccurate estimation of preload. Specialized catheters with the ability to measure end-diastolic volume provide more accurate estimations of LV filling pressures.

2. Catheter artifact (whip) and high positive end-expiratory pressures may produce inaccurate measurements.

3. Catheters may be difficult to "float" in patients with cardiomegaly or low cardiac output. Placing the patient upright and with the left side down may alleviate this problem. Fluoroscopy may also be helpful.

4. Arrhythmias during insertion include ventricular irritability (premature ventricular complexes and ventricular tachycardia) and right bundle branch block. Catheter placement in a patient with previous left bundle branch block may produce complete heart block. If pulmonary artery monitoring is essential, preparation for emergency pacing should be made.

5. Pulmonary artery rupture

a. More common in elderly adults and those with pulmonary hypertension

b. Avoid overwedging the balloon and prolonged balloon inflation.

c. Continuous monitoring of pulmonary artery tracing—balloon inflation must be stopped once the waveform changes. If the tip has migrated distally, less than 1.5 ml will cause the balloon to wedge.

d. Daily chest radiographs should be reviewed to ensure proximal catheter placement.

TABLE 83-2

DETERMINANTS OF CARDIAC OUTPUT

| Determinant | Definition | Effect on Cardiac Output | Measurement | Treatment |
|---|---|---|---|---|
| Preload | Length of myocardial fibers at end diastole, which is the result of ventricular filling pressure | Direct, up to physiologic limit | End-diastolic volume and pressure of the ventricles<br>Pulmonary diastolic pressure<br>Pulmonary capillary wedge pressure<br>Direct left atrial pressure measurements CVP (right atrial) | Volume expansion<br>Pericardiocentesis<br>Reduction of PEEP |
| Contractility | The inotropic state of the myocardium; length/tension/velocity relationship of the myocardium independent of initial length and afterload | Direct | Ventricular function curves<br>Ejection fraction<br>$V_{max}$<br>Vcf<br>PEP/LVET<br>dP/dt | Dopamine<br>Norepinephrine<br>Epinephrine<br>Isoproterenol<br>Dobutamine<br>Digitalis<br>Glucagon<br>GKI<br>Milrinone |

| Afterload | Systolic ventricular wall stress, which is produced by the force against which the myocardial fibers must contract | Inverse, as long as coronary flow is maintained | Aortic pressure for left ventricle; Pulmonary artery pressure for right ventricle | Diuretics; Phentolamine; Sodium nitroprusside; Nitroglycerin; Intraaortic balloon pumping; External counterpulsation |
| Pulse rate | The number of cardiac systoles per minute | Direct, >60 and <180 beats/min | Electrocardiogram; Count pulse | Bradycardia; Atropine; Pacemaker; Epinephrine; Tachycardia; Digitalis; Lidocaine; Electroversion |

CVP = central venous pressure; PEEP = positive end-expiratory pressure; $V_{max}$ = peak velocity; Vcf = velocity of circumferential fiber shortening; PEP = prejection period; LVET = left ventricular ejection time; dP/dt = rate of change of left ventricular pressure; GKI = glucose-potassium-insulin. Adapted from Hardy JD: *Textbook of Surgery*. Philadelphia, JB Lippincott, 1983, p 54.

## PULMONARY ARTERY (SWAN–GANZ) CATHETER

83

e. Signs of rupture—hemoptysis or bleeding from endotracheal tube
f. Treatment
  (1) Deflate balloon and remove Swan–Ganz catheter.
  (2) Supportive care
    (a) Given low pressure within pulmonary vascular system, majority of patients will spontaneously cease bleeding.
    (b) Position patient in Trendelenburg (head down) and left lateral decubitus (right side up) to decrease risk for pulmonary air embolus. If high clinical suspicion, can aspirate air from right ventricle via central line or cardiocentesis if necessary.
  (3) If patient continues to bleed or becomes unstable, operative intervention (wedge resection, pneumonectomy) may be required. Endotracheal intubation with either single- or double-lumen tube should protect the uninjured lung (most ruptures occur in the right lower lobe).
    (a) Position patient with uninjured side up.

# Index

Page numbers followed by f refer to figure, t refer to table.

INDEX

INDEX

INDEX

INDEX